PROGRESS IN BRAIN RESEARCH

VOLUME 99

CHEMICAL SIGNALLING IN THE BASAL GANGLIA

Other volumes in PROGRESS IN BRAIN RESEARCH

PROGRESS IN BRAIN RESEARCH

VOLUME 99

CHEMICAL SIGNALLING IN THE BASAL GANGLIA

EDITED BY

G.W. ARBUTHNOTT

Department of Preclinical Veterinary Sciences, University of Edinburgh, United Kingdom

P.C. EMSON

Institute of Animal Physiology and Genetics Research, Cambridge, United Kingdom

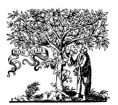

ELSEVIER
AMSTERDAM — OXFORD — NEW YORK — TOKYO
1993

ISBN 0-444-81562-7 (volume)
ISBN 0-444-80104-9 (series)

Elsevier Science Publishers B.V.
P.O. Box 211
1000 AE Amsterdam
The Netherlands

Library of Congress Cataloging-in-Publication Data

Chemical signalling in the basal ganglia / edited by G.W. Arbuthnott
  and P.C. Emson.
        p.   cm. -- (Progress in brain research : v. 99)
    Includes bibliographical references and index.
    ISBN 0-444-81562-7 (alk. paper)
    1. Basal ganglia. 2. Neurotransmitters. 3. Neurotransmitter
  receptors. 4. Basal Ganglia--chemistry--congresses. 5. Brain
  Chemistry--congresses. 6. Neural Transmission--congresses.
  7. Neurons--congresses. I. Arbuthnott, Gordon W. II. Emson, P. C.
  III. Series.
    [DNLM: W1 PR667J v.99 1993 / WL 307 C517 1993]
  QP376.P7 vol. 99
  [QP383.3]
  612.8'2 s--dc20
  [612.8'25]
  DNLM/DLC
  for Library of Congress   93-1791
                                                            CIP

Printed on acid-free paper

Printed in The Netherlands

List of Contributors

Marianne Amalric, Laboratoire de Neurosciences Fonctionelles, Unité de Neurochimie, Marseille, France.

Paul Apicella, University of Fribourg, Department of Physiology, Blvd. Perrolles, CH 1700 Fribourg, Switzerland.

Gordon Arbuthnott, MRC Group, Preclinical Veterinary Sciences, University of Edinburgh, Summerhall, Edinburgh EH9 1QH, U.K.

Sarah Augood, Institute of Animal Physiology and Genetics Research, Cambridge Research Station, Babraham, Cambridge CB2 4AT, U.K.

G. Bernardi, Clinica Neurologica, Dipartimento Sanita Universita di Roma "Tor Vergato", Via O. Raimondo no. 8, 00173 Rome, Italy.

S. Berretta, MIT, Department of Brain and Cognitive Sciences, Cambridge, MA 02139, U.S.A.

J.P. Bolam, MRC, Anatomical Neuropharmacology Unit, Mansfield Road, Oxford OX1 3TH, U.K.

Jon Brotchie, Experimental Neurology Group, Department of Cell and Structural Biology, Medical School, University of Manchester, Manchester M13 9PT, U.K.

L.L. Brown, Albert Einstein College of Medicine, Bronx, NY 10461, U.S.A.

P. Calabresi, Dipartimento di Sanita Pubblica e Biologica Cellulaire, Universita degli studi di Roma, Via Orazio Raimondo, 00173 Rome, Italy.

M.F. Chesselet, School of Medicine, Department of Pharmacology, University of Pennsylvania, 36th Street and Hamilton Walk, Philadelphia, PA 19104-6084, U.S.A.

Piers Emson, Institute of Animal Physiology and Genetics Research, Cambridge Research Station, Babraham, Cambridge CB2 4AT, U.K.

R.L.M. Faull, School of Medicine, Department of Anatomy, University of Auckland, Private Bag 92019, Auckland, New Zealand.

Chantal Francois, Institut National de la Santé et de la Recherche Medicale, INSERM U 106, Pav. INSERM Cl. Bernard, Hôpital de la Salpétrière, 47 Blvd. de l'Hôpital, F 75651 Paris, Cedex 13, France.

Anouk Garnier, Institute National de la Santé et de la Recherche Medicale, INSERM U 106, Pav. INSERM Cl. Bernard, Hôpital de la Salpetriere, 47 Blvd. de l'Hôpital, F 75651 Paris, Cedex 13, France.

Cathleen Gonzales, Department of Pharmacology, Wyeth-Ayerst Pharmaceutics, CN 8000, Princeton, NJ 08543, U.S.A.

A. Graybiel, Graybiel Laboratory, MIT, Department of Brain and Cognitive Sciences, E25-618 45 Carleton Street, Cambridge, MA 02139, U.S.A.

H.J. Groenewegen, Department of Anatomy, Vrije Universiteit, PO Box 7161, 1007 MC Amsterdam, The Netherlands.

R. Guevra Guzman, Department of Neurobiology, Institute of Animal Physiology, Research Station, Babraham, Cambridge CB2 4AT, U.K.

Lili-Naz Hazrati, Laboratoire de Neurobiologie, Hôpital de l'Enfant Jesus, 1401 18e Rue Quebec, Canada G1J 1Z4.

C.A. Ingham, MRC Group, PVS, R(D)SVS, University of Edinburgh, Summerhall, Edinburgh EH9 1QH, U.K.

K. Kadowaki, MRC Group, Institute of Animal Physiology and Genetics Research, Cambridge Research Station, Babraham, Cambridge CB2 4AT, U.K.

K.M. Kendrick, Department of Neurobiology, Institute of Animal Physiology, Research Station, Babraham, Cambridge CB2 4AT, U.K.

J. Kishimoto, MRC Group, Institute of Animal Physiology and Genetics Research, Cambridge Research Station, Babraham, Cambridge, CB2 4AT, U.K.

H. Kita, Department of Anatomy and Neurobiology, University of Tennessee Health Sciences Center, 875 Monroe Avenue, Memphis, TN 38163, U.S.A.

S.T. Kitai, Department of Anatomy and Neurobiology, University of Tennessee Health Sciences Center, 875

Monroe Avenue, Memphis, TN 38163, U.S.A.

George F. Koob, The Scripps Research Institute, 10666 N. Torrey Pines Road, Blake Building CVN 7, La Jolla, CA 92037, U.S.A.

Michael Lacey, Department of Pharmacology, University of Birmingham, The Medical School, Edgbaston, Birmingham B15 2TT, U.K.

Tomas Ljungberg, University of Fribourg, Department of Physiology, Blvd. Perrolles, CH 1700 Fribourg, Switzerland.

Marianne Mercugliano, Neurosciences Research, The Children's Seashore House, 3405 Civic Ctr. Blvd., Philadelphia, PA 19104, U.S.A.

Nicola B. Mercuri, Clinica Neurologica, Dipartimento Sanita Universita' di Roma "Tor Vergato", Via O. Raimondo no. 8, 00173 Rome, Italy.

G. Meredith, Department of Anatomy, Vrije Universiteit, PO Box 7161, 1007 MC Amsterdam, The Netherlands.

L.F.B. Nicholson, Department of Anatomy, School of Medicine, University of Auckland, Private Bag 92019, Auckland, New Zealand.

P. Norris, MRC Group, Institute of Animal Physiology and Genetics Research, Cambridge Research Station, Babraham, Cambridge CB2 4AT, U.K.

A. Parent, Centre Recherche Neurobiologie, Hôpital l'Enfant Jesus, 1401 18e Rue Quebec, Quebec, Canada, G1K 1Z4.

C.M.A. Pennartz, Department of Zoology, Vrije Universiteit, Kruislaan 320, SM 1098 Amsterdam, The Netherlands.

G. Percheron, Laboratoire de Neuromorphologie, Informationnelle et de Neurologie Experimentale du Mouvement, INSERM U 106, Pav. INSERM Cl. Bernard, Hôpital de la Salpétrière, 47 Blvd. de l'Hôpital, F 75651 Paris, Cedex 13, France.

Ying Quin, Department of Pharmacology, University of Pennsylvania, 36th and Hamilton Walk, Philadelphia, PA 19104, U.S.A.

H.A. Robertson, Dalhousie University, Department of Pharmacology, Halifax, Nova Scotia, Canada.

Ranulfo Romo, Department of Neuroscience, UNAM, Institute of Cellular Physiology, Apartado Postal 70-600, Mexico.

Pascal P. Salin, Laboratoire de Neurosciences Fonctionelles, CNRS, 31 Chemin Joseph Aiguier, BP 71, Marseille, Cedex 13402, France.

Eugenio Scarnati, University of Fribourg, Department of Physiology, Blvd. Perrolles, CH 1700 Fribourg, Switzerland.

W. Schultz, University of Fribourg, Department of Physiology, Blvd. Perrolles, CH 1700 Fribourg, Switzerland.

R. Senaris, MRC Group, Department of Neurobiology, Institute of Animal Physiology, Research Station, Babraham, Cambridge, CB2 4AT, U.K.

A.D. Smith, MRC, Anatomical Neuropharmacology Unit, Mansfield Road, Oxford OX1 3TH, U.K.

Y. Smith, Laboratoire de Neurobiologie, Hôpital de l'Enfant Jesus, 1401 18e Rue Quebec, Quebec, Canada G1J 1Z4.

Jean-Jacques Soghomonian, Centre Recherche Neurobiologie, Hôpital de l'Enfant Jesus, 1401 18e Rue Quebec, Quebec, Canada G1J 1Z4.

Philip G. Strange, Biological Laboratory, The University, Canterbury, Kent CT2 7NJ, U.K.

D.J. Surmeier, College of Medicine, The University of Tennessee, The Health Science Center, Department of Anatomy and Neurobiology, 875 Monroe Avenue, Memphis, TN 38163, U.S.A.

B.J.L. Synek, Department of Pathology, School of Medicine, University of Auckland, Private Bag 92019, Auckland, New Zealand.

James Tepper, Rutgers, The State University of New Jersey, Center for Molecular and Behavioural Neuroscience, University Heights, 195 University Avenue, Newark, NJ 07102, U.S.A.

Francine Trent, Rutgers, The State University of New Jersey, Aidekman Research Center, 197 University Avenue, Newark, NJ 07102, U.S.A.

Marcus von Krosigk, Section of Neurobiology, Yale University Medical school, 333 Cedar Street, New Haven, CT 06510, U.S.A.

H.J. Waldvogel, Department of Anatomy, School of Medicine, University of Auckland, Private Bag 92019,

Auckland, New Zealand.

K. Westmore, MRC Group, Department of Neurobiology, Institute of Animal Physiology, Research Station, Babraham, Cambridge, CB2 4AT, U.K.

J.R. Wickens, Department of Anatomy and Theoretical Neuroscience Research Group, Otago University Medical School, P.O. Box 913, Dunedin, New Zealand.

C. Wilson, Department of Anatomy and Neurobiology, University of Tennessee Health Sciences Center, 875 Monroe Avenue, Memphis, TN 38163, U.S.A.

Jerome Yelnik, Institut National de la Santé et de la Recherche Medicale, INSERM U 106, Pav. INSERM Cl. Bernard, Hôpital de la Salpétrière, 47 Blvd. de l'Hôpital, F 75651 Paris, Cedex 13, France.

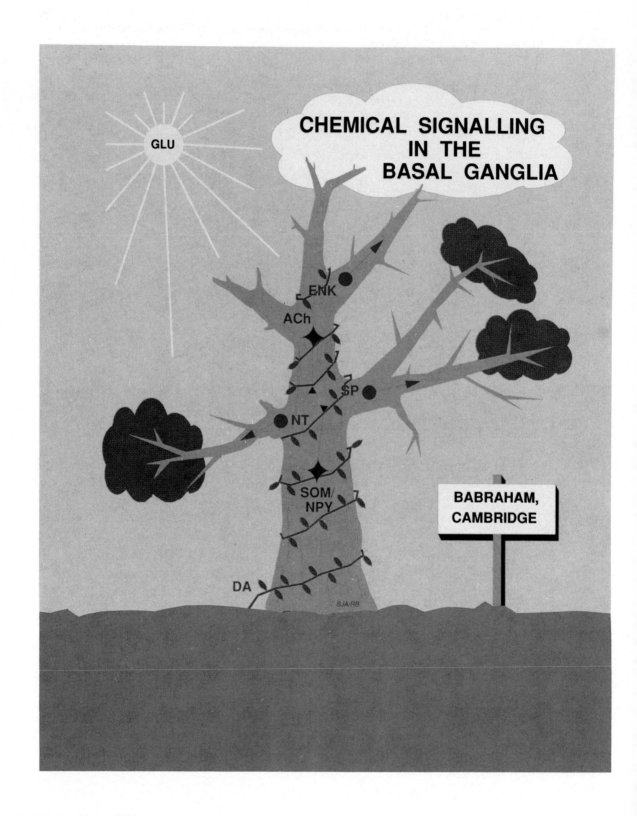

Preface

This volume in the Progress in Brain Research series grew from a conference held in Cambridge from 6 – 8 September 1991, in association with the European Neuroscience Association meeting which followed it. I had a great deal of fun helping Piers Emson, Sarah Augood and Paul Bolam organise the event − but I missed it myself. The meeting coincided with a trip to the antipodes whose dates could not be changed − so I missed it. By way of penance − or more honestly, because I couldn't bear to miss out on all of the information which became available at the meeting − I agreed to edit an extended and improved version of the proceedings as an overview of current research on the basal ganglia.

Not all the chapters come from participants and I am grateful to Drs. Tepper, Brown and Strange for responding to my request for contributions with such detailed and thoughtful reviews. I have also included two contributions of my own which represent firstly, what I would have said, had I been able to attend (Chapter 22), and secondly, what I was up to in New Zealand (Chapter 21) with Jeff Wickens in the Department of Anatomy in Dunedin. However, it is crazy to start to describe the contents of the book from the end. We have tried to make the order of the papers at least semi-logical. It is hard when so many of the contributions span several disciplines and cross between even the wide areas of basal ganglia research which we had chosen as headings.

We began with largely anatomical topics. Not that other papers do not make anatomical points, nor exclude new anatomical input; for example, among the chemical signals in the basal ganglia it seems that GABA was a special topic at the meeting. Not only is the neuronal distribution discussed in Chapter 4 but the molecular biology of the GABA neurones is the topic of Chapter 9, and their electrophysiology is explored both in Chapter 4 and Chapters 18 and 19. Even in New Zealand the influence was felt − Professor Faull (who was at the meeting) considers the effects of disease states on the GABA receptors, while Wickens discusses the possible functional importance of GABA-mediated feed forward inhibition in his Chapter (21) on the computer model that I went to study with him instead of attending the meeting.

The anatomical study was not at all confined to GABA, however, and there is an excellent discussion of the microcircuits in the nucleus accumbens by Meredith et al. (Chapter 1), a comparison of monkey and rat cholinergic neurones (Chapter 2), and two studies of striatal output pathways via globus pallidus (Chapters 5 and 6). This section of the book also contains a detailed study of the development of striatal neurones studied both with anatomical and with electrophysiological methods (Chapter 3). Their description of the development of the spines on medium-sized densely spiny neurones is an important new piece of work relevant to the studies I wanted to present at the meeting on the loss of spines which occurs with age and with loss of dopamine (Chapter 22). The 'anatomical part' of the book finishes with two chapters with a medical focus in which Faull et al. (Chapter 7) discuss some consequences of Huntington's disease, and Brotchie et al. (Chapter 8) discuss the consequences of the loss of dopamine as it occurs in Parkinson's disease.

We begin the molecular neurobiology section of the book with two chapters on the interneurones of the striatum. Chesselet et al. (Chapter 9) discuss the presence and control of two genes for glutamic acid decarboxylase which help to separate the interneuronal GABA from the GABA made in the output cells. Emson et al. (Chapter 10) on the other hand concentrate on the other interneurones as well, with discussions not only of the molecular biology but also on the release of acetylcholine by substance P — which is almost certainly released by the output neurone collaterals in the striatum. A masterly summary of the state of the art of distinguishing between dopamine receptors follows (Chapter 11) and that is in turn followed by papers illustrating the actions of blocking those same receptors (Chapter 12) or of stimulating them (Chapter 13) upon the expression of mRNAs within striatal cells.

In the third section, we tried to look at the responses of the whole animal and of the individual basal ganglia neurones to changes in the chemical signals supplied to them. The analysis includes behavioural studies (Chapter 14), studies of energy use in the striatum (Chapter 16) and an elegant correlation of behavioural and neuronal responses in Chapter 15. Electrophysiological studies which address the action of dopamine and other transmitters on cells in substantia nigra (Chapter 17) and on the cells of the neostriatum (Chapters 18, 19, 20) summarise clearly the complexity of such responses. The variety of the mixtures of channels present on different cells in the system matches the anatomical complexity in a bewildering array of possible actions and reactions so that it feels as if it is beyond the capacity of mere humans to comprehend the details sufficiently to actually apply this mass of information to the basal ganglia as a whole. The power of computer modelling to help us in this task and at the very least to refine the kind of question which we need to ask of the biology is obvious in Chapter 21.

Finally we suggest the possibility that, as well as having electrophysiological actions, dopamine may have a role in the maintenance of striatal neuronal structure. Such a role is suggested by ultrastructural studies of the spines on striatal neurones after 6-hydroxydopamine lesions and we have used the final chapter to float the suggestion that such a structural consequence of long term dopamine receptor blockade may well underlie the therapeutic action of neuroleptics while the electrophysiological consequences could perhaps be the basis for the extrapyramidal side effects.

So I am sorry to have missed the conference but glad to have had the chance to 'read all about it'. To that extent the book is already a success, for I am certain that others who, like me, missed the event will still find here the excitement and delight of excellent scientific work, described clearly and discussed with vision. The book is more than the meeting — not only because it includes work which was not presented at the meeting — but because here are the themes of current interest in the basal ganglia, discussed in full with excellent illustrations, and now there is time to study the results at leisure and draw one's own conclusions. Not only the confirmed 'basalgangliophile' but also the neuroanatomist, neurobiologist, neurologist, or electrophysiologist will find here some important questions posed and even a few of them answered to everyone's satisfaction. Here too are described some new tools, with which to tackle the remaining questions, tried for size on basal ganglia systems. There may not be a SINGLE function of the basal ganglia but the search for a way to describe their role in pathology is a problem which will continue to be vital to modern biology and medicine long after the book and its authors are equally dog-eared and worn out.

G.W. Arbuthnott

Contents

SECTION I

The Sources of the Signals

G.W. Arbuthnott and P.C. Emson (Eds.)
Progress in Brain Research, Vol. 99
© 1993 Elsevier Science Publishers B.V. All rights reserved.

CHAPTER 1

The cellular framework for chemical signalling in the nucleus accumbens

Gloria E. Meredith[1], Cyriel M.A. Pennartz[2] and Henk J. Groenewegen[1]

[1] *Department of Anatomy and Embryology, Free University Faculty of Medicine and* [2] *Department of Experimental Zoology, University of Amsterdam, Amsterdam, The Netherlands*

Introduction

Since the classical account of Heimer and Wilson (1975), in which they discussed the striatal nature of the nucleus accumbens and certain parts of the olfactory tubercle and coined the term "ventral striatum", many authors have stressed the similarities in cytoarchitecture, histochemistry and fibre connections between the ventral striatum and its dorsal neighbour, i.e., the caudate-putamen complex (e.g., Nauta et al., 1978; Domesick, 1981; Chronister et al., 1981). With regard to the connections, current data (Alexander et al., 1986; Groenewegen, 1988; Groenewegen et al., 1990) suggest that dorsal and ventral striatal sectors are involved in parallel pathways that lead from the cerebral cortex through the basal ganglia to the thalamus and back to the cortex. Corticofugal fibres from functionally distinct prefrontal cortical areas terminate in different parts of the ventral striatum (Sesack et al., 1989; Berendse et al., 1992a) where they converge with inputs from the hippocampus, the parahippocampal cortex, the amygdala, the midline and intralaminar thalamic nuclei and the ventral tegmental area (VTA)/medial substantia nigra (SN; for reviews, see Groenewegen et al., 1990, 1991). These inputs show a clear topographical organisation which is largely maintained in the outputs of the ventral striatum to the ventral pallidum (e.g., Kelley et al., 1982; Kelley and Domesick, 1982; Groenewegen and Russchen, 1984; Jayaraman, 1985; Phillipson and Griffiths, 1985; Groenewegen et al., 1987; Groenewegen and Berendse, 1990; Zahm and Heimer, 1990; Berendse and Groenewegen, 1990; Heimer et al., 1991a).

One part of the ventral striatum, the nucleus accumbens consists of two territories, the *shell* and the *core*, each with different input/output relationships (Berendse and Groenewegen, 1990; Zahm and Heimer, 1990; Heimer et al., 1991a; Berendse et al., 1992a,b). Shell and core were first described on the basis of the differential distribution of CCK-immunoreactivity (Zàborszky et al., 1985) and have now been recognized in the staining pattern of several other neurochemical substances (Herkenham et al., 1984; Voorn et al., 1986, 1989; Zahm and Heimer, 1988; Meredith et al., 1989; Groenewegen et al., 1989, 1991).

There is accumulating evidence that shell and core also differ in pharmacological features. For example, transmitter interactions shown to exist throughout the dorsal striatum, such as those between dopamine and acetylcholine, appear to be graded in the ventral striatum (Stoof et al., 1987, 1992; Henselmans and Stoof, 1991). The regulation of the expression of the opioid peptide enkephalin by the dopaminergic system appears to differ regionally in nucleus accumbens (Voorn and Docter, 1992). Further, the shell and core are affected differentially by 6-OHDA lesions of the midbrain dopamine cells

(Zahm, 1991); and lastly, pharmacological and environmental challenges produce significant differences in dopamine metabolism in the two regions (Deutch and Cameron, 1991). All interactions must ultimately occur at the cellular level which means that shell and core distinctions could be due to differences in, for example, the intrinsic circuitry, synaptic interactions or neuronal excitability.

The purpose of this chapter is to review some of the morphological and electrophysiological features of the nucleus accumbens paying particular attention to the predominant neuron, i.e., the spiny projection cell. We will focus on the synaptic and functional relationships of certain neurotransmitter systems, i.e., GABA, glutamate, dopamine and acetylcholine. The functional aspects of modulatory peptides are equally relevant, but relatively few studies have been dedicated to understanding these systems. Only the role of enkephalins will be discussed. Where possible and relevant, connectional, neurochemical and functional differences between shell and core neurons will be highlighted in order to provide a cellular basis for distinguishing the two regions. Unfortunately, only a few studies have explicitly noted the part of the nucleus under analysis which makes the assignment of features to either shell or core difficult.

Organisation of shell and core: neurochemical composition and afferent and efferent relationships

The shell consists of the peripheral zone of the nucleus accumbens, whereas the core comprises its central part, surrounding the rostral limb of the anterior commissure. However, considering that the differential patterns of various neuroactive substances are not completely coincident, an unequivocal definition of shell and core cannot be provided.

In the caudal part of the nucleus, the shell is clearly distinguishable medially and ventrally as most neurochemical markers show a higher immunoreactivity in the shell than in the core (Zàborszky et al., 1985; Voorn et al., 1986, 1989; Meredith et al. 1989; Groenewegen et al., 1989, 1991). In Nissl-stained sections, the shell is characterized by clusters of relatively small neurons that dominate the medial, ventral and lateral periphery of the shell and demarcate the border with the core. Cell density in the shell is lower than in the core. Herkenham et al., (1984) already emphasised these cytoarchitectonic characteristics and distinguished between medial and central parts of nucleus accumbens, which in retrospect might be interpreted as shell and core regions. Naloxone binding sites are very high in the cell clusters (Herkenham et al., 1984; Jongen-Rêlo et al., 1993) and, at the same caudal level, are considerably higher in the shell than in the core. More rostrally in the nucleus accumbens, cell clusters are less conspicuous. Naloxone binding densities are relatively high in the medial part of the nucleus, whereas ventrally and laterally, binding densities are much lower (Herkenham et al., 1984; Jongen-Rêlo et al., 1993). Yet, dense patches of naloxone binding mark the presumptive border between shell and core at these rostral levels. Neurochemical substances, such as substance P (Zahm and Heimer, 1988; Fig. 1A,C) or acetylcholinesterase (Meredith et al., 1989), are distributed in the nucleus in a manner similar to naloxone binding but the degree of overlap between these substances and naloxone has not been analysed. Although, in transverse sections, it is difficult to judge where the shell begins rostrally, horizontal sections through the

---

Fig. 1. Photomicrographs of the distribution of substance P immunoreactivity in the nucleus accumbens in transverse (A – C, rostral to caudal) and horizontal sections (D,E; levels just ventral to the anterior commissure and through the anterior limb of the anterior commissure, respectively). In the transverse sections, the darkly stained medial and ventral parts of the nucleus (B,C) mark the shell. Note that the rostral pole is (A) also strongly immunoreactive. In the horizontal sections, it is clear that the darkly stained area, which characterizes the shell, includes much of the rostral pole (cf. also Fig. 2). Arrows in E mark the levels of the transverse sections in A – C. Scale bar in C = 1 mm and also refers to A and B; Scale bar in D = 500 μm and is also valid for E. Abbreviations: ac, anterior commissure; aca, anterior limb of the anterior commissure; AcbC, core of the nucleus accumbens; acp, posterior limb of the anterior commissure; AcbSh, shell of the nucleus accumbens; CP, caudate-putamen.

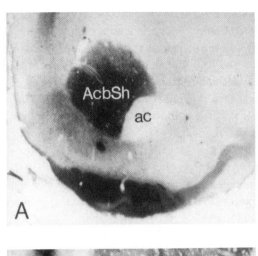

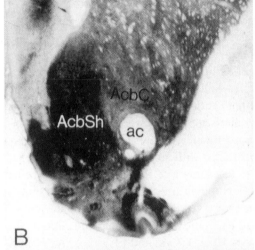

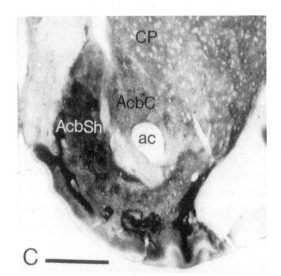

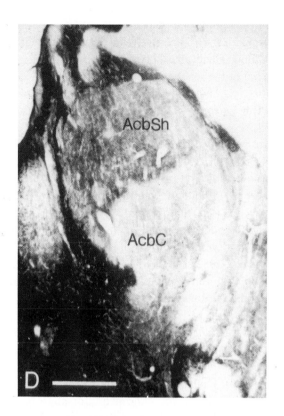

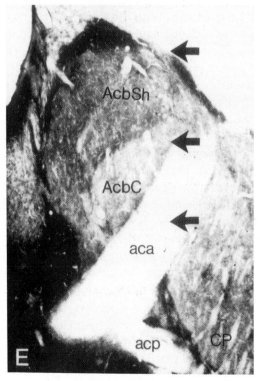

nucleus accumbens published by Herkenham et al. (1984; their fig. 7) show that the relatively high naloxone binding, which characterizes the caudal shell, is included in the rostral pole of the nucleus. A similar pattern can be appreciated in horizontal sections of substance P-stained material (Fig. 1D,E). Therefore, we consider the shell to extend into the rostral pole of the nucleus.

The shell is characterized by inputs from the hippocampal formation (Kelley and Domesick, 1982; Groenewegen et al., 1982): the ventral subiculum projects to its medial part, mainly caudally, and the dorsal subiculum projects to its lateral and ventral parts with a predominance rostrally (Fig. 2; Groenewegen et al., 1982, 1987). Interestingly, the intermediate subiculum projects to the dorsal part (not illustrated) and the dorsal subiculum to the ventral part (Fig. 2A) of the rostral pole, which we consider to be part of the shell (see above). Another distinctive input to the shell comes from the paraventricular nucleus of the thalamus (Berendse and Groenewegen, 1990). Thalamic afferents to the core arise predominantly from the intermediodorsal midline and the central medial intralaminar nuclei (Berendse and Groenewegen, 1990). Prefrontal cortical afferents to the shell originate mainly from the infralimbic and the medial orbital areas, whereas the caudal cell clusters in the shell receive fibres from the ventral prelimbic area (Berendse et al., 1992a). The core of the nucleus is supplied by prefrontal fibres from the dorsal and ventral parts of the prelimbic area and from the lateral prefrontal areas, i.e., the dorsal and ventral agranular insular areas (Berendse et al., 1992a). The dopaminergic fibres to the nucleus originate in the VTA and the medial SN. The input to the shell that arises in the medial VTA is particularly dense. The core is supplied by the more lateral VTA and medial SN (Beckstead et al., 1979; Phillipson and Griffiths, 1985; unpublished observations).

The differential outputs of the shell and core have been described recently by Heimer et al. (1991a) and efferents of the rostral pole have been investigated by Zahm and Heimer (1993). The core projects to, among other targets, a restricted part of the globus pallidus and the SN, whereas the shell, in addition,

has several target areas outside conventional basal ganglia structures. Thus, the shell appears to project not only to the subcommissural part of the ventral pallidum and the VTA, but also to widespread areas in the hypothalamus and the sublenticular part of the "extended amygdala" (Heimer et al., 1991a). The nature of the inputs and outputs of the shell points to an involvement in visceral and autonomic functions of this part of the nucleus. The core is more heterogeneous and may be involved in complex associational functions, related to those of the prelimbic and agranular insular prefrontal areas (cf. Kolb, 1984, 1990).

Morphological and electrophysiological characteristics of projection neurons

Morphology

Spiny neurons in the nucleus accumbens, identified with respect to their extrastriatal target, i.e., the ventral tegmental area or substantia nigra of the ventral mesencephalon, were intracellularly injected with Lucifer yellow (LY) and subsequently immunoreacted with an antiserum to this dye (Fig. 3A – C). The somata of the cells were found to be small to medium in size and round to oval in shape. Their perikarya have a mean cross sectional area of $104 \pm 30 \ \mu m^2$ and mean major and minor diameters of $10 \pm 1.8 \ \mu m$ and $14 \pm 2.2 \ \mu m$, respectively (Arts and Groenewegen, 1992); some somata may be coupled with gap junctions since O'Donnell and Grace (1991) report dye-coupling in 30% of spiny projection neurons following intracellular injection of LY in vivo.

The dendrites of spiny projection neurons are initially free of spines (Fig. 3B,C) but subsequently become densely spined (Meredith et al., 1992a). The axons branch extensively within the parent dendritic domain before exiting the nucleus (Chang and Kitai, 1985; Pennartz and Kitai, 1991).

If antibodies raised against γ-aminobutyric acid (GABA; Pickel et al., 1988a) or its synthetic enzyme, glutamate decarboxylase (GAD; Meredith et al., 1990), are applied to the nucleus after colchicine treatment, numerous positively stained neurons become visible. Most GAD- and GABA-immuno-

7

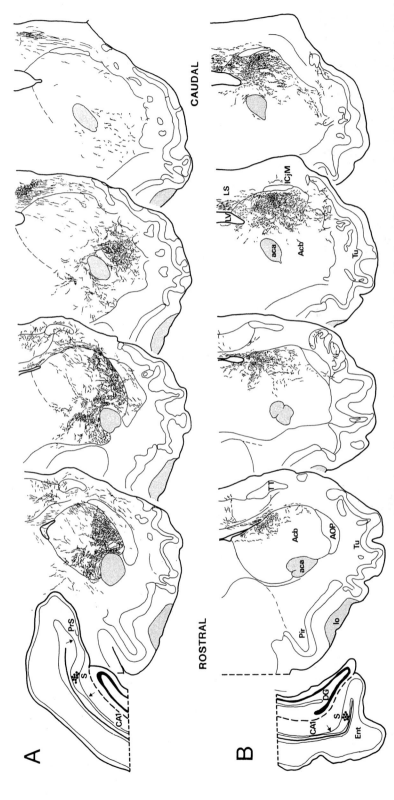

Fig. 2. Charts of anterogradely labelled fibres and terminals in the nucleus accumbens following injections of the tracer *Phaseolus vulgaris*-leucoagglutinin in the dorsal (*A*) and the ventral (*B*) subiculum of the hippocampal formation. Note that following the ventral injection (*B*), the labelling is concentrated in the medial part of the shell of the nucleus accumbens. Following the dorsal injection (*A*), the labelling is concentrated more rostrally and laterally in the nucleus. The ventral half of the rostral pole is covered by dorsal subicular afferents.

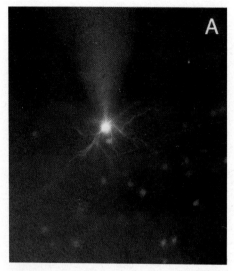

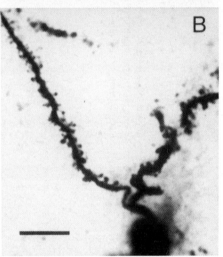

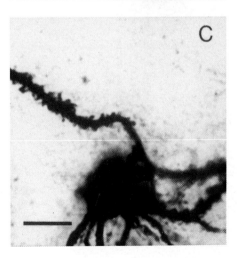

reactive perikarya are round with unindented nuclei and moderate amounts of cytoplasm; ultrastructurally, they resemble the spiny projection neuron (Pickel et al., 1988a; Meredith et al., 1990). A few GAD-immunoreactive perikarya have deeply indented nuclei and narrow rims of cytoplasm (Pickel et al., 1988a; Meredith et al., 1990). These may be aspiny GABAergic interneurons as described in the dorsal striatum (Bolam et al., 1983; Kita and Kitai, 1988).

Membrane properties

Membrane properties were studied by microelectrode recordings either in current-clamp or in voltage-clamp mode. Virtually all in vitro recordings appear to have been made from spiny projection neurons (Chang and Kitai, 1985; Pennartz et al., 1991; Pennartz and Kitai, 1991). The most conspicuous active membrane property that distinguishes these neurons from, for example, cortical pyramidal cells, is a strong inward rectification (Chang and Kitai, 1986; Uchimura et al., 1989a; Pennartz et al., 1991). In the depolarizing range of membrane potentials, several additional features were distinguished, such as a short-lasting spike after-hyperpolarization (Uchimura et al., 1989b; Pennartz et al., 1991), a relative lack of frequency adaptation in prolonged spike trains, and a slow ramp-like potential preceding spikes (Pennartz et al., 1991). The ionic properties of the intrinsic currents underlying these characteristics have not yet been investigated except for the inward rectifier (Uchimura et al., 1989a).

The behaviour of the K^+-permeable, inward-rectifying channel is considered anomalous, since its conductance is largest at hyperpolarized potentials

Fig. 3. *A*. Photomicrograph that shows a FB-labelled neuron impaled by a micropipette and filled with LY. This neuron was labelled with FB from the ventral mesencephalon. *B*. Ventral striatomesencephalic projection neuron that was intracellularly injected and then immunoreacted with antibodies against LY. This neuron is located in the shell of nucleus accumbens. Compare the density of spines on the dendritic shaft of this cell with that on the dendrite in *C*. *C*. Ventral striatomesencephalic neuron located in the core of the nucleus. Scale bars: 10 μm.

and decreases with depolarization, contrary to the behaviour of most K^+ channels. Uchimura et al. (1989a) estimated the inward rectifier to make up 44% of the resting conductance of the neuron. Their findings imply that a considerable fraction of inward-rectifying K^+ channels in neurons of the nucleus accumbens are open at rest and tend to keep the cell continuously in a strongly polarized state. This property may account for the relatively negative resting membrane potentials (-90 to -70 mV) of spiny projection neurons in slices (Uchimura et al., 1989b; Pennartz et al., 1991) as compared, for example, to pyramidal cells in slices of the hippocampus and neocortex. Furthermore, it may explain the low level of spontaneous unit activity recorded from accumbal units in awake or anaesthetized animals (Boeijinga et al., 1990; West and Michael, 1990; Apicella et al., 1991). Moreover, inward rectification lowers the probability that random synaptic inputs to the cell will cause firing, and requires that there is a certain degree of cooperativity and synchrony in the input patterns to trigger action potentials from the postsynaptic neuron (Wilson, 1991, this volume).

Shell – core differences

The morphology of spiny projection neurons differs significantly between shell and core (Meredith et al., 1992a). Neurons in the shell (Fig. 3B) have fewer primary dendrites that branch less often and are less heavily laden with spines than cells in the core (Fig. 3C). Among shell cells, those with the highest number of dendritic branches, highest spine density and greatest total dendritic length are found laterally. Further, core neurons have approximately 50% more surface area available for synaptic contacts than do cells in the shell (Meredith et al., 1992a).

To date, we have insufficient quantitative information on active membrane properties for comparison of spiny projection neurons in the shell and core. With regard to the passive membrane properties, however, shell and core neurons differ in at least two ways: the mean resting membrane potential is more negative and the mean input resistance is smaller in core than in shell neurons (Pennartz et al., 1992b). The nature of these differences is not yet clear. One of the underlying mechanisms could be that the inward-rectifying conductance in shell neurons is less prominent than in those of the core. Alternatively, the difference in input resistance may be related to the difference in total membrane area of core and shell neurons (see paragraph above). Irrespective of the precise mechanism, the data indicate that shell neurons, because of their passive membrane properties, are more excitable than core cells. This implication is in line with in vivo work that shows a larger percentage of spontaneously active units in the shell as compared to the core (P.H. Boeijinga, personal communication).

Neurochemical systems

The γ-aminobutyric acid (GABAergic) system

GABA has been recognized as playing a paramount role in fast synaptic transmission in the nucleus accumbens (Chang and Kitai, 1986; Uchimura et al., 1989b; Pennartz and Kitai, 1991; Pennartz et al., 1991). This neurotransmitter is utilized by the common, spiny projection neurons and by one category of aspiny interneurons (see above and Pickel et al., 1988a; Meredith et al., 1990). As has been reported for their dorsal striatal neighbours, the two cell types seem to have extensive intrastriatal axon collaterals (Bolam et al., 1983, 1985; Kita and Kitai, 1988).

Pickel and colleagues (1988a) describe the postsynaptic targets of GABA-immunoreactive terminal boutons in medial parts of the shell, and Meredith and Wouterlood (1991) report on glutamate decarboxylase (GAD)-immunoreactive synapses throughout the nucleus. Both GABA-containing and GAD-positive terminals form almost exclusively symmetrical junctions. They synapse with dendritic shafts about twice as often as with spines and 6% of GAD-immunoreactive and 2% of GABA-positive terminals contact cell somata (Pickel et al., 1988a; Meredith and Wouterlood, 1991). Table I summarizes the post-synaptic targets for GAD-immunoreactive synaptic boutons in the nucleus.

Both GABA-immunoreactive and GAD-positive endings synapse with other GABAergic elements (Pickel et al., 1988a; Meredith and Wouterlood, 1991) including cell bodies, dendrites and spines. Meredith and Wouterlood (1991) reported that GAD-immunoreactive endings occasionally synapse on the axon hillock of GAD-immunoreactive cells that resemble the common spiny projection neuron, a location that would place them in a strategic position to influence other projection neurons. GABA-positive terminal boutons in the nucleus have also been reported in close apposition to GABA- or TH-positive endings; however, these close appositions seem to lack recognizable densities (Pickel et al., 1988a).

Electrophysiologically, the GABAergic system of the ventral striatum appears to sustain at least three types of action (Table II). Firstly, according to intracellular recordings in spiny projection neurons of the shell, an EPSP evoked by fornix/fimbria or local stimulation is rapidly followed by a bicuculline- and picrotoxin-sensitive potential that reverses polarity at about -70 mV (Fig. 4, Pennartz and Kitai, 1991; Pennartz et al., 1991; Yuan et al., 1992; see, however, Uchimura et al., 1989b). These properties justify identification of this synaptic potential as a $GABA_A$ receptor-mediated IPSP. In view of the preponderant axonal arborizations of spiny projection neurons, we expected this IPSP to be mediated by lateral or recurrent inhibition. Surprisingly, however, its dynamic and pharmacological characteristics are better interpreted as a feed-

TABLE I

Characterized synaptic relationships in the nucleus accumbens

Chemical identity of synaptic bouton	Source of bouton	Location and identity of postsynaptic elements		
		Spines	Shafts	Perikarya
EAA ($n = 130$)	Midline thalamus[1]	Shell / core 33% / ?	Shell / core 56% / ?	Shell / core 4% / ?
EAA ($n = 274$[2]; $n = 107$[3])	Cortex: hippocampus[2] prefrontal cortex[3]	Shell < core 86% < 97%	Shell > core 10% > 1%	Shell > core 2% > 0%
Substance P ($n = 114$)	Local axon collaterals[4]	Medial n. accumbens 8%	Medial n. accumbens 30%	Medial n. accumbens 4%
ENK ($n = 409$)	Local axon collaterals[5]	Shell > core 19% > 11%	Shell < core 71% < 78%	Shell = core 5% = 6%
TH (presumed dopaminergic) ($n = 100$)	VTA/SN[6]	Shell < core 29% < 51%	Shell > core 68% > 37%	Shell = core 2% = 1%
GAD (presumed GABAergic) ($n = 107$)	Local axon collaterals[7]	N. accumbens 15%	N. accumbens 35%	N. accumbens 6%
ChAT (presumed cholinergic) ($n = 113$)	Local axon collaterals[8]	Substriatal grey lateral shell (?) 13%	Substriatal grey lateral shell (?) 61%	Substriatal grey lateral shell (?) 26%

n = total number of synaptic boutons analysed.

[1] Meredith and Wouterlood (1990); [2] Meredith et al. (1990); [3] Sesack and Pickel (1992); [4] Pickel et al. (1988b); [5] Meredith et al. (1992); [6] Zahm (1992); [7] Meredith and Wouterlood (1991); [8] Phelps and Vaughn (1986).

forward type of inhibition, which suggests the involvement of GABAergic interneurons in the response to fornix stimulation (Pennartz and Kitai, 1991). GABA$_A$ receptor-mediated IPSPs of similar time course and reversal potential were also found in the core (Pennartz et al., 1991) which means that the same type of spatiotemporal organisation of fast inhibition as postulated for the shell, is present.

Secondly, in addition to the fast GABA$_A$ receptor-mediated IPSP, GABA actions mediated by GABA$_B$ receptors have been reported in nucleus accumbens (Uchimura and North, 1991). The GABA$_B$ receptor agonist baclofen inhibited both the glutamatergic EPSP and the GABA$_A$ receptor-mediated IPSP mentioned above. Thirdly, a modest hyperpolarizing effect mediated by an increase in potassium conductance was also observed during baclofen application.

Thus, the GABAergic system of nucleus accum-

bens can sustain a fast inhibition, probably mediated by a feed-forward circuit onto spiny projection neurons, a modulation of both the fast excitation and inhibition, and a modulation of membrane potential and resting conductance in spiny projection neurons (see Table II). Altogether, the functional characteristics of the GABAergic system in this nucleus resemble those in many other brain structures, e.g., hippocampus (Dutar and Nicoll, 1988).

The glutamatergic system

Synaptic terminals releasing glutamate or related excitatory amino acids in the nucleus accumbens are thought to originate from thalamic, amygdaloid and cortical neurons, i.e., the hippocampal formation and prefrontal cortex (Altschuler et al., 1985; Christie et al., 1987; Fuller et al., 1987).

Axons arising from the ventral subiculum and

TABLE II

Electrophysiological actions of transmitters and modulators in the nucleus accumbens

Neuroactive substance	Receptor(s)	Origin	Presumed action	Target
Glutamate	AMPA/Kain	HPF, Amy, Th, PFCx	fast excitation	spiny projection neuron GABA interneuron
Glutamate	NMDA	HPF, Amy, Th, PFCx	slow excitation LTP-induction	spiny projection neuron
GABA	GABA$_A$	interneuron, spiny projection neuron	fast inhibition	spiny projection neuron
GABA	GABA$_B$	interneuron, spiny projection neuron	hyperpolarization, reduction EPSP and IPSP	spiny projection neuron
Dopamine	D1	VTA	reduction of EPSP and IPSP	spiny projection neuron
Dopamine	D2	VTA	reduction of EPSP	??
Acetylcholine	M1	ACh interneuron	depolarization, reduction of IPSP	??
Acetylcholine	M3	ACh interneuron	reduction of EPSP	??
ENK	δ, α	spiny projection neuron	reduction of EPSP and IPSP	??

Abbreviations: ACh, acetylcholine; AMPA, α-amino-3-hydroxy-5-methyl-4-isoxazolepropionic acid; Amy, amygdala; HPF, hippocampal formation; Kain, kainate; PFCx, prefrontal cortex; Th, thalamus; VTA, ventral tegmental area.

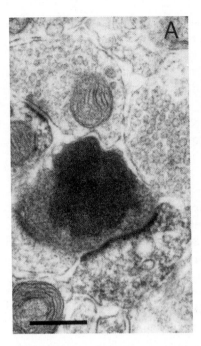 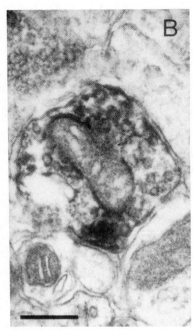 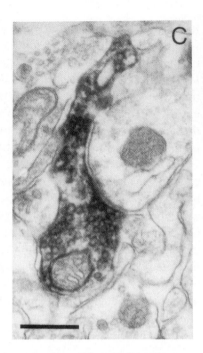

Fig. 4. Electron micrographs of (A) a degenerating hippocampal terminal in the shell of nucleus accumbens. This terminal is in asymmetric contact with a GAD-immunoreactive spine; (B) an enkephalin-immunoreactive bouton in the shell that is in symmetric synaptic contact with a spine; and (C) an enkephalin-immunoreactive bouton that forms a symmetric synapse with a dendrite in the core. Scale bars: 0.25 μm.

CA1 of the hippocampal formation project via the fornix to nucleus accumbens and terminate mainly in the shell region (see above and Kelly et al., 1982; Groenewegen et al., 1982, 1987; Meredith et al., 1990). The synapses are asymmetrical in configuration and are primarily formed with spines (Fig. 4A; Table I). However, approximately 10% are axodendritic and a further 2% axosomatic. Ventral subicular axon terminals often contact GAD-immunoreactive elements (Meredith et al., 1990). Indeed, all axosomatic contacts are made with GAD-immunoreactive perikarya that had the ultrastructural characteristics of the spiny projection neurons (Meredith et al., 1990).

Prefrontal cortical fibres also form asymmetrical junctions and nearly 100% of them terminate on spines in the core of nucleus accumbens (see Table I for summary; Sesack and Pickel, 1992). Such an extensive input to spines is similar to that reported for cortical fibres in the dorsal striatum (Somogyi et al., 1981; Dubé et al., 1988).

Corticostriatal afferent fibres appear to converge with dopaminergic inputs on the same element in both the shell and core of nucleus accumbens. Totterdell and Smith (1989) first reported the convergence of hippocamal and TH-positive endings on spiny neurons in the shell and Meredith (1992) identified the target neurons as projection cells in this region. Sesack and Pickel (1992) have demonstrated prefrontal cortical fibres and TH-immunoreactive terminals in contact with the same element in the core.

Close appositions between cortical and TH-containing terminals have been reported in both the shell (Sesack and Pickel, 1990) and the core (Sesack and Pickel, 1992) and the incidence seems high. Indeed, Sesack and Pickel (1992) report that axo-axonic appositions comprise 30% of the total terminal juxtapositions they examined. Close appositions could provide the morphological substrate for presynaptic interactions in this nucleus (see Discussion).

Terminals from the paraventricular nucleus of the thalamus form asymmetrical synaptic specializations but, in contrast to cortical terminals, the majority contact dendritic shafts (see Table I and Meredith and Wouterlood, 1990). Only one-third of these terminals end on spines and a further 4% on somata. Thalamic inputs may have a direct impact on the excitability of cholinergic interneurons since choline acetyltransferase (ChAT)-immunoreactive proximal dendrites and perikarya are among their postsynaptic targets (Meredith and Wouterlood, 1990).

From an electrophysiologist's point of view, the glutamatergic afferent fibres to nucleus accumbens play an important role in that they provide for both fast excitatory transmission and synaptic plasticity in accumbal neurons (Table II). In vitro experiments have shown that electrical stimulation of the hippocampal (Fig. 5) and prefrontal afferents and of the accumbal neuropil itself, elicits monosynaptic EPSPs in the spiny projection neurons. These appear to be mediated by α-amino-3-hydroxy-5-methyl-4-isoxazolepropionic acid (AMPA)/kainate receptors (Pennartz et al., 1990, 1991; Horne et al., 1990; Pennartz and Kitai, 1991; see, however, Uchimura et al., 1989b). When GABAergic inhibition is intact, NMDA receptor-mediated contributions to these EPSPs appear to be small and are restricted to the decay phase. In the absence of $GABA_A$ receptor-mediated inhibition, however, the NMDA component can grow to considerable amplitudes and its contribution can be enlarged even more following paired-pulse stimulation (Pennartz et al., 1991).

Long-term potentiation has now been shown to occur in three pathways to the nucleus accumbens: amygdaloid afferent inputs (Uno and Ozawa, 1991), subicular afferent pathway (Boeijinga et al., 1992) and prefrontal-cortical afferent fibres (Pennartz et al., 1993). The induction of LTP in the prefrontal cortex-accumbens projection depends strongly on NMDA receptor activity (Pennartz et al., 1993). From these findings it appears that NMDA receptors play a dual role in this nucleus: firstly, they contribute to fast excitation and amplification of short-term facilitation phenomena under conditions of reduced GABAergic inhibition, and secondly, they mediate a long-lasting potentiation of fast excitatory responses.

Despite the fact that several recording series have been conducted under similar conditions and in similarly prepared slices, no consistent shell/core

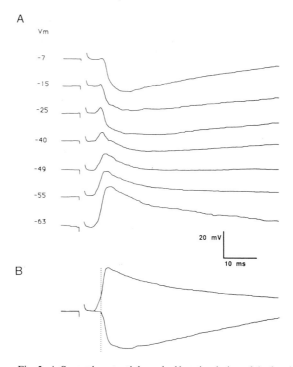

Fig. 5. A. Synaptic potentials evoked by stimulation of the fornix in an in vitro slice preparation. The fornix response was examined at several levels of membrane potential (indicated on the left) with the use of intracellular current injection. At membrane potentials more negative than −45 mV, a depolarizing response was recorded. At membrane potentials depolarized to −45 mV, a biphasic response emerged, consisting of an early depolarizing and a slightly delayed, hyperpolarizing component (reproduced from the *Journal of Neuroscience,* with permission; copyright: Society of Neuroscience). B. The onset latency of the hyperpolarizing component, recorded at −2 mV, was slightly longer than the onset latency of the depolarizing response, recorded at resting membrane potential. The onset of the hyperpolarizing component typically coincided with the mid-rising phase of the depolarizing response. Pharmacological experiments showed that the early, depolarizing response could be identified as an AMPA/kainate receptor-mediated EPSP and the delayed, hyperpolarizing response as a $GABA_B$ receptor-mediated IPSP. A and B were recorded from the same spiny neuron (resting membrane potential: −71 mV).

differences in glutamatergic excitation have been found to date (Pennartz et al., 1990, 1991; Pennartz and Kitai, 1991).

The dopaminergic system

Both the shell and core of nucleus accumbens receive a dense afferent dopaminergic innervation from the ventral mesencephalon (Voorn et al., 1986). Ultrastructurally, dopamine-immunoreactive and TH-positive (presumably dopaminergic) boutons are similar in appearance and pattern of termination. Synaptic boutons form mainly symmetric contacts, mainly with dendrites (see Table I; Voorn et al., 1986; Pickel et al., 1988a). Recently, however, a regional study of TH-positive terminals in accumbens revealed that, in the shell, TH-immunoreactive terminals contact dendritic shafts twice as often as spines, whereas in the core they synapse on shafts and spines in equal numbers (Zahm, 1992; summarized in Table I). These differences in synaptic arrangement may be related to the differential action of dopamine in the shell and the core (see below and Deutch and Cameron, 1991; Pennartz et al., 1992b).

In the shell, both perikarya and proximal dendrites of GABAergic neurons are among the targets of TH-positive axon terminals (Pickel et al., 1988a). Indeed, according to Pickel and colleagues (1988a), all axosomatic targets of TH-containing endings may be GABAergic. Our recent experiments show that numerous TH-positive terminals appose the proximal dendrites and somata of spiny projection neurons in the shell (Fig. 6$A-D$; Meredith and Wouterlood, 1993). Further, the convergence of TH-positive, presumably dopaminergic, endings with cortical terminals on the same postsynaptic element in both the shell and core, as we reported above in the section on the glutamatergic system, may underlie the dopamine-mediated attenuation of the cortical response (see below).

Most electrophysiological studies have emphasized the attenuating effect of dopamine on excitatory inputs coming from the hippocampal formation (Fig. 7; DeFrance et al., 1985; Yang and Mogenson, 1986; Pennartz et al., 1992a), the amygdala (Yim and Mogenson, 1988), thalamus (Hara et al., 1989) and the prefrontal cortex (Fig. 7; Pennartz et al., 1992a). In addition, inhibitory effects of dopamine on spontaneous firing activity in the nucleus have been reported (White and Wang, 1986; Clark and White, 1987; White, 1987). There is less agreement in the literature about the effects of dopamine on membrane properties of accumbal neurons studied in vitro. Uchimura et al. (1986) reported hyperpolarizing and depolarizing actions of D1 and D2 receptors respectively; others, however, have not observed such effects consistently (Pennartz et al., 1992a).

The effect of dopamine on synaptic transmission can be attributed to presynaptic mechanisms in nucleus accumbens (Yang and Mogenson, 1986; Yim and Mogenson, 1988; Higashi et al., 1989; Pennartz et al., 1992a), but different dopamine receptor subtypes have been held responsible for the attenuating effect on excitatory inputs. The findings of Yang and Mogenson (1986) indicate an involvement of the D2 receptor subtype in the attenuation of unit firing in response to fornix stimulation, whereas the results of pharmacological experiments support a role for the D1 receptor in modulating subicular, thalamic and prefrontal inputs (DeFrance et al., 1985; Hara et al., 1989; Higashi et al., 1989; Pennartz et al., 1992a).

The primary effect of dopamine is to inhibit the firing of accumbal neurons, particularly spiny projection neurons. However, dopamine inhibits GABAergic IPSPs to a similar extent as EPSPs and thus, it may also exert a disinhibitory effect on these neurons (Yim and Mogenson, 1988; Pennartz et al.,

Fig. 6. *A*. Electron micrograph illustrating a LY-injected spiny projection neuron in the shell of nucleus accumbens. The neuron was immunoreacted with antibodies to LY and the DAB reaction product was silver-enhanced. The material was further reacted with antibodies against TH. *B*. Correlated light micrograph of the neuron pictured in *A*. Region marked with the star is the fibre bundle seen to the right of the cell in *A*. *C*, *D* and *E* are high power electron micrographs showing a series of TH-immunoreactive boutons (b_1, b_2, b_3) in apposition to the soma and proximal dendrites of the striato-mesencephalic cell. Scale bars, 0.25 μm.

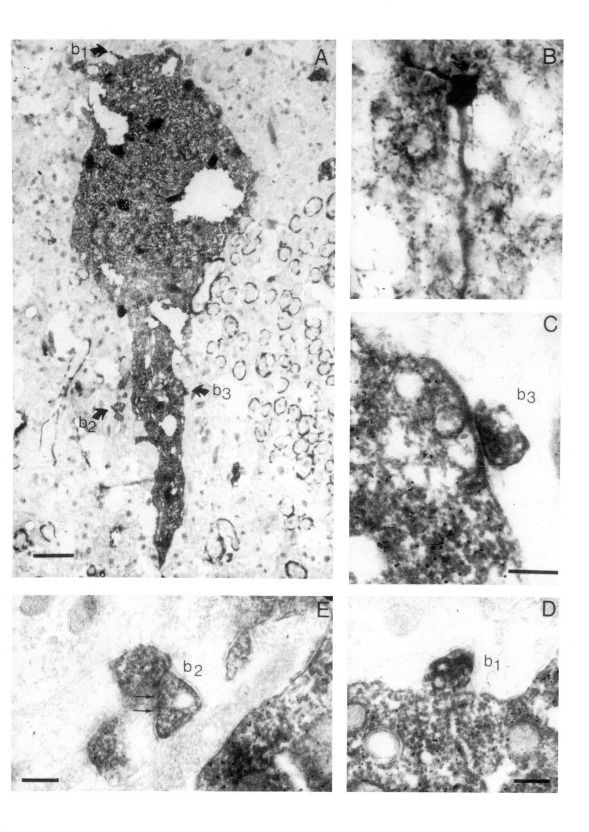

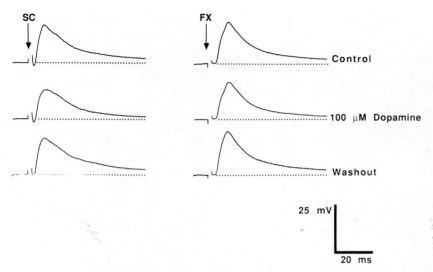

Fig. 7. In this accumbal neuron, dopamine (100 μM) reduced synaptic responses evoked by fornix (FX, right) as well as subcortical stimulation (SC, left). Electrical stimulation of the fornix excited hippocampal fibres, whereas subcortical stimulation primarily excited prefrontal afferent fibres to the nucleus accumbens. In control conditions (upper traces), prefrontal and hippocampal afferent fibres are shown to converge upon the same recorded neuron, evoking synaptic responses of considerable amplitude. In the middle traces, the synaptic responses were reduced by 100 μM dopamine. This modulatory effect was reversed after washout (lower traces).

1992a). Depending on the relative size of the EPSP and IPSP, either the inhibitory (EPSP-suppressing) or disinhibitory (IPSP-suppressing) influence of dopamine may prevail in a particular state of the striatal network. In addition to possible metabotropic and postsynaptic membrane effects of dopamine, this dual influence on synaptic inputs makes it difficult to regard dopamine as a purely inhibitory neuromodulator in nucleus accumbens.

Shell/core differences have only been investigated in in vitro slices where the D1 receptor-mediated attenuation of cortical inputs to spiny projection neurons seems to be present only in the shell (Pennartz et al., 1992b). Interestingly, D1 receptor mRNA is strongly expressed in the ventral subiculum (Fremeau et al., 1991) which primarily projects to the caudal shell (see the section on the organisation of shell and core, p. 4). Certainly, any regional differences in dopamine receptor-mediated affects should also be investigated in vivo. Another highly relevant issue for future research is the function of D3 dopamine receptors which seem to be selectively concentrated in the caudomedial part of the shell (Sokoloff et al., 1990).

The cholinergic system

The acetylcholine (ACh)-containing neurons in the nucleus accumbens form a small but important population of intrinsic cells (Phelps and Vaughn, 1986). These neurons which are more densely distributed in the shell than in the core (Meredith et al., 1989), have large perikarya (measuring 20 μm in diameter), aspiny dendrites and an extensive axonal network that terminates in the nucleus (Phelps and Vaughn, 1986). We have recently analyzed the perikaryal sizes of ChAT-immunoreactive neurons in the shell and core (Meredith and Wilmsen, unpublished observations) and found that cholinergic somata are significantly smaller (paired Student's t-test, $t = 1.41$, $P < 0.05$) in the shell ($n = 199$; mean $= 128.70 \pm$ S.D. 29.34 μm^2) than in the core ($n = 200$; mean $= 176.20 \pm$ S.D. 46.02 μm^2).

Ultrastructurally, the cholinergic cell can be distinguished from the projection neuron in that it has a large nucleus with a deeply indented nuclear membrane (Phelps and Vaughn, 1986; Meredith et al., 1989). Cholinergic terminals are found throughout the nucleus but there are insufficient data to note regional differences either in the density of endings or in the distribution of their postsynaptic targets. According to Phelps and Vaughan (1986), most ChAT-immunoreactive junctions are symmetrical. Approximately 60% of all ChAT-positive synaptic boutons form contacts with dendritic shafts, a further one-fourth with somata and the rest with spines. Ultrastructurally, the targets of axosomatic synapses resemble the spiny projection neurons (Phelps and Vaughn, 1986). Furthermore, cholinergic terminals have been seen in contact with somata and dendritic shafts of neurons containing enkephalin which presumably project out of the nucleus (see below and Meredith et al., 1992b). Although axo-axonic synaptic contacts could not be recognized with any certainty, ChAT-immunoreactive terminals occasionally appose other terminals directly (Meredith and Wouterlood, 1991).

Acetylcholine affects the overall excitability of accumbal neurons by modulating synaptic responses as well as membrane properties. In slice preparations, it is capable of strongly attenuating both EPSPs and IPSPs evoked by muscarinic receptor stimulation (Fig. 8; Pennartz and Lopes da Silva, 1994). It achieves this dual modulation by activating two different muscarinic receptors subtypes (M1 for IPSPs and probably M3 for EPSPs; Sugita et al., 1991). The site of muscarinic receptor action is inferred to be on glutamatergic (for EPSPs) and GABAergic (for IPSPs) terminals (Sugita et al., 1991; Pennartz and Lopes da Silva, unpublished observations). This type of muscarinic modulation is not limited to this nucleus or even to the entire striatal complex (cf. Malenka and Kocsis, 1988) and has also been found in, for example, the amygdala and the hippocampus (Valentino and Dingledine, 1981; Sugita et al., 1991). When comparing the action of muscarinic receptor agonists to the action of dopamine in nucleus accumbens, one is struck by the similarities in the synaptic modulatory mechanisms. There appears to be a difference between acetylcholine and dopamine, however, in their modulation of membrane properties. Uchimura and North (1990) reported that muscarinic agonists reduce the inward-rectifying K^+ conductance, giving rise to membrane depolarization and enhanced excitability (cf. Woodruff et al., 1976), whereas this conductance is probably not affected by dopamine (Uchimura et al., 1986; Pennartz et al., 1992b, 1993)

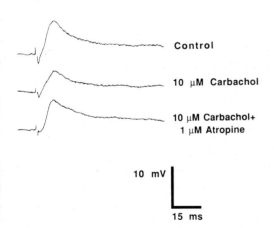

Fig. 8. Under control conditions (upper trace), local electrical stimulation in nucleus accumbens evoked a depolarizing response, which mainly consisted of an EPSP. Bath application of the cholinergic agonist carbachol (10 μM, middle trace) depressed the EPSP, and subsequent addition of 1 μM atropine (lower trace) antagonized the modulatory action of carbachol, indicating involvement of muscarinic receptors.

The enkephalinergic system

Enkephalinergic (ENK) endings in nucleus accumbens are predominantly symmetrical in configuration. Dendritic shafts are the principal targets throughout the nucleus (Fig. 5C); however, as Table I shows, ENK-positive endings in the shell contact nearly twice as many spines as in the core and, therefore, fewer dendrites than those in the core. The number of axosomatic contacts is approximately the same in shell and core (Meredith et al., 1993). Axosomatic contacts are generally made with medium-sized, round to oval perikarya with unindented nuclei that resemble the spiny projection neurons. Although axo-axonic synapses have not been seen, close appositions between enkephalin-containing terminals and other boutons have been reported (Meredith et al., 1992b).

Enkephalinergic neurons appear to be under the control of dopamine and if deprived of this input, the levels of enkephalin and preproenkephalin mRNA increase (Voorn and Docter, 1992). Dopamine depletion in the dorsal striatum results in morphological changes in local enkephalinergic terminals (Ingham et al., 1991).

In vivo electrophysiological studies have suggested that enkephalins and related opioid receptor agonists inhibit unit activity in nucleus accumbens (McCarthy et al., 1977; Hakan and Henriksen, 1989). In intracellular recordings in the core studied in vitro, Yuan et al. (1992) identified a cellular action of μ- and δ-opioid receptor agonists possibly underlying the inhibitory effects observed in vivo. These agonists reduced both IPSPs and EPSPs while leaving the membrane properties of accumbal neurons unaffected. Naloxone effectively antagonized these depressant effects on synaptic excitability, confirming an involvement of opioid receptors (Yuan et al., 1992). It remains to be investigated whether enkephalins and related substances suppress all afferent inputs to accumbens, or affect only specific pathways, as suggested by the demonstration that morphine does not inhibit unit activity evoked by fornix-fimbria stimulation (Hakan and Henriksen, 1989). Certainly, ENK analogues injected into the VTA stimulate a motor response and increase extracellular dopamine levels in nucleus accumbens (Kalivas and Duffy, 1990). Insufficient data are available to comment on shell/core differences in enkephalinergic modulation.

Chemical signalling in nucleus accumbens: morphological and physiological substrates

The morphological and electrophysiological data reviewed in this chapter indicate that the synaptic connections and function of nucleus accumbens spiny projection neurons are similar to those of caudate-putamen cells (for reviews, see Chang and Wilson, 1990; Smith and Bolam, 1990). Despite the general striatal-like character of the structure and neurotransmitter interactions in this nucleus, some important variations on the basic theme have been noted in comparisons of shell and core. Before embarking on the discussion of these differences and their possible functional implications, we want to

examine a discrepancy between the ultrastructural and electrophysiological data. Although a number of the physiological findings readily find their counterpart in the relationships of neuronal elements at the ultrastructural level, other electrophysiological phenomena are not easily correlated with morphological data – in particular, the presynaptic mechanisms that seem to play an important role in modulating glutamatergic and GABAergic transmission.

Reconciling morphology and electrophysiology: the diffusion hypothesis

Electrophysiological studies have demonstrated that GABA$_B$, dopamine D1 and D2, muscarinic, μ- and δ-opioid receptors can reduce glutamatergic and GABAergic transmission by presynaptic mechanisms. However, ultrastructural studies have failed to demonstrate the expected axo-axonal contacts. In the case of dopaminergic modulation of EPSPs, however, close appositions between dopaminergic and glutamatergic terminals (Pickel et al., 1988a,b; Sesack and Pickel, 1990, 1992; Meredith and Wouterlood, 1991) in the vicinity of projection neurons (Meredith, 1992) could provide an anatomical substrate that would allow for substance diffusion over relatively small distances. Diffusion-dependent or "paracrine" neuromodulation, a mechanism proposed much earlier to explain presynaptic actions (Tennyson et al., 1974; Beaudet and Descarries, 1978; Lehman and Langer, 1983), probably occurs when the firing activity of dopaminergic fibres gives rise to a local release of dopamine which, subsequently, diffuses into the surrounding intercellular space, sometimes arriving in sufficient concentration at a neighbouring (glutamatergic) terminal. The concentration of dopamine at such a terminal is likely to depend on several factors, e.g., the discharge frequency in the parent VTA neurons, the activity of dopamine uptake mechanisms and the precise diffusion distance (cf. Grace, 1991, for review). In this context, it may be relevant to note that during high-frequency stimulation of the median forebrain bundle, extracellular dopamine concentrations in nucleus accumbens, as quantified by in vivo voltammetry, may rise to micromolar concentrations (Wightman and Zimmerman, 1990). With due caution, then, we hypothesize that burst discharges in the dopaminergic VTA neurons can lead to short-range interactions with the release of amino acids mediating fast synaptic transmission onto spiny projection neurons. For the case of presynaptic modulation of EPSPs and/or IPSPs by acetylcholine, enkephalins and $GABA_B$ receptors, many relevant anatomical and neurochemical details are lacking, making it difficult to evaluate the possibility of diffusion-dependent neuromodulation.

Spiny projection neurons: a comparison between shell and core

In this report we have pointed out that the flow of information through nucleus accumbens is dependent upon the activity and modulation of a central neuron: the GABAergic, spiny projection cell which presumably contributes to the excitability of the nucleus and forms an important substrate for neuromodulation. Essentially the same types of chemical signals may influence this cell in the shell and in the core, but at least for dopamine, shell – core differences have been noted in the arrangement of the synaptic terminals (Zahm, 1992) and in the modulation of EPSPs (Pennartz et al., 1992b). Furthermore, when comparing our morphometric and electrophysiological data on spiny projection neurons in the shell and core, an interesting, albeit speculative, parallel can be drawn. The fact that core neurons have significantly more surface area than shell cells (Meredith et al., 1992a) may explain the larger passive input resistance of shell neurons in in vitro slice preparations (Pennartz et al., 1992b), and hence, may be related to the higher level of spontaneous activity of those units in vivo (Boeijinga et al., 1990). However, there are probably more factors that can explain the shell – core differences in passive membrane properties, one of which may be a difference in the inward-rectifying K^+ conductance.

Core neurons are significantly spinier than their counterparts in the shell (Meredith et al., 1992a),

which suggests that spines and their integrative properties play a greater role in determining the output of the core. Spines, when acting in concert, seem to be able to influence dendritic cable properties effectively (Perkel and Perkel, 1985; Jaslove, 1992), presumably through current spread to neighbouring spines (Shepherd et al., 1985). Distal excitatory synapses, which in nucleus accumbens are formed primarily by cortical axon terminals that impinge on spines, may cause an increase in synaptic conductance of dendrites. Spines presumably play a role in this event by amplifying local changes in intracellular calcium (Koch et al., 1992). Differences in spine density could have important consequences since lower densities may impose spatial restrictions on the actions of second messengers (Müller and Connor, 1991) in accumbal projection neurons.

Many questions remain before we can unravel the synaptic circuitry, its activation and operation, in the shell and core of nucleus accumbens. Certainly, differences between these two regions exist in the spatial segregation of inputs to spiny projection cells from cortical, dopaminergic and enkephalinergic neurons, but we lack sufficient data to comment on any differences in the synaptic arrangement of other terminals, such as ACh, GABA, or peptides, such as substance P. Although we have some evidence for the action of dopamine in the shell and core, regional differences in the action of cortical (glutamatergic), GABAergic, cholinergic and peptidergic inputs have yet to be identified.

Concluding remarks

The precise delineation of shell and core should prove invaluable to many research disciplines investigating nucleus accumbens. On the basis of the distribution of naloxone-binding sites, substance P immunoreactivity and hippocampal innervation patterns, the rostral pole of nucleus accumbens has been assigned primarily to the shell for the purposes of this review. However, more research is needed to determine whether the demarcation of shell and core, as proposed here, reflects a functional partitioning. Electrophysiological and behavioural approaches to the shell – core distinction are still in their infancy, but will, nevertheless, be crucial for gaining an understanding of such functional differences.

Anatomical analysis allows us to predict the synaptic circuitry of a region, yet alone gives no indication of the relative importance of any one input or set of inputs. There are several levels at which a neuron's function can be related to its structure, e.g., presynaptic, postsynaptic, electrotonic. The partitioning of nucleus accumbens into shell and core can only have significance when we establish, in detail, not only the synaptic connections but also the pre- and postsynaptic interactions of these two zones. Anatomically, we need to study quantitatively the spatial relationships of synaptic terminals and electrophysiologically, it would be useful to make quantal analyses of miniature EPSCs and IPSCs in order to dissect the precise mechanisms of presynaptic modulation. A particularly powerful approach would be to combine voltammetric detection of extracellular dopamine levels and recordings of unit activity, as this would enable us to assess the extracellular concentrations of endogenously released dopamine that may be necessary for the modulation of firing activity in this nucleus. Further investigation of any of the fundamental issues covered in this report will serve to advance our understanding of this nucleus and the mechanisms that underlie related neurological and psychiatric disorders (Heimer et al., 1991b).

Acknowledgements

We are grateful to Drs. A.H.M. Lohman and B.L. Roberts for critically reading the manuscript. We also wish to acknowledge the excellent technical assistance of A. Pattiselanno and expert photographic assistance of D. de Jong and S. Paniry. This work was supported by a Netherlands Organisation for Scientific Research (N.W.O.) program grant 900-550-093 and a Joint Scientific Research grant to G.E.M. from the British Council and N.W.O.

References

Alexander, G.E., DeLong, M.R. and Strick, P.L. (1986) Parallel organization of functionally segregated circuits linking basal ganglia and cortex. *Annu. Rev. Neurosci.,* 9: 357 – 381.

Alger, B.E. and Nicoll, R.A. (1982) Feed-forward dendritic inhibition in rat hippocampal pyramidal cells studied in vitro. *J. Physiol. (Lond.),* 328: 105 – 123.

Altschuler, R.A., Monaghan, D.T., Haser, W.G., Wenthold, R.J., Curthoys, N.P. and Cotman, C.W. (1985) Immunocytochemical localization of glutaminase-like and aspartate aminotransferase-like immunoreactivities in the rat and guinea pig hippocampus. *Brain Res.,* 330: 225 – 233.

Apicella, P., Ljungberg, T., Scarnati, E. and Schultz, W. (1991) Responses to reward in monkey dorsal and ventral striatum. *Exp. Brain Res.,* 85: 491 – 500.

Arts, M.P.M. and Groenewegen, H.J. (1992) Relationships of the dendritic arborizations of ventral striato-mesencephalic projection neurons with boundaries of striatal compartments. An in vitro intracellular study in the rat. *Eur. J. Neurosci.,* 4: 574 – 588.

Beaudet, A. and Descarries, L. (1978) The monoamine innervation of rat cerebral cortex: synaptic and non-synaptic terminals. *Neuroscience,* 3: 851 – 860.

Beckstead, R.M., Domesick, V.B. and Nauta, W.J.H. (1979) Efferent connections of the substantia nigra and ventral tegmental area in the rat. *Brain Res.,* 175: 191 – 217.

Berendse, H.W. and Groenewegen, H.J. (1990) Organization of the thalamostriatal projections in the rat, with special emphasis on the ventral striatum. *J. Comp. Neurol.,* 299: 187 – 228.

Berendse, H.W., Galis-de Graaf, Y. and Groenewegen, H.J. (1992a) Topographical organization and relationship with ventral striatal compartments of prefrontal corticostriatal projections in the rat. *J. Comp. Neurol.,* 316: 314 – 347.

Berendse, H.W., Groenewegen, H.J. and Lohman, A.H.M. (1992b) Compartmental distribution of ventral striatal neurons projecting to the mesencephalon in the rat. *J. Neurosci.,* 12: 2079 – 2103.

Boeijinga, P.H., Pennartz, C.M.A. and Lopes da Silva, F.H. (1990) Paired-pulse facilitation in the nucleus accumbens following stimulation of subicular inputs in the rat. *Neuroscience,* 35: 301 – 311.

Boeijinga, P.H., Mulder, A.B., Pennartz, C.M.A., Manshanden, I. and Lopes da Silva, F.H. (1992) Responses of the nucleus accumbens following fornix/fimbria stimulation in the rat. Identification and long-term potentiation of mono- and polysynaptic pathways. *Neuroscience,* 53: 1049 – 1058.

Bolam, J.P., Clarke, D.J., Smith, A.D. and Somogyi, P. (1983) A type of aspiny neuron in the rat neostriatum accumulates [^{3}H]γ-aminobutyric acid: combination of Golgi-staining, autoradiography and electron microscopy. *J. Comp. Neurol.,* 213: 121 – 134.

Glutamate decarboxylase-immunoreactive structures in the rat neostriatum: a correlated light and electron microscopic study including a combination of Golgi impregnation with immunocytochemistry. *J. Comp. Neurol.,* 237: 1 – 20.

Buzsaki, G. (1984) Feed-forward inhibition in the hippocampal formation. *Prog. Neurobiol.,* 22: 131 – 153.

Chang, H.T. and Kitai, S.T. (1985) Projection neurons of the nucleus accumbens: an intracellular labeling study. *Brain Res.,* 347: 112 – 116.

Chang, H.T. and Kitai, S.T. (1986) Intracellular recordings from rat nucleus accumbens neurons in vitro. *Brain Res.,* 366: 392 – 396.

Chang, H.T. and Wilson, C.J. (1990) Anatomical analysis of electrophysiologically characterized neurons in the rat striato-pallidal system. In: A. Björklund, T. Hökfelt, F.G. Wouterlood and A.N. Van Den Pol (Eds.), *Handbook of Chemical Neuroanatomy. Analysis of Neuronal Microcircuits and Synaptic Interactions, Vol. 8,* Elsevier, Amsterdam, pp. 351 – 402.

Christie, M.J., Summers, R.J., Stephenson, J.A., Cook, C.J. and Beart, P.M. (1987) Excitatory amino acid projections to the nucleus accumbens septi in the rat: a retrograde transport study utilizing D[^{3}H]aspartate and [^{3}H]GABA. *Neuroscience,* 22: 425 – 439.

Chronister, R.B., Sikes, R.W., Trow, T.W. and DeFrance, J.F. (1981) The organization of nucleus accumbens. In: R.B. Chronister and J.F. DeFrance (Eds.), *The Neurobiology of the Nucleus Accumbens,* The Haer Institute for Electrophysiological Research, Brunswick, ME, pp. 147 – 172.

Clark, D. and White, F.J. (1987) Review: D1 dopamine receptor – the search for a function: a critical evaluation of the D1/D2 dopamine receptor classification and its functional implications. *Synapse,* 1: 347 – 388.

DeFrance, J.F., Sikes, R.W. and Chronister, R.B. (1985) Dopamine action in the nucleus accumbens. *J. Neurophysiol.,* 54: 1568 – 1577.

Deutch, A.Y. and Cameron, D.S. (1991) Pharmacological characterization of dopamine systems in the nucleus accumbens core and shell. *Neuroscience,* 46: 49 – 56.

Domesick, V.B. (1981) Further observations on the anatomy of the nucleus accumbens and caudate-putamen in the rat: similarities and contrasts. In: R.B. Chronister and J.F. DeFrance (Eds.), *The Neurobiology of the Nucleus Accumbens,* The Haer Institute for Electrophysiological Research, Brunswick, ME, pp. 7 – 39.

Dubé, L., Smith, A.D. and Bolam, J.P. (1988) Identification of synaptic terminals of thalamic or cortical origin in contact with distinct medium-sized spiny neurons in the rat neostriatum. *J. Comp. Neurol.,* 267: 455 – 471.

Dutar, P. and Nicoll, R.A. (1988) Pre- and postsynaptic GABA$_B$-receptors in the hippocampus have different pharmacological properties. *Neuron,* 1: 585 – 591.

Fremeau, R.T., Duncan, G.E., Fornaretto, M.G., Dearry, A., Gingrich, J.A., Breese, G.R. and Caron, M.G. (1991) Localization of D1 dopamine receptor mRNA in brain supports a role in cognitive, affective, and neuroendocrine aspects of dopaminergic transmission. *Proc. Natl. Acad. Sci. U.S.A.,* 88: 3772 – 3776.

Fuller, T.A., Russchen, F.T. and Price, J.L. (1987) Sources of presumptive glutamergic/aspartergic afferents to the rat ventral striatopallidal region. *J. Comp. Neurol.,* 258: 317 – 338.

Grace, A.A. (1991) Phasic versus tonic dopamine release and the modulation of dopamine system responsivity: a hypothesis for the etiology of schizophrenia. *Neuroscience,* 41: 1 – 24.

Groenewegen, H.J. (1988) Organization of the afferent connections of the mediodorsal thalamic nucleus in the rat, related to the mediodorsal-prefrontal topography. *Neuroscience,* 24: 379 – 431.

Groenewegen, H.J. and Berendse, H.W. (1990) Parallel arrangement of forebrain circuits in the rat. 2. Ventral striatum, ventral pallidum, and mediodorsal thalamic nucleus. *Soc. Neurosci. Abstr.,* 16: 426.

Groenewegen, H.J. and Russchen, F.T. (1984) Organization of the efferent projections of the nucleus accumbens to pallidal, hypothalamic, and mesencephalic structures: a tracing and immunohistochemical study in the cat. *J. Comp. Neurol.,* 223: 347 – 367.

Groenewegen, H.J., Room, P., Witter, M.P. and Lohman, A.H.M. (1982) Cortical afferents of the nucleus accumbens in the cat, studied with anterograde and retrograde transport techniques. *Neuroscience,* 7: 977 – 996.

Groenewegen, H.J., Vermeulen-Van der Zee, E., Te Kortschot, A. and Witter, M.P. (1987) Organization of the projections from the subiculum to the ventral striatum in the rat. A study using anterograde transport of *Phaseolus vulgaris* leucoagglutinin. *Neuroscience,* 23: 103 – 120.

Groenewegen, H.J., Meredith, G.E., Berendse, H.W., Voorn, P. and Wolters, J.G. (1989) The compartmental organization of the ventral striatum in the rat. In: A.R. Crossman and M.A. Sambrook (Eds.), *Neural Mechanisms in Disorders of Movement. Current Problems in Neurology, Vol. 9,* John Libbey, London, pp. 45 – 54.

Groenewegen, H.J., Berendse, H.W., Wolters, J.G. and Lohman, A.H.M. (1990) The anatomical relationship of the prefrontal cortex with the striatopallidal system, the thalamus and the amygdala: evidence for a parallel organization. In: H.B.M. Uylings, C.G. Van Eden, J.P.C. De Bruin, M.A. Corner and M.G.P. Feenstra (Eds.), *The Prefrontal Cortex: Its Structure, Function, and Pathology – Progress in Brain Research, Vol. 85,* Elsevier, Amsterdam, pp. 95 – 118.

Groenewegen, H.J., Berendse, H.W., Meredith, G.E., Haber, S.N., Voorn, P., Wolters, J.G. and Lohman, A.H.M. (1991) Functional anatomy of the ventral, limbic system-innervated striatum. In: P. Willner and J. Scheel-Krüger (Eds.), *The Mesolimbic Dopamine System: from Motivation to Action,* John Wiley, Chicester, pp. 19 – 59.

Hakan, R.L. and Henriksen, S.J. (1989) Opiate influences on nucleus accumbens neuronal electrophysiology: dopamine and non-dopamine mechanisms. *J. Neurosci.,* 9: 307–312.

Hara, M., Sasa, M. and Takaori, S. (1989) Ventral tegmental area-mediated inhibition of neurons of the nucleus accumbens receiving input from the parafascicular nucleus of the thalamus is mediated by dopamine D1 receptors. *Neuropharmacology,* 28: 1203–1209.

Heimer, L. and Wilson, R.D. (1975) The subcortical projections of the allocortex: similarities in the neural associations of the hippocampus, the piriform cortex, and the neocortex. In: M. Santini (Ed.), *Golgi Centennial Symposium: Perspectives in Neurobiology,* Raven Press, New York, pp. 177–193.

Heimer, L., Zahm, D.S., Churchill, L., Kalivas, P.W. and Wohltman, C. (1991a) Specificity in the projection patterns of accumbal core and shell in the rat. *Neuroscience,* 41: 89–125.

Heimer, L., de Olmos, J., Alheid, G.F. and Zaborszky, L. (1991b) "Perestroika" in the basal forebrain: opening the border between neurology and psychiatry. In: G. Holstege (Ed.), *Progress in Brain Research, Vol. 87,* Elsevier, Amsterdam, pp. 109–165.

Henselmans, J.M.L. and Stoof, J.C. (1991) Regional differences in the regulation of acetylcholine release upon D-2 dopamine and *N*-methyl-D-aspartate receptor activation in rat nucleus accumbens and neostriatum. *Brain Res.,* 566: 8–12.

Herkenham, M., Moon Edley, S. and Stuart, J. (1984) Cell clusters in the nucleus accumbens of the rat, and the mosaic relationship of opiate receptors, acetylcholinesterase and subcortical afferent terminations. *Neuroscience,* 11: 561–593.

Higashi, H., Inanaga, K., Nishi, S. and Uchimura, N. (1989) Enhancement of dopamine actions on rat nucleus accumbens neurones in vitro after methamphetamine pre-treatment. *J. Physiol. (Lond.),* 408: 587–603.

Horne, A.L., Woodruff, G.N. and Kemp, J.A. (1990) Synaptic potentials mediated by excitatory amino acid receptors in the nucleus accumbens of the rat, in vitro. *Neuropharmacology,* 29: 917–921.

Ingham, C.A., Hood, S.H. and Arbuthnott, G.W. (1991) A light and electron microscopical study of enkephalin-immunoreactive structures in the rat neostriatum after removal of the nigrostriatal dopaminergic pathway. *Neuroscience,* 42: 715–730.

Jaslove, S.W. (1992) The integrative properties of spiny distal dendrites. *Neuroscience,* 47: 495–519.

Jayaraman, A. (1985) Organization of thalamic projections in the nucleus accumbens and the caudate nucleus in cats and its relation with hippocampal and other subcortical afferents. *J. Comp. Neurol.,* 231: 396–420.

Jongen-Rêlo, A.L., Groenewegen, H.J. and Voorn, P. (1993) Evidence for a multi-compartmental histochemical organization of the ventral striatum in the rat. *J. Comp. Neurol.,* in press.

Kalivas, P.W. and Duffy, P. (1990) Effect of acute and daily neurotensin and enkephalin treatments on extracellular dopamine in the nucleus accumbens. *J. Neurosci.,* 10: 2940–2949.

Kelley, A.E. and Domesick, V.B. (1982) The distribution of the projection from the hippocampal formation, to the nucleus accumbens in the rat: an anterograde- and retrograde-horseradish peroxidase study. *Neuroscience,* 7: 2321–2335.

Kelley, A.E., Domesick, V.B. and Nauta, W.J.H. (1982) The amygdalostriatal projection in the rat – an anatomical study by anterograde and retrograde tracing methods. *Neuroscience,* 7: 615–630.

Kita, H. and Kitai, S.T. (1988) Glutamate decarboxylase immunoreactive neurons in rat neostriatum: their morphological types and populations. *Brain Res.,* 447: 346–352.

Koch, C., Zador, A. and Brown, T.H. (1992) Dendritic spines: convergence of theory and experiment. *Science,* 256: 973–974.

Kolb, B. (1984) Functions of the frontal cortex of the rat: a comparative review. *Brain Res. Rev.,* 8: 65–98.

Kolb, B. (1990) Prefrontal cortex. In: B. Kolb and R.C. Tees (Eds.), *The Cerebral Cortex of the Rat,* MIT Press, Cambridge, MA, pp. 437–458.

Lehmann, J. and Langer, S.Z. (1983) The striatal cholinergic interneuron: synaptic target of dopaminergic terminals? *Neuroscience,* 10: 1105–1120.

Malenka, R.C. and Kocsis, J.D. (1988) Presynaptic actions of carbachol and adenosine on corticostriatal synaptic transmission studied in vitro. *J. Neurosci.,* 8: 3750–3756.

McCarthy, P.S., Walker, R.J. and Woodruff, G.N. (1977) Depressant action of enkephalins on neurons in the nucleus accumbens. *J. Physiol. (Lond.),* 267: 40P.

Meredith, G. (1992) Is there a striatal-V.T.A. feedback loop from the shell of nucleus accumbens? Anatomical observations. *7th International Catecholamine Symposium, Abstr.,* p. 208.

Meredith, G. and Wouterlood, F. (1990) Hippocampal and midline thalamic fibers and terminals in relation to the choline acetyltransferase-immunoreactive neurons in nucleus accumbens of the rat: a light and electron microscopic study. *J. Comp. Neurol.,* 296: 204–221.

Meredith, G. and Wouterlood, F. (1991) Synaptic organization of nucleus accumbens (ventral striatum). In: G. Bernardi, M.B. Carpenter, G.D. Chiara, M. Morelli and P. Stanzione (Eds.), *The Basal Ganglia III – Advances in Behavioral Biology, Vol. 39,* Plenum Press, New York, pp. 167–176.

Meredith, G. and Wouterlood, F. (1993) Identification of synaptic interactions of intracellularly injected neurons in fixed brain slices by means of dual-label electron microscopy. *J. Microsc. Res. Technol.,* 24: 31–42.

Meredith, G.E., Blank, B. and Groenewegen, H.J. (1989) The distribution and compartmental organization of the cholinergic neurons in nucleus accumbens of the rat. *Neuroscience,* 31: 327–345.

Meredith, G., Wouterlood, F.G. and Pattiselanno, A. (1990) Hippocampal fibers make synaptic contacts with glutamate decarboxylase-immunoreactive neurons in the rat nucleus accumbens. *Brain Res.,* 513: 329–334.

Meredith, G., Agolia, R., Arts, M.P.M., Groenewegen, H.J.

and Zahm, D.S. (1992a) Morphological differences between projection neurons of the core and shell in the nucleus accumbens of the rat. *Neuroscience, 50:* 149–162.

Meredith, G., Stitou, Z., Korf, E. and Chang, H.T. (1992b) Cholinergic-enkephalinergic synaptic relationships in the ventral striatum of the rat. *International Basal Ganglia Society IVth International Meeting, Abstr.*

Meredith, G., Ingham, C., Voorn, P. and Arbuthnott, G. (1993) Ultrastructural characteristics of enkephalin-immunoreactive boutons and their postsynaptic targets in the shell and core of the nucleus accumbens of the rat. *J. Comp. Neurol., 332:* 224–236.

Müller, W. and Connor, J.A. (1991) Dendritic spines as individual neuronal compartments for synaptic Ca^{2+} responses. *Nature, 354:* 73–76.

Nauta, W.J.H., Smith, G.P., Faull, R.L.M. and Domesick, V.B. (1978) Efferent connections and nigral afferents of the nucleus accumbens septi in the rat. *Neuroscience, 3:* 385–401.

O'Donnell, P. and Grace, A.A. (1991) Physiology and incidence of dye coupling in nucleus accumbens neurons. *IBRO World Congress of Neuroscience, Abstr., 3:* 146.

Pennartz, C.M.A. and Kitai, S.T. (1991) Hippocampal inputs to identified neurons in an in vitro slice preparation of the rat nucleus accumbens: evidence for feed-forward inhibition. *J. Neurosci., 11:* 2838–2847.

Pennartz, C.M.A. and Lopes da Silva, F.H. (1994) Muscarinic modulation of synaptic transmission in the rat nucleus accubens studied in vitro: frequency-dependence and block by 4-aminopyridine. (Submitted.)

Pennartz, C.M.A., Boeijinga, P.H. and Lopes da Silva, F.H. (1990) Locally evoked potentials in slices of the rat nucleus accumbens: NMDA and non-NMDA receptor mediated components and modulation by GABA. *Brain Res., 529:* 30–41.

Pennartz, C.M.A., Boeijinga, P.H., Kitai, S.T. and Lopes da Silva, F.H. (1991) Contribution of NMDA receptors to postsynaptic potentials and paired-pulse facilitation in identified neurons of the rat nucleus accumbens in vitro. *Exp. Brain Res., 86:* 190–198.

Pennartz, C.M.A., Dolleman-Van der Weel, M.J., Kitai, S.T. and Lopes da Silva, F.H. (1992a) Presynaptic dopamine D1 receptors attenuate excitatory and inhibitory limbic inputs to the shell region of the rat nucleus accumbens studied in vitro. *J. Neurophysiol., 67:* 1325–1334.

Pennartz, C.M.A., Dolleman-Van der Weel, M.J. and Lopes da Silva, F.H. (1992b) Differential membrane properties and dopamine effects in the shell and core of the rat nucleus accumbens studied in vitro. *Neurosci. Lett., 136:* 109–112.

Pennartz, C.M.A., Ameerun, R.F., Groenewegen, H.J. and Lopes da Silva, F.H. (1993) Synaptic plasticity in the rat prefrontal-accumbens pathway studied in vitro: relation to NMDA receptor activity, tetanic depolarization and dopamine. *Eur. J. Neurosci., 5:* 107–117.

Perkel, D.H. and Perkel, D.J. (1985) Dendritic spines: role of active membrane in modulating synaptic efficacy. *Brain Res.,* 325: 331–335.

Phelps, P.E. and Vaughn, J.E. (1986) Immunocytochemical localization of choline acetyltransferase in rat ventral striatum: a light and electron microscopic study. *J. Neurocytol.,* 15: 595–617.

Phillipson, O.T. and Griffiths, A.C. (1985) The topographic order of inputs to nucleus accumbens in the rat. *Neuroscience,* 16: 275–296.

Pickel, V.M., Towle, A.C., Joh, T.H. and Chan, J. (1988a) Gamma-aminobutyric acid in the medial rat nucleus accumbens: ultrastructural localization in neurons receiving monosynaptic input from catecholaminergic afferents. *J. Comp. Neurol., 272:* 1–14.

Pickel, V.M., Joh, T.H. and Chan, J. (1988b) Substance P in the rat nucleus accumbens: ultrastructural localization in axon terminals and their relation to dopaminergic afferents. *Brain Res., 444:* 247–264.

Sesack, S.R. and Pickel, V.M. (1990) In the rat medial nucleus accumbens, hippocampal and catecholaminergic terminals converge on spiny neurons and are in apposition to each other. *Brain Res., 527:* 266–279.

Sesack, S.R. and Pickel, V.M. (1992) Prefrontal cortical efferents in the rat synapse on unlabeled neuronal targets of catecholamine terminals in the nucleus accumbens septi and on dopamine neurons in the ventral tegmental area. *J. Comp. Neurol., 320:* 145–160.

Sesack, S.R., Deutch, A.Y., Roth, R.H. and Bunney, B.S. (1989) Topographical organization of the efferent projections of the medial prefrontal cortex in the rat: an anterograde tract-tracing study with *Phaseolus vulgaris* leucoagglutinin. *J. Comp. Neurol., 290:* 213–242.

Shepherd, G.M., Brayton, R.K., Miller, J.P., Segev, I., Rinzel, J. and Rall, W. (1985) Signal enhancement in distal cortical dendrites by means of interactions between active dendritic spines. *Proc. Natl. Acad. Sci. U.S.A., 82:* 2192–2195.

Smith, A.D. and Bolam, J.P. (1990) The neural network of the basal ganglia as revealed by the study of synaptic connections of identified neurones. *Trends Neurosci., 13:* 259–265.

Sokoloff, P., Giros, B., Martres, M.-P., Bouthenet, M.-L. and Schwartz, J.-C. (1990) Molecular cloning and characterization of a novel dopamine (D_3) as a target for neuroleptics. *Nature, 347:* 146–151.

Somogyi, P., Bolam, J.P. and Smith, A.D. (1981) Monosynaptic cortical input and local axon collaterals of identified striatonigral neurons. A light and electron microscopic study using the Golgi-peroxidase transport-degeneration procedure. *J. Comp. Neurol., 195:* 567–584.

Stoof, J.C., Russchen F.T., Verheijden, P.F.H.M. and Hoogland, P.V. (1987) A comparative study of the dopamine-acetylcholine interaction in telencephalic structures of the rat and of a reptile, the lizard *Gekko gecko. Brain Res., 404:* 273–281.

Stoof, J.C., Druckarch, B., De Boer, P., Westerink, B.H.C. and Groenewegen, H.J. (1992) Regulation of the activity of striatal neurons by dopamine. *Neuroscience,* 47: 755 – 770.

Sugita, S., Uchimura, N., Jiang, Z.-G. and North, R.A. (1991) Distinct muscarinic receptors inhibit release of γ-aminobutyric acid and excitatory amino acids in mammalian brain. *Proc. Natl. Acad. Sci. U.S.A.,* 88: 2608 – 2611.

Tennyson, V.M., Heikkila, R., Mytilineou, C., Coté, L. and Cohen, G. (1974) 5-hydroxydopamine "tagged" neuronal boutons in rabbit neostriatum; interrelationship between vesicles and axonal membrane. *Brain Res.,* 82: 341 – 348.

Totterdell, S. and Smith, A.D. (1989) Convergence of hippocampal and dopaminergic input onto identified neurons in the nucleus accumbens of the rat. *J. Chem. Neuroanat.,* 2: 285 – 298.

Uchimura, N. and North, R.A. (1990) Muscarine reduces inwardly rectifying potassium conductance in rat nucleus accumbens neurones. *J. Physiol. (Lond.),* 422: 369 – 380.

Uchimura, N. and North, R.A. (1991) Baclofen and adenosine inhibit synaptic potentials mediated by γ-aminobutyric acid and glutamate release in rat nucleus accumbens. *J. Pharmacol. Exp. Ther.,* 258: 663 – 668.

Uchimura, N., Higashi, H. and Nishi, S. (1986) Hyperpolarizing and depolarizing actions of dopamine via D-1 and D-2 receptors on nucleus accumbens neurons. *Brain Res.,* 375: 368 – 372.

Uchimura, N., Cherubini, E. and North, R.A. (1989a) Inward rectification in rat nucleus accumbens neurons. *J. Neurophysiol.,* 62: 1280 – 1286.

Uchimura, N., Higashi, H. and Nishi, S. (1989b) Membrane properties and synaptic responses of the guinea pig nucleus accumbens neurons in vitro. *J. Neurophysiol.,* 61: 769 – 779.

Uno, M. and Ozawa, N. (1991) Long-term potentiation of the amygdala-striatal synaptic transmission in the course of development of amygdaloid kindling in cats. *Neurosci. Res.,* 12: 251 – 262.

Valentino, R.J. and Dingledine, R. (1981) Presynaptic inhibitory effect of acetylcholine in the hippocampus. *J. Neurosci.,* 1: 784 – 792.

Voorn, P. and Docter, G.J. (1992) A rostrocaudal gradient in the synthesis of enkephalin in the nucleus accumbens. *Neuroreport,* 3: 161 – 164.

Voorn, P., Jorritsma-Byham, B., Van Dijk, C. and Buijs, R.M. (1986) The dopaminergic innervation of the ventral striatum in the rat: a light- and electron-microscopical study with antibodies against dopamine. *J. Comp. Neurol.,* 251: 84 – 99.

Voorn, P., Gerfen, C.R. and Groenewegen, H.J. (1989) The compartmental organization of the ventral striatum of the rat: immunohistochemical distribution of enkephalin, subtance P, dopamine, and calcium binding protein. *J. Comp. Neurol.,* 289: 189 – 201.

West, C.H.K. and Michael, R.P. (1990) Responses of units in the mesolimbic system to olfactory and somatosensory stimuli: modulation of sensory input by ventral tegmental stimulation. *Brain Res.,* 532: 307 – 316.

White, F.J. (1987) D-1 dopamine receptor stimulation enables the inhibition of nucleus accumbens neurons by a D-2 receptor agonist. *Eur. J. Pharmacol.,* 135: 101 – 105.

White, F.J. and Wang, R.Y. (1986) Electrophysiological evidence for the existence of both D-1 and D-2 receptors in the rat nucleus accumbens. *J. Neurosci.,* 6: 274 – 280.

Wightman, R.M. and Zimmerman, J.B. (1990) Control of dopamine extracellular concentration in rat striatum by impulse flow and uptake. *Brain Res. Rev.,* 15: 135 – 144.

Wilson, C.J. (1991) Synaptic cooperativity may arise from the fast inward rectification in neostriatal spiny cells. *Soc. Neurosci. Abstr.,* 17: 1217.

Woodruff, G.N., McCarthy, P.S. and Walker, R.J. (1976) Studies on the pharmacology of neurones in the nucleus accumbens of the rat. *Brain Res.,* 115: 233 – 242.

Yang, C.R. and Mogenson, G.J. (1986) Dopamine enhances terminal excitability of hippocampal-accumbens neurons via D2 receptor: role of dopamine in presynaptic inhibition. *J. Neurosci.,* 6: 2470 – 2478.

Yim, C.Y. and Mogenson, G.J. (1988) Neuromodulatory action of dopamine in the nucleus accumbens: an in vivo intracellular study. *Neuroscience,* 26: 403 – 415.

Yuan, X., Madamba, S. and Siggins, G.R. (1992) Opioid peptides reduce synaptic transmission in the nucleus accumbens. *Neurosci. Lett.,* 134: 223 – 228.

Zàborszky, L., Alheid, G.F., Beinfeld, M.C., Eiden, L.E., Heimer, L. and Palkovits, M. (1985) Cholecystokinin innervation of the ventral striatum: a morphological and radioimmunological study. *Neuroscience,* 14: 427 – 453.

Zahm, D.S. (1991) Compartments in rat dorsal and ventral striatum revealed following injection of 6-hydroxydopamine into the ventral mesencephalon. *Brain Res.,* 552: 164 – 169.

Zahm, D.S. (1992) An electron microscopic morphometric comparison of tyrosine hydroxylase immunoreactive innervation in the neostriatum and the nucleus accumbens core and shell. *Brain Res.,* 575: 341 – 346.

Zahm, D.S. and Heimer, L. (1988) Ventral striatopallidal parts of the basal ganglia in the rat: I. Neurochemical compartmentation as reflected by the distributions of neurotensin and substance P immunoreactivity. *J. Comp. Neurol.,* 272: 516 – 535.

Zahm, D.S. and Heimer, L. (1990) Two transpallidal pathways originating in nucleus accumbens. *J. Comp. Neurol.,* 302: 437 – 446.

Zahm, D.S. and Heimer, L. (1993) Specificity in the efferent projections of the nucleus accumbens in the rat: comparison of the rostral pole projection patterns with those of the core and shell. *J. Comp. Neurol.,* 327: 220 – 232.

G.W. Arbuthnott and P.C. Emson (Eds.)
Progress in Brain Research, Vol. 99
© 1993 Elsevier Science Publishers B.V. All rights reserved.

CHAPTER 2

Cholinergic neurons of the rat and primate striatum are morphologically different

Jérôme Yelnik, Gérard Percheron, Chantal François and Anouk Garnier

Laboratoire de Neuromorphologie informationnelle et de Neurologie expérimentale du mouvement, INSERM U106, Hôpital de la Salpêtrière, 75013 Paris, France

Introduction

It is well-established that the striatum contains a population of cholinergic neurons which can be revealed by using either acetylcholinesterase (AChE) histochemistry or choline acetyltransferase (ChAT) immunohistochemistry (Levey et al., 1983; Eckenstein and Sofroniew, 1983; Mesulam et al., 1984; Woolf, 1991). Cholinergic neurons have been identified in the striatum of rats (Lynch et al., 1972; Butcher and Bilezikjian, 1975; Butcher and Hodge, 1976; Armstrong et al., 1983; Levey et al., 1983; Eckenstein and Sofroniew, 1983; Satoh et al., 1983; Bolam et al., 1984b; Phelps et al., 1985), cats (Kimura et al., 1981; Parent and O'Reilly-Fromentin, 1982), monkeys (Mesulam et al., 1984; Smith and Parent, 1984; Satoh and Fibiger, 1985; DiFiglia, 1987) and humans (Nagai et al., 1983). In order to disclose the dendritic and axonal morphology of cholinergic neurons, comparisons were made with previous classifications based on Golgi-impregnated material. These classifications were in fact elaborated in different animal species: rats (Lu and Brown, 1977; Danner and Pfister, 1979; Dimova et al., 1980; Chang et al., 1982), mice (Rafols et al., 1989), cats (Kemp and Powell, 1971), dogs (Tanaka, 1980; Leontovich, 1983), monkeys (Fox et al., 1971a,b; DiFiglia et al., 1976) and humans (Leontovich, 1954; Braak and Braak, 1982; Graveland et al., 1985). In addition, a variety of

different criteria such as cell body size, dendritic morphology, number of spines or axon length were used for identifying and classifying neurons. Finally, striatal cholinergic neurons were assumed to be similar in all animal species and their characterization became obscure. The goal of this paper is to compare the morphology of cholinergic neurons in primates and non-primates using data of our recent morphological taxonomy of the neurons of the primate striatum (Yelnik et al., 1991).

The dendritic morphology of striatal neurons in primates

Neurons of the striatum of monkey and human were analyzed in adult brains impregnated following the Golgi method of Anderson (1954) or Davenport and Combs (1954). Dendritic arborizations were reconstructed from serial sections and digitized in three dimensions with the aid of a computer-aided technique (Yelnik et al., 1981). Their morphological features were described using topological, metrical and geometrical quantitative parameters. Topological parameters comprised the number of stems and tips, the dendritic formula, the branching index and the stature (Percheron, 1979, 1982). Metrical parameters comprised the mean length of dendritic segments (all segments, stems, internodes, twigs), the total dendritic length and the longest dendrite. Geometrical parameters consisted of the dimensions of

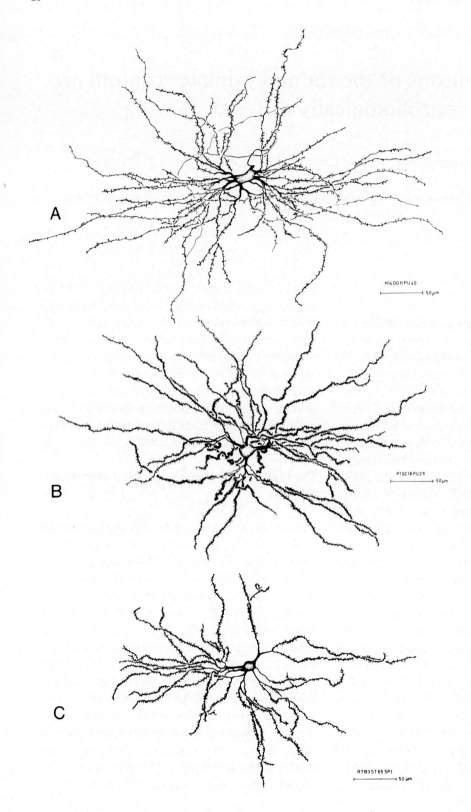

A   H14DG11PU40
                              ⊢────⊣ 50µm

B   P1GC18PU29
                              ⊢────⊣ 50µm

C   R7B3ST65SPI
                       ⊢────⊣ 50 µm

the dendritic arborization (length, width, thickness) as measured with reference to its principal system of axes (Yelnik et al., 1983). Neuronal species, defined as sets of neurons having statistically similar morphological features, were isolated on the basis of multidimensional statistical tests.

Four neuronal species were identified in primates (Yelnik et al., 1991). *Spiny neurons* (Fig. 1) represent the bulk (96%) of striatal neurons. They have different topological and metrical parameters in monkeys and humans: a dendritic formula of 5 – 35 (5 stems, 35 tips) in monkeys and 6 – 42 in humans, a mean length of dendritic segments of 93 μm in monkeys and 75 μm in humans. They have also a higher density of dendritic spines in monkeys (8 per 10 μm) than in humans (2.6 per 10 μm). Conversely, the geometry of dendritic arborizations (430 × 330 × 230 μm) is remarkably similar in both species. *Leptodendritic neurons* (2%) do not differ in monkeys and humans and are statistically undistinguishable from pallidal (Yelnik et al., 1984) and nigral pars reticulata (Yelnik et al., 1987) neurons. They are mainly characterized by very long and sparsely ramified dendrites (Fig. 2*B*): the dendritic formula is 4 – 20, the dendritic segments are 196 μm long and the dendritic arborization is 1200 μm long (up to 1600 μm). *Spidery neurons* (1%) are immediately recognizable with their large, globular cell body and their very thick dendritic stems which branch profusely into varicose processes which curve back toward the soma (Fig. 2*C*). They have a dendritic formula of 12 – 129, a mean length of dendritic segments of 95 μm and a dendritic arborization of 600 μm long. *Microneurons* (1%) have a dendritic formula of 6 – 64, a mean length of dendritic segments of 40 μm and a dendritic arborization of 240 μm long.

These four neuronal species can be found, under different namings, in previous studies (table 2 in Yelnik et al., 1991). Differences bear mainly on the classification of large neurons. Fox et al. (1971b) illustrate leptodendritic neurons (their figs. 3, 16) and spidery neurons (their figs. 4, 8) but classified both types as "large aspiny neurons". DiFiglia et al. (1976) classified leptodendritic neurons as "large version of spiny type II" and spidery neurons as "aspiny type II". In the classification of Braak and Braak (1982), they appear as type III and type IV respectively.

Characterization of cholinergic neurons in the primate striatum

The brain of one monkey (*Macaca irus*) was sectioned on a freezing microtome and processed according to the DFP-histochemical technique of Poirier et al. (1977) to reveal AChE-containing neurons. Sections were couterstained with neutral red or cresyl violet. Samples of both AChE-containing and unlabeled cell bodies were selected for quantitative analysis. The largest contour of each cell body was digitized on an XY digitizer and its area was measured using the formula of Pullen (1984). The biggest and smallest diameters were determined by program. A shape index (biggest/smallest diameter) was calculated. This procedure was also applied to the cell bodies of Golgi-impregnated neurons. By this way, AChE-containing cell bodies could be correlated quantitatively with the neuronal species defined previously on the basis of dendritic features.

Only three types of cell bodies are identifiable on the basis of their size and shape in the primate striatum. Indeed, spiny neurons and microneurons have both small and round cell bodies and are not distinguishable on these somatic criteria. Spidery neurons have round cell bodies which are the largest cell bodies of the primate striatum. Leptodendritic neurons have an elongated cell body whose size is intermediate. Finally the three types of cell bodies are: small round, medium elongated and large round. This is

Fig. 1. Spiny neurons of the striatum of human (*A*), monkeys (*B*) and rats (*C*). Each dendritic arborization was reconstructed from serial sections and drawn through the × 100 immersion objective. Note that the overall dimensions of arborizations are not significantly different in the three species. Conversely, there are differences in the number of dendritic segments and in their density of dendritic spines (see text). Golgi method.

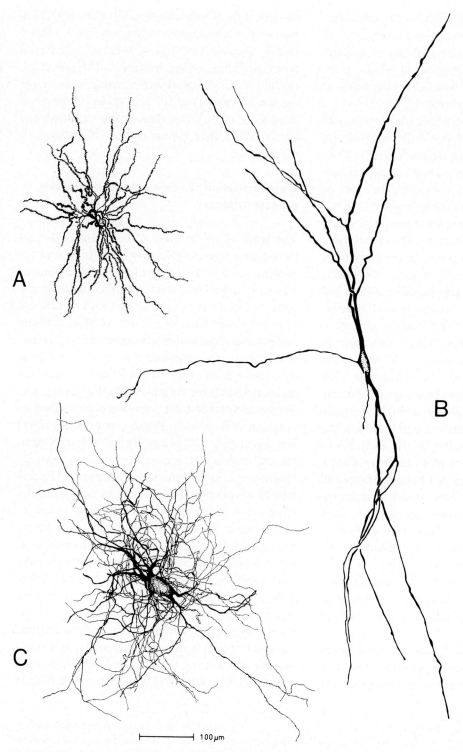

Fig. 2. Three of the four neuronal species of the monkey (*Papio papio*) striatum: spiny neuron (*A*), leptodendritic neuron (*B*), spidery neuron (*C*). Golgi method. Same magnification for the three neurons. Note that the spidery neuron has the largest cell body (1406 μm^2), the leptodendritic neuron is medium-sized (684 μm^2) and the spiny neuron has a small round cell body (254 μm^2).

in agreement with the distribution of cell bodies as it appears in Nissl-stained sections (fig. 1 in Pasik et al., 1979; fig. 11 in Yelnik et al., 1991). In material processed for revelation of AChE, positive cell bodies were large and round. They were larger than all non-labeled counterstained neurons including both medium elongated and small round cell bodies (Yelnik et al., 1991). As AChE histochemistry has been demonstrated to closely correspond to ChAT immunoreactivity in the striatum of macaques (Mesulam et al., 1984), it can be concluded that AChE-positive neurons are the cholinergic neurons of the striatum of monkeys. As they have the largest cell bodies of the striatum, it can be concluded that they correspond to spidery neurons. This conclusion, suggested by Smith and Parent (1984), is in agreement with the electron microscope analysis of DiFiglia (1987).

Cholinergic neurons, or spidery neurons, of the primate striatum are thus characterized by a voluminous and globular cell body which is the largest one of all other striatal neurons in primates. They correspond to the larger achromatic cells of cytoarchitectonic preparations. They have a large number (12) of very thick (up to 10 μm) dendritic stems. These stems branch rapidly into numerous branches which become thinner and thinner at each bifurcation. Distal branches are very numerous (129) and most of them are thin and varicose. They often curve back toward the soma. As a whole, the dendritic arborization of spidery neurons is highly recognizable on its high density and the curved and varicose aspect of its distal processes (Fig. 2C).

The dendritic morphology of striatal neurons in rats

Golgi-impregnated brains of adult rats were also examined for this study. Rats were perfused through the aorta with 1% paraformaldehyde and 1% glutaraldehyde in 0.1 M phosphate buffer. Brains were processed by the Golgi method according to the modification of Van der Loos (1956). Neurons were drawn through the camera lucida (× 100 immersion objective) and analyzed qualitatively. Some of

them, which could be reconstructed from serial sections, were analyzed quantitatively according to our computer-aided method.

The overall distribution of striatal neurons in the rat is the same as in primates, i.e., comprising about 96% spiny neurons and a few neurons having a larger cell body than spiny neurons. Spiny neurons of the rat striatum (Fig. 1C) have lower topological and metrical parameters than spiny neurons of monkey and human. The longest dendrite in rats was 220 μm (Fig. 1C), 200 – 250 μm (Kitai et al., 1979), 280 μm (Wilson and Groves, 1980), 200 – 220 μm (Dimova et al., 1980), 220 μm (Bishop et al., 1982), which is smaller than the 275 μm measured in primates (Yelnik et al., 1991). The mean length of dendritic segments (67 μm in Fig. 1C) is also smaller than in monkeys (93 μm) and humans (75 μm), and so is the dendritic formula: 6 – 30 for the rat, 5 – 35 for the monkey and 6 – 42 for the human. Conversely, the dimensions of dendritic arborizations were 360 × 230 × 180 μm in Fig. 1C and 260 – 530 × 240 – 425 × 260 – 350 in Preston et al. (1980), which is similar to the 430 × 330 × 230 μm that we measured in primates (Yelnik et al., 1991). Spine distribution (5 per 10 μm in Fig. 1C) was intermediate.

Two different types of large neurons were identifiable in our material. Neurons of the first type (Fig. 3B) had a fusiform cell body and 3 – 4 dendritic trees with long, smooth and sparsely branched dendrites (9 – 11 dendritic tips). They correspond to the large type I of Chang et al. (1982) and Chang and Kitai (1982) and resemble the leptodendritic neurons of primates. However, their dendrites were definitely thinner and shorter (400 μm for the longest one) than their primate counterpart (compare Figs. 2B and 3B). This observation is consistent with previous measurements in the rat: up to 150 μm (Takagi et al., 1984), 250 μm (Bolam et al., 1984a), 350 μm (Rafols et al., 1989), 400 μm (Chang et al., 1982) and 450 μm (Bishop et al., 1982). As the longest dendrite was 1270 μm in primates (Yelnik et al., 1991), this could suggest that large neurons of rats constitute a particular type. However, as they have a low dendritic formula and relatively long dendrites, they fit with the criteria of Ramon-Moliner

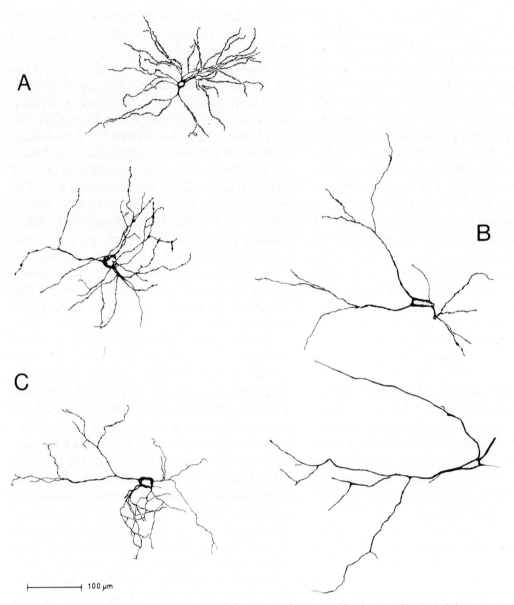

Fig. 3. Three neuronal types of the rat striatum. Golgi method. Same magnification as in Fig. 2. *A*. Spiny neuron with a small cell body (135 μm^2). *B*. Two large neurons (497 and 392 μm^2) with elongated cell bodies and sparsely ramified dendrites. Note that the cell bodies are smaller and the dendrites far shorter than for leptodendritic neurons of primates (Fig. 2*B*). *C*. Two large neurons (471 and 430 μm^2) with round cell bodies and more numerous, varicose and tortuous dendrites. Note that these neurons strongly differ from the spidery neurons of primates shown in Fig. 2*C*.

(1969) and are likely to represent the leptodendritic neurons of the rat striatum.

The second type of large neurons that we observed (Fig. 3*C*) had a round or polygonal cell body with 4 – 6 dendritic trees. As a whole the dendritic arborization had 21 – 28 dendritic tips. The mean length of segments was 40 – 60 μm, the longest dendrite was 200 – 250 μm, the total dendritic length 1400 – 2500 μm. This type is similar to the large type II of Chang et al. (1982) and Chang and Kitai (1982). According to Bolam et al. (1984a), this type would be similar to the type IV of Braak and Braak (1982) in humans and the aspiny type II of DiFiglia et al. (1976) in monkeys, i.e., our spidery neurons. In our opinion, however, this comparison does not hold true because of significant differences, both qualitative (compare Figs. 2C and 3C) and quantitative: 21 – 28 tips vs. 129 in primates, a total dendritic length of 1400 – 2500 μm vs. 23400 μm in primates. This strongly suggests that there are no spidery neurons in the rat striatum, which raises the question of the morphology of the rat cholinergic neurons.

Characterization of cholinergic neurons in the rat striatum

The first studies of cholinergic neurons in non-primate species were based on AChE histochemistry (Lynch et al., 1972; Butcher and Bilezikjian, 1975; Butcher and Hodge, 1976; Henderson, 1981; Armstrong et al., 1983) and concluded that two populations of neurons, one with medium-sized cell bodies, the other with large fusiform or multipolar cell bodies, were AChE-positive. Later, however, Eckenstein and Sofroniew (1983), Levey et al. (1983) and Phelps et al. (1985) using immunohistochemical detection of ChAT concluded that the apparent heterogeneity of ChAT-positive cell bodies might be explained by different orientations of elongated cell bodies and that cholinergic neurons constituted a single population of large neurons. Moreover, Bolam et al. (1984b) demonstrated, by combining Golgi impregnation, electron microscopy, AChE histochemistry and ChAT immunohistochemistry, that only one out of three populations of AChE-positive neurons (Bolam et al., 1984a) were immunoreactive to ChAT.

For Bolam et al. (1984b), cholinergic neurons have a large triangular or multipolar cell body, "long infrequently branching dendrites", and correlate with the giant neurons of Kemp and Powell (1971), the type V of Dimova et al. (1980), the giant neurons of Danner and Pfister (1981) and the type I large of Chang et al. (1982). These different types correspond to the leptodendritic neuron of Fig. 3B.

Bolam et al. (1984b) specify that cholinergic neurons are not "the same as the large neurons with a 'spidery' appearance and 'swirling' dendrites", i.e., their type 2 which comprises the type II large of Chang et al. (1982) and their large version type 3 AChE-positive (Bolam et al., 1984a). Phelps et al. (1985) described ChAT-immunoreactive neurons as having large oval or multipolar somata and "three to four primary dendrites that branch and extend long distance". Such a description is also that of a leptodendritic neuron. Kubota et al. (1987) described ChAT-immunoreactive neurons as having a large, oval, spindle, triangular or multipolar cell body, 3 – 5 dendritic trees emerging from the poles of the soma, and long and sparsely branched dendrites. They correlated these cholinergic neurons with the giant neurons of Kemp and Powell (1971) and the type I large of Chang et al. (1982), thus, also with leptodendritic neurons.

Conclusions

Finally it appears from our results and from the data of the literature that: (1) cholinergic neurons of the striatum have the largest cell bodies of this cerebral region in both primate and non-primate species; (2) those striatal neurons having the largest cell body in the striatum are leptodendritic neurons in non-primate species whereas they are spidery neurons in monkeys and man; (3) cholinergic neurons of non-primate species are leptodendritic neurons whereas they are spidery neurons in primates; and (4) spidery neurons do not exist in non-primate species.

The morphological difference between striatal cholinergic neurons of the rat and primate is considerable and raises several questions. One concerns the differentiation of the neuronal species of the striatum through phylogenesis. A first important point is that the dimensions of the dendritic arborizations of spiny neurons do not change from rats to humans. This implies that the grain of the dendritic lattice does not change (Yelnik et al., 1991), which is likely to be a fundamental feature of the striatal organization. Conversely, the present results demonstrate that leptodendritic neurons are subject to a considerable increase of dendritic length from rats to primates. Such an increase was also observed for the leptodendritic neurons of the globus pallidus (700 μm in rats, 1200 μm in primates; Yelnik et al., 1984) and substantia nigra pars reticulata (900 μm in rats, 1100 μm in macaques, 1600 μm in humans; Yelnik et al., 1987) but it does not represent a general rule of phylogenesis. For example, subthalamic neurons, as well as spiny neurons, remain unchanged from rats and cats to monkey and human (Yelnik and Percheron, 1979; Hammond and Yelnik, 1983). In rats, cholinergic neurons of the striatum are of the same morphological type as the cholinergic neurons of the nucleus basalis of Meynert and the peripallidal laminae (Ingham et al., 1985) and even of other brain regions (Woolf, 1991). Thus, in rats, there is a correlation between morphology and chemical content. In primates, conversely, cholinergic neurons of the striatum are definitely different from the cholinergic neurons of the basal forebrain. They have highly specific morphological features which are not observed in other regions of the nervous system. Pasik et al. (1991) have recently raised the question of the axonal nature of the cholinergic neurons of the striatum. As cholinergic neurons in rats are leptodendritic neurons and as leptodendritic neurons in primates (their large spiny II) are projection neurons, they deduce that cholinergic neurons of rats should be projection neurons. However, the interneuronal nature of cholinergic neurons has been demonstrated by fluorescent tracer experiments (Woolf and Butcher, 1981). In addition, leptodendritic neurons projecting to the substantia nigra have been shown in only the ventral part of the rat striatum (Bolam et al., 1981), which suggests that the remaining leptodendritic neurons of the rat striatum, i.e., the cholinergic neurons, could be interneurons.

An abundant literature has been devoted to the functional role of cholinergic neurons but it has never taken into account interspecific morphological differences. In Woolf's (1991) review for example, cholinergic neurons are considered as a global system contrasting with the modularity of sensory systems. While this is likely to be true for the cholinergic neurons of the rat striatum, it does not seem to be applicable to spidery neurons, the cholinergic neurons of the primate striatum, which have relatively small but very dense arborizations. As they represent only 1% of striatal neurons, they constitute a dendritic lattice which is characterized by zones of high dendritic density alternating with zones which are almost free of cholinergic processes (see fig. 12 in Yelnik et al., 1991). This implies that groups of spiny neurons could be strongly controlled by the activity of cholinergic neurons while others could not. Therefore, the anatomical organization of the cholinergic system of the striatum is submitted to a considerable transformation from rats to humans. An evolution from a globally organized system to a fine-grain modular system is certainly a highly significant feature of the primate striatum, which should be carefully considered in the analysis of the function of the striatum.

References

Anderson, A.D. (1954) Alcoholic thionin counterstaining following Golgi dichromate-silver impregnation. *Stain Technol.*, 29: 179 – 184.

Armstrong, D.M., Saper, C.B., Levey, A.I., Wainer, B.H. and Terry, R.D. (1983) Distribution of cholinergic neurons in rat brain: demonstrated by the immunocytochemical localization of choline acetyltransferase. *J. Comp. Neurol.*, 216: 53 – 68.

Bishop, G.A., Chang, H.T. and Kitai, S.T. (1982) Morphological and physiological properties of neostriatal neurons: an intracellular horseradish peroxidase study in the rat. *Neuroscience*, 7: 179 – 191.

Bolam, J.P., Somogyi, P., Totterdell, S. and Smith, A.D. (1981) A second type of striatonigral neuron: a comparison between retrogradely labelled and Golgi-stained neurons at the light and electron microscopic levels. *Neuroscience*, 6: 2141 – 2157.

Bolam, J.P., Ingham, C.A. and Smith, A.D. (1984a) The section-Golgi-impregnation procedure, 3. Combination of Golgi-impregnation with enzyme histochemistry and electron microscopy to characterize acetylcholinesterase-containing neurons in the rat striatum. *Neuroscience*, 12: 687 – 709.

Bolam, J.P., Wainer, B.H. and Smith, A.D. (1984b) Characterization of cholinergic neurons in the rat neostriatum. A combination of choline acetyltransferase immunocytochemistry, Golgi impregnation and electron microscopy. *Neuroscience*, 12: 711 – 718.

Braak, H. and Braak, E. (1982) Neuronal types in the striatum of man. *Cell Tissue Res.*, 227: 319 – 342.

Butcher, L.L. and Bilezikjian, L. (1975) Acetylcholinesterase-containing neurons in the neostriatum and substantia nigra revealed after punctate intracerebral injection of di-isopropylfluorophosphate. *Eur. J. Pharmacol.,* 34: 115 – 125.

Butcher, L.L. and Hodge, G.K. (1976) Postnatal development of acetylcholinesterase in the caudate-putamen nucleus and substantia nigra of rats. *Brain Res.,* 106: 223 – 240.

Chang, H.T. and Kitai, S.T. (1982) Large neostriatal neurons in the rat: an electron microscopic study of gold-toned Golgi-stained cells. *Brain Res. Bull.,* 8: 631 – 643.

Chang, H.T., Wilson, C.J. and Kitai, S.T. (1982) A Golgi study of the rat neostriatal neurons: light microscopic analysis. *J. Comp. Neurol.,* 208: 107 – 126.

Danner, H. and Pfister, C. (1979) Untersuchungen zur Struktur der Neostriatum des Ratte. *J. Hirnforsch.,* 20: 285 – 301.

Danner, H. and Pfister, C. (1981) 4 Spine-lose Neurontypen im Neostriatum der Ratte. *J. Hirnforsch.,* 22: 465 – 477.

Davenport, H.A. and Combs, C.M. (1954) Golgi's dichromate-sivler method. 3. Chromating fluids. *Stain Technol.,* 29: 165 – 173.

DiFiglia, M. (1987) Synaptic organization of cholinergic neurons in the monkey neostriatum. *J. Comp. Neurol.,* 255: 245 – 258.

DiFiglia, M., Pasik, P. and Pasik, T. (1976) A Golgi study of neuronal types in the neostriatum of monkeys. *Brain Res.,* 114: 245 – 256.

Dimova, R., Vuillet, J. and Seite, R. (1980) Study of the rat neostriatum using a combined Golgi electron microscope technique and serial sections. *Neuroscience,* 5: 1581 – 1596.

Eckenstein, F. and Sofroniew, M.V. (1983) Identification of central cholinergic neurons containing both choline acetyltransferase and acetylcholinesterase and of central neurons containing only acetylcholinesterase. *J. Neurosci.,* 3: 2286 – 2291.

Fox, C.A., Andrade, A.N., Hillman, D.E. and Schwyn, R.C. (1971a) The spiny neurons in the primate striatum: a Golgi and electron microscopic study. *J. Hirnforsch.,* 13: 181 – 201.

Fox, C.A., Andrade, A.N., Schwyn, R.C. and Rafols, J.A. (1971b) The aspiny neurons and the glia in the primate striatum: a Golgi and electron microscopic study. *J. Hirnforsch.,* 13: 341 – 362.

Graveland, G.A., Williams, R.S. and DiFiglia, M. (1985) A Golgi study of the human neostriatum: neurons and afferent fibers. *J. Comp. Neurol.,* 34: 317 – 333.

Hammond, C. and Yelnik, J. (1983) Intracellular labelling of rat subthalamic neurones with horseradish peroxidase: computer analysis of dendrites and characterization of axon arborization. *Neuroscience,* 8: 781 – 790.

Henderson, Z. (1981) Ultrastructure and acetylcholinesterase content of neurons forming connections between the striatum and substantia nigra of rat. *J. Comp. Neurol.,* 197: 185 – 196.

Ingham, C.A., Bolam, J.P., Wainer, B.H. and Smith, A.D. (1985) A correlated light and electron microscopic study of identified cholinergic basal forebrain neurons that project to the cortex in the rat. *J. Comp. Neurol.,* 239: 176 – 192.

Kemp, J.M. and Powell, T.P.S. (1971) The structure of the caudate nucleus of the cat: light and electron microscopy. *Phil.*

Trans. R. Soc. Lond. (Biol.), 262: 383 – 401.

Kimura, H., McGeer, P.L., Peng, J.H. and McGeer, E.G. (1981) The central cholinergic system studied by choline acetyltransferase immunohistochemistry in the cat. *J. Comp. Neurol.,* 200: 151 – 201.

Kitai, S.T., Preston, R.J., Bishop, G.A. and Kocsis, J.D. (1979) Striatal projection neurons: morphological and electrophysiological studies. In: L.J. Poirier, T.L. Sourkes and P.J. Bédard (Eds.), *Advances in Neurology, Vol. 24,* Raven Press, New York, pp. 45 – 51.

Kubota, Y., Inagaki, S., Shimada, S., Kito, S., Eckenstein, F. and Tohyama, M. (1987) Neostriatal cholinergic neurons receive direct synaptic inputs from dopaminergic axons. *Brain Res.,* 413: 179 – 184.

Leontovich, T.A. (1954) Fine structure of subcortical ganglia (in Russian). *Z. Nevropat. Psikh.,* 54: 168 – 178.

Leontovich, T.A. (1983) Spatial arrangement of tissue elements of nucleus caudatus in dog (in Russian). *Neurophysiology,* 15: 474 – 484.

Levey, A.I., Wainer, B.H., Mufson, E.J. and Mesulam, M.-M. (1983) Co-localization of acetylcholinesterase and choline acetyltransferase in the rat cerebrum. *Neuroscience,* 9: 9 – 22.

Lu, E.J. and Brown, W.J. (1977) The developing caudate nucleus in the euthyroid and hypothyroid rat. *J. Comp. Neurol.,* 171: 261 – 284.

Lynch, G.S., Lucas, P.A. and Deadwyler, S.A. (1972) The demonstration of acetylcholinesterase containing neurones within the caudate nucleus of the rat. *Brain Res.,* 45: 617 – 621.

Mesulam, M.-M., Mufson, E.J., Levey, A.I. and Wainer, B.H. (1984) Atlas of cholinergic neurons in the forebrain and upper brainstem of the macaque based on monoclonal choline acetyltransferase immunohistochemistry and acetylcholinesterase histochemistry. *Neuroscience,* 12: 669 – 686.

Nagai, T., Pearson, T., Peng, F., McGeer, E.G. and McGeer, P.L. (1983) Immunohistochemical staining of the human forebrain with monoclonal antibody to human choline acetyltransferase. *Brain Res.,* 265: 300 – 306.

Parent, A. and O'Reilly-Fromentin, J. (1982) Distribution and morphological characteristics of acetylcholinesterase-containing neurons in the basal forebrain of the cat. *Brain Res. Bull.,* 8: 183 – 196.

Pasik, P., Pasik, T. and DiFiglia, M. (1979) The internal organization of the neostriatum of mammals. In: I. Divac and R.G.E. Oberg (Eds.), *The Neostriatum,* Pergamon Press, New York, pp. 5 – 36.

Pasik, P., Pasik, T. and Holstein, G.R. (1991) The ultrastructural chemoanatomy of the basal ganglia: 1984-1989. I. The neostriatum. In: G. Bernardi et al. (Eds.), *The Basal Ganglia III,* Plenum, New York, pp. 187 – 197.

Percheron, G. (1979) Quantitative analysis of dendritic branching. I. Simple formulae for the quantitative analysis of dendritic branching. *Neurosci. Lett.,* 14: 287 – 293.

Percheron, G. (1982) Principles and methods of the graph theo-

34

retical analysis of natural binary arborescences. *J. Theor. Biol.*, 99: 509 – 552.

Phelps, P.E., Houser, C.R. and Vaughn, J.E. (1985) Immunocytochemical localization of choline acetyltransferase within the rat neostriatum: a correlated light and electron microscopic study of cholinergic neurons and synapses. *J. Comp. Neurol.*, 238: 286 – 307.

Poirier, L.J., Parent, A., Marchand, R. and Butcher, L.L. (1977) Morphological characteristics of the acetylcholinesterase-containing neurons in the CNS of DFP-treated monkeys. Part 1. Extrapyramidal and related structures. *J. Neurol. Sci.*, 31: 181 – 198.

Preston, R.J., Bishop, G.A. and Kitai, S.T. (1980) Medium spiny neuron projection from the rat neostriatum: an intracellular horseradish peroxidase study. *Brain Res.*, 183: 253 – 263.

Pullen, A.H. (1984) A structured program in Basic for cell morphometry: its application to the spinal motoneurone. *J. Neurosci. Methods,* 12: 155 – 178.

Rafols, J.A., Cheng, H.W. and McNeill, T.H. (1989) Golgi study of the mouse striatum: age-related dendritic changes in different neuronal populations. *J. Comp. Neurol.*, 279: 212 – 227.

Ramon-Moliner, E. (1969) The leptodendritic neuron: its distribution and significance. *Ann. N.Y. Acad. Sci.*, 167: 65 – 70.

Satoh, K. and Fibiger, H.C. (1985) Distribution of central cholinergic neurons in the baboon (*Papio papio*). I. General morphology. *J. Comp. Neurol.*, 236: 197 – 214.

Satoh, K., Staines, W.A., Atmadja, S. and Fibiger, H.C. (1983) Ultrastructural observations of the cholinergic neuron in the rat striatum as identified by acetylcholinesterase pharmacohistochemistry. *Neuroscience*, 10: 1121 – 1136.

Smith, Y. and Parent, A. (1984) Distribution of acetylcholinesterase-containing neurons in the basal forebrain and upper brainstem of the squirrel monkey (*Saimiri sciureus*). *Brain Res. Bull.*, 12: 95 – 104.

Takagi, H., Somogyi, P. and Smith, A.D. (1984) Aspiny neurons and their local axons in the neostriatum of the rat: a correlated light and electron microscopic study of Golgi-impregnated material. *J. Neurocytol.*, 13: 239 – 265.

Tanaka Jr., D. (1980) Development of spiny and aspiny neurons in the caudate nucleus of the dog during the first postnatal month. *J. Comp. Neurol.*, 192: 247 – 263.

Van der Loos, H. (1956) Une combinaison de deux vieilles méthodes histologiques pour le système nerveux central. *Mschr. Psychiatr. Neurol.*, 132: 330 – 334.

Wilson, C.J. and Groves, P.M. (1980) Fine structure and synaptic connections of the common spiny neuron of the rat neostriatum: a study employing intracellular injection of horseradish peroxidase. *J. Comp. Neurol.*, 194: 599 – 616.

Woolf, N.J. (1991) Cholinergic systems in mammalian brain and spinal cord. *Prog. Neurobiol.*, 37: 475 – 524.

Woolf, N.J. and Butcher, L.L. (1981) Cholinergic neurons in the caudate-putamen complex proper are intrinsically organized: a combined Evans Blue and acetylcholinesterase analysis. *Brain Res. Bull.*, 7: 487 – 507.

Yelnik, J. and Percheron, G. (1979) Subthalamic neurons in primates: a quantitative and comparative analysis. *Neuroscience,* 4: 1117 – 1143.

Yelnik, J., Percheron, G., Perbos, J. and François, C. (1981) A computer-aided method for the quantitative analysis of dendritic arborizations reconstructed from serial sections. *J. Neurosci. Methods,* 4: 347 – 364.

Yelnik, J., Percheron, G., François, C. and Burnod, Y. (1983) Principal component analysis: a suitable method for the three-dimensional study of the shape, dimensions and orientation of dendritic arborizations. *J. Neurosci. Methods,* 9: 115 – 125.

Yelnik, J., Percheron, G. and François, C. (1984) A Golgi analysis of the primate globus pallidus. II. Quantitative morphology and spatial orientation of dendritic arborizations. *J. Comp. Neurol.*, 227: 200 – 213.

Yelnik, J., François, C., Percheron, G. and Heyner, S. (1987) Golgi study of the primate substantia nigra I. Quantitative morphology and typology of nigral neurons. *J. Comp. Neurol.*, 265: 455 – 472.

Yelnik, J., François, C., Percheron, G. and Tande, D. (1991) Morphological taxonomy of the neurons of the primate striatum. *J. Comp. Neurol.*, 313: 273 – 294.

G.W. Arbuthnott and P.C. Emson (Eds.)
Progress in Brain Research, Vol. 99

CHAPTER 3

In vivo studies of the postnatal development of rat neostriatal neurons

James M. Tepper and Francine Trent

Center for Molecular and Behavioral Neuroscience, Rutgers, The State University of New Jersey, Newark, 07102 NJ, U.S.A.

Introduction

The electrophysiological and morphological properties of the mammalian neostriatum have been the subject of numerous studies over the past 25 years. Of the many different cell types in the neostriatum identified by Golgi staining or intracellular labeling (e.g., Kemp and Powell, 1971a; DiFiglia et al., 1976; Bishop et al., 1982; Chang et al., 1982), the most information is known about the medium spiny neuron, the principal output neuron of the nucleus, and the neuron that comprises up to 95% of the cell population in the rat neostriatum (for review, see Wilson, 1990). The spontaneous activity and synaptic responses of the medium spiny neuron have been shown to be dominated by certain aspects of its passive membrane properties as well as by the morphological and physiological organization of its extrinsic excitatory inputs. The relatively low input impedance and sparse and bursty spontaneous activity of these neurons result in large part from a very considerable fast anomalous rectification (Wilson, 1992, this volume). The characteristic response of neostriatal neurons to stimulation of their principal excitatory cortical or thalamic afferents is complex, consisting of an early EPSP composed of both mono- and polysynaptic components, a subsequent long-lasting hyperpolarization, and a late depolarization, and is virtually identical in all spe-

cies studied (Buchwald et al., 1973; Wilson et al., 1983; Herrling, 1984; Wilson, 1986; Calabresi et al., 1990).

Despite the considerable literature on the neurophysiology of neostriatal neurons in the adult rat, relatively little is known about the electrophysiological properties of neostriatal neurons in neonates, or the time course of the postnatal development of mature physiology and morphology. There are some data from extracellular recording experiments which suggest that there is little or no spontaneous activity in rat neostriatum prior to postnatal day 10 (P10; Napier et al., 1985; Tepper et al., 1990a,b), and in vitro intracellular recording experiments have revealed important differences in passive membrane properties and synaptic responses to local stimulation in neonates versus adults (Misgeld et al., 1986). There have also been a number of studies of the postnatal development of the basal ganglia in kittens (Adinolfi, 1977; Morris et al., 1979; Hull et al., 1981; Levine et al., 1982); compared to rat, however, the feline basal ganglia is considerably more developed at birth, and displays a more protracted postnatal development.

There have been almost no reports of the postnatal development of the neurophysiological properties of rat neostriatal neurons in vivo. Such information is important for several reasons. The rat is the most common experimental subject for studies of the anatomy and physiology of the basal ganglia, and more is known about the basal ganglia of the adult rat than that of any other species. In addition, in recent years there has been intensive research in the field of neuronal grafting. The most successful grafting experiments have been performed in rats, in which suspensions of embryonic neurons have been transplanted into the brains of adult hosts (see Gage and Fisher, 1991, for a recent review). Such grafts have been demonstrated to survive in the host, and to establish both afferent and efferent synaptic connections with host neurons (Rutherford et al., 1987; Walsh et al., 1988; Wictorin et al., 1989, 1990; Fisher et al., 1991; Xu et al., 1989, 1991a,b). Although early studies of the neurophysiological and morphological properties of fetal neurons grafted to adult hosts emphasized the similarity of the electrophysiological properties among the grafted neurons and their in situ counterparts (e.g., Wuerthele et al., 1981; Arbuthnott et al., 1985; Rutherford et al., 1987), more recent studies have found significant differences between various types of neurons in situ and those that were transplanted, even after the grafts have been allowed to mature for several months in the host (Walsh et al., 1988; Fisher et al., 1991; Xu et al., 1991b). It is possible that the differences between in situ and graft cells may arise from a functional immaturity on the part of the graft neurons themselves, but before concluding this, a characterization of the physiological and morphological properties of early postnatal neurons in vivo is required. In this chapter, we will review some recent experiments detailing the electrophysiological and morphological characteristics of neostriatal neurons in neonatal rats, and compare and contrast these properties to those observed in the neostriatum of adults.

Methods

The subjects for all experiments were Sprague-Dawley rat pups ranging in age from postnatal day 6 (P6) through P49, and adult male Sprague-Dawley rats. All rats were bred at the Institute of Animal Be-

havior at Rutgers from stock obtained from Charles River. Both pups and adults were anesthetized with urethane ($1.2-1.5$ g/kg, i.p.). When necessary, adults were supplemented with ketamine ($20-30$ mg/kg, i.m.), and pups were supplemented by inhalation of metofane. Adults and pups greater than 21 days of age were installed into a stereotaxic frame and prepared for intracellular recording by conventional means (see Tepper et al., 1987, for details). Younger neonates were affixed to a modified stereotaxic apparatus by a modification of the method originally described by Nakamura et al. (1987). Briefly, pups were placed on a custom stage designed to hold their head parallel to the stereotaxic frame bars. After removal of the scalp, a small 3 cm stainless steel rod which had short lengths of 3 mm o.d. stainless steel tubing soldered to the ends was affixed to the top of the skull in the coronal plane approximately 3.5 mm anterior to lambda with cyanoacrylate glue and dental cement. Standard stereotaxic earbars were inserted into the hollow tubes, and the pups' four extremities were affixed to the stage with cyanoacrylate glue. To minimize respiratory artifacts and stabilize the preparation, pups were suspended with a small tail clamp. Body temperature was maintained at $37 \pm 1°C$ by a solid state feedback-controlled heating pad.

Microelectrodes were pulled from 2.0 mm o.d. capillary tubing, filled with 1 M potassium acetate containing 3% biocytin (Horikawa and Armstrong, 1988) and possessed in vivo impedances between 75 and 90 MΩ. All other aspects of stimulating and recording have been described in detail previously (Tepper et al., 1987, 1990a,b).

Following the electrophysiological experiments, an overdose of urethane was administered, and rats were perfused with $20-50$ ml of isotonic saline followed by $50-250$ ml of 4% paraformaldehyde/0.2% glutaraldehyde in 0.15 M sodium phosphate buffer, pH 7.4. The brains were removed, left in the same fixative overnight, and sectioned on a Vibratome® at 60 μm and reacted for the presence of biocytin by the methods of Horikawa and Armstrong (1988).

Results

Membrane properties

Neostriatal medium spiny neurons recorded in vivo or in vitro display a prominent, fast inward rec-tification in response to both depolarizing and hyperpolarizing current pulses (Kita et al., 1984; Kawaguchi et al., 1989; Calabresi et al., 1990) that contributes significantly to the electrophysiological responses of these neurons in the adult (see Wilson,

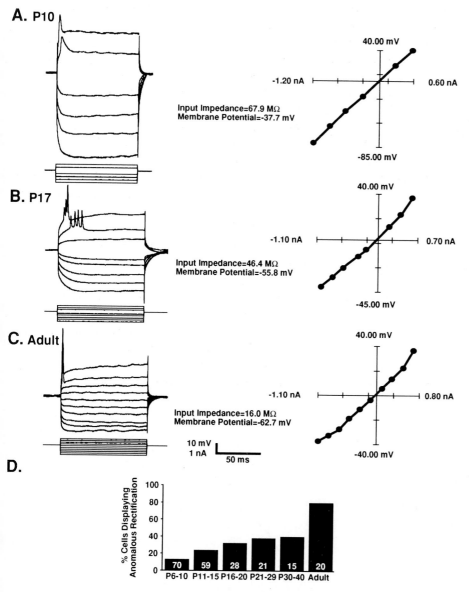

Fig. 1. Neonatal neostriatal medium spiny neurons do not display anomalous rectification. *A*. Typical membrane responses evoked by intracellular current pulses in a P10 pup. Note the linear current – voltage relation. *B*. Neuron from a P17 pup displays a modest anomalous rectification in both depolarizing and hyperpolarizing directions. *C*. Adult medium spiny neuron exhibits marked anomalous rectification. Note trend towards decreasing input resistance and increasing resting membrane potential over development. *D*. Summary graph of the postnatal development of anomalous rectification. Numbers within bars indicate number of neurons per group. Each trace is the average of four single sweeps.

38

1992, for a recent review). One of the most striking aspects of the membrane characteristics of neonatal neostriatal neurons is the complete absence of this anomalous rectification in a large majority of the neurons (Trent and Tepper, 1991). Prior to P11, less than 13% of neostriatal neurons ($n = 70$) exhibit the marked inward rectification in either hyperpolaring or depolarizing directions, and most of the neurons display fairly linear current – voltage relations, as illustrated for one representative neuron in Fig. 1A. There is steady increase in the proportion of neurons that exhibit anomalous rectification over the next three weeks, with approximately 40% of neurons from the P21 – P29 ($n = 21$) and P30 – P40 ($n = 15$) groups showing this property compared to over 80% ($n = 20$) in adults as summarized in Fig. 1D.

A smaller fraction (i.e., 22%) of neostriatal neurons from the first and second postnatal weeks exhibit I – V curves that are dominated by a marked *outward* rectification in both the depolarizing and hyperpolarizing directions. In many cases the outward rectification in response to hyperpolarizing current injections was so extreme that the apparent input resistance rose above 100 MΩ, as illustrated for one neuron in Fig. 2A. This was not due to a gross electrode non-linearity as routine extracellular checks of microelectrode linearity performed both

prior to impalement and after exiting neurons showed that these electrodes were very linear over a range exceeding ± 1.5 nA. This outward rectification is extremely atypical for adult neostriatal neurons recorded either in vivo or in vitro, as mentioned above, and was never observed in the present studies in animals older than P20.

A third difference in membrane properties between neonatal and mature medium spiny cells is the presence of a transient depolarizing potential (TDR) that appeared as a hump near the onset of intracellularly evoked membrane depolarizations (Trent et al., 1992) as shown in Fig. 3A. The mean maximal amplitude of the TDR evoked from rest was 18.1 ± 1.6 mV (mean ± S.E.M.) ($n = 40$) and mean duration was 23 ± 1 msec ($n = 44$). The TDR was observed in 56% of neurons from P6 – P10 pups ($n = 73$), 47% in P11 – P15 pups ($n = 68$), 6% in P16 – P29 pups ($n = 49$), and was never observed in older pups or adults as summarized in Fig. 3C. The TDR was voltage-sensitive; in vivo it was activated at membrane potentials more negative than – 37 mV, and could be inactivated by holding the membrane potential more positive than – 40 mV. The frequency and maximal amplitude of the TDR was increased by hyperpolarizing prepulses, suggesting that the conductance(s) responsible are partially inactivated at rest. Preliminary

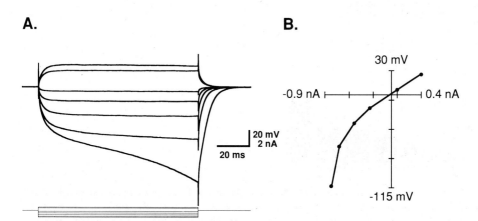

A.　　　　　　　　　　**B.**

Fig. 2. Less typical type of current – voltage relation displayed by 22% of early neonatal neostriatal neurons. A. Responses to intracellular current injections in a P11 pup reveals an extraordinary degree of outward rectification in response to modest hyperpolarizing current pulses. B. I – V plot of the data in A. Each trace is the average of six single sweeps.

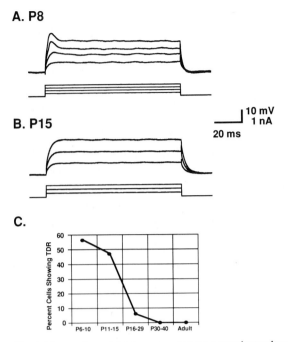

A. P8

B. P15

10 mV
1 nA
20 ms

C.

Fig. 3. Neonatal neostriatal neurons possess a transient voltage-dependent conductance that is activated by intracellular injection of depolarizing current. *A*. This transient depolarizing potential (TDR) is indicated by the ''hump'' present near the start of the pulse in a P8 pup while the same paradigm fails to evoke a TDR in neostriatal neurons from older animals. *C*. The proportion of neostriatal neurons exhibiting the TDR decreases over the first postnatal month and is never observed in animals ≥ P30. Each trace is the average of four single sweeps.

results from in vitro experiments indicate that the TDR is not affected by 1 μm tetrodotoxin, but is abolished by 500 μm cadmium, suggesting that it represents an inward calcium current. A calcium-dependent phenomenon very similar to the TDR has been observed in recordings from 10-day-old rat dorsal horn neurons in vitro (Murase and Randic, 1983); the nearly identical amplitude (13.8 + 3.1 mV) and duration (26.5 + 4.0 msec) suggest that the TDR may be a manifestation of a low threshold calcium spike in neonatal neostriatal neurons. It is interesting to note that most neurons that exhibit the TDR also exhibit a long duration spike following relaxation of strong hyperpolarizing current pulses that is similar to the low threshold spike described for mature thalamic neurons in vitro (Jahnsen and Llinás, 1984). Although mature neostriatal neurons do exhibit some calcium-dependent physiological properties (e.g., Galarraga et al., 1989), neither low threshold spikes nor TDR-like phenomena are commonly observed under normal physiological conditions. The apparent loss of the TDR over development may be related to a more general phenomenon in which voltage-activated currents carried by calcium are prominent in the early development of neurons but disappear during pre- and postnatal development (Spitzer, 1982).

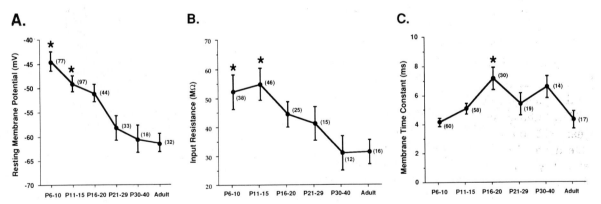

Fig. 4. The resting membrane potential, input resistance and time constant of neostriatal neurons are developmentally regulated. *A,B*. There is a progressive increase in the resting membrane potential over the first three postnatal weeks concomitant with a decrease in membrane input resistance. *C*. The membrane time constant, τ, develops non-linearly. In early neonates, τ initially increases steadily and reaches a peak during the third postnatal week and subsequently decreases to values observed in adults. Numbers within bars indicate number of neurons per group. Error bars represent S.E.M. Asterisks indicate significant difference from adult groups (Schéffé, $P < 0.1$).

The resting membrane potential shows a marked dependence on development, as shown in Fig. 4A. From a mean around − 44 mV during the first post-natal week, the average resting membrane potential increases by almost 50% by the end of the fourth week when it no longer differs from that of adults. This change in membrane potential and the appearance of anomalous rectification described above appear along with a progressive decrease in membrane input resistance as illustrated in Fig. 4B, although this measurement, and that of the time constant may be complicated by the anomalous rectification itself as well as a significant somatic shunt encountered in recording these neurons (Wilson, 1984; Bargas et al., 1988). The membrane time constant, measured by peeling exponents from small intracellularly injected hyperpolarizing transients, also varies significantly during postnatal development from around 4 msec at P6−P10 to a maximum over 7 msec at P16−P20 compared to an adult value around 4 msec, as shown in Fig. 4C.

Responses to cortical and thalamic stimulation

Excitatory responses to both cortical and thalamic stimuli could be observed by P6, the earliest age at which good quality intracellular recordings could be obtained. As shown in Fig. 5, the most typical response to cortical or thalamic stimulation in young neonates (< P21) consisted of a relatively simple EPSP, lacking both the subsequent long-lasting hyperpolarization and late depolarization that is characteristic of responses to identical stimuli in the adult (Buchwald et al., 1973; Wilson et al., 1983). Although never observed in animals younger than P12, the long-lasting hyperpolarization and late depolarization were simultaneously first observed near the middle of the third postnatal week in a small proportion (i.e., 15%; n = 41) of neurons. The proportion of neurons exhibiting this triphasic response to cortical or thalamic input increased steadily but still had not reached adult frequencies by the end of the sixth postnatal week as shown in Fig. 5B.

The initial EPSP itself showed both age-dependent and age-independent features, as illustrated in

Fig. 6. Although neither the mean maximal amplitude (about 10 mV) nor duration (about 50 msec) changed as a function of postnatal development, the onset latency was significantly longer in neonates than adults (F = 17.8, df = 5,216, P < 0.001), and the rise time was significantly shorter in pups less than P15 than in older neonates or adults (F = 3.4, df = 5,159, P < 0.01). Even in the youngest neonates, the initial EPSP consisted of both monosynaptic and polysynaptic components as previously described for adult neostriatal neurons (Wilson, 1986). In contrast to the situation obtained in adult neostriatum, the cortically evoked EPSP

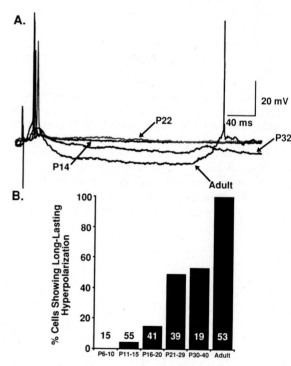

Fig. 5. Cortically evoked responses elicited by neostriatal neurons increase in complexity over the postnatal period. *A.* Stimulation of ipsilateral prefrontal cortex evokes a simple EPSP lacking the late long-lasting hyperpolarization and rebound depolarization in young neonates (P14, P22) that later develops into the characteristic triphasic response (P32, adult). *B.* The late long-lasting hyperpolarization in response to cortical stimulation does not appear in a significant proportion of neurons until the third postnatal week. Numbers within bars indicate numbers of cells tested.

could be completely reversed by intracellular injection of depolarizing current in many neonates.

Approximately one-third of the neostriatal neurons recorded in pups less than P15 ($n = 94$) exhibited an anomalous hyperpolarizing response to cortical stimulation, as illustrated for three representative neurons in Fig. 7. One of the response's most distinguishing characteristics was its time dependence, illustrated in Fig. 7A. If it was observed at all, the hyperpolarization was apparent immediately upon cell penetration. Over the next 5–10 min, the amplitude of the hyperpolarizing potential became progressively smaller until it disappeared altogether. This was not due to any apparent deterioration of the recording conditions as the input impedance did not change over this interval, nor to an increase in membrane polarization. It was likewise not dependent on repeated stimulation; the hyperpolarization decayed even if the neuron was not subjected to continuous stimulation from cortex or thalamus.

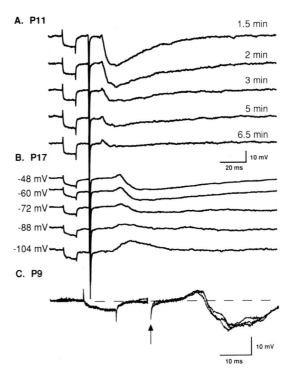

Fig. 7. Many neonatal neostriatal neurons display an anomalous hyperpolarizing response to cortical stimulation. A. Cortically evoked hyperpolarizations were transient phenomena that attained maximal amplitude immediately upon impalement and decayed in a time-dependent fashion over the next 5–10 min. B. The hyperpolarization could be decreased and reversed by intracellular injection of hyperpolarizing current indicating that it is a true IPSP. C. In most cases the IPSP was preceded by an EPSP that occurred several milliseconds prior to the IPSP's onset and at the expected latency for a cortically evoked EPSP. In A and B, each trace is the average of four single sweeps. C consists of the superimposition of three single sweeps.

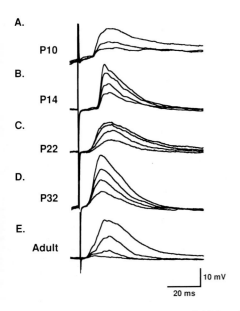

Fig. 6. Power series illustrating that the initial cortically elicited EPSP displays both age-dependent and age-independent characteristics. Although the mean maximal amplitude and duration remained constant over development, the rise time increased and the onset latency decreased as a function of age. Each trace is the average of four single sweeps.

This hyperpolarization was considered to be an IPSP since it exhibited a reversal potential of approximately -68 mV ($n = 3$), considerably more hyperpolarized than the spike threshold of these neurons, and consistent with its mediation by chloride ions shown in Fig. 7B. Most ($> 80\%$) of these hyperpolarizing responses were clearly preceded by a small amplitude EPSP with a mean onset latency (9.1 ± 0.6 msec; $n = 22$) that was the same as that of the typical cortically evoked EPSP (9.3 ± 0.4 msec; $n = 70$) shown at high gain in Fig. 7C. The IPSP onset latency (13.1 ± 0.8 msec; $n = 27$) followed that of the initial EPSP by approximately 4 msec. The IPSP was observed less and less frequently in older pups, and was never observed in pups greater than P23 or in adults.

Spontaneous activity

In adults, medium spiny neurons fire slowly and irregularly in a bursty pattern (Wilson and Groves, 1981). In vivo intracellular recordings show that the membrane potential alternates between a relatively hyperpolarized state, the "disabled" state around − 80 mV and a depolarized or "enabled" state near − 50 mV, and it has been argued that these two states result from afferent input and not intrinsic mechanisms (Wilson, this volume). In neonates, there is virtually no spontaneous activity until around P15. When spontaneous activity first appears, it is in the form of randomly occurring single spikes separated by long (up to several minutes) intervals. At this developmental stage, each neuron's resting membrane potential is extremely stable; the prolonged enabled and disabled periods are completely absent, and shorter duration fluctuations in membrane potential are greatly reduced in frequency. Over the next three weeks, the rate of spontaneous activity increases, and the neurons begin to fire in a bursty pattern typical of adult neostriatal neurons. The increase in firing rate and the change in firing pattern is accompanied by a gradual increase in the frequency and amplitude of "spontaneous" shifts in resting membrane potential, and by the fifth postnatal week the spontaneous activity appears essentially as it does in adults.

It is interesting to note that the manifestation of enabled and disabled states is concomitant with the development of the long-lasting hyperpolarization following cortical or thalamic stimulation. That is, through the end of the third postnatal week, the membrane potential remains relatively stable, and, as noted above, the long-lasting hyperpolarization following afferent excitation is absent. Over the next few weeks, some of the neurons begin to exhibit prolonged depolarizing and hyperpolarizing shifts in membrane potential and concomitant bursting activity, while others do not. Invariably, those neu-

rons that displayed the shifts in membrane potential also exhibited a long-lasting hyperpolarization in response to cortical stimulation, whereas those neurons that failed to show prolonged depolarizing and hyperpolarizing episodes also failed to exhibit a long-lasting hyperpolarization, as illustrated for four representative neurons in Fig. 8.

As has been described previously for neostriatal and other central nervous system neurons (Misgeld et al., 1986; McCormick and Prince, 1987; Nakamura et al., 1987; Williams and Marshall, 1987; Michelson and Lothman, 1989; Tepper et al., 1990a,b), both spontaneous and evoked action potentials in early neonates exhibited longer dura-

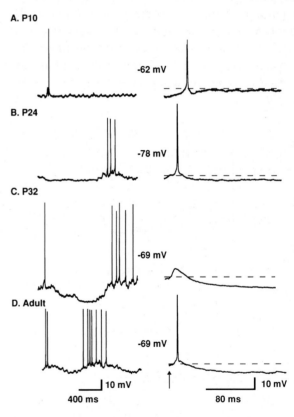

Fig. 8. There is a correlation between the occurrence of enabled and disabled states of membrane potential described by Wilson (this volume) (left) and the manifestation of the long-lasting hyperpolarization following cortical stimulation (right) over development. Arrow denotes application of cortical stimulus. Dashed line indicates pre-stimulus resting membrane potential. Numbers indicate resting membrane potential.

tions and decreased amplitudes compared to those in adults.

Neuronal morphology

Although the basic cell size and shape, and dendritic configuration of early postnatal neostriatal medium spiny neurons is very similar to that of adults (Kemp and Powell, 1971a; Wilson and Groves, 1980), intracellular labeling of electrophysiologically characterized neurons with biocytin has revealed two additional developmental events that were not well-detected by earlier Golgi studies of developing basal ganglia neurons (Adinolfi, 1977; Hull et al., 1981), as well as allowing a correlation between the morphological properties of the neurons and their physiological characteristics. As has been known for some time, neonatal medium spiny neurons in a number of species are essentially aspiny, and possess rather thin and varicose dendrites compared to adults. Although in adults, the vast majority of cortical and thalamic afferents form asymmetric synapses onto the heads of dendritic spines (Kemp and Powell, 1971b,c), in early postnatal neurons intracellularly labeled with biocytin in vivo, there are very few spines prior to P10 as shown in Fig. 8A. Between P11 and P20, the spine density increases dramatically, and the dendrites assume the non-varicose morphology that they possess in the adult, illustrated in Fig. 8. It is interesting to note that the most marked increases in spine density take place between P15 and P20, precisely the time during which the majority of cortical and thalamic afferents reach the neostriatum and form asymmetric axo-spinous synaptic connections (Hattori and McGeer, 1973). It is also during this period that the IPSP response to cortical stimulation disappears, suggesting that the appearance of the IPSP is dependent upon some developmentally transient aspect of the postnatal maturation of the cortical and/or thalamic innervation.

In contrast to the dendritic immaturity of neonatal neostriatal neurons, the local axon collateral plexus that characterizes the morphology of the mature medium spiny neuron and which has been proposed to play a major role in neostriatal information processing (e.g., Groves, 1983) is already present in the youngest animals in which we were able to obtain good intracellular filling, shown in Fig. 8E. There were no obvious differences between the local axon collateral systems from neurons early in the second postnatal week and in those in adults (Trent and Tepper, 1991).

Discussion

The rat neostriatum undergoes an extended postnatal development, both in terms of the membrane properties of individual neurons as well as their synaptic connectivity. Many of the properties of immature neostriatal neurons, for example, decreased average spontaneous firing rate, unusually wide action potentials, relatively depolarized resting membrane potential and lack of anomalous rectification are not specific to neostriatal neurons, and have been reported previously for a number of different neurons in central nervous system neurons in neonates including those of the spinal cord (Murase and Randic, 1983), hippocampus (Michelson and Lothman, 1989; Segal, 1990), midbrain (Pitts et al., 1990; Tepper et al., 1990a,b) and neocortex (McCormick and Prince, 1987; Lorenzon and Foehring, 1991; Fukuda and Prince, 1992).

Although one of the most characteristic features of adult neostriatal medium spiny neuron neurophysiology, both in vivo and in vitro, is the prominent fast inward rectification seen in response to both de- and hyperpolarizing current injection (Wilson, 1992, this volume), the vast majority of neostriatal medium spiny neurons in neonates did not exhibit anomalous rectification. The absence of anomalous rectification early in the neonatal period has been previously reported in in vitro preparations of neostriatum (Misgeld et al., 1986) and hippocampus (Segal, 1990), and the results of the present study confirm that this absence is due to an intrinsic difference in membrane properties of neonatal versus adult neurons, and not to some artifact of the slice preparation. A lack of anomalous rectification has also been reported in grafted fetal rat neostriatal medium spiny neurons in in vitro

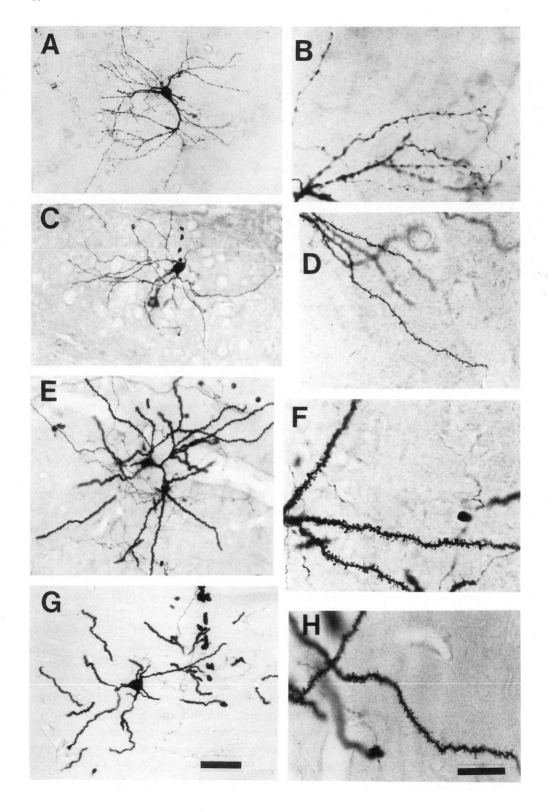

recording experiments (Walsh et al., 1988), and even after many months' survival in the host brain in in vivo recordings (Xu et al., 1991b). The absence of this type of rectification is likely to contribute to the increased stability of the resting membrane potential of neonatal neostriatal neurons compared to those of adults, and the absence of the long depolarizing episodes which generate bursts of spikes in mature neostriatal neurons (Wilson and Groves, 1980; Wilson, this volume). A secondary effect of the lack of anomalous rectification is that it fixes the membrane time and space constants by removing their dependence on membrane potential (Wilson, 1992), thereby causing the response of neonatal spiny neurons to excitatory afferent input to be essentially independent of the membrane state of the neuron.

Although even the youngest neonatal neurons in this study responded to cortical and/or thalamic input, there were several differences among the responses to afferent excitatory input in neonates and adults. In neonates younger than P12, the characteristic sequence of depolarization – long-lasting hyperpolarization – depolarization was absent, and the most common response to cortical stimulation was a simple EPSP.

Although some have claimed that the long-lasting hyperpolarization seen in adult neostriatal neurons following stimulation of excitatory afferents is an IPSP resulting from activation of the inhibitory recurrent axon collateral system of the medium spiny neuron (e.g., Buchwald et al., 1973; Hull et al., 1973; Levine et al., 1986), there is strong evidence that this phenomenon is due to a disfacilitation of excitatory cortical inputs. Wilson and colleagues have shown that unlike other synaptic

A. P 12

B. ADULT

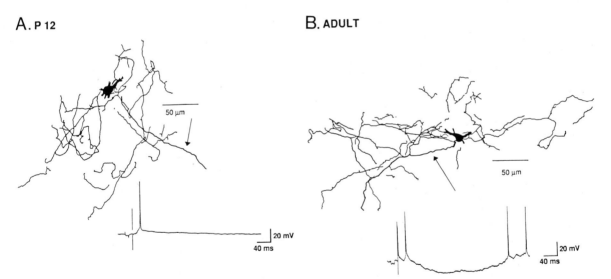

Fig. 10. *A*. The local axon collateral system of the P12 neuron shown in Fig. 9*A* is well-developed as indicated by the partial camera lucida reconstruction (120 μm in depth) and does not differ markedly from that observed in adults (*B*). Despite the well-developed local axon collateral system, cortical stimulation fails to elicit the long-lasting hyperpolarization in the P12 pup, but does so in the adult.

Fig. 9. Neonatal neostriatal medium spiny neurons are morphologically immature and bear thin, varicose and virtually aspiny dendrites as revealed by intracellular labeling with biocytin. *A,C,E,G*. Low magnification photomicrographs of medium spiny neurons intracellularly labeled with biocytin from P12 (*A*), P20 (*C*), P27 (*E*) and adult rats (*G*). *B,D,F,H*. Higher magnification photomicrographs of the dendrites of the neurons shown on the left. The density of dendritic spines increases up through P21 – P29. Note that even at P12, portions of the local axon collaterals are visible as fine beaded processes in *A* and *B*. Calibration marker = 50 μm in *A,C,E* and *G*, and 20 μ in *B,D,F* and *H*.

potentials in neostriatal neurons, the long-lasting hyperpolarization: (1) is accompanied by a small decrease in membrane conductance instead of a significant increase; (2) shows only a minimal dependence on experimentally induced alterations in membrane potential in a direction that indicates a reversal potential that is the same as that for the early and late EPSP components of the response; and (3) is abolished by lesions of the corticostriatal or the thalamostriatal pathways (Wilson et al., 1983). This conclusion is supported by the absence of the two later components of the response to cortical stimulation in early neonates in the present study. Although there are clearly some corticostriatal and thalamostriatal fibers present even in the youngest neonates examined since stimulation of cortex or thalamus could evoke EPSPs in these animals, the bulk of the cortical and thalamic inputs do not arrive, ramify and form axospinous synapses in neostriatum until the middle of the third postnatal week (Hattori and McGeer, 1973). Prior to this time, although a limited number of anterogradely labeled corticostriatal fibers can be observed in neostriatum at the level of the electron microscope, many of the boutons appear to be less densely packed with synaptic vesicles than in the adult, and were not observed in synaptic contact. Of those that do form synapses, the vast majority formed asymmetric synapses with dendritic shafts, not spine heads (Sharpe et al., 1992). Furthermore, in the present experiments, when descending through cortex en route to neostriatum, very little spontaneous activity was detected in cortex until late in the third postnatal week, the time at which the long-lasting hyperpolarization and rebound excitation first appeared in a significant proportion of neurons (cf. Fig. 6). Finally, as discussed below, the axon collateral plexus of biocytin-filled medium spiny neurons is already well-developed at least by the first postnatal week when the neurons do not exhibit the long-lasting hyperpolarization but when others have shown that these neurons do exhibit adult-like sensitivity to GABA agonists (Levine et al., 1990). None of the findings in the present study are consistent with the notion that the long-lasting hyper-

polarization following afferent excitation derives from intrastriatal inhibition; rather these data support the disfacilitation hypothesis of Wilson and colleagues (Wilson et al., 1983).

It is of interest to note that the development of the "enabled" and "disabled" states, the prolonged depolarizing and hyperpolarizing shifts in membrane potential that characterize the spontaneous activity of the adult medium spiny neuron, coincided with the appearance of the long-lasting hyperpolarization in response to cortical and/or thalamic stimulation. This observation supports Wilson's contention that these states derive, at least in part, from afferent input from cortex and/or thalamus (Wilson and Groves, 1980; Wilson, this volume). Although they are virtually devoid of spontaneous activity, the neonatal neurons do not appear to be in the "disabled" state, however, since their average resting membrane potential is significantly more depolarized than in adults. It is unlikely that this depolarization derives from tonic cortical or thalamic input, since the lack of disfacilitation following cortical or thalamic stimulation indicates that there is little or no tonic activity in the corticostriatal pathway during the first two postnatal weeks. Furthermore, other types of neurons in neonatal rats also appear to be depolarized early in postnatal development (e.g., Tepper et al., 1990a,b). It may be that the depolarized state arises from intrinsic cellular factors, for example, a generally reduced activity of an electrogenic Na^+/K^+ ATPase in neonates, as has recently been demonstrated for neonatal hippocampal neurons (Atsuo and Prince, 1992).

The prominent IPSP that was evoked by cortical stimulation in neonates is particularly interesting, and very similar to one reported by Misgeld et al. (1986) following intrastriatal stimulation in slices of neonatal rat neostriatum, although they did not comment on its transient nature. This potential was clearly distinct from the long-lasting hyperpolarization that succeeds the initial cortically evoked EPSP in adult neostriatal neurons in that it was of considerably shorter duration, was sensitive to experimentally induced alterations in membrane potential, and exhibited a reversal potential near that which would be expected for a chloride-mediated IPSP. It is quite likely that this IPSP represents the action of the inhibitory recurrent axon collateral plexus and/or the effects of feedforward inhibition through striatal interneurons. One could speculate that one of the major reasons that this IPSP is so much more apparent in neonates than in adults is because of the low density and sparse nature of the corticostriatal inputs in the neonates in contrast to the more diffuse and widespread innervation in adults (Hattori and McGeer, 1973; Sharpe et al., 1992). This could result in the occurrence of patchy "hot spots" of cortical and/or thalamic input, which would increase the probability of encountering neurons that are less densely innervated directly by cortical and/or thalamic afferents than their nearby neighbors. Under these conditions, the relative input resulting from recurrent or feedforward inhibition may outweigh that from direct excitation allowing the IPSP to be manifest more clearly than in the normal adult striatum. It is interesting to note that this type of innervation pattern has recently been reported for cortical inputs to intrastriatal grafts of neostriatal neurons (Xu et al., 1989; Wilson et al., 1990), and these grafted neurons, but not adjacent host neurons, have also been shown to exhibit cortically and thalamically evoked IPSPs (Xu et al., 1991b) that are similar in many respects to those observed in neonates in situ.

The disappearance of this IPSP over the first few minutes of recording is puzzling; the same transience has been described by Xu and colleagues in grafted neostriatal neurons (Xu et al., 1991b). As they suggest, perhaps the intracellular penetration damages or alters the intracellular environment in such a way as to block the manifestation of the IPSP. In any event, it appears that the physiology of spiny neurons in the immature neostriatum is more significantly affected by intrinsic or feedforward inhibition than that of the mature striatum, and this may contribute to the extremely low levels of spontaneous activity observed in the first few postnatal weeks.

The morphology of neonatal neostriatal medium spiny neurons differs significantly from that of mature medium spiny neurons. Although the size and appearance of the somata is essentially the same as in adults, the most characteristic feature of these neurons, the densely spine-laden dendrites, appear varicose and almost spine-free up through the first two postnatal weeks, consistent with an earlier report based on Golgi staining (Chronister et al., 1976). The dendritic arbor is also less expansive during this time. During the third postnatal week, coincident with the elaboration of the cortical and thalamic afferents and their corresponding synaptogenesis (Hattori and McGeer, 1973), the dendrites become heavily invested with spines and lose their varicose appearance. A similar developmental sequence has been described for feline neostriatal medium spiny neurons, although they are considerably more mature at birth than rodent neostriatal neurons and exhibit a prolonged postnatal maturation compared to that of the rat (Adinolfi, 1977). Nevertheless, even the dendrites of feline medium spiny neurons are only sparsely invested with spines in the first postnatal week (Hull et al., 1981). Based on modeling studies of spiny dendrites (Wilson, 1984, 1992), the paucity of dendritic spines and the lack of anomalous rectification in the early neonatal period should make neonatal medium spiny neurons more electrotonically compact than adult neurons. This is likely the explanation for the relative ease with which cortically evoked EPSPs could be reversed by intracellular current injection in the early neonates in the present study, and suggests that during postnatal development, medium spiny neurons should be more sensitive to the effects of individual synaptic inputs than is the case in the adult. This phenomenon may explain why the magnitude of the maximal cortically evoked EPSP does not change over postnatal development despite the fact that the number of excitatory afferent synapses increases substantially.

One of the more interesting observations to emerge from these studies is the striking similarity (and difference from in situ adult neurons) among many of the electrophysiological and morphological characteristics of neonatal neostriatal neurons and those of fetal neostriatal neurons grafted to ibo-

TABLE I

Comparison among adult, neonatal and grafted neostriatal neurons

	Adult	Neonate	Graft
Anomalous rectification	Yes	No	No
Enabled-disabled states	Yes	No	No
Transient IPSP	No	Yes	Yes
EPSP latency	Short	Long	Long
Spine density	High	Low	Intermediate-low

tenic or kainic acid-treated neostriatum (Zemanick et al., 1987; Walsh et al., 1988; Xu et al., 1991b; see Table I). These similarities include: lack of anomalous rectification, increased membrane resistance, decreased spine density, increased latency to cortically evoked EPSPs, lack of a long-lasting hyperpolarization and subsequent late depolarization following afferent excitation, presence of an early fast IPSP following cortical or thalamic stimulation that decays over time, and absence of discrete enabled and disabled states of the resting membrane potential. Some of these shared features may arise from the reduced extrinsic excitatory input existing in both the immature neostriatum and in grafted fetal neurons and imply that as with nigral dopaminergic neurons (Fisher et al., 1990; Tepper et al., 1990a), grafted neostriatal neurons remain in a developmentally arrested state, both physiologically and morphologically, even several months after transplantation.

Acknowledgements

This work was supported by UPHS grants MH-45286 and NS-30679. We thank Dr. C.J. Wilson for generously supplying us with his software for the time constant analyses (Oscilloscope®) and for making a preprint of his chapter in this volume available to us.

References

Adinolfi, A.M. (1977) The postnatal development of the caudate nucleus: a Golgi and electron microscopic study of kittens. *Brain Res.,* 133: 251 – 266.

Arbuthnott, G., Dunnett, S. and MacLeod, N. (1985) Electrophysiological properties of single units in dopamine-rich mesencephalic transplants in rat brain. *Neurosci. Lett.,* 57: 205 – 210.

Atsuo, F. and Prince, D.A. (1992) Postnatal development of electrogenic sodium pump activity in rat hippcampal neurons. *Dev. Brain Res.,* 65: 101 – 114.

Bargas, J., Galarraga, E. and Aceves, J. (1988) Electrotonic properties of neostriatal neurons are modulated by extracellular potassium. *Exp. Brain Res.,* 72: 390 – 398.

Bishop, G.A., Chang, H.T. and Kitai, S.T. (1982) Morphological and physiological properties of neostriatal neurons: an intracellular horseradish peroxidase study in the rat. *Neuroscience,* 7: 179 – 191.

Buchwald, N.A., Price, D.D., Vernon, L. and Hull, C.D. (1973) Caudate intracellular responses to thalamic and cortical inputs. *Exp. Neurol.,* 38: 311 – 323.

Calabresi, P., Mercuri, N.B., Stefani, A. and Bernardi, G. (1990) Synaptic and intrinsic control of membrane excitability of neostriatal neurons. I. An in vivo analysis. *J. Neurophysiol.,* 63: 651 – 662.

Chang, H.T., Wilson, C.J. and Kitai, S.T. (1982) A Golgi study of rat neostriatal neurons: light microscopic analysis. *J. Comp. Neurol.,* 208: 107 – 126.

Chronister, R.B., Farnell, K.E., Marco, L.A. and White Jr., L.E. (1976) The rodent neostriatum: a Golgi analysis. *Brain Res.,* 108: 37 – 46.

DiFiglia, M., Pasik, P. and Pasik, T. (1976) A Golgi study of neuronal types in the neostriatum of monkeys. *Brain Res.,* 114: 245 – 256.

Fisher, L.J., Young, S.J., Tepper, J.M., Groves, P.M. and Gage, F.H. (1991) Electrophysiological characteristics of cells within mesencephalon suspension grafts. *Neuroscience,* 40: 109 – 122.

Fukuda, A. and Prince, D.A. (1992) Postnatal development of electrogenic sodium pump activity in rat hippocampal pyramidal neurons. *Dev. Brain Res.,* 65: 101 – 114.

Gage, F.H. and Fisher, L.J. (1991) Intracerebral grafting: a toll for the neurobiologist. *Neuron,* 6: 1 – 12.

Galarraga, E., Bargas, J., Sierra, A. and Aceves, J. (1989) The role of calcium in the repetitive firing of neostriatal neurons. *Exp. Brain Res.,* 75: 157 – 168.

Groves, P.M. (1983) A theory of the functional organization of the neostriatum and the neostriatal control of voluntary movement. *Brain Res. Rev.,* 5: 109 – 132.

Hattori, T. and McGeer, P.L. (1973) Synaptogenesis in the corpus striatum of infant rat. *Exp. Neurol.,* 38: 70 – 79.

Herrling, P.L. (1984) Evidence for GABA as the transmitter for early cortically evoked inhibition of cat caudate neurons. *Exp.*

Brain Res., 55: 528 – 534.

Horikawa, K. and Armstrong, W.E. (1988) A versatile means of intracellular labeling: injection of biocytin and its detection with avidin conjugates. *J. Neurosci. Methods,* 25: 1 – 11.

Hull, C.D., Bernardi, G., Price, D.D. and Buchwald, N.A. (1973) Intracellular responses of caudate neurons to temporally and spatially combined stimuli. *Exp. Neurol.,* 38: 324 – 336.

Hull, C.D., McAllister, J.P., Levine, M.S. and Adinolfi, A.M. (1981) Quantitative developmental studies of feline neostriatal spiny neurons. *Dev. Brain Res.,* 1: 309 – 332.

Jahnsen, H. and Llinás, R. (1984) Electrophysiological properties of guinea-pig thalamic neurones: an in vitro study. *J. Physiol. (Lond.),* 349: 205 – 226.

Kawaguchi, Y., Wilson, C.J. and Emson, P.C. (1989) Intracellular recording of identified neostriatal patch and matrix spiny cells in a slice preparation preserving cortical inputs. *J. Neurophysiol.,* 62: 1052 – 1069.

Kemp, J.M. and Powell, T.P.S. (1971a) The structure of the caudate nucleus of the cat: light and electron microscopy. *Phil. Trans. R. Soc. (Lond.) (B),* 262: 383 – 401.

Kemp, J.M. and Powell, T.P.S. (1971b) The synaptic organization of the caudate nucleus. *Phil. Trans. R. Soc. (Lond.) (B),* 262: 403 – 412.

Kemp, J.M. and Powell, T.P.S. (1971c) The site of termination of afferent fibers in the caudate nucleus. *Phil. Trans. R. Soc. (Lond.) (B),* 262: 413 – 427.

Kita, T., Kita, H. and Kitai, S.T. (1984) Passive membrane properties of rat neostriatal neurons in an in vitro slice preparation. *Brain Res.,* 300: 129 – 139.

Levine, M.S., Fisher, R.S., Hull, C.D. and Buchwald, N.A. (1982) Development of spontaneous neuronal activity in the caudate nucleus, globus pallidus-entopeduncular nucleus, and substantia nigra of the cat. *Dev. Brain Res.,* 3: 429 – 441.

Levine, M.S., Fisher, R.S., Hull, C.D. and Buchwald, N.A. (1986) Postnatal development of identified medium-sized caudate spiny neurons in the cat. *Dev. Brain Res.,* 24: 47 – 62.

Levine, M.S., Adams, C.E., Hannigan, J.H., Hull, C.D. and Buchwald, N.A. (1990) Caudate neurons respond to excitatory and inhibitory amino acids in early postnatal periods in the cat. *Dev. Neurosci.,* 12: 196 – 203.

Lorenzon, N.M. and Foehring, R.C. (1991) Ontogeny of sensitivity to neuromodulators in rat neocortical neurons. *Soc. Neurosci. Abstr.,* 17: 746.

McCormick, D.A. and Prince, D.A. (1987) Post-natal development of electrophysiological properties of rat cerebral cortical pyramidal neurones. *J. Physiol. (Lond.),* 393: 743 – 762.

Michelson, H.B. and Lothman, E.W. (1989) An in vivo electrophysiological study of the ontogeny of excitatory and inhibitory processes in the rat hippocampus. *Dev. Brain Res,* 47: 113 – 122.

Misgeld, U., Dodt, H.U. and Frotscher, M. (1986) Late development of intrinsic excitation in the rat neostriatum: an in vitro study. *Dev. Brain Res.,* 27: 59 – 67.

Morris, R., Levine, M.S., Cherubini, E., Buchwald, N.A. and Hull, C.D. (1979) Intracellular analysis of the development of responses of caudate neurons to stimulation of cortex, thalamus, and substantia nigra in the kitten. *Brain Res.,* 173: 471 – 487.

Murase, K. and Randic, M. (1983) Electrophysiological properties of rat spinal dorsal horn neurones in vitro: calcium-dependent action potentials. *J. Physiol. (Lond.),* 334: 141 – 153.

Nakamura, S., Kimura, F. and Sakaguchi, T. (1987) Postnatal development of electrical activity in the locus ceruleus. *J. Neurophysiol.,* 58: 510 – 524.

Napier, T.C., Coyle, S. and Breese, G.R. (1985) Ontogeny of striatal unit activity and effects of single or repeated haloperidol administration in rats. *Brain Res.,* 333: 35 – 44.

Pitts, D.K., Freeman, A.S. and Chiodo, L.A. (1990) Dopamine neuron ontogeny: electrophysiological studies. *Synapse,* 6: 309 – 320.

Rutherford, A., Garcia-Munoz, M., Dunnett, S.B. and Arbuthnott, G.W. (1987) Electrophysiological demonstration of host cortical inputs to striatal grafts. *Neurosci. Lett.,* 83: 275 – 281.

Segal, M. (1990) Developmental changes in serotonin actions in rat hippocampus. *Dev. Brain Res.,* 52: 247 – 252.

Sharpe, N., Trent, F. and Tepper, J.M. (1992) Postnatal changes in neostriatal synaptic input. *Soc. Neurosci. Abstr.,* 18: 697.

Spitzer, N.C. (1982) The development of electrical excitability. In: T.A. Sears (Ed.), *Neuronal-Glial Cell Interrelationships,* Springer, New York, pp. 77 – 91.

Tepper, J.M., Sawyer, S.F. and Groves, P.M. (1987) Electrophysiologically identified nigral dopaminergic neurons intracellulary labeled with HRP: light microscopic analysis. *J. Neurosci.,* 7: 2794 – 2806.

Tepper, J.M., Trent, F. and Nakamura, S. (1990a) Postnatal development of the electrical activity of rat nigrostriatal dopaminergic neurons. *Dev. Brain Res.,* 54: 21 – 33.

Tepper, J.M., Trent, F. and Nakamura, S. (1990b) In vivo development of the spontaneous activity of rat nigrostriatal neurons. In: G. Bernardi, M.B. Carpenter and G. Di Chiara (Eds.), *Basal Ganglia III,* Plenum, New York, pp. 251 – 260.

Trent, F. and Tepper, J.M. (1991) Postnatal development of synaptic responses, membrane properties and morphology of rat neostriatal neurons in vivo. *Soc. Neurosci. Abstr.,* 17: 938.

Trent, F., Xu, Z.C., Wilson, C.J. and Tepper, J.M. (1992) A cadmium-sensitive voltage-dependent conductance is transiently expressed during development of neostriatal neurons. *Soc. Neurosci. Abstr.,* 18: 697.

Walsh, J.P., Zhou, F.C., Hull, C.D., Fisher, R.S., Levine, M.S. and Buchwald, N.A. (1988) Physiological and morphological characterization of striatal neurons transplanted into the striatum of adult rats. *Synapse,* 2: 37 – 44.

Wictorin, K., Clarke, D.J., Bolam, J.P. and Björklund, A. (1989) Host corticostriatal fibres establish synaptic connections with grafted striatal neurons in the ibotenic acid lesioned striatum. *Eur. J. Neurosci.,* 1: 189 – 195.

Wictorin, K., Clarke, D.J., Bolam, J.P. and Björklund, A. (1990) Fetal striatal neurons grafted into the ibotenate lesioned adult striatum: efferent projections and synaptic contacts in the host globus pallidus. *Neuroscience,* 37: 301 – 315.

Williams, J.T. and Marshall, K.C. (1987) Membrane properties of adrenergic responses in locus coeruleus neurons of young rats. *J. Neurosci.,* 7: 3687 – 3694.

Wilson, C.J. (1984) Passive cable properties of dendritic spines and spiny neurons. *J. Neurosci.,* 4: 281 – 297.

Wilson, C.J. (1986) Postsynaptic potentials evoked in spiny neostriatal projection neurons by stimulation of ipsilateral and contralateral neocortex. *Brain Res.,* 367: 201 – 213.

Wilson, C.J. (1990) Basal ganglia. In: G. Shephard (Ed.), *The Synaptic Organization of the Brain,* third edition, Oxford University Press, New York, pp. 279 – 316.

Wilson, C.J. (1992) Dendritic morphology, inward rectification, and the functional properties of neostriatal neurons. In: P. McKenna, J. Davis and S.F. Zornetzer (Eds.), *Single Neuron Computation,* Academic Press, Orlando, FL, pp. 141 – 172.

Wilson, C.J. and Groves, P.M. (1980) Fine structure and synaptic connections of the common spiny neuron of the rat neostriatum. A study employing intracellular injection of horseradish peroxidase. *J. Comp. Neurol.,* 194: 599 – 615.

Wilson, C.J. and Groves, P.M. (1981) Spontaneous firing patterns of identified spiny neurons in the rat neostriatum. *Brain Res.,* 220: 67 – 80.

Wilson, C.J., Chang, H.T. and Kitai, S.T. (1983) Disfacilitation and long-lasting inhibition of neostriatal neurons in the rat. *Exp. Brain Res.,* 51: 227 – 235.

Wilson, C.J., Xu, Z.C., Emson, P.C. and Feler, C. (1990) Anatomical and physiological properties of the cortical and thalamic innervations of neostriatal tissue grafts. *Prog. Brain Res.,* 87: 417 – 426.

Wuerthele, S.M., Freed, W.J., Olson, L., Morihisa, J., Spoor, L., Wyatt, R.J. and Hoffer, B.J. (1981) Effect of dopamine agonists and antagonists on the electrical activity of substantia nigra neurons transplanted into the lateral ventricle of the rat. *Exp. Brain Res.,* 44: 1 – 10.

Xu, Z.C., Wilson, C.J. and Emson, P.C. (1989) Restoration of the corticostriatal projection in rat neostriatal grafts: electron microscopic analysis. *Neuroscience,* 29: 539 – 550.

Xu, Z.C., Wilson, C.J. and Emson, P.C. (1991a) Restoration of thalamostriatal projections in rat neostriatal grafts: an electron microscopic analysis. *J. Comp. Neurol.,* 303: 22 – 34.

Xu, Z.C., Wilson, C.J. and Emson, P.C. (1991b) Synaptic potentials evoked in spiny neurons in rat neostriatal grafts by cortical and thalamic stimulation. *J. Neurophysiol.,* 65: 477 – 493.

Zemanick, M.C., Walker, P.D. and McAllister II, J.P. (1987) Quantitative analysis of dendrites from transplanted neostriatal neurons. *Brain Res.,* 414: 149 – 152.

G.W. Arbuthnott and P.C. Emson (Eds.)
Progress in Brain Research, Vol. 99
© 1993 Elsevier Science Publishers B.V. All rights reserved.

CHAPTER 4

GABAergic circuits of the striatum

Hitoshi Kita

Department of Anatomy and Neurobiology, College of Medicine, The University of Tennessee at Memphis, Memphis, TN 38163,
U.S.A.

Introduction

The neostriatum contains a large number of neurons and terminals which contain γ-aminobutyric acid (GABA), an inhibitory transmitter. GABAergic inhibition has been thought to play a major role in regulating the neuronal activities of the striatum. In this chapter, I will summarize our studies on the GABAergic circuits and their functions in the striatum. I will first describe the anatomical organizations and then discuss the functional implications of GABAergic elements.

Anatomical organization of GABA-containing elements in the striatum

The neostriatum contains two types of GABAergic neurons. They are GABAergic spiny projection neurons (which have extensive axon collaterals within the striatum) and GABAergic interneurons. The striatum also receives GABAergic afferents from the globus pallidus and the substantia nigra.

Spiny projection neurons of the striatum

Approximately 90% of the neurons in the striatum are projection neurons to the pallidum and/or substantia nigra. The somatodendritic and axonal morphology of these neurons has been extensively studied by Golgi and intracellular labeling techniques (Kemp and Powell, 1971; Fox et al., 1971a; DiFiglia et al., 1976; Kitai et al., 1979; Wilson and Groves, 1980; Somogyi et al., 1981; Chang et al.,

1982; Graveland et al., 1985). These neurons have a medium-sized soma with a large, centrally located smooth nucleus and a thin rim of cytoplasm. The primary dendrites are smooth, whereas secondary and tertiary dendrites are covered by a large number of spines. Thus, they are often referred to as medium spiny neurons. The spiny projection neuron has local axon collaterals which terminate on neighboring spiny neurons (Kitai et al., 1979; Wilson and Groves, 1980; Somogyi et al., 1981). The local axon collaterals form feedback circuits within the striatum. About twenty years ago the nature of striato-pallidal and striato-nigral projections was shown to be GABAergic inhibitory (Yoshida and Precht, 1971; Precht and Yoshida, 1971). Since that time, striatal projection neurons are assumed to contain GABA. Immunohistochemical studies have demonstrated that glutamate decarboxylase (GAD, the synthetic enzyme of GABA) or γ-aminobutyric transaminase can be localized in medium-sized projection neurons (Ribak et al., 1979; Oertel and Mugnaini, 1984; Afsharpour et al., 1985; Penny et al., 1986). However, it was not certain if either a subpopulation or most of spiny neurons contain GABA. Some immunohistochemical studies indicated a majority of medium neurons exhibited GAD immunoreactivity (Oertel and Mugnaini, 1984) or numerous medium-sized somata were GAD-positive (Ribak et al., 1979). On the other hand, other reports indicated only about 20% of striato-nigral neurons were immunoreactive for γ-aminobutyric transaminase (Araki et al., 1985), or

47% of the total striatal neurons were immunoreactive for GAD (Penny et al., 1986) and about 20% of striato-pallidal and 45% of striato-nigral neurons were immunoreactive for GAD (Afsharpour et al., 1985).

We have attempted to resolve the discrepancy in the percentage of the GABA-containing neurons in the rat striatum by means of GAD immunohistochemistry. The major problem associated with a quantitative immunohistochemical study is the incidence of a false positive or negative in labeling. False labeling may occur when non-specific antibodies or inadequate immunohistochemical procedures (e.g., inadequate buffer solutions and concentrations of antibodies) are used. We, therefore, tried several buffer fixative configurations and different dilutions of antibodies. We found that the phosphate-buffered fixative with picric acid and 1 : 2000 dilution of the primary antiserum (developed and characterized by Oertel et al., 1983) produced the best GAD immunoreactivity. There are two other sources of false negatives for GAD immunoreactivity. One is poor penetration of the antibodies through the tissue. It is our experience that using Triton-X obscures GAD immunoreactivity of the somata but increases the fiber and terminal labeling. We also noted that freeze-thawing of tissues using liquid nitrogen does not necessarily increase penetration of the GAD antibody (Fig. 2A; see also Kosaka et al., 1987). To combat the first problem, we analyzed only the neurons located at the surface of the sections. The second problem is that the intensity of immunostaining tends to be too low to be recognized as positive. We injected colchicine, an axonal transport blocker, into the lateral ventricle, a procedure known to greatly increase the intensity of GAD immunostaining. Previous studies, including our own, have consistently shown that the population of GAD-immunoreactive neurons in the striatum was relatively small when animals were not treated with colchicine (Bolam et al., 1983; Afsharpour et al., 1985; Penny et al., 1986).

The striatum contains a high density of neurons immunoreactive for GAD (Fig. 1A). These neurons are divided into three types based on their somatic morphology and the intensity of reaction products. The first type are medium-sized neurons with a somatic diameter of 10 – 15 μm and moderate intensity for GAD immunoreactivity. These have a narrow ring of cytoplasm surrounding a nucleus. The morphological characteristics of the somata of these neurons are identical to those of the medium-spiny projection neurons (Kitai et al., 1979; Chang et al., 1981). The population of this type of GAD-immunoreactive neurons is very high, over 80%. The second type are small to medium-sized neurons that were intensely immunoreactive for GAD. Their somata are round or oval and contain a narrow ring of cytoplasm surrounding the nucleus (Fig. 2B – E). These neurons range from 3 to 5% of the total neurons in the striatum. The somatic morphology of these neurons appears to be similar to the high GABA-uptake, local-circuit neurons that are small to medium in size and have nuclear invaginations (Bolam et al., 1983). Further morphological details of this neuron type will be discussed in the next section.

The third type are the intensely stained large neurons. These are polygonal and have a large volume of cytoplasm surrounding the nucleus (Fig. 2F,G). These neurons are extremely rare and only a few cells were found in the entire surface of each striatal section. A possible corresponding type for these neurons may be large neurons having somatic spines (Chang et al., 1982) or large striato-nigral projection neurons (Bolam et al., 1981).

Our study revealed that the proportion of GABAergic neurons in the rat striatum, including all three types, is at least 85% of the total neurons. This number is much higher than previous estimations. The high percentage of GABAergic neurons in this study is the result of pretreating the animals with colchicine and observing only the surface of vibratome sections in order to avoid the problem of false negative counts associated with poor penetration of antibodies. Judging from previous morphological studies, we can argue that more than 80% of the observed GAD-positive neurons are medium-sized projection neurons and about 4% are local-

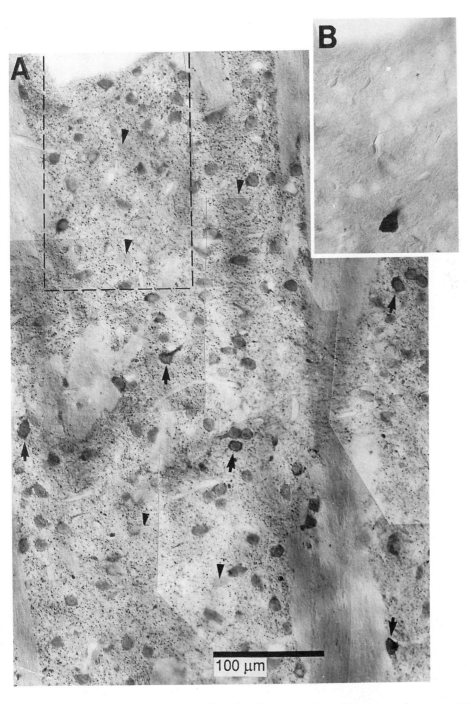

Fig. 1. *A*. A photomontage showing the surface of a vibratome section of the striatum immunoreacted for GAD. Several intensely stained, medium-sized cells (e.g., arrows) and a few unstained cells (e.g., arrowheads) among a large population of moderately stained, medium-sized cells can be seen. *B*. A ChAT-immunoreacted section which is next to the section shown in *A* (marked by dotted lines). The area contains two GAD-negative cells, of which one is immunoreacted for ChAT (Kita and Kitai, 1988).

54

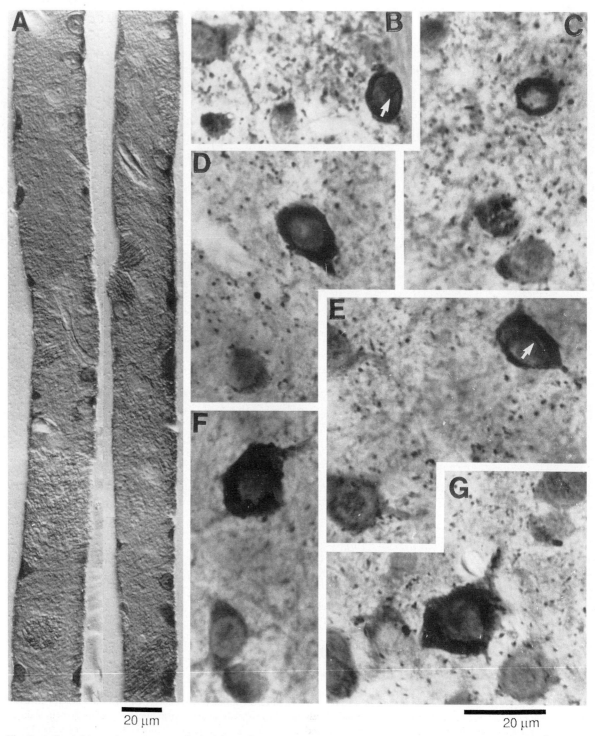

Fig. 2. *A.* Semi-thin sections cut perpendicularly to a vibratome section of striatum. Most of the cells located on the edges (i.e., the surface of the vibratome section) of sections were immunoreactive for GAD. However, most of the cells located in the middle of the vibratome section were not stained. *B – E.* Small to medium-sized neurons intensely immunoreactive for GAD. The nucleus of these neurons often had deep nuclear invaginations (e.g., arrows in *B* and *E*). *F,G.* Large polygonal neurons intensely immunoreactive for GAD. The neurons have a large volume of cytoplasm surrounding the nucleus (Kita and Kitai, 1988).

circuit neurons, and that most striatal projection neurons are GABAergic. A similar observation has been made by Oertel and Mugnaini (1984). It is also reasonable to assume that several neuropeptides (e.g., enkephalins, substance P and dynorphins), localized in medium-sized striatal neurons (Graybiel et al., 1981; Oertel et al., 1981, 1983; Afsharpour et al., 1985), coexist with GABA projection neurons.

GABAergic interneurons of the striatum

As mentioned earlier, a small population of neu-

rons expressed a very strong immunoreactivity for GABA and GAD in the striatum (Oertel and Mugnaini, 1984; Kita and Kitai, 1988; Cowan et al., 1990). They have been considered GABAergic interneurons. Studies with GABA or GAD immunohistochemistry and the Golgi impregnation method indicate that GABAergic interneurons have medium-sized somata with aspiny varicose dendrites (Bolam et al., 1985; Pasik et al., 1988). The morphological details of these neurons were not known until the recent finding that the immuno-

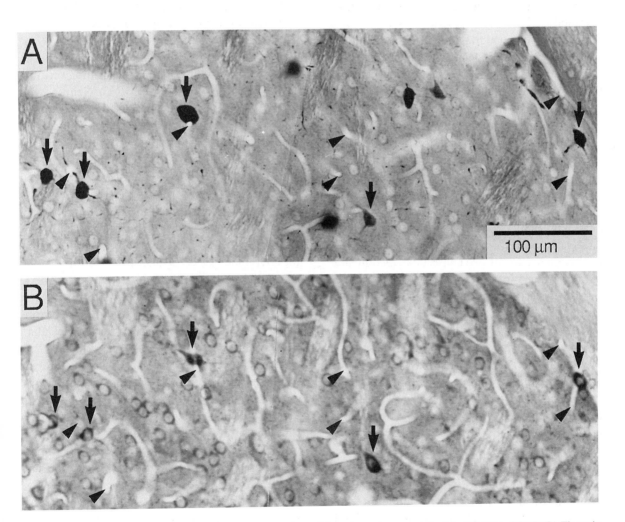

Fig. 3. *A* and *B*. Paired surfaces of two consecutive striatal sections of the striatum immunostained for PV *(A)* and GAD *(B)*. The staining is limited to the surface of the sections. Arrows point to neurons immunoreactive for PV which are also strongly immunoreactive for GAD. The striatum contains a large number of neurons immunonegative for PV but moderately or slightly immunoreactive for GAD. Arrow heads in *A* and *B* point to corresponding cut ends of capillaries (Kita et al., 1990).

histochemistry for the Ca-binding protein parvalbumin (PV) stains subpopulations of GABAergic neurons in many areas of the mammalian central nervous system including the GABAergic interneurons in the striatum (Celio and Heizmann, 1981; Heizmann, 1984; Gerfen et al., 1985; Celio, 1986; Kosaka et al., 1987; Cowan et al., 1990; Kita et al., 1990).

It has been suggested that PV participates in Ca^{2+} translocation and Ca^{2+} buffering in the neurons (Heizmann, 1984). PV is found in neurons which are known to have the ability to generate a continuous high-frequency firing (e.g., cortical interneurons, reticular thalamus neurons, and substantia nigra pars reticulata neurons). These neurons are known to generate Ca spikes upon activation of neurons. A high-frequency firing may also cause a large flow of Ca^{2+} into their nerve terminals. It is conceivable that PV plays an important role in buffering these transient rises of Ca^{2+}.

A small number of neurons in the striatum were immunoreactive for PV (Fig. 3A). Immunohistochemistry for GAD revealed a small number of intensely stained neurons and a large number of light or unstained neurons (Fig. 3B). In order to determine if most PV neurons in the striatum were GABAergic, pairs of two consecutive sections were immunostained for GAD and PV, respectively. Because these sections were not treated with Triton-X, staining was limited to elements on the surface of the sections including the somata which were cut and separated into two sections. By observing the surfaces of the paired plastic embedded sections with a Nomarski light microscope, matching parts of the split somata were found (for details, see Kosaka et al., 1985). Ninety-four percent of the strongly GAD-immunoreactive neurons in the striatum were identified as PV neurons. Similarly, 96% of PV neurons were strongly immunoreactive for GAD. The results were consistent with the observation by Cowan and associates that most PV-immunoreactive neurons are strongly immunoreactive for GABA (Cowan et al., 1990). The data indicate that most, if not all, strongly GAD-immunoreactive neurons in the striatum contain PV.

Because PV immunohistochemistry stains primarily the GABAergic interneurons rather than the GABAergic spiny projection neurons, it offers an opportunity to study the morphology of striatal interneurons in detail at both light and electron microscopic levels. In the sections treated with Triton-X, the staining intensity of neurons varied considerably (Fig. 4). Entire somatodendritic profiles were visible in strongly immunoreactive neurons, whereas only somata and proximal dendrites were visible in moderately immunoreactive neurons and only somata can be observed in slightly immunoreactive neurons (Fig. 4A). These PV neurons had somata with a fusiform or polygonal shape (Fig. 4A,B). The dendrites, when visible, were smooth and cylindrical at the proximal portion but were varicose at the distal portion (Fig. 4B,C). Neurons with similar somato-dendritic morphology have been described in Golgi studies of rat, cat, monkey and human striatum (Kemp and Powell, 1971; Fox et al., 1971a,b; DiFiglia et al., 1976; Chang et al., 1982; Graveland et al., 1985). While we have not counted the number of PV neurons, we can safely estimate that 3 – 5% of rat striatal neurons are immunoreactive for PV since most neurons which are immunoreactive for PV are strongly immunoreactive for GAD (and vice versa) and that 3 – 5% of striatal neurons were strongly immunoreactive for GAD (Kita and Kitai, 1988). Fig. 5 shows a drawing of a coronal section of the striatum in which PV neurons were plotted using three different marks depending on the staining intensity. The drawing indicates that the distribution of PV neurons is not even; areas containing many PV neurons and small areas devoid of PV neurons are intermingled in the striatum. Fig. 5 also shows that strongly PV-immunoreactive neurons tend to locate in the lateral part of the striatum which receives heavy projections from the motor and the somatosensory cortices (Donoghue and Herkenham, 1986). Moderately immunoreactive PV neurons are located in the middle part of the striatum. The medial part of the striatum facing the lateral ventricle or the pallidum and the caudal part of the nucleus accumbens were nearly devoid of PV neurons. The general distribution pattern seen in the coronal as well as in the horizontal sections was that the density of strongly immunoreactive neurons decreased as the distance from the subcortical white matter increased. The distribution of PV fibers was similar to that of darkly stained neurons probably because the intensely labeled fibers belong to darkly stained neurons.

The size of the PV neurons was estimated from

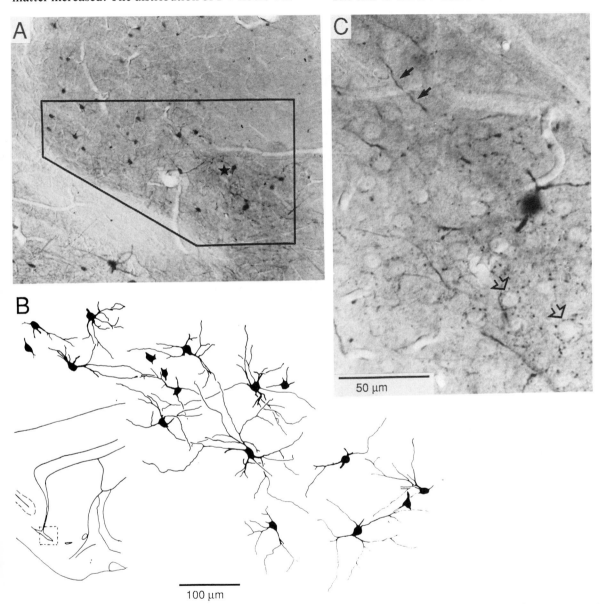

Fig. 4. *A*. A sagittal section of the striatum shows PV-immunoreactive neurons in the rostroventral striatum. The section was treated with Triton-X in order to increase penetration of immunoreagents into the section. *B*. A drawing of PV-immunoreactive neurons in the area marked in *A*. The staining intensity of neurons varies considerably; in some neurons only somata are stained but somata and dendrites are clearly seen in other neurons. *C*. A higher magnification photomicrograph of the area marked by a star in *A*. PV-immunoreactive boutons are unevenly distributed in the striatum. Open arrows point to PV-immunonegative neurons which are in a PV bouton-rich area and are outlined by PV-immunoreactive boutons. Black arrows point to an example of varicose distal dendrites of PV neurons (Kita et al., 1990).

the somatic area (i.e., the area occupied by the outline of the somata seen under the light microscope). The somatic area ranged from 120 to 522 μm^2 with a mean of 240 μm^2 (S.D. = 78) and had a single peak. The somatic area of spiny projection neurons and cholinergic interneurons range from 100 to 300 μm and from 300 to 600 μ, respectively (Chang et al., 1982). Thus, most of the PV neurons can be classified as medium in size and are slightly larger than the spiny neurons.

PV-immunoreactive fibers with boutons were observed in the striatum under the light microscope. The fibers were usually thin, however, the boutons were large (i.e., most of them were over 1 μm) in diameter. The fibers and boutons were unevenly distributed in the striatum (Fig. 4C). The somata of spiny projection neurons which were characterized as medium in size and round in shape with a thin rim of cytoplasm, are often outlined by a number of PV boutons (Fig. 4C). The number of PV boutons seen in the vicinity of somata varied considerably from neuron to neuron. Some of the somata appeared not to be contacted by any PV boutons. The results imply that most spiny projection neurons receive various degrees of innervation from GABAergic interneurons, while some of them are free from the innervation.

PV-immunoreactive neurons and fibers were

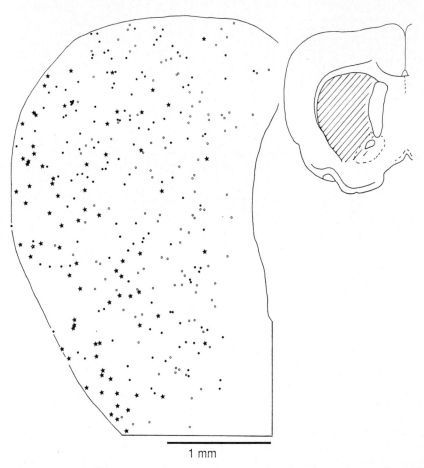

1 mm

Fig. 5. A plot of PV-immunoreactive neurons in a coronal section of the striatum. Three different marks are used depending on the staining intensity; stars represent darkly stained neurons with visible distal dendrites, filled circles represent neurons with soma and proximal dendrites, and open circles represent neurons where only somata are visible. These PV-immunoreactive neurons are unevenly distributed in the striatum (Kita et al., 1990).

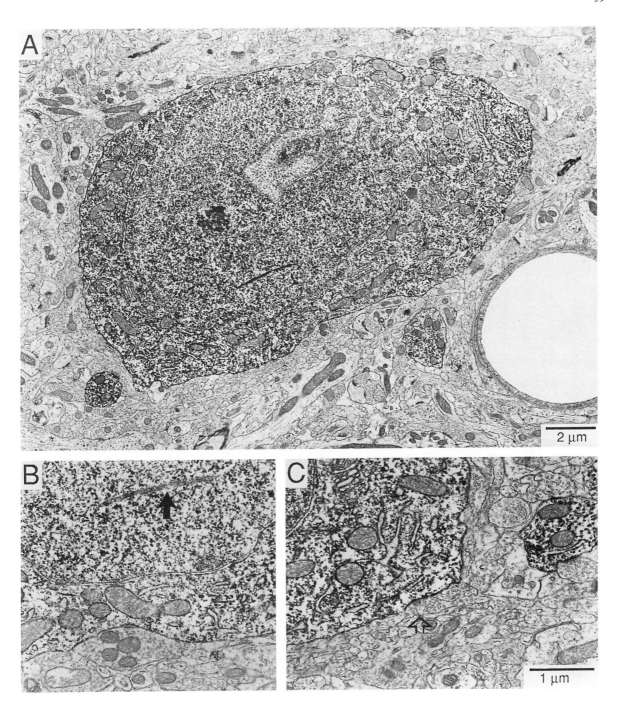

Fig. 6. The soma of a PV-immunoreactive neuron. *A*. The soma contains cytoplasm rich in organelles and a deeply indented nucleus with an intranuclear rod and a nucleolus. *B*. A higher magnification of the intranuclear rod (marked by an arrow) and a large PV-immunonegative bouton forming a punctum adherens on the soma. *C*. An example of a small PV-immunonegative bouton with relatively large vesicles forming symmetrical synapses with a PV-immunopositive soma (marked by an arrow) and a PV-immunoreactive dendrite with a PV-immunonegative synaptic bouton (Kita et al., 1990).

examined under the electron microscope. The somata of PV neurons have a deeply indented nucleus and often an intranuclear rod (Fig. 6*A,B*). While the cytoplasm entrapped in the indentations contains only ribosomes, the remaining cytoplasm is rich in organelles including endoplasmic reticulum, Golgi apparatus, mitochondria and vesicles with various sizes. Multivesicular bodies and vesicles are more numerous in the cytoplasm near the origin of dendrites and the dendritic cytoplasm (Figs. 6*A*, 7). Many PV-immunoreactive dendrites with a diameter of 0.4 – 1.5 μm were observed in the neuropile of the striatum. Dendritic spines were rarely found. Of 120 electron micrographs of dendrites sampled, only four had a short spine-like appendage (Fig. 9*C*).

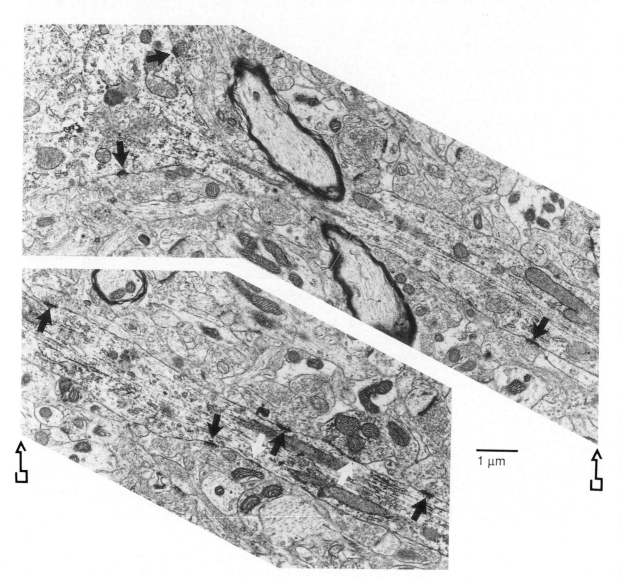

Fig. 7. A part of the soma and a proximal dendrite of a PV-immunoreactive neuron receiving a large number of asymmetrical (marked by black arrows) and a few symmetrical synapses (white arrows). The two electron micrographs are continuous (arrows in the margin mark the cut point) (Kita et al., 1990).

On the other hand, we observed eight close membrane appositions, most likely the gap junctions, formed between two neighboring PV dendrites (Fig. 8). The appositions were seen either on the smooth dendritic shaft or on small protrusions. Although dye-coupling between processes of spiny neurons has been reported (Cepeda et al., 1989; Kawaguchi et al., 1989), gap junctions are rarely found in ultrastructure studies of the striatum (as they were not mentioned in most of the previous electron microscopic studies). However, it is likely that they may be formed frequently between GABAergic interneurons, as we were able to find eight of them by searching areas where two PV dendrites came in close proximity. The gap junction is known to function as a low-resistance electrical path. Unlike the chemical synapse, electrical signals can conduct the junction without delay. It is possible that GABAergic interneurons connected through gap junctions are activated synchronously by their inputs and simultaneously inhibit a large number of their target neurons.

Boutons forming synapses with somata and dendrites of PV neurons were studied. About two-thirds of the randomly sampled boutons formed asymmetrical synapses and the others formed symmetrical synapses. The somata of PV neurons were contacted by only a few synaptic boutons; usually 2 – 4 synapses were identified on a single section of the somata. The dendrites of PV neurons had more frequent synapses; 20 – 50% of the length outlining sectioned dendrites were covered with synaptic boutons. Both symmetrical and asymmetrical synapses were found on the PV dendrites of all sizes and the number of asymmetrical synapses was larger than the number of symmetrical ones on any dendrite, especially on the smaller dendrites.

The boutons forming asymmetrical synapses were small in diameter (less than 1 μm) and contained densely packed round vesicles (Figs. 7, 9C). Our study of combined PV immunohistochemistry and PHA-L anterograde labeling indicates that fibers from the sensorimotor cortex terminate on PV neurons. However, it was very rare to observe thalamo-striatal fibers terminating on PV neurons even after injection of PHA-L into a large area of the intralaminar nuclei in the rat (unpublished observation). A recent pre-embedding double-labeling immunohistochemical study indicates that axon terminals of cholinergic interneurons of the striatum form synapses with somata and dendrites of PV neurons (Chang and Kita, 1992). The boutons forming

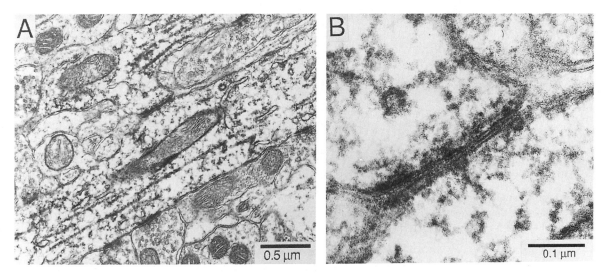

Fig. 8. *A*. A gap junction formed between two PV-immunoreactive dendrites. *B*. A higher magnification of the junction. A gap can be seen between the two opposing membranes (Kita et al., 1990).

symmetrical synapses included more than one type. Some of these boutons were immunoreactive for PV (e.g., Fig. 10B) and were found on both the somata and dendrites of PV neurons. This observation indicates that PV neurons receive strong inhibitory inputs from other PV neurons. Boutons with a morphology similar to the previously reported tyrosine hydroxylase-immunoreactive boutons also formed synapses mainly with somata and large proximal dendrites of PV neurons. These boutons were small in size (i.e., less than 0.5 μm) and contained large vesicles, 50 – 80 nm in diameter (e.g., Fig. 6C). A

previous immunohistochemical study suggests the existence of dopamine innervation to the GABAergic interneurons of the striatum (Kubota et al., 1987). These observations imply that dopamine may change the activity of GABAergic interneurons. The other PV-immunonegative boutons forming symmetric synapses with PV neurons displayed a variety of morphological features.

A large number of PV-immunoreactive myelinated and unmyelinated axons with boutons were seen in the striatum (Fig. 9A,B). The PV-immunoreactive boutons had a diameter of

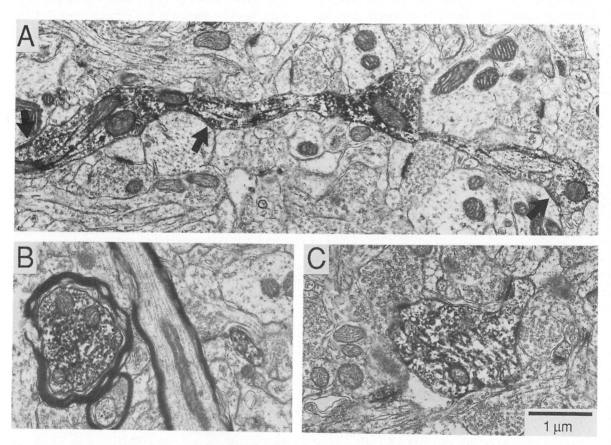

Fig. 9. A bouton forming a synapse en passant. *A*. Arrows point to symmetrical synapses on unstained dendrites. *B*. A cross view of myelinated and unmyelinated axons. *C*. A PV-immunoreactive dendrite with a short, spine-like appendage receiving asymmetrical synapses (Kita et al., 1990).

Fig. 10. *A – D*. PV-immunoreactive boutons forming symmetrical synapses with a spiny dendrite *(A)* and a PV-immunoreactive dendrite *(B)*. A PV-immunoreactive dendrite *(C)* and a varicose dendrite *(D)*. The PV-immunoreactive bouton in *C* also formed punctum adherens with a postsynaptic dendrite (marked by arrows) (Kita et al., 1990).

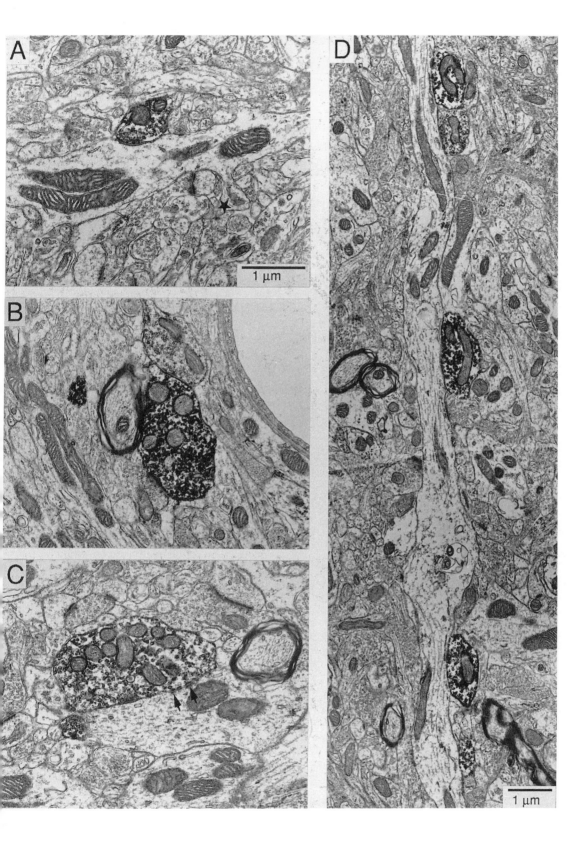

0.3 – 2 μm, contained round or elongated vesicles that were about 35 nm in diameter, and often had more than one mitochondria (Fig. 10, 11). Some of the boutons formed punctum adherentia with a postsynaptic element (Fig. 10*C*). All the PV-immunoreactive boutons formed symmetrical synapses. There were no differences between the boutons forming synapses with PV-immunopositive elements and those forming synapses with immunonegative elements. Approximately half of the PV boutons were found on somata and proximal dendrites of PV-immunonegative medium-sized neurons containing a large, round, centrally located nucleus (Fig. 11). When the areas containing dense PV-immunoreactive fibers were observed, several PV-immunoreactive synaptic boutons on the soma

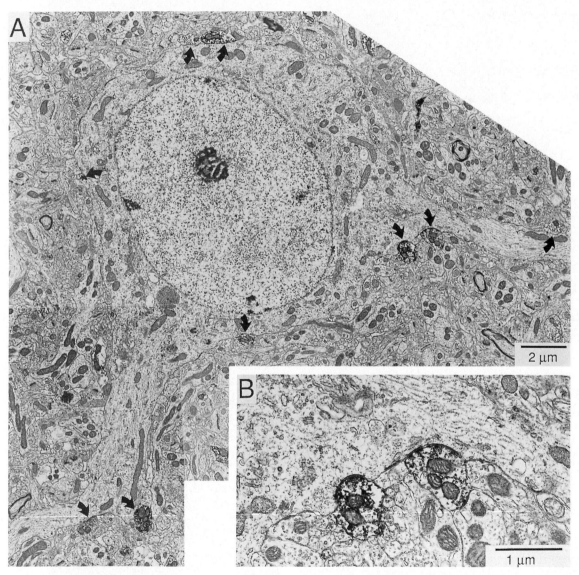

Fig. 11. A medium-sized neuron contacted with a large number of PV-immunoreactive boutons (marked by arrows). The somatic morphology is typical of spiny projection neuron. All of these boutons were confirmed to form synapses with the neuron by observing adjacent sections (Kita et al., 1990).

and proximal dendrites of immunonegative neurons in a single section were commonly seen (Fig. 11). The others formed synapses with dendrites of various sizes. Some of the dendrites forming synapses with PV boutons had spines (Fig. 10*A*). It is evident that one of the postsynaptic targets of PV neurons is the spiny projection neurons. These projection neurons may receive a powerful inhibition upon activation of the GABAergic interneurons. It was occasionally observed that a large number of PV-immunoreactive boutons form synapses on varicose dendrites (Fig. 10*D*). While the neuron type of the dendrites has yet to be identified, possible candidates include somatostatin-containing neurons of the striatum. It has been shown recently that PV boutons seldom form synapses with cholinergic interneurons of the striatum (Chang and Kita, 1992). An ultrastructural study of somatostatin neurons in the rat striatum reports that relatively large boutons with numerous pleomorphic vesicles (which were very similar to PV-immunoreactive ones) form symmetrical synapses on proximal dendrites of somatostatin-immunoreactive neurons (DiFiglia and Aronin, 1982).

The anatomical studies indicate that, in the striatum, immunohistochemistry for PV selectively stains GABAergic interneurons that are medium to large in size with aspiny dendrites. The GABAergic interneurons are incorporated into a feed-forward inhibitory circuit in which they receive both extrinsic excitatory (i.e., mainly from the cortex) and intrinsic inhibitory inputs and their outputs inhibit both spiny projection neurons and interneurons (i.e., GABAergic and probably somatostatin-containing neurons) of the striatum.

GABAergic afferents of the striatum

The GABAergic afferents to the striatum arise from the globus pallidus and the substantia nigra pars reticulata. These projections are considered minor and sparse. Our recent study in the rat, however, indicates that a large number of pallidal neurons project to the striatum and some of them contain PV (Kita et al., 1991). Staines and his associates have shown that somatostatin-containing interneurons of the striatum receive heavy innervation from the pallidum (Staines and Hincke, 1991). The details of the nigro-striatal GABAergic projection are unknown. It is, however, apparent now that the PV-immunoreactive axon terminals mentioned above include those extrinsic sources. The PV-immunoreactive boutons which formed synapses with the varicose dendrites may belong to the pallidal afferent fibers.

GABAergic responses in the striatum

The importance of the inhibitory response in the striatum was recognized in early electrophysiological studies (Malliani and Purpura, 1967; Buchwald et al., 1973; Hull et al., 1973). For example, stimulation of the sensorimotor cortex, which projects heavily to the striatum, evokes a very short duration of excitation followed by a long duration (200 – 500 msec) of inhibition in striatal neurons. Recent intracellular recording studies demonstrate a sequence of postsynaptic responses involved in the responses, including a short duration EPSP, a short duration IPSP, and a disfacilitation of cortical inputs (Herrling, 1984; Wilson, 1986). The IPSPs appear to have an important role in that they limit the firing of striatal neurons by reducing (e.g., shunting) the amplitude and duration of the EPSP after cortical stimulation.

The nature of the IPSP was studied in great detail by using brain slice preparations (Misgeld et al., 1982; Lighthall and Kitai, 1983; Kita et al., 1985a,b). Rat brain slices approximately 500 μm thick, including the striatum, were placed in a chamber in which chemical and physical environments were maintained to allow the slices to live for several hours. In brain slice preparations, stimulation of the striatum or the cortex evokes a depolarization in the nearby striatal neurons (Misgeld et al., 1982; Lighthall and Kitai, 1983; Kita et al., 1985a,b; Kawaguchi et al., 1989). Fig. 12*A* shows responses of striatal neurons to local (i.e., about 1 mm from recording site in the striatum) electrical stimulation. Local stimulation evoked short latency depolarizing potentials without subsequent hyperpolarizing components. The initial part of the depolarization was considered EPSP, because it could trigger spikes on its crest. While the responses to local stimulation did not include hyperpolarizing components, the following experiment indicated IPSPs existed in the later part of the depolarizing responses. When neurons were depolarized by intracellular current injections local stimulation appeared to

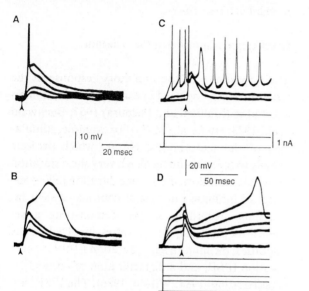

Fig. 12. Effects of intracellular injection of a Na-channel blocker QX-314 on local stimulation-induced postsynaptic responses in the striatal neuron in a brain slice preparation. A. Superimposed records of depolarizing postsynaptic potentials to local stimulation at four different intensities before QX-314 injection. Stronger stimulations trigger fast spike potentials (spikes are truncated). Arrowheads in this and subsequent figures indicate the onset of local stimulation. B. Superimposed records of responses to local stimulation given at the same stimulus intensity as in A after injection of QX-314. Only a slow spike potential is triggered from the large depolarizing postsynaptic response. C. Responses to local stimulation were examined at the resting condition and two levels of the depolarizing condition before the QX-314 injection. At higher intensity of depolarizing current, small hyperpolarizations can be seen following the initial depolarizing response. Spike potentials are generated from the initial depolarizing response in each case. D. Local stimulation-induced responses are examined at the resting and four levels of depolarized condition after QX-314 injections. Hyperpolarizing synaptic potentials succeeding depolarizing postsynaptic potentials become more apparent at higher levels of depolarization. Calibration in A also applies in B, calibration in C also applies in D (modified from Kita et al., 1985a).

evoke a depolarization followed by a hyperpolarization while repetitive spiking obscured these responses (Fig. 12C). Injection of QX-314, an Na-channel blocker, abolished generation of Na spikes but preserved depolarizing responses to local stimulation. Large depolarizing potentials in this condition evoked slow Ca spikes (Fig. 12B). Intracellular injection of a depolarizing current of approximately 0.6 nA clearly disclosed hyperpolarizing responses following the EPSPs after local stimulation (Fig. 12D). The latency of the IPSPs was estimated from responses of the neurons which were depolarized to the level of the reversal potential of the EPSPs by current injections (Fig. 13A). The mean latency of the hyperpolarizations was 3.8 msec ($n = 30$) which was slightly longer than that of EPSPs (i.e., 2.6 msec). The duration of the IPSPs was less than 130 msec. The IPSPs can follow relatively short interstimulus intervals and summate (Fig. 13B). The duration and the amplitude of the IPSPs can be enhanced by addition of pentobarbital into the perfusing medium (Fig. 14). The reversal potential of the IPSPs estimated under these conditions was approx-

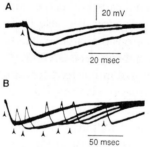

Fig. 13. Properties of the local stimulation-induced hyperpolarizing synaptic potentials of a striatal neuron injected with a Na-channel blocker QX-314 in order to eliminate spike generation. A. Hyperpolarizing synaptic potentials induced by local stimulation at three different intensities recorded from a neuron continuously depolarized by a current with the intensity of 2.9 nA. The duration of hyperpolarizing synaptic potentials is altered by stimulus intensity, but the latency appears to be constant. B. Effects of double stimulation on hyperpolarizing synaptic potentials. This neuron was continuously depolarized with 2.9 nA current application. The duration of test hyperpolarizing synaptic potentials are larger than that of the control at interstimulus intervals of less than 60 msec. Voltage calibration in A also applies in B (Kita et al., 1985a).

imately −60 mV. Misgeld and his associates have used the K-channel blocker 4-aminopyridine in order to enhance the release of the neurotransmitter. Local stimulation of that slice preparation evoked relatively long lasting GABAergic IPSPs with a reversal potential of about −60 mV (Misgeld et al., 1982).

The neurotransmitter and the ionic channels involved in the generation of the IPSP were also studied using brain slice preparations. The experiments include intracellular Cl⁻ injection, substitution of extracellular NaCl with Na-acetate, and extracellular application of picrotoxin or bicuculline. Intracellular Cl⁻ injection was accomplished by using a recording microelectrode containing 3M KCl through which Cl⁻ was applied with a passage of hyperpolarizing current pulses (duration of 500 msec, intensity of 0.5−2.0 nA, injection period of more than 5 min). Injection of Cl⁻ increased the amplitude of EPSPs without a noticeable change in the resting membrane potentials (Fig. 15). Fig. 15*A*

shows control responses to local stimulation at two different intensities recorded immediately after a neuron was penetrated. Weak, local stimulation induces an EPSP from which an action potential is triggered and a strong local stimulation produces a larger EPSP from which two action potentials are triggered (Fig. 15*A* and *C*). After Cl⁻ is injected intracellularly there is an increase in the amplitude and duration of EPSPs induced by local stimulation (Fig. 15 *B* and *D*). Under these conditions, multiple action potentials are triggered on the falling phase of EPSPs (Fig. 15*B* and *D*). A similar increase in the amplitude of EPSPs is observed after NaCl in the Ringer's solution was replaced with sodium acetate.

Increase in the Cl⁻ permeability during EPSPs was also tested by application of picrotoxin or bi-

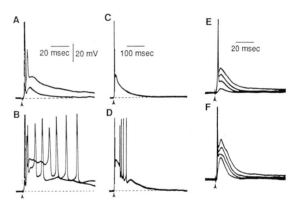

Fig. 15. Effects of intracellular Cl⁻ injection and bicuculline application on depolarizing postsynaptic potentials induced in striatal neurons by local stimulation in slice preparations. *A* and *C*. Responses evoked by local stimulation immediately after penetration of the neuron by a KCl filled electrode. In *A*, two levels of stimulation intensity were used. *B* and *D*. Responses evoked by the same stimulus intensities used in *A* and *C*, respectively, after Cl⁻ injection. Cl⁻ was injected into the neuron by 500 msec hyperpolarizing current pulses at 1 Hz for 10 min. A clear increase in the amplitude of the depolarizing postsynaptic potentials and firing of several action potentials can be noted. *E*. Control recordings of responses evoked by local stimulation given at four different intensities. *F*. Responses evoked by the same stimulus intensity in *E* after application of bicuculline methiodide (100 μM for 30 min). A clear increase in the amplitude of depolarizing postsynaptic potentials can be seen. Voltage calibration in *A* also applies to *B*−*F*. Time calibration in *A*, *C* and *E* also applies to *B*, *D* and *F*, respectively (modified from Kita et al., 1985a).

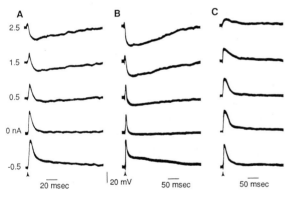

Fig. 14. Effects of pentobarbital and bicuculline on the local stimulation-induced responses of the striatum in a slice preparation. *A*. Control records of local stimulation-induced responses to hyper- and depolarizing current injection. This neuron has been injected with a Na-channel blocker QX-314 in order to eliminate spike generation. *B*. Similar analysis taken after addition of pentobarbital (100 μM) to the Ringer's solution. The amplitude and duration of hyperpolarization responses were augmented. *C*. The addition (200 μM) of bicuculline to the medium containing pentobarbital abolishes the hyperpolarizing responses. Remaining are initial depolarizing responses with a duration of about 50 msec followed by a long-lasting small depolarization. Voltage calibration in *A* also applies in *B* and *C* (Kita et al., 1985b).

cuculline in the Ringer's solution. In these experiments, recordings were made with K-methylsulfate filled electrodes. Fig. 15E shows the response to local stimulation at four different intensities recorded in normal Ringer's solution. Recordings obtained after application of bicuculline methiodide (100 μM, 30 min) in the Ringer's solution are seen in Fig. 15F). The amplitude of EPSPs is much larger than before bicuculline application.

The above mentioned studies all indicate that the IPSPs are GABAergic and involve an increase in Cl^- conductance. It is also evident that electrical stimulation of the cortex or the striatum evokes an EPSP and an IPSP which overlap each other with a small latency difference. Because the reversal potential of the GABAergic IPSP is about -60 mV and the resting membrane potential of the striatal neurons often is more negative than that, the IPSP is seen as a depolarizing potential. The IPSP inhibits firing activity of striatal neurons by decreasing the amplitude and the duration of EPSPs (i.e., shunting the excitatory postsynaptic currents).

The neurons responsible for the IPSPs

As mentioned before, the spiny neurons in the neostriatum possess an extensive network of axon collaterals within the striatum (Preston et al., 1980; Wilson and Groves, 1980). Because most spiny projection neurons contain GABA (Oertel and Mugnaini, 1984; Kita and Kitai, 1988), it is reasonable to assume that the collaterals of striatal projection neurons are responsible for the GABAergic responses evoked by cortical or local stimulation. This possibility was examined by antidromic stimulation of spiny neurons both in slice preparations and in anesthetized rats (Wilson et al., 1989). No IPSP comparable to those associated with excitatory orthodromic stimulation could be observed under these conditions. These studies indicate that collaterals of spiny neurons are not the main source of the IPSP. In order to further determine whether orthodromic inhibition could occur in the absence of action potentials in the spiny neurons, cortical stimulation was applied in a slice with intact connections from a portion of the cerebral cortex. Conditions were arranged in order to evoke small subthreshold synaptic potentials in spiny neurons, but not to cause any spiny neurons to fire action potentials. Under these circumstances, we were still able to detect the IPSP. Thus, excitation of spiny projection neurons is neither necessary nor sufficient for the observation of the GABAergic IPSP in spiny cells. The GABAergic IPSP must therefore arise from the action of another GABAergic cell type in the striatum. The alternative origin for the IPSPs are GABAergic interneurons of the striatum. The anatomical features of these aforementioned interneurons are in accordance with this possibility. It has been recorded both in vivo and in brain slice preparations that a small number of striatal neurons responded with a burst of high-frequency spikes after stimulation of the sensorimotor cortex. Fig. 16 shows intracellular recordings of a neuron in the striatum of an anesthetized rat. Stimulation of the sensorimotor cortex induced short-latency depolarizations of which the amplitude and the duration increased with an increase in stimulus intensity (Fig. 16A). Fig. 16B shows responses to cortical stimulation obtained during intracellular current injections to alter the membrane potential of the neurons. The amplitude of the responses either decreased or increased when the neuron was depolarized or hyperpolarized, respectively, indicating that the depolarizations are EPSPs. The EPSPs with a large amplitude triggered multiple sharp spikes on their crest. Fig. 16C shows responses to paired stimulation. The EPSPs to two short interval stimulations showed temporal summation. When two stimulations with a longer interval (e.g., about 120 msec in Fig. 16C) were given, the amplitude of the EPSP to the second stimulation was larger than the initial one, indicating that the mechanism of short-term potentiation exists in the pathway. The neuron was intracellularly injected with horseradish peroxidase after acquisition of physiological data. This neuron had a relatively large soma (i.e., about 20×30 μm) and six primary dendrites. The primary dendrites are short and divided into secondary and tertiary dendrites which often are free of spines, long and varicosed (Fig. 16D). The morphology is very similar to

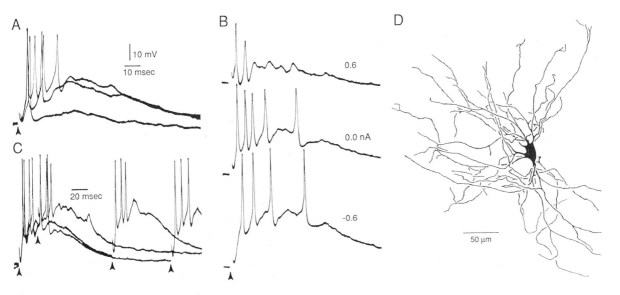

Fig. 16. *A – C*. Strong excitatory responses recorded in a striatal aspiny neuron (that was revealed by intracellular staining) after stimulation of the sensorimotor cortex of an anesthetized rat. *A*. Responses to three different intensity stimulations. Large and long-duration depolarizations evoked by strong stimulation triggered a burst of spikes. *B*. The amplitude of the long-duration depolarization was increased by a hyperpolarizing current and was decreased by a depolarizing current injection (current intensity indicated at right of each trace). The observation indicates the depolarizing potentials are EPSPs. *C*. Responses to paired stimulation with various intervals. The EPSPs to short-interval stimulation summate. It can also be seen in the responses to about 100 msec interval stimulation that the responses to second stimulation are larger than those of initial stimulation. *D*. Drawing of the neuron from which recordings *A – C* were obtained. The neuron was injected with horseradish peroxidase and was reconstructed from 50 μm serial brain sections under a light microscope equipped with a drawing tube.

those of PV-immunoreactive neurons of the striatum.

Summary and concluding remarks

The neostriatum contains many GABAergic neurons and GABAergic synaptic terminals which are considered to be major elements in regulating the neuronal activities of the striatum. Fig. 17 is the summary diagram indicating the existence of a feedforward and a feed-back GABAergic inhibitory circuit within the striatum which can be activated by cortical inputs. Anatomical and physiological studies indicate that GABAergic interneurons play a major role in the regulation of the firing activity of the spiny projection neurons through their feedforward connection. It is also suggested by anatomical studies that cholinergic and dopaminergic inputs affect the activity of GABAergic interneurons.

There are still many issues to be resolved before understanding the functional importance of GABAergic circuits in the striatum. It is not known if the GABAergic interneurons and spiny projection neurons receive the same inputs from the cortex. We also do not know the extent of axonal arborization of individual GABAergic interneurons. Another important and obvious question is the nature of the functional roles of intra-striatal collaterals of spiny projections neurons. It is tempting to speculate that the release of GABA from the collateral axons of spiny neurons is tightly regulated by some neuroactive substance(s) in the striatum. We were able to evoke IPSPs in the spiny projection neurons by antidromically activating their descending axons when 4-aminopyridine (i.e., a K-channel blocker which increases neurotransmitter release from terminals by increasing the duration of the action potential) was infused into the recording site (Kita,

70

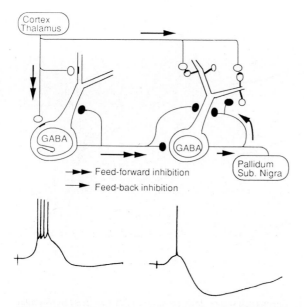

Fig. 17. Schematic drawing of striatal GABAergic circuits. Inputs from the sensorimotor cortex and/or thalamus can produce a strong excitation (a burst discharge) in GABAergic interneurons (which are characterized by having an invaginated nucleus). The cortical or thalamic inputs, on the other hand, will generate a short-duration excitation with one or two spikes followed by an inhibitory period in the spiny neurons projecting to the globus pallidus and substantia nigra. The projection neurons have uninvaginated nuclei and spiny dendrites. Axons of GABAergic interneurons form synapses on some dendrites of spiny projection neurons, thus forming a feed-forward inhibitory circuit in the striatum. The local axon collaterals of spiny projection neurons form synapses on neighboring spiny projections neurons and form feed-back inhibitory circuits.

unpublushed data). Although some basic knowledge of striatal GABAergic circuits has been obtained, obviously more studies are required to understand how these circuits contribute in processing the information which arrives from the cortex and other parts of the brain and how they form their inputs.

Acknowledgements

This work was supported by the USPHS grants NS-25783 and NS-26473, and the Human Frontier Science Program grant.

References

Afsharpour, S., Kita, H., Penny, G.R. and Kitai, S.T. (1985) Glutamic acid decarboxylase, substance P and Leu-enkephalin-immunoreactive neurons in the rat neostriatum that project to the globus pallidus and substantia nigra. Soc. Neurosci. Abstr., 11: 110.

Araki, M., McGeer, P.L. and McGeer, E.G. (1985) Striatonigral and pallidonigral pathways studied by a combination of retrograde horseradish peroxidase tracing and a pharmaco-histochemical method for γ-aminobutyric acid transaminase. Brain Res., 331: 17 – 24.

Bolam, J.P., Powell, J.F., Totterdell, S. and Smith, A.D. (1981) The proportion of neurons in the rat neostriatum that project to the substantia nigra demonstrated using horseradish peroxidase conjugated with wheatgerm agglutinin. Brain Res., 220: 339 – 343.

Bolam, J.P., Clarke, D.J., Smith, A.D. and Somogyi, P. (1983) A type of aspiny neuron in the rat neostriatum accumulates [3H] γ-aminobutyric acid: combination of Golgi-staining, autoradiography, and electron microscopy. J. Comp. Neurol., 213: 121 – 134.

Bolam, J.P., Powell, J.F., Wu, J.-Y. and Smith, A.D. (1985) Glutamate decarboxylase-immunoreactive structures in the rat neostriatum: a correlated light and electron microscopic study including a combination of Golgi-impregnation with immunocytochemistry. J. Comp. Neurol., 237: 1 – 20.

Buchwald, N.A., Price, D.D., Vernon, L. and Hull, C.D. (1973) Caudate intracellular response to thalamic and cortical inputs. Exp. Neurol., 38: 311 – 323.

Celio, M.R. (1986) Parvalbumin in most gamma-aminobutyric acid-containing neurons of the rat cerebral cortex. Science, 231: 995 – 997.

Celio, M.R. and Heizmann, C.W. (1981) Calcium-binding protein parvalbumin as a neuronal marker. Nature, 293: 300 – 302.

Cepeda, C., Walsh, J.P., Hull, C.D., Howard, S.G., Buchwald, N.A. and Levine, M.S. (1989) Dye-coupling in the neostriatum of the rat: 1. Modulation by dopamine-depleting lesions. Synapse, 4: 229 – 237.

Chang, H.T. and Kita, H. (1992) Interneurons in the rat striatum: relationships between parvalbumin neurons and cholinergic neurons. Brain Res., 574: 307 – 311.

Chang, H.T. and Kitai, S.T. (1982) Large neostriatal neurons in the rat: an electron microscopic study of gold-toned Golgi-stained cells. Brain Res. Bull., 8: 631 – 643.

Chang, H.T., Wilson, C.J. and Kitai, S.T. (1981) Single neostriatal efferent axons in the globus pallidus: a light and electron microscopic study. Science, 213: 915 – 918.

Chang, H.T., Wilson, C.J. and Kitai, S.T. (1982) A Golgi study of rat neostriatal neurons: light microscopic analysis. J. Comp. Neurol., 208: 107 – 126.

Cowan, R.L., Wilson, C.J., Emson, P.C. and Heizmann, C.W. (1990) Parvalbumin-containing GABAergic interneurons in the rat neostriatum. *J. Comp. Neurol.,* 302: 198 – 205.

DiFiglia, M. and Aronin, N. (1982) Ulstrastructural features of immunoreactive somatostatin neurons in the rat caudate nucleus. *J. Neurosci.,* 2: 1267 – 1274.

DiFiglia, M., Pasik, P. and Pasik, T. (1976) A Golgi study of neuronal types in the neostriatum of monkeys. *Brain Res.,* 114: 245 – 256.

Donoghue, J.P. and Herkenham, M. (1986) Neostriatal projections from individual cortical fields conform to histochemically distinct striatal compartments in the rat. *Brain Res.,* 365: 397 – 403.

Fox, C.A., Andrade, A.N., Schwyn, R.C. and Rafols, J.A. (1971a) The spiny neurons in the primate striatum: a Golgi and electron microscopic study. *J. Hirnforsch.,* 13: 181 – 201.

Fox, C.A., Andrade, A.N., Schwyn, R.C. and Rafols, J.A. (1971b) The aspiny neurons and the glia in the primate striatum: a Golgi and electron microscopic study. *J. Hirnforsch.,* 13: 341 – 362.

Gerfen, C.R., Baimbride, K.G. and Miller, J.J. (1985) The neostriatal mosaic: compartmental distribution of calcium-binding protein and parvalbumin in the basal ganglia of the rat and monkey. *Proc. Natl. Acad. Sci. U.S.A.,* 82: 8780 – 8784.

Graveland, G.A., Williams, R.S. and DiFiglia, M.A. (1985) A Golgi study of the human neostriatum: neurons and afferent fibers. *J. Comp. Neurol.,* 234: 317 – 333.

Graybiel, A.M., Ragsdale, C.W., Yoneoka, E.S. and Elde, R.P. (1981) An immunohistochemical study of enkephalins and other neuropeptides in the striatum of the cat with evidence that opiate peptides are arranged to form mosaic patterns in register with the striosomal compartments visible by acetylcholinesterase staining. *Neuroscience,* 6: 377 – 397.

Heizmann, C.W. (1984) Parvalbumin and intracellular calcium-binding protein: distribution, properties and possible roles in mammamian cells. *Experientia,* 40: 910 – 921.

Herrling, P.L. (1984) Evidence for GABA as the transmitter for early cortically evoked inhibition of cat caudate neurons. *Exp. Brain Res.,* 55: 528 – 534.

Hull, C.D., Bernardi, G., Price, D.D. and Buchwald, N.A. (1973) Intracellular responses of caudate neurons to temporally and spatially combined stimuli. *Exp. Neurol.,* 38: 324 – 336.

Kawaguchi, Y., Wilson, C.J. and Emson, P.C. (1989) Intracellular recording of identified neostriatal patch and matrix spiny cells in a slice preparation preserving cortical inputs. *J. Neurophysiol.,* 62: 1052 – 1068.

Kemp, J.M. and Powell, T.P.S. (1971) The structure of caudate nucleus of the cat: light and electron microscopy. *Phil. Trans. R. Soc. Lond. (Biol.),* 262: 383 – 401.

Kita, H. and Kitai, S.T. (1988) Glutamate decarboxylase immunoreactive neurons in rat neostriatum: their morphological types and populations. *Brain Res.,* 447: 346 – 352.

Kita, H., Kita, T. and Kitai, S.T. (1985b) Active membrane properties of rat neostriatal neurons in an in vitro slice preparation. *Exp. Brain Res.,* 60: 54 – 62.

Kita, H., Kosaka, T. and Heizmann, C.W. (1990) Parvalbumin-immunoreactive neurons in the rat neostriatum: a light and electron microscopic study. *Brain Res.,* 536: 1 – 15.

Kita, H., Chang, H.T. and Fujimoto, K. (1991) Pallidoneostriatal projections of the rat. *Soc. Neurosci. Abstr.,* 17: 453.

Kita, T., Kita, H. and Kitai, S.T. (1985a) Local stimulation induced GABAergic response in rat striatal slice preparations: intracellular recordings on QX-314 injected neurons. *Brain Res.,* 360: 304 – 310.

Kitai, S.T., Preston, R.J., Bishop, G.A. and Kocsis, J.D. (1979) Striatal projection neurons: morphological and electrophysiological studies. In: L.J. Poirier, T.L. Sourkes and P.J. Bedard (Eds.), *Advances in Neurology, Vol. 24,* Raven Press, New York, pp. 45 – 51.

Kosaka, T., Kosaka, K., Tateishi, K., Hamaoka, Y., Yanaihara, N., Wu, J.-Y. and Hama, K. (1985) GABAergic neurons containing CCK-8-like and/or VIP-like immunoreactivities in the rat hippocampus and dentate gyrus. *J. Comp. Neurol.,* 239: 420 – 430.

Kosaka, T., Katsumaru, H., Hama, K., Wu, J.-Y. and Heizmann, C. (1987) GABAergic neurons containing the Ca^{2+}-binding protein parvalbumin in the rat hippocampus and dentate gyrus. *Brain Res.,* 419: 119 – 130.

Kubota, Y., Inagaki, S. and Wu, Jang-Yen (1987) Dopaminergic axons directly make synapses with GABAergic neurons in the rat neostriatum. *Brain Res.,* 416: 147 – 156.

Lighthall, J.W. and Kitai, S.T. (1983) A short duration GABAergic inhibition in identified neostriatal medium spiny neurons: in vitro slice study. *Brain Res. Bull.,* 11: 103 – 110.

Malliani, A. and Purpura, D.P. (1967) Intracellular studies of the corpus striatum: II. Patterns of synaptic activities in lenticular and entopeduncular. *Brain Res.,* 6: 341 – 354.

Misgeld, U., Wagner, A. and Ohno, T. (1982) Depolarizing IPSPs and depolarization by GABA of rat neostriatum cells in vitro. *Exp. Brain Res.,* 45: 108 – 114.

Oertel, W.H. and Mugnaini, E. (1984) Immunocytochemical studies of GABAergic neurons in rat basal ganglia and their relations to other neuronal systems. *Neurosci. Lett.,* 47: 233 – 238.

Oertel, W.H., Schmechel, D.E., Mugnaini, E., Tappax, M.L. and Kopin, I.J. (1981) Immunocytochemical localization of glutamate decarboxylase in cerebellum with a new antiserum. *Neuroscience,* 6: 2715 – 2735.

Oertel, W.H., Riethmuller, G., Mugnaini, E., Schmechel, D.E., Weindl, A., Gramsch, C. and Herz, A. (1983) Opioid peptide-like immunoreactivity localized in GABAergic neurons of rat neostriatum and central amygdaloid nucleus. *Life Sci.* (Suppl. I), 33: 73 – 76.

Pasik, P., Pasik, T., Holstein, G.R. and Hamori, J. (1988) GABAergic elements in the neuronal circuits of the monkey neostriatum: a light and electron microscopic immunocytochemical study. *J. Comp. Neurol.,* 187: 261 – 284.

Penny, G.R., Afsharpour, S. and Kitai, S.T. (1986) The glutamate decarboxylase-, leucine enkephalin-, methionine enkephalin- and substance P-immunoreactive neurons in the neostriatum of the rat and cat: evidence for partial population overlap. *Neuroscience,* 17: 1011 – 1045.

Precht, W. and Yoshida, M. (1971) Blockage of caudate-evoked inhibition of neurons in the substantia nigra by picrotoxin. *Brain Res.,* 32: 229 – 233.

Preston, R.J., Bishop, G.A. and Kitai, S.T. (1980) Medium spiny neuron projection from the rat striatum: an intracellular peroxidase study. *Exp. Brain Res.,* 183: 253 – 263.

Ribak, C.E., Vaughn, J.E. and Roberts, E. (1979) The GABA neurons and their axon terminals in rat corpus striatum as demonstrated by GAD immunocytochemistry. *J. Comp. Neurol.,* 187: 261 – 284.

Somogyi, P., Bolam, J.P. and Smith, A.D. (1981) Monosynaptic cortical input and local axon collaterals of identified striatonigral neurons. A light and electron microscopic study using the Golgi-peroxidase transport-degeneration procedure. *J. Comp. Neurol.,* 195: 567 – 584.

Staines, W.A. and Hincke, M.T.C. (1991) Substantial alterations in neurochemical and metabolic indices in select basal ganglia neurons follow lesions of globus pallidus neurons in rats. *Soc. Neurosci. Abstr.,* 17(1): 456.

Wilson, C.J. (1986) Postsynaptic potentials evoked in spiny neostriatal projection neurons by stimulation of ipsilateral and contralateral neocortex. *Brain Res.,* 367: 201 – 213.

Wilson, C.J. and Groves, P.M. (1980) Fine structure and synaptic connections of the common spiny neuron of the rat neostriatum: a study employing intracellular injection of horseradish peroxidase. *J. Comp. Neurol.,* 194: 599 – 615.

Wilson, C.J., Kita, H. and Kawaguchi, Y. (1989) GABAergic interneurons, rather than spiny cell axon collaterals, are responsible for the IPSP responses to afferent stimulation in neostriatal spiny neurons. *Soc. Neurosci. Abstr.,* 15(1): 907.

Yoshida, M. and Precht, W. (1971) Monosynaptic inhibition of neurons of substantia nigra by caudatonigral fibers. *Brain Res.,* 32: 225 – 228.

G.W. Arbuthnott and P.C. Emson (Eds.)
Progress in Brain Research, Vol. 99
© 1993 Elsevier Science Publishers B.V. All rights reserved.

CHAPTER 5

Convergence of synaptic terminals from the striatum and the globus pallidus onto single neurones in the substantia nigra and the entopeduncular nucleus

J.P. Bolam, Y, Smith[1], C.A. Ingham[2], M. von Krosigk and A.D. Smith

MRC Anatomical Neuropharmacology Unit, Oxford, U.K.; [1] Laboratoire de Neurobiologie, Hôpital de l'Enfant Jésus, Québec, Canada; and [2] Department of Preclinical Veterinary Sciences, Royal School of Veterinary Studies, University of Edinburgh, Edinburgh, U.K.

Introduction

It is now well established that the output signal of the basal ganglia under resting conditions is one of inhibition. The targets of the basal ganglia in the thalamus, superior colliculus or brain-stem are inhibited and, immediately preceding movement, these regions are released from inhibition, in other words disinhibited (see Chevalier and Deniau, 1990, for review). This disinhibition is brought about by a two neurone chain, both components of which use GABA as a transmitter. The first component of this chain is a GABAergic projection that arises in the striatum and terminates in the output stations of the basal ganglia, i.e., the substantia nigra pars reticulata (SNr) and the entopeduncular nucleus (internal pallidal segment in primates). Secondly, the projections from the output stations to the target regions of the basal ganglia (thalamus, superior colliculus and brain-stem) are also GABAergic. The former pathways, under resting conditions are electrically quiescent, whereas the latter pathways are tonically active. Therefore at rest, the neurones in the target regions of the basal ganglia are tonically inhibited by the SNr and entopeduncular nucleus. Immediately preceding movement, the striatum is activated, the striatofugal neurones fire and the tonically active neurones in the SNr or entopeduncular

nucleus are inhibited. The consequence of inhibiting these cells is that the neurones in the target regions are released from the tonic inhibition, i.e., they are disinhibited. The disinhibition is then associated with movement. This scheme of disinhibition of the target neurones of the basal ganglia has been most elegantly demonstrated in relation to eye movement in the behaving monkey (Hikosaka and Wurtz, 1985a,b; Hikosaka and Sakamoto, 1986). The anatomy at the synaptic level for this phenomenon is well established, since striatal output neurones make direct synaptic contact with the projection neurones of the SNr (Somogyi et al., 1979; Williams and Faull, 1985; Smith and Bolam, 1991) and the entopeduncular nucleus (M. Bevan, personal communication).

As well as the inhibition of neurones in the output stations of the basal ganglia which leads to the disinhibition of neurones in the target regions, activation of the striatum can also lead to the opposite effects (Chevalier and Deniau, 1990). i.e., *increased* firing of neurones in the output stations and therefore *increased* inhibition of neurones in the target regions. Two microcircuits, that are not mutually exclusive, have been proposed to underlie this phenomenon. First, an indirect pathway from the striatum to the output stations that includes the globus pallidus and the subthalamic nucleus; activation of this pathway leads to increased firing of neurones in the subthalamic nucleus. The neurones of the subthalamic nucleus are excitatory (Nakanishi et al., 1987; Smith and Parent, 1988; Albin et al., 1989; Robledo and Féger, 1990), and their increased firing leads to increased firing of neurones in the output stations and therefore greater inhibition of neurones in the target regions. This pathway is currently under investigation from both functional and anatomical angles and is not dealt with in this paper. The second possibility is a pathway from the striatum to the globus pallidus (external globus pallidus in primates) which then projects directly to the output stations. It is well known that in addition to the SNr and entopeduncular nucleus, the globus pallidus is the other major target of the striatum, which in turn projects to the SNr and entopeduncular nucleus. Since pallidal neurones are GABAergic and tonically active (Ribak et al., 1979; Oertel et al., 1984; Ottersen and Storm-Mathisen, 1984; Beckstead and Kersey, 1985; Mugnaini and Oertel, 1985; Smith et al., 1987; Schmued et al., 1989) activation of striatal neurones that project to the globus pallidus will lead to inhibition of pallidal neurones which in turn will lead to a disinhibition (in effect excitation) of neurones in the output stations and therefore a greater inhibition of neurones in the target regions of the basal ganglia. One of the objects of this paper is to describe experiments that test anatomically whether this pathway can account for the excitation of the output neurones of the substantia nigra following striatal stimulation. Thus, the following questions were addressed. (1) Do pallidal output neurones make synaptic contact with the projection neurones of the substantia nigra? (2) Is the synaptology of this input suitable to produce an inhibition of the SNr neurones? (3) Do the terminals of pallidal neurones in the SNr contain GABA?

As mentioned above the internal segment of the globus pallidus (GPi) or entopeduncular nucleus is also one of the major output stations of the basal ganglia. The neurones in this region receive a major input from the striatum, which presumably accounts for the inhibition of GPi neurones that oc-curs during behaviour or following striatal stimulation (DeLong and Georgopoulos, 1981; Tremblay and Filion, 1989; Mink and Thach, 1991). As with the SNr, neurones in the entopeduncular nucleus or GPi may also respond during behaviour or following striatal stimulation with excitation (Tremblay and Filion, 1989; Mink and Thach, 1991). The second objective of the present paper is therefore to review experiments that were designed to test whether input from the globus pallidus to the entopeduncular nucleus could account for the increased firing of neurones in this region. The questions that were addressed are similar to those that were applied to the SNr. (1) Do pallidal output neurones make synaptic contact with neurones in the entopeduncular nucleus? (2) Is the synaptology of this input suitable to produce an inhibition of the neurones in the entopeduncular nucleus? (3) Do the terminals of pallidal neurones in the entopeduncular nucleus contain GABA?

On the basis of electrophysiological analyses it appears that a significant proportion of neurones in the SNr or entopeduncular nucleus respond to striatal stimulation with both excitation and inhibition following activation of the striatum (Tremblay and Filion, 1989; Chevalier and Deniau, 1990; Mink and Thach, 1991). If our proposals are correct about the projections from the globus pallidus to the SNr and entopeduncular nucleus (see above), then these physiological responses may be explained by a *convergence* of striatal and pallidal inputs onto individual neurones in the output stations. The third objective of this paper is therefore to review those experiments designed to test anatomically whether single neurones in the SNr and entopeduncular nucleus receive convergent synaptic input from the striatum and the globus pallidus.

The data presented in this manuscript have been described in detail in several communications dealing with the output of the globus pallidus to the substantia nigra and the entopeduncular nucleus in the rat (Smith and Bolam, 1989, 1990, 1991; Bolam and Smith, 1992; von Krosigk et al., 1992).

TABLE I

Number of animals, localization of injection sites and areas examined for the double anterograde labelling experiments

Number of animals	Injection sites			Areas examined
	PHA-L	Biocytin	WGA-HRP	
13	Globus pallidus (dorsal)	Striatum (dorsomedial)	Superior colliculus	EPN, SNr GP
26	Globus pallidus (ventro-lateral)	Striatum (ventrolateral)	Parvicellular reticular formation	SNr (lateral), GP

Materials and methods

Double anterograde labelling combined with the retrograde transport of lectin-conjugated horseradish peroxidase (WGA-HRP)

Thirty-nine Wistar rats (180 – 250 g) were used in this series of experiments (Table I). They were anaesthetised with a mixture of chloral hydrate and pentobarbital (Equithesin) before receiving iontophoretic injections of *Phaseolus vulgaris* leucoagglutinin (PHA-L) in the globus pallidus (Gerfen and Sawchenko, 1984), pressure injections of biocytin in the striatum and pressure injections of WGA-HRP in the superior colliculus or the parvicellular reticular formation (PcRT) (see Table I). The stereotaxic coordinates were chosen according to the atlases of König and Klippel (1963) and Paxinos and Watson (1986). Once the appropriate survival periods (7 – 10 days for PHA-L; 48 h for biocytin and WGA-HRP) terminated, the animals were deeply anaesthetised with an overdose of Equithesin and perfuse-fixed with a mixture of paraformaldehyde and glutaraldehyde. The brains were then dissected from the skull, sectioned into 60 μm-thick transverse sections on a vibrating microtome and processed for the localisation of the different tracers according to the protocols that have been described in detail in previous communications (Smith and Bolam, 1991;

Bolam and Smith, 1992; von Krosigk et al., 1992) (see Fig. 1). Briefly, the sections were first processed for the localisation of the retrogradely transported WGA-HRP by means of the tetramethylbenzidine (TMB) method (Olucha et al., 1985). They were then prepared for the histochemical localisation of biocytin followed by the immunohistochemical reaction to reveal PHA-L. In the sections prepared for light microscopy, biocytin was localised using diaminobenzidine (DAB) whereas PHA-L was revealed using nickel-enhanced DAB (Ni-DAB) (Wouterlood et al., 1987). In the sections prepared for electron microscopy, the WGA-HRP and biocytin were localised as in the light microscopic sections but PHA-L was revealed using benzidine dihydrochloride (BDHC) (Levey et al., 1986; see also Smith and Bolam, 1991, for more details). Once the different tracers were revealed, the sections prepared for light microscopy were mounted onto gelatin-coated slides and examined in the light microscope. The sections prepared for electron microscopy were post-fixed in osmium tetroxide, dehydrated in a graded series of alcohol and embedded in electron microscope resin on microscope slides (for more details, see Bolam and Ingham, 1990; Smith and Bolam, 1991).

Analysis of the material and post-embedding immunocytochemistry

The sections containing the injection sites were examined in the light microscope to determine the extent of the tracers in their respective targets. Sections containing the substantia nigra or the entopeduncular nucleus were analysed in the light microscope for the presence of retrogradely labelled neurones (nigrocollicular or nigroreticular) or non-retrogradely labelled neurones apposed by striatal (biocytin-labelled) and/or pallidal (PHA-L-labelled) terminals. Regions where the two sets of terminals converged onto single elements were drawn and photographed before being cut from the slides and stuck to the top of a resin block with cyanoacrylate glue. Serial ultrathin sections were cut with an ultramicrotome and collected on single-slot copper or nickel grids. They were then examined

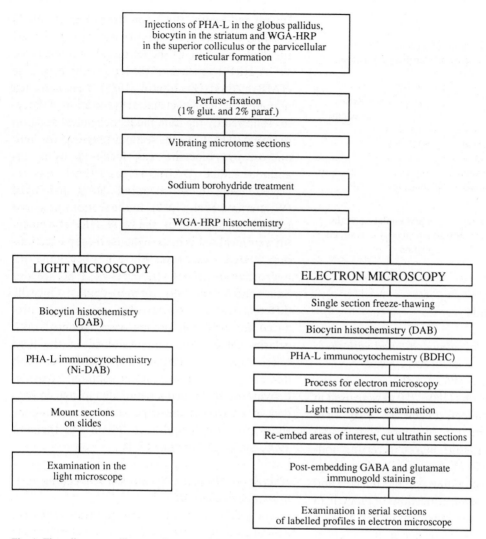

Fig. 1. Flow diagram to illustrate the steps of the experimental protocol for the double anterograde labelling method combined with the retrograde transport of WGA-HRP.

in the electron microscope for the presence of retrogradely and non-retrogradely labelled elements receiving convergent synaptic inputs from striatal (biocytin-labelled, DAB as chromogen) and pallidal (PHA-L-labelled, BDHC as chromogen) terminals. A series of ultrathin sections adjacent to those containing both sets of anterogradely labelled terminals were processed according to the post-embedding immunogold staining protocol using antisera raised against glutamate (Ottersen, 1987, 1989) or GABA (Hodgson et al., 1985; Somogyi and Hodgson, 1985; Somogyi et al., 1985), the details of which are described in previous communications (see Bolam and Ingham, 1990). In the electron microscope, the GABA- or glutamate-immunoreactive terminals were recognised by the presence of a high density of immunogold particles associated with them. An element was considered immunoreactive for GABA when the density of gold particles associated with it was at least five times higher than the density of gold particles overlying non-immunoreactive elements in the same tissue. For the glutamate immunostaining, a bouton was considered positive if it had a relatively high density of immunogold particles overlying it in at least two serial sections and the same bouton was GABA-negative in an adjacent section (see Fig. 4).

Results and discussion

Convergence of striatal and pallidal terminals onto single output neurones in the substantia nigra

Light microscopic observations   In the light microscope the two sets of anterogradely labelled terminals and the retrogradely labelled neurones were easily distinguished from each other and from the non-labelled elements by the colour and texture of the peroxidase reaction products associated with them. The biocytin-labelled striatal terminals contained the brown amorphous DAB reaction product whereas the PHA-L-labelled pallidal terminals contained the dark blue Ni-DAB reaction product. The retrogradely labelled nigrocollicular and nigroreticular cells were recognised by the presence of large blue granules of TMB reaction product that were randomly dispersed throughout the perikaryon and proximal dendrites (for more details see Smith and Bolam, 1991; von Krosigk et al., 1992).

Following WGA-HRP injections in the superior colliculus or the PcRT, numerous retrogradely labelled cells were found in the SNr. The nigrocollicular cells were distributed throughout the entire rostrocaudal and mediolateral extent of the SNr whereas the nigroreticular cells were confined to the caudal half of the dorsolateral SNr (von Krosigk and Smith, 1990; von Krosigk et al., 1992). This pattern of distribution of the two populations of nigrofugal neurones is in keeping with previous findings obtained in different species (see Parent, 1986).

The striatum has long been known as the major source of afferents to the substantia nigra in mammals (Parent, 1986, 1990). In keeping with this, biocytin injections in the rat striatum led to the anterograde labelling of rich plexuses of fibres and terminals in the SNr (Smith and Bolam, 1991; von Krosigk et al., 1992). These fibres arborized in the SNr

according to the topography of the striatonigral projection that has been described previously (Gerfen, 1985). Briefly, after injections of biocytin in the dorsomedial part of the striatum, the anterogradely labelled striatonigral terminals were found predominantly in the ventromedial two-thirds of the ipsilateral SNr (Smith and Bolam, 1991). On the other hand, injections of biocytin confined to the ventrolateral part of the caudal striatum led to profuse axonal labelling within the dorsolateral third of the SNr (von Krosigk et al., 1992).

The existence of a pallidonigral projection was first demonstrated by means of retrograde transport methods (see Smith and Bolam, 1991, for references). These findings are extended by the results of the anterograde labelling studies (Smith and Bolam, 1989, 1990). A large number of anterogradely labelled varicose fibres were visualised in the ipsilateral SNr (Smith and Bolam, 1991). The PHA-L-immunoreactive pallidonigral fibres were distributed in the SNr according to a topography similar to that described for the striatonigral fibres. In contrast to the striatonigral terminals which were small and did not show any particular neuronal association, the pallidonigral varicosities were large and formed pericellular baskets around both retrogradely and non-retrogradely labelled neurones (see Smith and Bolam, 1989, 1990, 1991). In the areas of the SNr where the two fields of anterogradely labelled terminals and the retrogradely labelled cells overlapped, the perikaryon and the proximal dendrites of single nigrocollicular and nigroreticular cells were found to be apposed by both PHA-L-positive terminals (pallidal) and biocytin-labelled terminals (striatal) (Smith and Bolam, 1991; von Krosigk et al., 1992). On occasions it was evident that single pallidal fibres gave rise to numerous varicosities that were apposed to the same retrogradely labelled perikaryon.

Electron microscopic observations   In the sections prepared for electron microscopy, the biocytin-labelled striatal and the PHA-L-immunoreactive pallidal terminals were differentiated from one another on the basis of the texture of the peroxidase

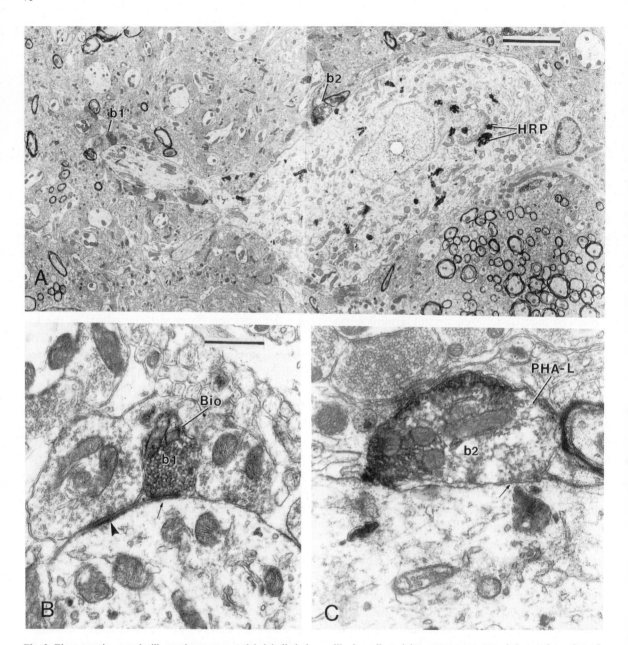

Fig. 2. Electron micrographs illustrating a retrogradely labelled nigrocollicular cell receiving convergent synaptic inputs from the striatum and the globus pallidus. *A*. Low power view of a SNr neurone that has been retrogradely labelled with WGA-HRP after injection
in the superior colliculus. This cell is contacted by two anterogradely labelled boutons (b1 and b2) which are shown at higher magnification in *B* and *C*. The bouton b1 (*B*) has been anterogradely labelled with biocytin (Bio) after injection in the dorsomedial striatum. It
contains the amorphous DAB reaction product and is in symmetric synaptic contact (arrow in *B*) with the proximal dendrite of the retrogradely labelled cell. An unlabelled bouton that forms an asymmetrical synaptic contact with the nigrocollicular cell is indicated by an
arrowhead in *B*. The bouton b2 (*C*) was labelled following the injection of PHA-L in the globus pallidus. It contains the crystalline
BDHC reaction product and is in symmetric synaptic contact (arrow in *C*) with the perikaryon of the retrogradely labelled neurone.
Scale markers: 5μm in *A* and 0.5 μm in *B* (valid for *C*).,

reaction product associated with them. The striatal terminals contained the amorphous DAB reaction product whereas the pallidal terminals contained the crystalline BDHC reaction product. The two sets of anterogradely labelled terminals were easily distinguished from the retrogradely labelled nigrocollicular and nigroreticular neurones that contained granules of TMB reaction product (Fig. 2).

In keeping with previous ultrastructural studies, the biocytin-labelled terminals that were visualised in the substantia nigra displayed typical ultrastructural features of striatonigral terminals that have been described previously (Grofová and Rinvik, 1970; Rinvik and Grofová, 1970; Somogyi et al., 1981; Williams and Faull, 1985; Nitsch and Riesenberg, 1988), i.e., they were small, poor in mitochondria and packed with round or oval synaptic vesicles (Fig. 2). They formed symmetric synapses predominantly with distal dendrites and much less frequently with the proximal dendritic shafts and perikarya of SNr neurones (Table II). In many cases the dendritic shafts and the perikarya that were postsynaptic to the striatal terminals contained granules of TMB reaction product indicating that they were projection neurones innervating the superior colliculus or the PcRT (Fig. 2). In the areas where the anterogradely labelled terminals and the retrogradely labelled cells overlapped, the nigrocollicular and the nigroreticular cells were frequently contacted by striatal terminals (Smith and Bolam, 1991; von Krosigk et al., 1992). Post-embedding immunostaining revealed that the anterogradely labelled striatonigral terminals display GABA immunoreactivity (von Krosigk et al., 1992). These data are in keeping with previous anatomical (Ribak et al., 1980; Fisher et al., 1986; Nitsch and Riesenberg, 1988) and physiological (see Chevalier and Deniau, 1990, for a review) results suggesting that the striatonigral pathway uses GABA as a transmitter. This part of the study suggests therefore: (1) the existence of a GABAergic striato-nigro-collicular pathway (see also Williams and Faull, 1985) which is presumably involved in the control of visual saccades (see Chevalier and Deniau, 1990); and (2) the existence of a GABAergic striato-nigro-reticular pathway which is likely to be involved in the control of orofacial movements (for references, see von Krosigk and Smith, 1990; von Krosigk et al., 1992).

In contrast to the striatal boutons, the PHA-L-immunoreactive pallidal terminals that were visualised in the substantia nigra were large, contained many mitochondria and formed symmetric synapses predominantly with the perikarya and proximal dendrites of nigral neurones (Table II). In addition, a few PHA-L-positive terminals were found to form asymmetric synapses with dendritic shafts. In those cases where the PHA-L-labelled pallidal terminals occurred in areas of the substantia nigra that contained retrogradely labelled nigrocollicular and nigroreticular neurones, frequent symmetric synapses were observed between the pallidal terminals and the nigrofugal cells (Fig. 2; Smith and Bolam, 1990; von Krosigk et al., 1992). Furthermore, numerous unlabelled perikarya and dendritic shafts found in the vicinity of the retrogradely labelled neurones were also contacted by anterogradely labelled pallidal terminals. The PHA-L-immunoreactive pallidal terminals were found to display GABA immunoreactivity (Smith and Bolam, 1989, 1990; von Krosigk et al., 1992).

Regions of the SNr containing the biocytin-labelled striatal terminals, the PHA-L-immunoreactive pallidal terminals and the retrogradely labelled nigrocollicular or nigroreticular neurones were selected to test the possibility of convergence of striatal and pallidal terminals onto single nigrofugal cells. The electron microscopic examination of twelve nigrocollicular and twelve nigroreticular cells that were found to be apposed by both sets of anterogradely labelled terminals in the light microscope, revealed that both of these populations of SNr output neurones receive *convergent* synaptic inputs from the striatum and the globus pallidus (Fig.2; Smith and Bolam, 1991; von Krosigk et al., 1992). In many cases, the PHA-L-labelled pallidal terminals formed symmetric synapses with the perikaryon of the retrogradely labelled cells whereas the biocytin-labelled striatal terminals were found to form symmetric synapses on the dendritic shaft of the same neurone (Fig. 2).

In the surrounding neuropil, numerous non-retrogradely labelled perikarya and dendritic shafts also received synapses from both sets of anterogradely labelled terminals (Smith and Bolam, 1991). Although the nigrothalamic and nigrotegmental cells have not been examined for the possibility of receiving convergent synaptic inputs from the striatum and the globus pallidus, the fact that separate series of experiments have demonstrated the existence of striatal (Somogyi et al., 1979; Tokuno et al., 1989) and pallidal (Smith and Bolam, 1990) terminals forming synapses with these neurones suggests that the convergence of striatal and pallidal inputs onto single nigrofugal cells is a general phenomenon in the rat SNr. The functional significance of the convergent synaptic inputs from the striatum and the globus pallidus onto single nigral output neurones is briefly discussed in the last section of this report (see also Smith and Bolam, 1991; von Krosigk et al., 1992).

Striatal input to PHA-L-labelled cells in the globus pallidus

The existence of a striatopallidal connection has been demonstrated by means of various anatomical and physiological approaches (for reviews, see Parent, 1986, 1990). Although it is not fully elucidated, this projection appears to be organised according to a dorsoventral, rostrocaudal and mediolateral topography (Parent, 1986). In the present experiment, large plexuses of anterogradely labelled striatal terminals were found in the globus pallidus following biocytin injections in the striatum (Smith and Bolam, 1991; von Krosigk et al., 1992). In the light microscope, these plexuses appeared as numerous thin axons and small varicosities that were often apposed to the surface of pallidal neurones. In sections of the globus pallidus that contained the anterogradely labelled terminals and had been processed to reveal the injected PHA-L, the striatopallidal terminals were often apposed to the pallidal neurones that had taken up the PHA-L (Smith and Bolam, 1991; von Krosigk et al., 1992). In the electron microscope, the biocytin-labelled terminals that were visualised in the globus pallidus displayed features similar to those of the striatopallidal terminals that have been described in other studies (Kemp, 1970; Chang et al., 1981; Chung and Hassler, 1984) and similar to the striatal terminals in the substantia nigra. In those regions where the plexuses of anterogradely labelled terminals overlapped with the PHA-L injection site, frequent symmetric synapses between small biocytin-labelled striatal terminals and PHA-L-immunoreactive cells were found in the globus pallidus (see Smith and Bolam, 1991). Since the PHA-L-immunoreactive cells in the globus pallidus were labelled by the local uptake of the tracer, those neurones are part of the population that gave rise to the PHA-L-immunoreactive terminals in the substantia nigra (see Gerfen and Sawchenko, 1984). If this is the case, our findings are in keeping with previous data suggesting the existence of a direct striato-pallido-nigral pathway in rodent (Totterdell et al., 1984). An important question that still remains to be answered in order to better understand the way by which the striatum and the globus pallidus interact to control the activity of nigrofugal neurones, is whether it is the striatal and pallidal neurones that are synaptically connected in the globus pallidus that send convergent synaptic inputs onto single nigrofugal cells. Future experiments combining the intracellular injection of single striatal and pallidal neurones with electron microscopy should help to elucidate this problem.

Convergence of striatal and pallidal terminals onto neurones in the entopeduncular nucleus

Light microscopic observations In keeping with the known efferent connections of the striatum (see Parent, 1986, 1990), the injections of biocytin in this structure led to a multitude of anterogradely labelled fibres (DAB-labelled) that traversed the entopeduncular nucleus. Close to these fibre tracts the neuropil of the entopeduncular nucleus contained plexuses of anterogradely labelled varicose fibres and isolated boutons. In addition to the biocytin-labelled striatal fibres the entopeduncular nucleus also contained many PHA-L-labelled fibres and boutons derived from the globus pallidus. As in the

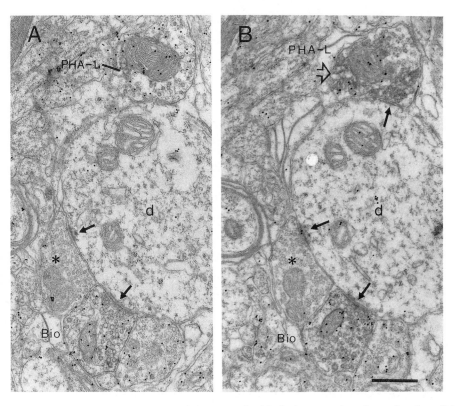

Fig. 3. Illustration of *convergent* synaptic input to a dendrite in the entopeduncular nucleus from GABA-containing terminals derived from the striatum and the globus pallidus. Electron micrographs of serial sections of a dendrite in the entopeduncular nucleus. The dendrite receives synaptic input from three boutons. One of the boutons (PHA-L) is anterogradely labelled with PHA-L from the globus pallidus (benzidine reaction product indicated by open arrow in *B*), forms symmetrical synaptic contact (arrow) and is GABA-immunoreactive as indicated by the high density of immunogold particles overlying it. A second bouton (Bio) is anterogradely labelled with biocytin from the striatum, forms symmetrical synaptic contact with the dendrite and is also GABA-positive. The third bouton (asterisk) is not anterogradely labelled, is GABA-negative and forms an asymmetrical synaptic contact with the dendrite. Scale: 0.5μm.

substantia nigra, the density of the pallidal fibres was less, but the boutons and axonal varicosities were much larger than those of striatal origin (see above). The pallidal fibres and varicosities, unlike those from the striatum, were often seen in association with unlabelled neuronal perikarya and dendrites. Furthermore, single pallidal fibres often gave rise to multiple boutons that were associated with single neurones. In many of the sections there was an overlap between the areas of anterogradely labelled striatal fibres and anterogradely labelled pallidal fibres; these regions were examined in the electron microscope (see Bolam and Smith, 1992, for more details).

Electron microscopic observations Consistent with other ultrastructural studies of anterogradely labelled striatal terminals in the globus pallidus and substantia nigra (Chang et al., 1981; Bolam and Smith, 1990; Smith and Bolam, 1991a; von Krosigk et al., 1991; see also above) the biocytin-labelled striatal boutons (DAB-containing) in the entopeduncular nucleus were of medium size and were generally packed with synaptic vesicles (round or oval) and occasional mitochondria. Synaptic specialisations were of the symmetrical type. The majority of the striatal terminals made synaptic contact with dendritic shafts of fairly small diameter but they also made synaptic contact with larger diameter den-

TABLE II

The postsynaptic targets of striatal and pallidal terminals in the rat substantia nigra reticulata and entopeduncular nucleus

Source of terminals	Postsynaptic targets					
	Perikarya		Large dendrites		Small dendrites (> 1.5 μm)	
	SNr	EPN	SNr	EPN	SNr	EPN
Striatum	7 (3.3%)	19 (4.4%)	47 (20.3%)	26 (6.0%)	177 (76.6%)	389 (89.6%)
Globus pallidus	57 (54.3%)	22 (12.8%)	33 (31.4%)	40 (23.3%)	15 (14.3%)	110 (64%)

drites and perikarya (see Fig. 3, Table II). The ultrathin sections of the entopeduncular nucleus also contained many structures that were labelled with the BDHC reaction product and thus identified as containing the PHA-L that was deposited in the globus pallidus. The anterogradely labelled pallidal terminals (Fig. 3) had characteristics similar to those described for labelled terminals in the substantia nigra after injection of PHA-L in the globus pallidus (Smith and Bolam, 1989, 1990a,b, 1991a; see above). Thus, they were large and usually contained several mitochondria. The vesicles did not fill the whole of the bouton but were congregated close to the active zone and were of irregular shape and size. Synaptic specialisations were of the symmetrical type and the proportion in contact with large diameter dendrites (i.e., proximal) and perikarya was higher than that for striatal terminals (Table II).

It was apparent that neurones that received input from either the anterogradely labelled pallidal terminals or the anterogradely labelled striatal terminals also received input from additional, unlabelled terminals that had the morphological characteristics of striatal or pallidal terminals. Examination of regions of the entopeduncular nucleus in which there was an overlap of the anterogradely labelled striatal and pallidal terminals revealed that these two sets of boutons converge onto single neurones in the entopeduncular nucleus. Convergent synaptic inputs from the globus pallidus and the striatum occurred both on perikarya and dendrites of neurones

in the entopeduncular nucleus. Post-embedding GABA immunostaining of the ultrathin sections revealed that the terminals from both the striatum and the globus pallidus display GABA immunoreactivity (Fig. 3) (Bolam and Smith, 1992).

Thus, in agreement with others (Shu and Peterson, 1988; Staines, 1988; Hazrati et al., 1990; Kincaid et al., 1991), our results demonstrate that the entopeduncular nucleus (or GPi in primates) receives a direct input from the globus pallidus. Furthermore our results show that individual neurones in the entopeduncular nucleus receive *convergent* synaptic inputs from the globus pallidus and the striatum. Finally they demonstrate that both the striatal and pallidal terminals that form synapses with neurones in the entopeduncular nucleus display GABA immunoreactivity and therefore probably use GABA as a transmitter.

A second type of terminal labelled with PHA-L in the entopeduncular nucleus

In addition to the terminals that were anterogradely labelled from the globus pallidus and formed symmetrical synaptic specialisations (see above), a second, but smaller population of terminals in the entopeduncular nucleus were labelled with the PHA-L (Bolam and Smith, 1992) that was deposited in the globus pallidus. These terminals were different in that they were smaller and formed asymmetrical synapses that were often associated with sub-junctional dense bodies (Fig. 4). This was

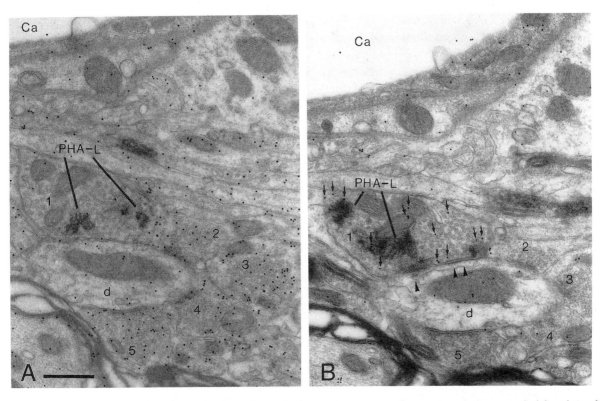

Fig. 4. GABA and glutamate immunostaining of a PHA-L-labelled terminal that forms an asymmetrical synapse. Serial sections of a PHA-L-labelled terminal (number 1) in the entopeduncular nucleus that were immunostained to reveal GABA (*A*) or glutamate (*B*). In *A* the PHA-L-labelled terminal apposed to a dendrite (d) is GABA-negative (eight gold particles per square micron) whereas four other boutons (numbers 2 – 5) have a high density of immunogold particles overlying them relative to unstained structures (40 – 80 gold particles per square micron), thus identifying them as GABA-positive. In *B* the PHA-L-labelled terminals forms an asymmetrical synaptic contact with the dendrite (arrowheads) that is associated with a subjunctional dense body (left arrowhead). In this micrograph the PHA-L bouton has a high density of immunogold particles overlying it relative to unstained structures (small arrows) (12 gold particles per square micron), indicating that it is glutamate-positive, whereas boutons 2, 3 and 5 are clearly glutamate-negative (0 – 5 gold particles per square micron). (Ca indicates a capillary in both micrographs). A total of eleven PHA-L-labelled terminals were identified that formed asymmetrical synaptic contact and displayed glutamate immunoreactivity but were GABA-negative. Scale bar in *A* indicates 0.5 μm.

also the case in the substantia nigra; a small population of terminals anterogradely labelled with PHA-L that was injected in the globus pallidus formed asymmetrical synapses (see Smith and Bolam, 1991; von Krosigk et al., 1992). Several lines of evidence lead us to the conclusion that these terminals are not derived from the globus pallidus but from the subthalamic nucleus. Thus, it is possible that the PHA-L was taken up by subthalamic terminals in the globus pallidus, retrogradely transported to the subthalamic nucleus and then anterogradely transported via collaterals, to the entopeduncular nucleus

and/or the SNr (see Bolam and Smith, 1992, for more details). Evidence in favour of this possibility comes from the fact that in the present material neurones that had retrogradely transported the PHA-L from the globus pallidus were present in the subthalamic nucleus (Smith et al., 1990). Further evidence comes from the immunostaining experiments. Although the post-embedding immunostaining for GABA clearly labelled biocytin-positive terminals from the striatum and the type of PHA-L-positive terminals that formed symmetrical synapses, those PHA-L-labelled terminals that formed asymmetrical synapses were GABA-negative. In contrast to this, post-embedding immunostaining for glutamate stained the PHA-L-labelled terminals that formed asymmetrical synapses but not those that formed symmetrical synapses nor the striatal terminals (Fig. 4). Since it is known that all neurones in the globus pallidus are GABAergic (for references, see Bolam and Smith, 1992), this observation implies that glutamate-positive terminals are not derived from the globus pallidus. Furthermore, since neurones of the subthalamic nucleus are glutamatergic (Nakanishi et al., 1987; Smith and Parent, 1988; Albin et al., 1989; Robledo and Féger, 1990) the immunostaining results are in favour of them being derived from the subthalamic nucleus. Finally, the morphology of the glutamate-positive PHA-L-labelled terminals visualised in the entopeduncular nucleus is similar to that of subthalamic terminals, identified by anterograde labelling, in the substantia nigra and globus pallidus of the rat (Kita and Kitai, 1987). The implication of these findings is that neurones in the entopeduncular nucleus and identified output neurones in the SNr receive direct synaptic input from the subthalamic nucleus and that there is a *convergence* of inputs from the striatum, the globus pallidus and the subthalamic nucleus onto individual neurones in the output stations of the basal ganglia (see Smith and Bolam, 1992).

Correlation with physiological observations

The present findings provide an anatomical basis for the physiological observations described in the Introduction, i.e., that the output neurones of the basal ganglia can respond to activation of the striatum with a decreased firing rate, an increased firing rate or a combination of the two. As mentioned above and discussed in detail by Chevalier and Deniau (1990), the decrease of activity of neurones in the output stations of the basal ganglia following striatal stimulation is mediated by a direct GABA-containing input from the striatum to the entopeduncular nucleus and the substantia nigra. The results summarised in the present paper provide a possible explanation for the increased firing. It is known that neurones in the globus pallidus are toni-

cally active, thus the projection from these neurones to the entopeduncular nucleus and SNr will provide a tonic inhibition of the neurones in these regions. Since one of the major outputs of the striatum is the globus pallidus (see above), then activation of the striatum will lead to an inhibition of neurones in the globus pallidus and therefore a release from inhibition of neurones in the SNr and the entopeduncular nucleus. Thus, activation of the striato-pallido-nigral/entopeduncular pathway will lead to increased firing of neurones in the substantia nigra or the entopeduncular nucleus. The consequence of this in the target regions of the basal ganglia is *increased* inhibition which may be associated with decreased movement (Alexander and Crutcher, 1990; DeLong, 1990). Given that the direct pathway from the striatum to the output stations leads to the inhibition of neurones in the SNr/entopeduncular nucleus complex, then the fact that these cells receive convergent input from both the striatum and the globus pallidus offers an anatomical substrate for the physiological observations of both inhibition and excitation of individual basal ganglia output neurones that occurs following striatal stimulation (Chevalier and Deniau, 1990).

In summary, our results demonstrate neuronal circuits at the synaptic level (Fig. 5) that can account for the excitation of neurones in the entopeduncular nucleus and SNr following stimulation of the striatum. The anatomical organisation of the basal ganglia thus supports two pathways by which striatal outflow can cause an excitation of basal ganglia output neurones and therefore a greater inhibition of their target neurones in the thalamus, superior colliculus and brain-stem. The relative functional significance of these two pathways remains to be established.

Concluding remarks

The anatomical findings and the implications arising from the data presented in this paper can be summarised as follows.

(1) They demonstrate the existence of a direct synaptic input from the globus pallidus to the neurones in the output stations of the basal ganglia.

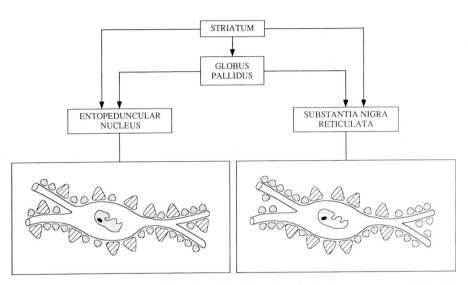

Fig. 5. Schematic diagram summarising the major findings described in the present report. The striatum and the globus pallidus send convergent synaptic inputs onto single neurones in the entopeduncular nucleus and the substantia nigra. The pattern of innervation of the entopeduncular and SNr cells is illustrated at the bottom of the diagram. The large pallidal boutons are illustrated by the hatched terminals whereas the small striatal boutons are depicted by the dotted terminals. In the SNr the pallidal boutons are confined to the proximal part of the neurone whereas in the entopeduncular nucleus they are more evenly distributed. In both structures the striatal boutons terminate preferentially on the distal dendrites.

(2) They show that this input is strategically placed in the proximal regions of the neurones, such that it is ideally situated to have a prominent control or influence over the output of the basal ganglia.

(3) They suggest that this control or influence is likely to be inhibitory since the terminals derived from the globus pallidus contain, and presumably use, GABA as a transmitter.

(4) They demonstrate that the neurones in the output stations of the basal ganglia (some of which have been identified as projection neurones) receive convergent synaptic input from the striatum and the globus pallidus.

(5) It is likely that administration of PHA-L to the globus pallidus results in the labelling of subthalamic terminals in the SNr and entopeduncular nucleus. These terminals display glutamate immunoreactivity and converge onto the same neurones that receive input from the striatum and the globus pallidus.

(6) The pallidal input to neurones in the substantia nigra at least, and the convergence with striatal terminals, appears to be a general phenomenon as

deposits of tracers in different regions of the striatum and globus pallidus gave rise to similar patterns of synaptic innervation in the substantia nigra.

(7) The present results emphasise the similarities at the synaptic level, between the two major output structures of the basal ganglia, the substantia nigra pars reticulata and the entopeduncular nucleus.

(8) The findings summarised herein also provide an antomical substrate for the physiological observations demonstrating that the output neurones of the basal ganglia respond to striatal stimulation by a decrease, increase or a combination of decrease/increase of their firing rates.

Acknowledgements

The authors would like to thank Sharon Gordon-Smith, Paul Jays, Frank Kennedy, Sue Hood and Frieda Christie for their technical assistance. Particular thanks are due to Caroline Francis for the quantification of the immunogold staining. We would also like to thank Dr. Peter Somogyi who kindly provided the antiserum to GABA and Drs. O.P. Ottersen and J. Storm-Mathisen for the antiserum to glutamate. During the period of the work described in this paper Y. Smith and M. von Krosigk were supported by the Medical Research Council of Canada.

References

Albin, R.L., Young, A.B. and Penney, J.B. (1989) The functional anatomy of basal ganglia disorders. *Trends Neurosci.*, 12: 366 – 375.

Alexander, G.E. and Crutcher, M.D. (1990) Functional architecture of basal ganglia circuits: neural substrates for parallel processing. *Trends Neurosci.*, 13: 266 – 271.

Beckstead, R.M. and Kersey, K.S. (1985) Immunohistochemical demonstration of differential substance P-, met-enkephalin-, and glutamic acid decarboxylase-containing cell body and axon distributions in the corpus striatum of the cat. *J. Comp. Neurol.*, 232: 481 – 498.

Bolam, J.P. and Ingham, C.A. (1990) Combined morphological and histochemical techniques for the study of neuronal microcircuits. In: A. Björklund, T. Hökfelt, F.G. Wouterlood and A.N. van den Pol (Eds.), *Handbook of Chemical Neuroanatomy, Analysis of Neuronal Microcircuits and Synaptic Interactions, Vol. 8,* Elsevier, Amsterdam, pp. 125 – 198.

Bolam, J.P. and Smith, Y. (1992) The striatum and the globus pallidus send convergent synaptic inputs onto single cells in the entopeduncular nucleus of the rat: a double anterograde labelling study combined with post-embedding immunocytochemistry for GABA. *J. Comp. Neurol.*, 321: 456 – 476.

Chang, H.T., Wilson, C.J. and Kitai, S.T. (1981) Single neostriatal efferent axons in the globus pallidus: a light and electron microscopic study. *Science,* 213: 915 – 918.

Chevalier, G. and Deniau, J.M. (1990) Disinhibition as a basic process in the expression of striatal functions. *Trends Neurosci.*, 13: 277 – 280.

Chung, Y.W. and Hassler, R.G. (1984) Types of synapses in the pallidum and their differential degeneration following lesions of pallidal afferents in squirrel monkey *(Saimiri sciureus)*. In: R.G. Hassler and J.F. Christ (Eds.), *Advances in Neurology, Vol. 40,* Raven Press, New York, pp. 21 – 27.

DeLong, M.R. (1990) Primate models of movement disorders of basal ganglia origin. *Trends Neurosci.*, 13: 281 – 285.

DeLong, M.R. and Georgopoulos, A.P. (1981) Motor functions of the basal ganglia. In: V.B. Brooks (Ed.), *APA Handbook of Physiology, The Nervous System, Vol. 2,* Am. Physiol. Soc., Bethesda, MD, pp. 1017 – 1061.

Fisher, R.S., Buchwald, N.A., Hull, C.D. and Levine, M.S. (1986) The GABAergic striatonigral neurons of the cat: demonstration by double peroxidase labelling. *Brain Res.*, 398: 148 – 156.

Gerfen, C.R. (1985) The neostriatal mosaic: I. Compartmental organization of projection from the striatum to the substantia nigra in the rat. *J. Comp. Neurol.*, 236: 454 – 476.

Gerfen, C.R. and Sawchenko, P.E. (1984) An anterograde neuroanatomical tracing method that shows the detailed morphology of neurons, their axons and terminals: immunohistochemical localization of an axonally transported plant lectin, *Phaseolus vulgaris* leucoagglutinin (PHA-L). *Brain Res.*, 290: 219 – 238.

Grofová, I. and Rinvik, E. (1970) An experimental electron microscopic study on the striatonigral projection in the cat. *Exp. Brain Res.*, 11: 249 – 262.

Hazrati, L-N., Parent, A., Mitchell, S. and Haber, S.N. (1990) Evidence for interconnections between the two segments of the globus pallidus in primates: a PHA-L anterograde tracing study. *Brain Res.*, 533: 171 – 175.

Hikosaka, O. and Sakamoto, M. (1986) Cell activity in monkey caudate nucleus preceding saccadic eye movement. *Exp. Brain Res.*, 63: 659 – 662.

Hikosaka, O. and Wurtz, R.H. (1985a) Modification of saccadic eye movements by GABA-related substances. I. Effect of muscimol and bicuculline in monkey superior colliculus. *J. Neurophysiol.*, 53: 266 – 291.

Hikosaka, O. and Wurtz, R.H. (1985b) Modification of saccadic eye movements by GABA-related substances. II. Effects of muscimol in monkey substantia nigra pars reticulata. *J. Neurophysiol.*, 53: 292 – 308.

Hodgson, A.J., Penke, B., Erdei, A., Chubb, I.W. and Somogyi, P. (1985) Antisera to γ-aminobutyric acid. I. Production and characterization using a new model system. *J. Histochem. Cytochem.*, 33: 229 – 239.

Kemp, J.M. (1970) The termination of striato-pallidal and striato-nigral fibres. *Brain Res.*, 17: 125 – 128.

Kincaid, A.E., Penney, J.B., Young, A.B. and Newman, S.W. (1991) Evidence for a projection from the globus pallidus to the entopeduncular nucleus in the rat. *Neurosci. Lett.*, 128: 121 – 125.

Kita, H. and Kitai, S.T. (1987) Efferent projections of the subthalamic nucleus in the rat: light and electron microscopic analysis with the PHA-L method. *J. Comp. Neurol.*, 260: 435 – 452.

König, J.F.R. and Klippel, R.A. (1963) *The Rat Brain. A Stereotaxic Atlas of the Forebrain and Lower Parts of the Brainstem,* Williams and Wilkins, Baltimore, MD.

Levey, A.I., Bolam, J.P., Rye, D.B., Hallanger, A.E., Demuth, R.M., Mesulam, M.-M. and Wainer, B.H. (1986) A light and electron microscopic procedure for sequential double antigen localization using diaminobenzidine and benzidine dihydrochloride. *J. Histochem. Cytochem.*, 34: 1449 – 1457.

Mink, J.W. and Thach, W.T. (1991) Basal ganglia motor control. I. Nonexclusive relation of pallidal discharge to five movement modes. *J. Neurophysiol.*, 65: 273 – 300.

Mugnaini, E. and Oertel, W.H. (1985) An atlas of the distribution of GABAergic neurons and terminals in the rat CNS as revealed by GAD immunocytochemistry. In: A. Björklund and T. Hökfelt (Eds.), *GABA and Neuropeptides in the CNS, Handbook of Chemical Neuroanatomy, Vol. 4, Part I,* Elsevier, Amsterdam, pp. 436 – 595.

Nakanishi, H., Kita, H. and Kitai, S.T. (1987) Intracellular study of rat substantia nigra pars reticulata neurons in an in vitro preparation: electrical properties and response characteristics to subthalamic stimulation. *Brain Res.,* 437: 45 – 55.

Nitsch, C. and Riesenberg, R. (1988) Immunocytochemical demonstration of GABAergic synaptic connections in rat substantia nigra after different lesions of the striatonigral projection. *Brain Res.,* 461: 127 – 142.

Oertel, W.H., Nitsch, C. and Mugnaini, E. (1984) Immunocytochemical demonstration of the GABA-ergic neurons in the rat globus pallidus and nucleus entopeduncularis and their GABA-ergic innervation. In: R.G. Hassler and J.F. Christ (Eds.), *Advances in Neurology, Vol. 40,* Raven Press, New York, pp. 91 – 98.

Olucha, F., Martinez-Garcia, F. and Lopez-Garcia, C. (1985) A new stabilizing agent for the tetramethyl benzidine (TMB) reaction product in the histochemical detection of horseradish peroxidase (HRP). *J. Neurosci. Methods,* 13: 131 – 138.

Ottersen, O.P. (1987) Postembedding light- and electron microscopic immunocytochemistry of amino acids: description of a new model system allowing identical conditions for specificity testing and tissue processing. *Exp. Brain Res.,* 69: 167 – 174.

Otterson, O.P. (1989) Quantitative electron microscopic immunocytochemistry of neuroactive amino acids. *Anat. Embryol.,* 180: 1 – 15.

Ottersen, O.P. and Storm-Mathisen, J. (1984) Glutamate- and GABA-containing neurons in the mouse and rat brain, as demonstrated with a new immunocytochemical technique. *J. Comp. Neurol.,* 229: 374 – 392.

Parent, A. (1986) *Comparative Neurobiology of the Basal Ganglia,* Wiley, New York, 335 pp.

Parent, A. (1990) Extrinsic connections of the basal ganglia. *Trends Neurosci.,* 13: 254 – 258.

Paxinos, G. and Watson, C. (1986) *The Rat Brain in Stereotaxic Coordinates,* Academic Press, London.

Penney, J.B., Young, A.B. and Newman, S.W. (1991) Evidence for a projection from the globus pallidus to the entopeduncular nucleus in the rat. *Neurosci Lett.,* 128: 121 – 125.

Ribak, C.E., Vaughn, J.E. and Roberts, E. (1979) The GABA neurons and their axon terminals in rat corpus striatum as demonstrated by GAD immunocytochemistry. *J. Comp. Neurol.,* 187: 261 – 284.

Ribak, C.E., Vaughn, J.E. and Roberts, E. (1980) GABAergic nerve terminals decrease in the substantia nigra following hemitransections of the striatonigral and pallidonigral pathways. *Brain Res.,* 192: 413 – 420.

Rinvik, E. and Grofová, I. (1970) Observations on the fine structure of the substantia nigra in the cat. *Exp. Brain Res.,* 11: 229 – 248.

Robledo, P. and Féger, J. (1990) Excitatory influence of rat subthalamic nucleus to substantia nigra pars reticulata and pallidal complex: electrophysiological data. *Brain Res.,* 518:

47 – 54.

Schmued, L., Phermsangngam, P., Lee, H., Thio, S., Chen, E., Truong, P., Colton, E. and Fallon, J. (1989) Collateralization and GAD immunoreactivity of descending pallidal efferents. *Brain Res.,* 487: 131 – 142.

Shu, S.Y. and Peterson, G.M. (1988) Anterograde and retrograde transport of *Phaseolus vulgaris* leucoagglutinin (PHA-L) from the globus pallidus to the striatum of the rat. *J. Neurosci. Methods,* 25: 175 – 180.

Smith, Y. and Bolam, J.P. (1989) Neurons of the substantia nigra reticulata receive a dense GABA-containing input from the globus pallidus in the rat. *Brain Res.,* 493: 160 – 167.

Smith, Y. and Bolam, J.P. (1990) The output neurones and the dopaminergic neurones of the substantia nigra receive a GABA-containing input from the globus pallidus in the rat. *J. Comp. Neurol.,* 296: 47 – 64.

Smith, Y. and Bolam, J.P. (1991) Convergence of synaptic inputs from the striatum and the globus pallidus onto identified nigrocollicular cells in the rat: a double anterograde labelling study. *Neuroscience,* 44: 45 – 73.

Smith, Y. and Parent, A. (1988) Neurons of the subthalamic nucleus in primates display glutamate but not GABA immunoreactivity. *Brain Res.,* 453: 353 – 356.

Smith, Y., Parent, A., Séguéla, P. and Descarries, L. (1987) Distribution of GABA-immunoreactive neurons in the basal ganglia of the squirrel monkey *(Saimiri sciureus). J. Comp. Neurol.,* 259: 50 – 64.

Smith, Y., Bolam, J.P. and von Krosigk, M. (1990) Topographical and synaptic organization of the GABA-containing pallidosubthalamic projection in the rat. *Eur. J. Neurosci.,* 2: 500 – 511.

Somogyi, P. and Hodgson, A.J. (1985) Antisera to γ-aminobutyric acid. III. Demonstration of GABA in Golgi-impregnated neurons and in conventional electron microscopic sections of cat striate cortex. *J. Histochem. Cytochem.,* 33: 249 – 257.

Somogyi, P., Hodgson, A.J. and Smith, A.D. (1979) An approach to tracing neuron networks in the cerebral cortex and basal ganglia. Combination of Golgi staining, retrograde transport of horseradish peroxidase and anterograde degeneration of synaptic boutons in the same material. *Neuroscience,* 4: 1805 – 1852.

Somogyi, P., Bolam, J.P., Totterdell, S. and Smith, A.D. (1981) Monosynaptic input from the nucleus accumbens-ventral striatum region to retrogradely labelled nigrostriatal neurones. *Brain Res.,* 217: 245 – 263.

Somogyi, P., Hodgson, A.J., Chubb, I.W., Penke, B. and Erdei, A. (1985) Antisera to γ-aminobutyric acid. II. Immunocytochemical application to the central nervous system. *J. Histochem. Cytochem.,* 33: 240 – 248.

Staines, W.A. (1988) PHA-L studies of the efferent connections of the rat globus pallidus. *Soc. Neurosci. Abstr.,* 16: 427.

Tokuno, H., Morizumi, T., Kudo, M., Kitao, Y. and Nakamura, Y. (1989) Monosynaptic striatal inputs to the nigrotegmental

88

neurons: an electron microscopic study in the cat. *Brain Res.,* 485: 189 – 192.

Totterdell, S., Bolam, J.P. and Smith, A.D. (1984) Characterization of pallidonigral neurons in the rat by a combination of Golgi impregnation and retrograde transport of horseradish peroxidase: their monosynaptic input from the neostriatum. *J. Neurocytol.,* 13: 593 – 616.

Tremblay, L. and Filion, M. (1989) Responses of pallidal neurons to striatal stimulation in intact waking monkeys. *Brain Res.,* 498: 1 – 16.

von Krosigk, M. and Smith, A.D. (1990) Descending projections from the substantia nigra and retrorubral field to the medullary and pontomedullary reticular formation. *Eur. J. Neurosci.,* 3: 260 – 273.

von Krosigk, M., Smith, Y., Bolam, J.P. and Smith, A.D. (1992) Synaptic organization of GABAergic inputs from the striatum and the globus pallidus onto neurons in the substantia nigra and retrorubral field which project to the medullary reticular formation. *Neuroscience,* 50: 531 – 549.

Williams, M.N. and Faull, R.L.M. (1985) The striatonigral projection and nigrotectal neurons in the rat. A correlated light and electron microscopic study demonstrating a monosynaptic striatal input to identified nigrotectal neurons using a combined degeneration and horseradish peroxidase procedure. *Neuroscience,* 14: 991 – 1010.

Wouterlood, F.G., Bol, J.G.J.M. and Steinbusch, H.W.M. (1987) Double-label immunocytochemistry: combination of anterograde neuroanatomical tracing with *Phaseolus vulgaris* leucoagglutinin and enzyme histochemistry of target neurons. *J. Histochem. Cytochem.,* 35: 817 – 823.

G.W. Arbuthnott and P.C. Emson (Eds.)
Progress in Brain Research, Vol. 99

CHAPTER 6

Striatal and subthalamic afferents to the primate pallidum: interactions between two opposite chemospecific neuronal systems

Lili-Naz Hazrati and André Parent

Centre de Recherche en Neurobiologie, Hôpital de l'Enfant-Jésus, Québec, Québec, Canada G1J 1Z4

Introduction

The pallidum or globus pallidus in primates plays a crucial role in the integration of neural information that flows through the cortico-basal ganglia-cortical loop (DeLong et al., 1985; Alexander et al., 1986; Alexander and Crutcher, 1990). This key structure of the basal ganglia is mostly composed of large projection neurons (Fox et al., 1974; DiFiglia et al., 1982; Park et al., 1982; Falls et al., 1983; Pasik and Pasik, 1983; Yelnik et al., 1984) that integrate information arising principally from the striatum (Papez, 1946; Szabo, 1962, 1967, 1970; Cowan and Powell, 1966; Nauta and Mehler, 1966; Johnson and Rosvold, 1971; Fox and Rafols, 1976; Chang et al., 1981; Percheron et al., 1984; Kawagushi et al., 1990; Hazrati and Parent, 1992a) and the subthalamic nucleus (Whittier and Mettler, 1949; Nauta and Cole, 1978; Carpenter et al., 1981a,b; Kita and Kitai, 1987; Smith et al., 1990; Hazrati and Parent, 1992a,b). These two major sources of pallidal afferents are the only basal ganglia components that receive massive and direct projections from the cerebral cortex (Kemp and Powell, 1970; Künzle, 1975, 1978; Künzle and Akert, 1977; Hartmann-von Monakow et al., 1978; Van Hoesen et al., 1981; Afsharpour, 1985; Selemon and Goldman-Rakic, 1985; Gerfen, 1989). The subthalamic nucleus is known to exert a glutamate-mediated excitation upon pallidal neurons (Kitai and Kita, 1987; Smith

and Parent, 1988), whereas the striatum inhibits pallidal cells through the use of γ-aminobutyric acid (GABA) as a neurotransmitter (McGeer et al., 1971; Jessel et al., 1978; Ribak et al., 1979; Oertel et al., 1984). Thus, a detailed knowledge of the anatomical framework for interactions between these two opposite chemospecific pallidal afferents is a prerequisite for a proper understanding of the functional organization of the basal ganglia.

Previous anterograde labeling studies have revealed that the subthalamic nucleus and the striatum project to both the internal (GPi) and the external (GPe) segment of the pallidum, where they arborize in the form of bands (Nauta and Cole, 1978; Parent et al., 1984; Parent, 1986; Smith et al., 1990). Furthermore, earlier light (Hazrati et al., 1987) and electron microscopic (Hassler and Chung, 1984) studies have provided indirect evidence for convergence of subthalamic and striatal afferents upon single pallidal neurons. The aim of the present paper is to summarize some of our most recent findings pertaining to the orginization of the striatopallidal and subthalamopallidal projections in the squirrel monkey. A special attention will be paid to recent data obtained with the double anterograde labeling method demonstrating that the excitatory glutamatergic subthalamopallidal projection and the inhibitory GABAergic striatopallidal projection converge upon single pallidal neurons in primates.

Methodological considerations

The results reported herein are derived from neuroanatomical studies undertaken in young adult squirrel monkeys (*Saimiri sciureus*) with the help of *Phaseolus vulgaris* leucoagglutinin (PHA-L) and biocytin (*N*-biotinyl-L-lysine $C_{16}H_{28}N_4O_4S$) as anterograde tracers. These two anterograde tracers are much more sensitive than tritiated amino acids or wheat germ agglutinin conjugated to horseradish peroxidase (WGA-HRP) to delineate neural pathways in the brain. Furthermore, they can provide a much more detailed view of axonal trajectories and terminal arborizations than other currently used anterograde tracers (Gerfen and Sawchenko, 1984; King et al., 1990).

In our studies, PHA-L and biocytin were used alone (Hazrati et al., 1987, 1990; Smith et al., 1990; Hazrati and Parent, 1991, 1992c), in combination with one another (Hazrati and Parent, 1992a,b), and in combination with various immunohistochemical procedures to reveal neurotransmitters or neurotransmitter-related enzymes (Hazrati and Parent, 1992c). In all cases the two tracers were iontophoretically injected with glass micropipettes that were stereotaxically driven following the coordinates of the atlas of Emmers and Akert (1963). The survival periods were 12 days after PHA-L injection and two days after biocytin delivery. The presence of the tracers was revealed according to the immunohistochemical protocol of Gerfen and Sawchenko (1984) for PHA-L and that of King et al. (1990) for biocytin, with some slight modifications for use in primates (Hazrati and Parent, 1992a – c). The chromogens employed for the visualization of the peroxidase end-product reaction were either diaminobenzidine (DAB), with or without nickel intensification (NiDAB, Hancock, 1982), or benzidine dihydrochloride (BDHC, Levey et al., 1986).

Furthermore, material prepared for the visualization of these two tracers is amenable to ultrastructural examination (Smith and Bolam, 1990; Hazrati and Parent, 1992c). In the present study, some pallidal sections were thus incubated without Triton-X-100, postfixed in osmium tetroxyde and dehydrated in a graded series of alcohols and propylene oxide. They were then embedded in Epon, mounted onto microscope slides, coverslipped and placed in an oven at 60°C for 72 h. After a careful analysis in the light microscope, areas of the GPi that contained woolly fibers composed of PHA-L- and/or biocytin-labeled axon varicosities were cut out from the slide and re-embedded in blocks. Serial ultrathin sections were cut from these blocks on a ultramicrotome and collected on copper grids. The sections were then stained with lead citrate and observed with a Phillips 300 electron microscope. The sections were scanned for PHA-L and/or biocytin-labeled terminal boutons that were in close contact with dendrites.

In most double anterograde labeling experiments designed for light microscopy, the chromogen combination was DAB and NiDAB. In such a case the two types of anterogradely labeled fibers and terminals could easily be distinguished by their color: brown for those displaying the DAB reaction product and dark-blue for those showing the NiDAB reaction product. However, in order to be able to differentiate between PHA-L and biocytin-labeled profiles at the electron microscopic level, PHA-L was revealed with BDHC and biocytin with DAB (see Levey et al., 1986; Smith and Bolam, 1990). In such a case DAB and BDHC could be distinguished mainly on the basis of texture and preferential location of the reaction products. The DAB reaction product was amorphous and rather uniformly distributed, whereas the BDHC reaction product appeared as granules or crystals randomly dispersed throughout the labeled profiles (Levey et al., 1986; Smith and Bolam, 1990).

Our studies have provided the first evidence that PHA-L and biocytin are as effective as anterograde tracers in primates as they are in rodents. Moreover, we found that biocytin labeling was as prominent as the PHA-L labeling with intensification (NiDAB). The permutation of the tracers during injection procedures led to anterograde labeling that was similar, with differences that appeared uniquely due to slight variations in the location and sizes of the injection sites. Moreover, the comparison of the quality of the anterograde labeling observed in sections immunostained for PHA-L or biocytin alone versus those treated for the visualization of both tracers revealed that there was no loss of sensitivity with the double-labeling technique. Likewise, the order in which the tracers were revealed, that is biocytin first and PHA-L second or vice-versa, did not affect the quality of the labeling.

The subthalamopallidal projection

The organization of the subthalamopallidal projection has been studied with PHA-L alone (Smith et al., 1990), or with PHA-L and biocytin in a double anterograde labeling study of the striatopallidal and subthalamopallidal projections (Hazrati and Parent, 1992a, see below). After injections of either PHA-L or biocytin into the subthalamic nucleus, numerous coarse and smooth fibers arise from the injection site. These fibers traverse the ventral part of the internal capsule via the subthalamic fasciculus and invade massively the caudomedial pole of the GPi. They ascended rostrally by coursing through the globus pallidus where they form at least two distinct vertical bands lying parallel and adjacent to the medullary laminae in each pallidal segment (Fig. 1E). The number and distribution of these bands vary according to the size and location of the injection sites, and a clear mediolateral and rostrocaudal topography in the organization of the subthalamopallidal projection can easily be demonstrated (Carpenter et al., 1981a,b; Parent and Smith, 1987).

These bands are composed of a multitude of axon collaterals that detach themselves at right angle from the main thick subthalamopallidal fibers that course caudorostrally throughout the pallidum. The axon collaterals entwine rather loosely the distal dendrites but closely surround the proximal dendrites and soma of pallidal neurons (Figs. 1F, 2). This pattern of organization does not significantly vary along the caudorostral extent of the bands. The fact that similar bands have been observed in the pallidum after injections of WGA-HRP or PHA-L in the putamen of the squirrel monkey (Parent et al.,

1984; Smith and Parent, 1986; Hazrati et al., 1987; see below) indicates that these band-like terminal fields are the most characteristic feature of the pattern of innervation of the pallidum in primates.

This typical band-like pattern most likely reflects the fact that the pallidal cell lying near the medullary laminae in both rodents and primates possess very long dendrites oriented in a radial fashion along the same narrow perpendicular plane (Park et al., 1982; Yelnik et al., 1984). The discoidal dendritic domains of these pallidal neurons are aligned parallel to the medullary laminae, so that their largest surface is facing the incoming striatal and subthalamic fibers (see Percheron et al., 1984). It is therefore likely that the bands of dense anterograde labeling that occur within the pallidum after injections of anterograde tracers in the subthalamic nucleus (and the striatum, see below) correspond to pallidal zones where such dendritic disks are particularly abundant. Interestingly, injections of HRP in the subthalamic nucleus of macaque monkeys have been shown to produce retrograde labeling of pallidal cells that are distributed in arrays parallel and adjacent to the medullary laminae (Carpenter, 1981b). This raises the possibility of a close reciprocal relationship between subthalamic and pallidal neurons. However, the fact that the pallidosubthalamic projections derived from the rostral and central divisions of the GPe terminate in distinct loci in the subthalamic nucleus (Carpenter et al., 1981a) argues against the existence of a strict point-to-point relationship between the subthalamic nucleus and the pallidum in primates.

Previous studies in the rat involving intracellular labeling of subthalamic nucleus neurons and PHA-L anterograde labeling of subthalamopallidal axons revealed that single subthalamic nucleus neurons innervate both the entopeduncular nucleus and the globus pallidus in rodents (Kita et al., 1983; Kita and Kitai, 1987). In contrast, HRP injections in either the GPe or the GPi of monkeys retrogradely label different cell populations in the subthalamic nucleus (Carpenter et al., 1981a). Furthermore, retrograde fluorescent double labeling studies of pallidal afferents in squirrel monkeys show that few subthalamic nucleus neurons innervate the two pallidal seg-

92

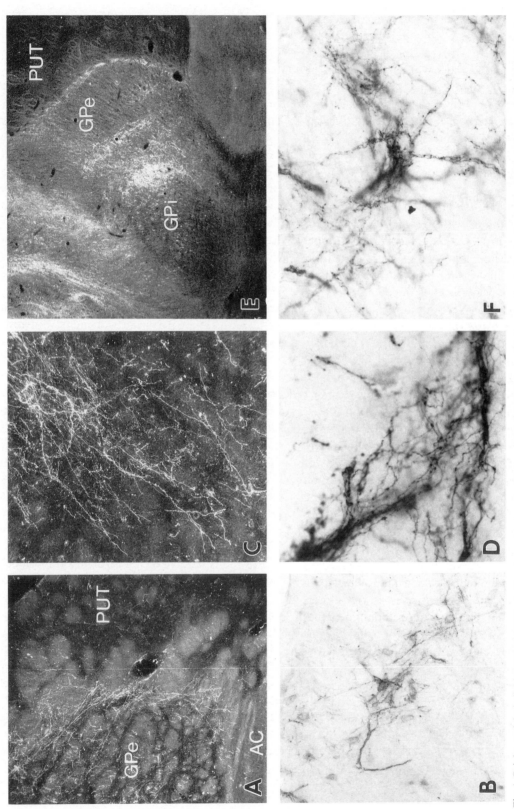

Fig. 1. Bright- and dark-field photomicrographs showing examples of anterogradely labeled fibers and their patterns of arborization in the pallidum as seen after PHA-L injections into the putamen (A – D) and into the subthalamic nucleus (E,F). A – D. Numerous, thin and straight varicose labeled fibers lying along the inner surface of the external medullary laminae (marginal band) are shown at low (A) and high (C) power magnification, whereas part of the dense network of woolly fibers encountered more caudally in the same band are illustrated in B and D. E,F. An overall view of pallidal bands formed by subthalamic afferents and a high power view of some of the labeled subthalamopallidal fibers forming one of these bands are shown in E and F, respectively. AC, anterior commissure; GPe, external segment of the globus pallidus; GPi, internal segment of the globus pallidus; PUT, putamen.

ments, the GPe and GPi receiving their innervation respectively from neurons in the lateral and medial portions of the subthalamic nucleus (Parent et al., 1989). However, it is not yet known if the two bands formed in each pallidal segment by the subthalamopallidal fibers arise from collaterals of the same subthalamic neurons or from separate neuronal populations.

The striatopallidal projection

The striatopallidal projection in the squirrel monkey displays a precise rostrocaudal, mediolateral and dorsoventral topography. Furthermore, as it is the case for the subthalamopallidal afferents, the striatopallidal fibers arborize in the form of elongated vertical bands lying parallel to the medullary laminae (Hazrati et al., 1987; Hazrati and Parent, 1992b). For example, fibers emerging from either PHA-L or biocytin injection sites in the putamen form a few large and compact bundles that penetrate the pallidum through its lateral border by directly piercing the external medullary lamina. Within the pallidum, thin and varicose fibers brake off from the main compact bundles, turn caudally and run for a certain distance along a rather straight rostrocaudal trajectory before terminating at levels caudal to that of the injection sites.

Two important features of the organization of the striatopallidal projections are worth noting here. First, the various bands of terminal arborization appear sequentially along the rostrocaudal axis of the pallidum. Bands occur first in the GPe and, as these GPe bands become less prominent, bands start to appear in the GPi. Second, the most laterally located band formed by putamen efferents is much larger than bands located more deeply in the pallidum. This marginal band occupies a very restricted mediolateral domain but extends dorsoventrally over most of the ventral two-thirds of the GPe. By comparison, the bands that occur more medially in both GPe and GPi are shorter and many of them are closely interdigitated but do not intermix.

Our findings are at variance with those from previous Golgi studies in which the striatopallidal fibers were described as a multitude of straight and poorly branched axons that pass across several layers of pallidal neurons with typical discoidal dendritic domains making synapse en passant with the dendrites of these neurons. This type of arrangement together with the funnel shape of the pallidum led some authors to consider the pallidal complex as a place of intense convergence, a sort of informational funnel where convergence between the sensorimotor and associative components of the striatopallidal projection system would lead to functional integration (Percheron et al., 1984). However, our data clearly reveal that striatopallidal axons arborize profusely, principally at a right angle to the radially aligned main bundles of striatofugal axons. These arborizations occupied a restricted mediolateral domain of the pallidum and are found only within specific sectors of the pallidum.

As is the case for the subthalamopallidal projection, the striatopallidal afferents provide at least two band-like terminal fields in each pallidal segment (Fig. 2E). However, the bands formed by striatopallidal fibers are much more heterogeneous than those deriving from subthalamopallidal fibers. Typically, a striatopallidal band is composed rostrally of several thin, varicose, and poorly branched fibers making only an en passant type of contact with the soma of pallidal neurons (Fig. 1A,C), whereas caudally the same fibers arborize profusely and closely entwine the dendrites of pallidal neurons, thus forming typical woolly fibers (Fig. 1B,D). The fact that striatopallidal fibers arborize in the form of twin bands is in agreement with results from previous radioautographic and intracellular HRP injection studies (Chang et al., 1981; Wilson and Phelan, 1982; Kawaguchi et al., 1990) who revealed that single striatal neurons in the rat formed two distinct terminal fields in the globus pallidus, which is the rodent homologue of the primate GPe. Striatopallidal fibers in rodents were found to arborize first in a band-like fashion along the external medullary lamina and, second, in a more diffuse, plexus-like manner in the more central portion of the globus pallidus (Wilson and Phelan, 1982). Our findings suggest that, as in the rat, the striatum in primates has a dual representation at pallidal levels, and that this dual representation exists in both GPe and GPi. Since a previous retrograde, double-labeling study in the squirrel monkey showed that the striatal innervation of each pallidal segment arises from separate neurons (Parent et al., 1989), it must be presumed that the twin bands in the GPe and the GPi originate from distinct striatal neuronal populations.

The fact that striatopallidal fibers arborize twice in each pallidal segment may be taken as an indication that specific groups of striatal neurons send two copies of the same information to two distinct subsets of pallidal neurons. This peculiar organization, which involves a fair amount of redundancy in the information processing at pallidal levels, may be of utmost importance in the functional organization of the basal ganglia. For instance, the two subsets of pallidal neurons receiving the same striatal information may project to different pallidal recipient structures or to different sectors in the same pallidal recipient structure. Each of these two subsets of pallidal neurons may also be under a different influence from other pallidal inputs such as the subthalamic nucleus, the dorsal raphe nucleus, the substantia nigra and the centromedian-parafascicular complex (see Parent, 1986, 1990, and references therein).

Previous anterograde tract-tracing studies with tritiated amino acids or WGA-HRP have reported that the pallidal projection field from a single injected region of the striatum was large, encompassing a greater proportion of the pallidum than the injection site did in the striatum (Hedreen and DeLong, 1991). Thus, it was concluded that there was necessarily a high degree of overlap in the pallidal projection territories of neighboring regions of the striatum (Hedreen and DeLong, 1991). In these studies, however, the use of tritiated amino acids or WGA-HRP as anterograde tracers did not easily allow a clear distinction between terminal fields and fibers of passage. Our results obtained with the highly sensitive anterograde tracers PHA-L and biocytin do not support the existence of such a marked convergence in the striatopallidal projection system. For example, injection of PHA-L at two differ-

ent anteroposterior levels in the striatum leads to dense innervation in the form of woolly fibers only at very specific points in the pallidum. Typically, two of these woolly fiber terminal fields occur within two rostrocaudally distant portions of the same band of terminal arborization, and each of these two fields are interconnected by weakly varicose fibers that do not appear to densely innervate pallidal neurons (Fig. 2E). Furthermore, injections of PHA-L and biocytin into two small areas of the striatum located side by side along the mediolateral plane lead to anterograde labeling in the form of distinct bands that are located one above the other in the marginal zone of the GPe, but are closely interdigitated in the medial sector of the GPe and in the GPi. Although located very near to one another these two types of band never intermixt (Hazrati and Parent, 1992b). These results reveal that projections from striatal cell groups, even groups that are quite close to one another, do not converge upon the same pallidal neuronal population. Instead, they terminate upon separate pallidal cell groups or layers that may represent important functional subunits in the pallidum. Taken together these results indicate that, in contrast to previous beliefs, the striatopallidal system in primates is highly ordered and displays a high degree of specificity with respect to its target sites in the pallidum. It appears that different complex anatomical strategies are used to exploit the relatively small pallidal volume and ensure that the finely tuned corticostriatal information is not blurred as it flows through the funnel-shaped pallidum.

Interactions between subthalamic and striatal pallidal afferents

The concomitant injections of PHA-L or biocytin into the putamen or the subthalamic nucleus result in profuse anterograde fiber labeling characterized by typical elongated terminal bands in the two pallidal segments. Interestingly, the bands formed by the subthalamopallidal and striatopallidal fibers are largely in register with one another and their location is in direct relation with the size and extent of the injections in the striatum and the subthalamic nucleus. These bands consist of dense intermingling of numerous thin or coarse, smooth or varicose fibers, that were labeled with one of the two tracers.

Detailed examination of the terminal arborizations of the two afferents revealed a high degree of convergence of striatal and subthalamic fibers upon single pallidal cells. The most common pattern of convergence consists of: (1) soma and proximal dendrites closely surrounded by numerous axonal varicosities of subthalamic origin and a few striatal varicosities; and (2) distal dendrites ensheathed by numerous striatopallidal fibers (woolly fibers) and only one or two thin subthalamopallidal fibers (Fig. 2A – D). Another pattern of convergence occurs, particularly in the rostral pole of both GPe and GPi and, to a lesser extent, in the dense zones of heavy labeling that occurred in band-like regions. It consists of a more diffuse, principally somatic, type of innervation deriving from very thin and varicose striatal and subthalamic fibers, that form diffuse plexuses over pallidal neurons (Fig. 2A). Furthermore, some pallidal cells located at the periphery of the main labeling zones are surrounded by only one type of fiber (either striatopallidal or subthalamopallidal). Whether or not this represents true divergence or simply reflects the fact that the injection sites involved parts of the striatum and subthalamic nucleus that are not functionally related remains to be investigated.

The results obtained after double anterograde labeling studies confirm that the subthalamopallidal and striatopallidal fibers travel in opposite direction along the rostrocaudal axis of the pallidum and display different patterns of innervation (Fig. 2E). Typically, the subthalamic fibers ensheathe rather loosely the distal dendrites but closely surround the proximal dendrites and soma of pallidal neurons, and this pattern remains virtually the same throughout the whole rostrocaudal extent of the labeling in the pallidum. In contrast, the proximal segment of the striatopallidal fibers contacts en passant the pallidal cells, whereas its distal portion branches abundantly and very closely entwines the dendrites of pallidal neurons in the more caudal areas of the anterograde labeling. The two inputs converge upon single pallidal cells at all rostrocaudal levels of the pallidum, but the convergence is particularly obvious in the GPi where the striatal fibers ensheathe nearly completely the dendrites of pallidal neurons and the subthalamic fibers form very tight pericellular arrangements around the soma of pallidal cells. These results suggest that the subthalamic fibers can uniformly excite a rather large collection of pallidal neurons aligned along the caudorostral axis of the pallidum, whereas the striatal fibers appear to exert a more specific inhibitory control upon selected subsets of these subthalamically driven pallidal neurons (Fig. 2E).

Differences between the two pallidal segments

Some important differences were noted between the GPe and the GPi in regard to the patterns of arborization of the striatopallidal and subthalamopallidal projections. For example, in material deriving from experiments in which PHA-L was used as single anterograde tracer, the subthalamopallidal fibers display axonal varicosities that are significantly larger around the soma and proximal dendrites of the GPi than they are in the same locations in the GPe. In fact, the axonal varicosities of the subthalamopallidal fibers appear to progressively increase in size as the fibers approach the cell bodies. In contrast, the striatopallidal fibers that closely ensheathe the dendrites of pallidal neurons bear varicosities of similar size and shape in the GPi and the GPe.

In material deriving from experiments undertaken with both PHA-L and biocytin as double anterograde tracers, these differences between GPi and GPe were even more striking. The striatopallidal fibers form characteristic woolly fibers with the dendrites of pallidal neurons in both the GPi and GPe. These woolly fibers comprise a multitude of rather small axonal varicosities ($0.5 - 1.5$ μm), separated from one another by relatively short intervaricose segments. A smaller number of similar striatopallidal varicosities are encountered over pallidal cell bodies in both the GPi and GPe (Fig. 3). In contrast, the subthalamopallidal afferents rarely form dense woolly fibers but appear as more diffuse

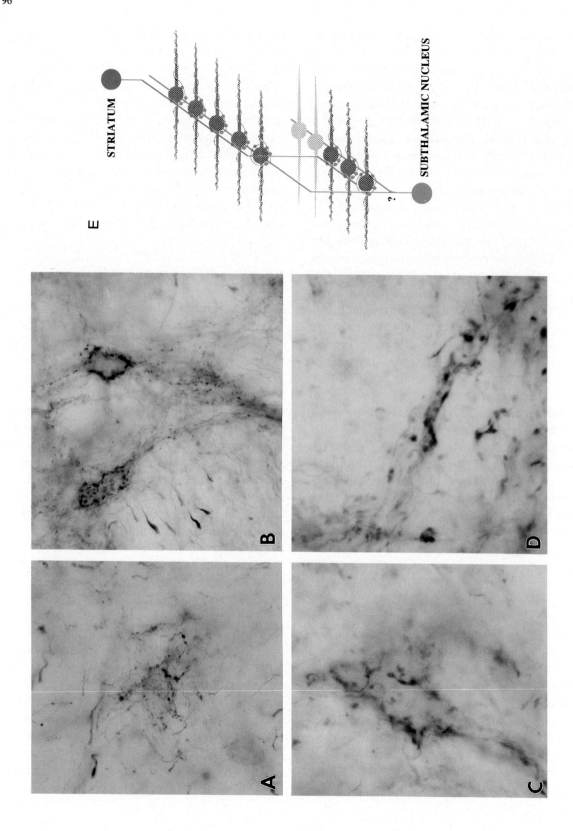

plexuses within the pallidal neuropil. Most often, a few subthalamopallidal fibers bearing varicosities that are slightly larger than those of the striatopallidal fibers can be seen to ascend along distal dendrites of pallidal neurons. These varicosities, which are separated from one another by intervaricose segments of variable length, are typically round with a diameter ranging from 1 to 2 μm (Fig. 3). As mentioned above, the subthalamopallidal axonal varicosities progressively enlarge and become more flattened as they reach the proximal dendrites and soma of pallidal neurons. The longest diameter of the perisomatic subthalamopallidal varicosities in the GPi ranges from 3 to 4 μm (Fig. 3). In the GPe, the perisomatic subthalamopallidal varicosities are similar in size and shape to those found along distal dendrites (Fig. 3).

The functional significance of these differences between the GPi and the GPe in respect to the pattern of arborization of the subthalamopallidal and striatopallidal afferents remains to be investigated. However, it is worth noting that the very characteristic perisomatic baskets formed by the large axonal varicosities of the subthalamopallidal fibers strikingly resemble the prominent pericellular contacts made by the GPe fibers terminating upon GPi neurons (Hazrati et al., 1990). Indeed, anterograde labeling studies with PHA-L have revealed the existence of interconnections between the two pallidal segments in the squirrel monkey. Fibers from the GPe were reported to form numerous large varicosities reminiscent of terminal boutons, which closely surround GPi cell bodies and primary dendrites. In contrast, fibers from the GPi that invaded the GPe display a rather linear course, have long intervaricose segments, and appear to contact en passant several GPe neurons (Hazrati et al., 1990). Since virtually all pallidal neurons in the squirrel monkey display GABA immunoreactivity (Smith et al., 1987), it can be assumed that these pallidopallidal interconnections are GABAergic. Therefore, it may be hypothesized that the strong pericellular GABAergic inhibitory input deriving from GPe neurons is there to counteract the powerful and similarly organized glutamatergic excitatory input from the subthalamic nucleus upon the GPi neurons, which are major output elements of the basal ganglia.

However, it must be admitted that the presence of large excitatory terminal boutons closely surrounding the soma of pallidal neurons is rather unexpected because in most brain areas boutons of the excitatory type are rather small and terminate principally upon distal dendrites (see Peter et al., 1991). Furthermore, although the presence of a small number of large boutons terminating upon the soma and proximal dendrites of pallidal neurons has been

Fig. 2. Color photomicrographs showing examples of the anterograde labeling observed in the pallidum after PHA-L and biocytin injections into the subthalamic nucleus and the striatum, respectively ($A-D$), and a schematic diagram illustrating the organization of the subthalamopallidal and striatal afferents (E). A. Loosely arranged plexuses composed of very thin subthalamopallidal (blue) and striatopallidal (brown) fibers covering pallidal neurons. $B-D$. Pallidal neurons whose cell bodies are closely surrounded by subthalamopallidal fibers (blue, B,C) and dendrites entwined with both subthalamopallidal (blue) and striatopallidal (brown) varicose fibers (B,D). E. Schematic illustration proposing a model of the organization of the subthalamic and striatal fibers at pallidal level based on data obtained with the anterograde double-labeling technique. The drawing emphasizes the pattern of convergence of the two inputs upon two distant series of rostrocaudally aligned pallidal cells. The soma of these pallidal cells are represented by gray circles, whereas their dendrites are indicated by horizontal gray lines. The large red circle represents a single striatal cell whose axon is illustrated by a red line with small red circles representing striatal varicosities making en passant type of contact with pallidal soma in the proximal segment of the axon. In its terminal portion, this striatal axon branches and closely entwines the dendrites of a more caudally located pallidal neuron. These terminal branches are illustrated as sinuous and dotted red lines. The same striatal fiber continues its rostrocaudal course to innervate in the same fashion a second more ventrally located set of pallidal cells. The large blue circle represents a single subthalamic cell whose main axon (blue line) bifurcates giving rise to two branches that course caudorostrally beneath each set of pallidal cells. These branches emit short collaterals (sinuous and dotted blue lines) that loosely entwine dendrites but closely surround the soma of pallidal neurons. The question mark indicates the uncertainty as to whether the innervation of the two sets of pallidal neurons derives from a single subthalamopallidal axon that branches, as illustrated here, or arises from two different axons deriving from separate subthalamic neurons.

documented in some electron microscopic studies of the primate and rodent globus pallidus (see DiFiglia et al., 1982; Falls et al., 1983), these boutons were shown to make symmetrical synaptic junctions, which is indicative of inhibitory rather than excitatory influence. Therefore, it is possible that the large labeled boutons encountered around the soma and proximal dendrites of pallidal neurons after subthalamic nucleus injections result from the fact that the tracer was first retrogradely transported from the subthalamic nucleus to GPe neurons and then anterogradely delivered to the GPi via the GPe-GPi

projection. However, in order to be possible, such an indirect labeling would require the GPe-GPi connection to be extremely massive, organized in a strict point-to-point manner and composed of axon collaterals of the pallidosubthalamic projection.

Ultrastructural observations

Observations made at the electron microscopic level confirm that PHA-L- or biocytin-labeled axonal varicosities visualized along the dendrites of pallidal neurons at the light microscopic level correspond to

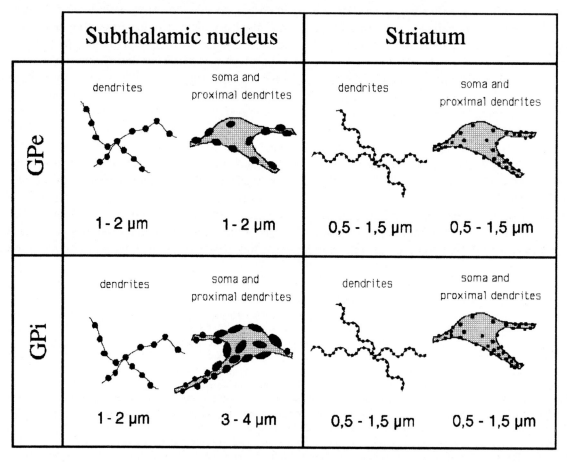

Fig. 3. Computer-generated drawings illustrating the differences between the external (GPe) and internal (GPi) segment of the pallidum in respect to the patterns of arborization of afferents from the subthalamic nucleus and the striatum. The diagram also gives a rough estimate of the sizes of the various terminal varicosities encountered along the distal dendrites as well as on the soma and proximal dendrites of pallidal neurons in both GPe and GPi. These values were obtained from materials prepared for the demonstration of both subthalamopallidal (PHA-L-labeled, NiDAB) and striatopallidal (biocytin-labeled, DAB) afferents on single sections examined with a light microscope.

well characterized terminal boutons. In fact, the BDHC (for PHA-L) and the DAB (for biocytin) reaction products in the pallidal neuropil were exclusively confined to axonal structures, including axon terminals. As mentioned above, the DAB reaction product appears as amorphous, electron-dense material attached to microtubules, mitochondria and small electron-lucent vesicles, whereas the BDHC reaction product stands as electron-dense granules or crystals randomly dispersed throughout the labeled elements (see Smith and Bolam, 1990).

Two types of terminal bouton could be easily identified in the few sectors of the GPi enriched in woolly fibers that were examined in the present study. The first type consists of small terminal boutons that display the characteristic amorphous DAB immunoprecipitate, indicating the presence of biocytin injected into the striatum (Fig. 4A,B). The second type consists of larger terminal boutons that display the granular BDHC immunoprecipitate, indicating the presence of PHA-L injected into the subthalamic nucleus. These large subthalamopallidal boutons often contain numerous mitochondria (Fig. 4C) and are much less frequent than the smaller striatopallidal boutons. Several subthalamopallidal axon terminals could be seen to make an asymmetrical type of synaptic contact with dendrites (Fig. 4C–E), whereas striatopallidal boutons appear to form a symmetrical type of synaptic contact with similar postsynaptic elements (Fig. 4A,B). Occasionally, two boutons of each type could be seen to contact the same dendrite (Fig. 4F), thus supporting the view that striatopallidal and subthalamopallidal axons converge upon the same pallidal neurons.

Previous electron microscopic studies of the globus pallidus in primates have revealed a rather homogeneous neuropil organization without marked variations between the two pallidal segments (see Fox and Rafols, 1976; DiFiglia et al., 1982; Pasik and Pasik, 1983; Hassler and Chung, 1984). This impression of homogeneity most probably derives from the fact that the exact origin of the various types of axon terminals could not be determined with certainty in these earlier studies. Therefore, instead of providing a detailed view of the synaptic articulation of a specific type of pallidal input, these investigations gave a rather overall account of all the possible synaptic interactions at pallidal level (see Hassler and Chung, 1984). Our light microscopic results obtained with single or double anterograde labeling methods clearly indicate that the organization of the striatopallidal and subthalamopallidal afferents, as well as the interactions between these two major pallidal inputs, are much more complex than could have been expected from previous studies. For example, we showed that the striatopallidal and the subthalamopallidal projections form at least two distinct band-like terminal fields in each pallidal segment and that these terminal fields are largely in register with one another. Furthermore, our data revealed that in contrast to the subthalamopallidal fibers, which arborize in a rather uniform manner throughout the pallidum, the striatopallidal fibers are organized in diffuse plexuses rostrally but form typical woolly fibers caudally in the same terminal band. These differences, added to the variations in the patterns of subthalamic and striatal innervation noted between the two pallidal segments, must be taken into account when sampling the pallidal complex for electron microscopic analysis.

In this context the few ultrastructural observations made above should be considered as very preliminary because the sampling was restricted to only a few regions of the GPi where dense woolly fibers could be visualized at the light microscopic level. A much more widespread and detailed survey is needed if one hopes to reach a more global understanding of the intimate aspect of the interactions between the striatopallidal and subthalamopallidal projections. Of particular interest would be the identification of the different types of axonal bouton contacting the cell body of pallidal neurons in both the GPe and the GPi. These terminals could be easily characterized by combining the use of PHA-L and biocytin for defining the origin of each type of bouton with GABA and glutamate post-embedding immunogold procedures for the identification of the neurotransmitter involved.

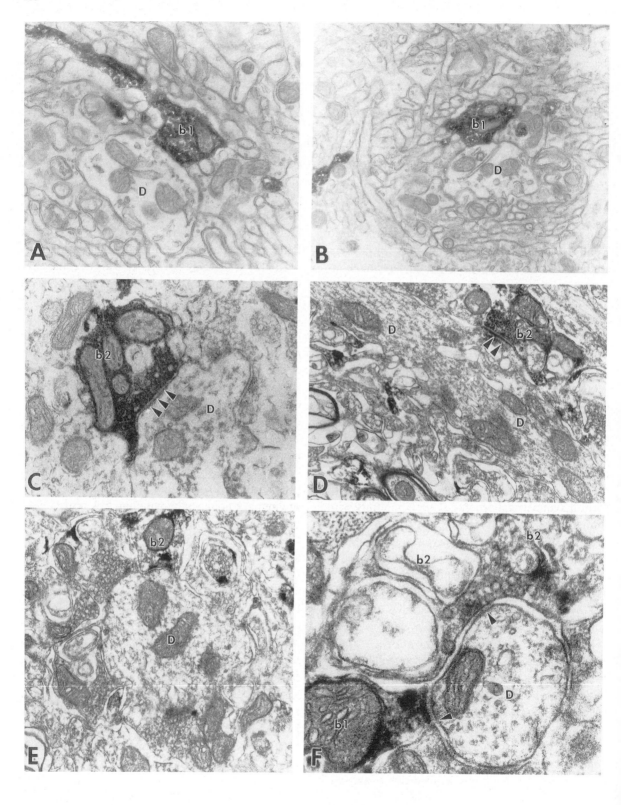

Concluding remarks

Studies undertaken in squirrel monkeys with PHA-L and biocytin as single or double anterograde tracers have revealed important aspects of the organization of the striatopallidal and subthalamopallidal projections in primates and provided the first evidence that these two major inputs to the globus pallidus converge upon the same pallidal neurons. The striatopallidal projection system was found to be highly ordered and to display a high degree of specificity with respect to its target sites in the pallidum. Different complex anatomical strategies appear to be used to maximally exploit the relatively small pallidal space and ensure that the finely tuned corticostriatal information is not blurred as it flows through the funnel-shaped pallidum. In contrast, the subthalamopallidal fibers were found to arborize in a rather uniform pattern throughout the rostrocaudal extent of the pallidum, although some important variations have been noted between the two pallidal segments.

The striatopallidal and subthalamopallidal fibers were shown to arborize at least twice in each pallidal segment, indicating that both the striatum and the subthalamic nucleus have multiple representations at pallidal level. The two types of fiber arborized in the form of vertical bands that were largely in register with one another. The striatopallidal and subthalamopallidal fibers were found to converge upon single pallidal cells at all rostrocaudal levels of the pallidum, but the convergence was particularly obvious caudally within each of these terminal bands. At this level, the striatal fibers ensheathed nearly completely the dendrites of pallidal neurons, whereas the subthalamic fibers formed very tight pericellular arrangements around the soma of pallidal cells.

Our results suggest that the subthalamic input can uniformly excite a rather large collection of pallidal neurons, while the striatal input appears to exert a more specific inhibitory control upon selected subsets of these subthalamically driven pallidal neurons. The inhibition at one point in time of a particular subset of GPi neurons that are normally under the tonic excitatory influence of the subthalamic nucleus is likely to lead to the disinhibition of the thalamocortical neurons receiving this pallidal input, thus allowing a certain aspect of movement to be executed. In such a scheme, the specificity of the globus pallidus involvement in the control of motor behavior heavily relies upon the highly ordered organization of the striatopallidal projection, whose principal function is to integrate and convey the finely tuned corticostriatal information with the highest possible degree of accuracy. Conversely, the subthalamic nucleus is considered as a structure that exerts a generalized excitatory influence upon the globus pallidus, thus acting as a "driving force" of the basal ganglia (see Kitai and Kita, 1987).

However, the role of the subthalamic nucleus is likely to be much more subtle. The subthalamic

Fig. 4. Examples of some ultrastructural features of subthalamopallidal (PHA-L-labeled, BDHC as chromogen) and striatopallidal (biocytin-labeled, DAB as chromogen) terminal boutons as seen in double anterograde labeling material. The sampling was restricted to only a few small areas of the GPi that were enriched with woolly fibers. *A,B.* Two typical striatopallidal labeled boutons (b1) making symmetrical type of contact with a dendrite (D). Part of the labeled axon giving rise to one of the terminal bouton can be seen in *A*. *C,D.* Typical subthalamopallidal labeled boutons (b2) making asymmetrical type of contact (arrowheads) with dendrites (D) that have been cut transversely (*C*) and longitudinally (*D*). Note the rather large size of these boutons, which characteristically contain numerous mitochondria. *E.* A smaller subthalamopallidal labeled bouton (b2) in contact with what appears to be a more distal dendrite. Note the numerous nearby unlabeled boutons filled with small, electron-lucent, synaptic vesicles. These unlabeled boutons contact the same dendrite in a typical rosette-like fashion. *F.* Two differently labeled terminal boutons (b1 and b2) in close contact (arrowheads) with the same dendrite (D). The smaller bouton (b1) contains amorphous, electron-dense reaction product mostly related to small electron-lucent vesicles, whereas the larger bouton (b2) displays a few randomly dispersed electron-dense granules or crystals. The former labeling appears typical of DAB immunoprecipitate whereas the latter is characteristic of BDHC reaction product. Thus, this electron photomicrograph is strongly suggestive of convergence of striatopallidal and subthalamopallidal terminals upon single dendrites of pallidal neurons.

nucleus, like the striatum, receives a prominent and topographically organized input from the sensorimotor cortex (see Hartmann-von Monakow and Künzle, 1978; Afsharpour, 1985). Therefore, the neurons of the subthalamic nucleus like those of the striatum can integrate and convey cortical information to the globus pallidus in a rather specific manner. Since the subthalamopallidal and striatopallidal projections converge upon the same pallidal neurons, it can be presumed that the functional state of each pallidal neuron is largely determined by the complex interplay of excitatory and inhibitory inputs deriving from subthalamic and striatal neurons, which are both under the direct glutamate-mediated excitatory influence of the cerebral cortex (Parent and Hazrati, 1993). Other less prominent pallidal inputs, such as the dopaminergic, serotoninergic and cholinergic projections deriving respectively from the substantia nigra, the dorsal raphe nucleus and the pedunculopontine nucleus, may also play a crucial role in the modulation of pallidal neurons. However, much remains to be known about the anatomical and functional organization of the brain-stem pallidal afferents.

Acknowledgements

The authors thank Carole Harvey and Lisette Bertrand for technical assistance, Suzanne Bilodeau for typing the manuscript, and Isabelle Daudelin for the artwork. This research was supported by Grant MT-5781 of the Medical Research Council of Canada to A. Parent. Lili-Naz Hazrati was the recipient of a Studentship from the Fonds de Recherche en Santé du Québec.

References

Afsharpour, S. (1985) Topographical projections of the cerebral cortex to the subthalamic nucleus. *J. Comp. Neurol.*, 236: 14–28.

Alexander, G.E. and Crutcher, M.D. (1990) Functional architecture of basal ganglia: neural substrate of parallel processing. *Trends Neurosci.*, 13: 266–271.

Alexander, G.E., DeLong, M.R. and Strick, P.L. (1986) Parallel organization of functionally segregated circuits linking basal ganglia and cortex. *Annu. Rev. Neurosci.*, 9: 357–381.

Carpenter, M.B., Batton III, R.R., Carleton, S.C. and Keller, J.T. (1981a) Interconnections and organization of pallidal and subthalamic nucleus neurons in the monkey. *J. Comp. Neurol.*, 197: 579–603.

Carpenter, M.B., Carleton, S.C., Keller, J.T. and Conte, P. (1981b) Connections of the subthalamic nucleus in the monkey. *Brain Res.*, 224: 1–29.

Chang, H.T., Wilson, C.J. and Kitai, S.T. (1981) Single neostriatal efferent axons in the globus pallidus: a light and electron microscopic study. *Science*, 213: 915–918.

Cowan, W.M. and Powell, T.P.S. (1966) Striatopallidal projection in the monkey. *J. Neurol. Neurosurg. Psychiatry*, 29: 426–439.

DeLong, M.R., Crutcher, M.D. and Georgopoulos, A.P. (1985) Primate globus pallidus and subthalamic nucleus: functional organization. *J. Neurophysiol.*, 53: 530–543.

DiFiglia, M., Pasik, P. and Pasik, T. (1982) A Golgi and ultrastructural study of the monkey globus pallidus. *J. Comp. Neurol.*, 212: 53–75.

Emmers, E. and Akert, K. (1963) *A Stereotaxic Atlas of the Brain of the Squirrel Monkey (Saimiri sciureus)*, The University of Wisconsin Press, Madison, WI.

Falls, W.M., Park, M.R. and Kitai, S.T. (1983) An intracellular HRP study of the rat globus pallidus. II. Fine structural characteristics and synaptic connections of medially located large GP neurons. *J. Comp. Neurol.*, 221: 229–245.

Fox, C.A. and Rafols, J.A. (1976) The striatal efferents in the globus pallidus and in the substantia nigra. In: M.D. Yahr (Ed.), *The Basal Ganglia,* Raven Press, New York, pp. 37–55.

Fox, C.A., Andrade, A.N., Lu Qui, I.J. and Rafols, J.A. (1974) The primate globus pallidus: a Golgi and electron microscopic study. *J. Hirnforsch.*, 15: 75–93.

Gerfen, C.R. (1989) The neostriatal mosaic: striatal patch-matrix organization is related to cortical lamination. *Science*, 246: 385–388.

Gerfen, C.R. and Sawchenko, P.E. (1984) An anterograde neuroanatomical tracing method that shows the detailed morphology of neurons, their axons and terminals: immunohistochemical localization of an axonally transported plant lectin, *Phaseolus vulgaris* leucoagglutinin (PHA-L). *Brain Res.*, 290: 219–238.

Hancock, M.B. (1982) A serotonin-immunoreactive fiber system in the dorsal columns of the spinal cord. *Neurosci. Lett.*, 31: 247–252.

Hartmann-von Monakow, K., Akert, K. and Künzle, H. (1978) Projections of the precentral motor cortex and other cortical areas of the frontal lobe to the subthalamic nucleus in the monkey. *Exp. Brain Res.*, 33: 395–403.

Hassler, R. and Chung, Y.-M. (1984) Identification of eight types of synapses in the pallidum externum and internum in squirrel monkey (*Saimiri sciureus*). *Acta Anat.*, 118: 65–81.

Hazrati, L.-N. and Parent, A. (1991) Projection from the external pallidum to the reticular thalamic nucleus in the squirrel monkey. *Brain Res.*, 550: 142–146.

Hazrati, L.-N. and Parent, A. (1992a) Convergence of subthalamic and striatal efferents at pallidal level in primates: an anterograde double-labeling study with biocytin and PHA-L. *Brain Res.*, 569: 336–340.

Hazrati, L.-N. and Parent, A. (1992b) The striatopallidal projection displays a high degree of anatomical specificity in the primate. *Brain Res.*, 592: 213–227.

Hazrati, L.-N. and Parent, A. (1992c) Projection from the deep cerebellar nuclei to the pedunculopontine nucleus in the squirrel monkey. *Brain Res.*, 585: 267–271.

Hazrati, L.-N., Parent, A. and Smith, Y. (1987) Organization of striatal and subthalamic nucleus afferents to pallidum in primates as revealed by PHA-L anterograde tracing method. *Soc. Neurosci. Abstr.*, 13: 1571.

Hazrati, L.-N., Parent, A., Mitchell, S. and Haber, S.N. (1990) Evidence for interactions between the two pallidal segments in primates: a PHA-L anterograde tracing study. *Brain Res.*, 533: 171–175.

Hedreen, J.C. and DeLong, M.R. (1991) Organization of striatopallidal, striatonigral, and nigrostriatal projections in the macaque. *J. Comp. Neurol.*, 304: 569–595.

Jessel, T.M., Emson, P.C., Paxinos, G. and Cuello, A.C. (1978) Topographic projections of substance P and GABA pathways in the striato- and pallido-nigral system: a biochemical and immunohistochemical study. *Brain Res.*, 152: 487–498.

Johnson, T.N. and Rosvold, H.E. (1971) Topographic projections on the globus pallidus and the substantia nigra of selectively placed lesions in the precommissural caudate nucleus and putamen in the monkey. *Exp. Neurol.*, 33: 584–596.

Kawaguchi, Y., Wilson, C.J. and Emson, P.C. (1990) Projection subtypes of rat neostriatal matrix cells revealed by intracellular injection of biocytin. *J. Neurosci.*, 10: 3421–3438.

Kemp, J.M. and Powell, T.P.S. (1970) The corticostriate projection in the monkey. *Brain*, 93: 525–546.

King, M.A., Louis, P.M., Hunter, B.E. and Walker, D.W. (1990) Biocytin: a versatile anterograde neuroanatomical tract-tracing alternative. *Brain Res.*, 497: 361–367.

Kita, H. and Kitai, S.T. (1987) Efferent projections of the subthalamic nucleus in the rat: light and electron microscopic analysis with the PHA-L method. *J. Comp. Neurol.*, 260: 435–452.

Kita, H., Chang, H.T. and Kitai, S.T. (1983) The morphology of intracellularly labeled rat subthalamic nucleus. *J. Comp. Neurol.*, 215: 245–257.

Kitai, S.T. and Kita, H. (1987) Anatomy and physiology of the subthalamic nucleus: a driving force of the basal ganglia. In: M.B. Carpenter and A. Jayaraman (Eds.), *The Basal Ganglia II – Structure and Function: Current Concepts*, Plenum Press, New York, pp. 357–373.

Künzle, H. (1975) Bilateral projections from precentral motor cortex to the putamen and other parts of the basal ganglia. An autoradiographic study in *Macaca fascicularis*. *Brain Res.*, 88:

195–209.

Künzle, H. (1978) An autoradiographic analysis of the efferent connections from premotor and adjacent prefrontal regions (areas 6 and 9) in *Macaca fascicularis*. *Brain Behav. Evol.*, 15: 185–234.

Künzle, H. and Akert, K. (1977) Efferent connections of cortical area 8 (frontal eye field) in *Macaca fascicularis*. *J. Comp. Neurol.*, 173: 147–164.

Levey, A.I., Bolam, J.P., Rye, D.B., Hallanger, A.E., Demuth, R.M., Mesulam, M.-M. and Wainer, B.H. (1986) A light and electron microscopic procedure for sequential double antigen localization using diaminobenzidine and benzidine dihydrochloride. *J. Histochem. Cytochem.*, 34: 1449–1457.

McGeer, P.L., McGeer, E.G., Wada, J.A. and Jung, E. (1971) Effects of globus pallidus lesions and Parkinson's disease on brain glutamic acid decarboxylase. *Brain Res.*, 32: 425–431.

Nauta, H.J.W. and Cole, M. (1978) Efferent projections of the subthalamic nucleus: an autoradiographic study in monkey and cat. *J. Comp. Neurol.*, 180: 1–16.

Nauta, H.J.W. and Mehler, W.R. (1966) Projections of the lentiform nucleus in the monkey. *Brain Res.*, 1: 3–42.

Oertel, W.H., Nitsch, C. and Mugnaini, E. (1984) Immunocytochemical demonstration of the GABAergic neurons in the rat globus pallidus and nucleus entopeduncularis and their GABA-ergic innervation. In: R.G. Hassler and J.F. Christ (Eds.), *Parkinson-specific Motor and Mental Disorders, Advances in Neurology, Vol. 40*. Raven Press, New York, pp. 91–98.

Papez, J.W. (1942) A summary of fiber connections of the basal ganglia with each other and with other portions of the brain. *Res. Publ. Assoc. Nerv. Ment. Dis.*, 21: 21–68.

Parent, A. (1986) *Comparative Neurobiology of the Basal Ganglia*, Wiley, New York.

Parent, A. (1990) Extrinsic connections of the basal ganglia. *Trends Neurosci.*, 13: 254–258.

Parent, A. and Hazrati, L.-N. (1993) Anatomical aspects of information processing in primate basal ganglia. *Trends Neurosci.*, 16: 111–116.

Parent, A. and Smith, Y. (1987) Organization of efferent projections of the subthalamic nucleus in the squirrel monkey as revealed by retrograde labeling methods. *Brain Res.*, 436: 296–310.

Parent, A., Bouchard, C. and Smith, Y. (1984) The striatopallidal and striatonigral projections: two distinct fiber systems in primate. *Brain Res.*, 303: 385–390.

Parent, A., Smith, Y., Filion, M. and Dumas, J. (1989) Distinct afferents to internal and external pallidal segments in the squirrel monkey. *Neurosci. Lett.*, 96: 140–144.

Park, M.R., Falls, W.M. and Kitai, S.T. (1982) An intracellular HRP of the rat globus pallidus. I. Response and light microscopic analysis. *J. Comp. Neurol.*, 211: 284–294.

Pasik, T. and Pasik, P. (1983) The internal organization of the pallidum in mammals. *J. Neural Transm.*, 19: 13–35.

Percheron, G., Yelnik, J. and François, C. (1984) A Golgi analy-

104

sis of the primate globus pallidus. III. Spatial organization of the striatopallidal complex. *J. Comp. Neurol.,* 227: 214 – 227.

Peter, A., Palay, S.L. and Webster, H. deF. (1991) *The Fine Structure of the Nervous System: Neurons and Their Supporting Cells,* 3rd edn., New York University Press, New York.

Ribak, C.E., Vaughn, J.E. and Roberts, E. (1979) The GABA neurons and their axon terminals in the rat corpus striatum as demonstrated by GAD immunocytochemistry. *J. Comp. Neurol.,* 187: 261 – 284.

Selemon, L.D. and Goldman-Rakic, P.S. (1985) Longitudinal topography and interdigitation of corticostriatal projections in the rhesus monkey. *J. Neurosci.,* 5: 776 – 794.

Smith, Y. and Bolam, J.P. (1990) Convergence of synaptic inputs from the striatum and the globus pallidus onto identified nigrocollicular cells in the rat: a double anterograde labeling study. *Neuroscience,* 44: 45 – 73.

Smith, Y. and Parent, A. (1986) Differential connections of caudate nucleus and putamen in the squirrel monkey (*Saimiri sciureus*). *Neuroscience,* 18: 347 – 371.

Smith, Y. and Parent, A. (1988) Neurons of the subthalamic nucleus in primates display glutamate but not GABA immunoreactivity. *Brain Res.,* 453: 353 – 356.

Smith, Y., Parent, A., Séguéla, P. and Descarries, L. (1987) Distribution of GABA immunoreactive neurons in the basal ganglia of the squirrel monkey (*Saimiri sciureus*). *J. Comp. Neurol.,* 259: 50 – 65.

Smith, Y., Hazrati, L.N. and Parent, A. (1990) Efferent projections of the subthalamic nucleus in the squirrel monkey as studied by the PHA-L anterograde tracing method. *J. Comp. Neurol.,* 294: 306 – 323.

Szabo, J. (1962) Topical distribution of the striatal efferents in the monkey. *Exp. Neurol.,* 5: 21 – 36.

Szabo, J. (1967) The efferent projections of the putamen in the monkey. *Exp. Neurol.,* 19: 463 – 476.

Szabo, J. (1970) Projections from the body of the caudate nucleus in the rhesus monkey. *Exp. Neurol.,* 27: 1 – 15.

Van Hoesen, G.W., Yeterian, E.H. and Lavizzo-Mourey, R. (1981) Widespread corticostriate projections from temporal cortex of rhesus monkey. *J. Comp. Neurol.,* 199: 205 – 219.

Whittier, J.R. and Mettler, F.A. (1949) Studies on the subthalamus of the rhesus monkey. I. Anatomy and fiber connections of the subthalamic nucleus of Luys. *J. Comp. Neurol.,* 90: 281 – 317.

Wilson, C.J. and Phelan, K.D. (1982) Dual topographic representation of neostriatum in the globus pallidus of rats. *Brain Res.,* 243: 354 – 359.

Yelnik, J., Percheron, G. and François, C. (1984) A Golgi analysis of the primate globus pallidus. II. Quantitative morphology and spatial orientation of dendritic arborization. *J. Comp. Neurol.,* 227: 200 – 213.

G.W. Arbuthnott and P.C. Emson (Eds.)
Progress in Brain Research, Vol. 99

CHAPTER 7

The distribution of GABA$_A$-benzodiazepine receptors in the basal ganglia in Huntington's disease and in the quinolinic acid-lesioned rat

R.L.M. Faull[1], H.J. Waldvogel[1], L.F.B. Nicholson[1] and B.J.L. Synek[2]

Departments of [1]Anatomy and [2]Pathology, School of Medicine, University of Auckland, Private Bag 92019, Auckland, New Zealand

Introduction

Huntington's disease is an inherited neurodegenerative disease which is characterised by progressive involuntary choreiform movements, psychological change and dementia (Hayden, 1981). The major neuropathological changes in Huntington's disease are found in the basal ganglia and comprise striatal neuronal cell loss and atrophy of the caudate nucleus and putamen (Martin and Gusella, 1986). The striatal cell loss typically involves the medium-sized GABAergic spiny efferent neurons (which also contain enkephalin or substance P) and striatal interneurons, but selectively spares the aspiny interneurons which contain the peptides somatostatin and neuropeptide Y and the enzyme NADPH-diaphorase (Dawbarn et al., 1985; Ferrante et al., 1985, 1987; Graveland et al., 1985; Martin and Gusella, 1986; Kowall et al., 1987). In addition to these neurotransmitter and neuronal changes, there are also marked neurotransmitter receptor changes in the basal ganglia in Huntington's disease (Penney and Young, 1982; Whitehouse et al., 1985). In particular, GABA$_A$-benzodiazepine receptors are markedly depleted in the caudate nucleus and putamen and increased in the globus pallidus and substantia nigra (Reisine et al., 1979, 1980; Penney and Young, 1982; Walker et al., 1984; Whitehouse et al., 1985).

Although the gene for Huntington's disease has been localized to the short arm of chromosome 4 (Gusella et al., 1983), the pathogenesis of the disease still remains unknown. Over recent years, however, excitotoxic mechanisms have been suggested as a possible factor in the neurodegenerative process (DiFiglia, 1990) and the excitotoxin quinolinic acid has been specifically implicated in the pathogenesis of Huntington's disease (Beal et al., 1986; Kowall et al., 1987). Quinolinic acid is an endogenous metabolite in the brain that produces axon-sparing lesions and neurochemical changes in the rat striatum similar to those in Huntington's disease (Schwarcz et al., 1983; Beal et al., 1986; Ellison et al., 1987; Kowall et al., 1987). In particular, intrastriatal injections of quinolinic acid in the rat brain result in a marked depletion of GABAergic efferent neurons with the apparent selective sparing of somato-statin-neuropeptide-Y-NADPH-diaphorase neurons (Beal et al., 1986, 1989; Kowall et al., 1987). Others have shown, however, that somatostatin-neuropeptide Y cells are not spared in quinolinic acid lesions of the striatum (Boegman et al., 1987; Davies and Roberts, 1987) and have questioned the validity of the proposed model.

In order to further investigate the validity of the quinolinic acid animal model of Huntington's disease, we have documented the GABA$_A$-benzodiazepine receptor changes in the striatum and globus pallidus in Huntington's disease and then investigated whether the same pattern of receptor changes occurs in the basal ganglia of the quinolinic acid-lesioned rat model of the disease. In both the human and animal studies, the distribution of $GABA_A$-benzodiazepine receptors was investigated using receptor autoradiography following in vitro labelling of cryostat sections with a tritiated $GABA_A$-benzodiazepine receptor ligand ([^{3}H]flunitrazepam) and immunohistochemical techniques with a monoclonal antibody (bd-17) to the $\beta_{2,3}$ subunits of the $GABA_A$-benzodiazepine receptor complex.

Material and methods

Tissue collection and preparation

Human tissue. A total of 40 post-mortem human brains were used in this study. Seventeen brains were obtained from patients with no history of neurological disease and 23 brains from patients with a family and clinical history of Huntington's disease. The neurologically normal control brains were from 7 females and 10 males, aged 20 – 71 years (average age of 51 years) and the interval between death and the receipt of the brain tissue (i.e., the post-mortem delay) ranged from 3.5 to 25.5 h (average delay of 13.0 h). The Huntington's disease brains were from 7 female and 16 male patients, aged 42 – 74 years (average age of 57 years) with a post-mortem delay of 2.5 – 35 h (average delay of 14.7 h).

On receipt of each brain, blocks of tissue were immediately selected from various regions of the basal ganglia for the autoradiographic and immunohistochemical localization of receptors and for neuropathological diagnostic studies. The blocks of tissue for the autoradiographic localization of receptors were frozen on dry ice. The tissue blocks for immunohistochemistry and neuropathology were fixed by immersion in freshly made 4% paraformaldehyde and 0.1 – 0.5% glutaraldehyde in 0.1 M phosphate buffer at pH 7.4 for 3 – 9 days.

Animal tissue. Twenty-two male albino Wistar rats were used in this study. The rats were anaesthe-

tized with sodium pentobarbital and an injection of 15 nl of quinolinic acid (dissolved in 0.1 ml NaOH at a concentration of 4 M) was stereotoxically placed in the dorsal region of the right striatum (coordinates: 0.8 mm anterior to bregma; 2.5 mm lateral to the midline; and 4 mm ventral to the pial-surface). The animals were killed at time intervals of 1, 2, 4, 8, 16 and 32 weeks following the injection of quinolinic acid. The animals used for the autoradiographic localization of receptors were killed by decapitation, the brains removed, frozen on dry ice and processed as detailed below. The animals to be used for the immunohistochemical localization of receptors were reanaesthetized and perfused through the heart with physiological saline (0.9% NaCl) followed by 500 ml of freshly prepared 4% paraformaldehyde and 0.1 – 2.5% glutaraldehyde in 0.1 M phosphate buffer at pH 7.4. The brains were removed from the skull, postfixed for 2 – 12 h and processed as detailed below.

Autoradiographic localization of $GABA_A$-benzodiazepine receptors

The frozen blocks of tissue from the control and Huntington's disease human basal ganglia and the frozen rat brains were mounted onto cryostat chucks, sectioned in the frontal plane at 16 μm using a cryostat, and the sections thaw-mounted onto gelatine/chrome-alum-coated slides. As detailed below, two adjacent series of slide-mounted sections were processed for the autoradiographic localization of benzodiazepine receptors: one series of sections was incubated with [^{3}H]flunitrazepam (a ligand with a high affinity for both Type I and Type II $GABA_A$-benzodiazepine receptors) in order to demonstrate the overall localization of $GABA_A$-benzodiazepine receptors and the second adjacent series of sections was incubated with [^{3}H]flunitrazepam in the presence of CL218,872 (a ligand with a high affinity for Type I and a low affinity for Type II $GABA_A$-benzodiazepine receptors (Klepner et al., 1979; Lo et al., 1982)) in order to show the localization of Type II $GABA_A$-benzodiazepine receptors. These autoradiographic receptor ligand binding studies were carried out as follows. Briefly, the sections were incubated in 50 mM Tris-HCl (pH 7.4) containing either 1 nM [^{3}H]flunitrazepam (84 Ci/mmole, Amersham) alone or in combination with 200 nM CL218,872 for 1 h. They were then washed (2 × 1 min in Tris-HCl buffer, dipped in distilled water) and dried under a stream of cold air. All the above steps were performed at 4°C. Non-specific [^{3}H]flunitrazepam binding was determined by incubation of slides in the presence if 1 μM clonazepam. Once dry, slides were brought to room temperature, taped into X-ray cassettes, apposed with [^{3}H]-sensitive Hyperfilm (Amersham) and exposed in the dark at 4°C for 6 – 10 weeks. The exposed films were developed in Kodak D19 for 4 min at 15°C, washed and fixed. The autoradiograms were printed using standard photographic procedures to yield reverse-image type autoradiograms where the autoradiographic labelled receptors appear as white dots on a black blackground (see Figs. 1, 3 and 5). Following development of the autoradiograms, the sections were counterstained for myelin and cell distribution.

A third adjacent series of slide-mounted sections was processed for acetylcholinesterase (AChE) histochemistry as previously described (Faull and Villiger, 1986).

Immunohistochemical localization of GABA$_A$-benzodiazepine receptors

The fixed blocks of human basal ganglia tissue and the fixed rat brains were sectioned in the coronal plane on a vibratome at a thickness of 50 – 70 μm. The sections were collected in phosphate-buffered saline (PBS) and processed for immunohistochemistry using a monoclonal antibody, bd-17, against the β$_{2,3}$ subunits of the GABA$_A$-benzodiazepine receptor complex. The preparation and characterization of this antibody has been previously described (Häring et al., 1985; Schoch et al., 1985; Richards et al., 1986, 1987b; Houser et al., 1988). The localization of the antibody was visualized using standard immunohistochemical methods as detailed below.

The sections were washed (3 × 10 min) in phosphate-buffered saline (PBS) containing 0.2%

Triton-X and then transferred to 50% methanol with 1% H$_2$O$_2$ for 30 min to aid penetration of the antibodies and to reduce non-specific background staining. The sections were then incubated for 1 h in 20% goat serum followed by incubation in the primary antibody (a hybridoma solution of bd-17 (Schoch et al., 1985)) for 2 – 3 days at 4°C (continuous agitation). The sections were then incubated in secondary antibody (biotinylated goat antimouse IgG, Sigma) at 1:500 overnight, then in ExtrAvidin® peroxidase conjugate (Sigma) at 1:1000 for 4 h. Following each of these steps the tissue was washed (3 × 10min) in PBS. The sections were then reacted for 15 min with 0.05% 3,3-diaminobenzidine tetrahydrochloride (Sigma) and 0.01% H$_2$O$_2$ (pH 7.4) in 0.1 M phosphate buffer, pH 7.4, to visualize the reaction product. The sections were then washed in PBS, mounted on chrome-alum slides, rinsed in distilled water and dehydrated through a graded alcohol series to xylene and coverslipped with DePeX (Serva).

Control sections to show non-specific labelling were processed as above except that the primary antibody was substituted by 1% goat serum.

Neuropathological analysis

In order to determine the extent and grade of the neuropathological changes in the basal ganglia and to confirm the chemical diagnosis of Huntington's disease, fixed tissue blocks from the basal ganglia of the Huntington's disease brains were routinely processed for histology and the sections stained and analysed according to the protocol and neuropathological grading criteria of Vonsattel and colleagues (Vonsattel et al., 1985; Myers et al., 1991).

Results

The aims of this study were two-fold. First, to compare the anatomical distribution of GABA$_A$-benzodiazepine receptors in the major nuclear complexes of the basal ganglia (the striatum and globus pallidus) in the normal and Huntington's disease human brain. Secondly, to investigate whether the same pattern of GABA$_A$-benzodiazepine receptor

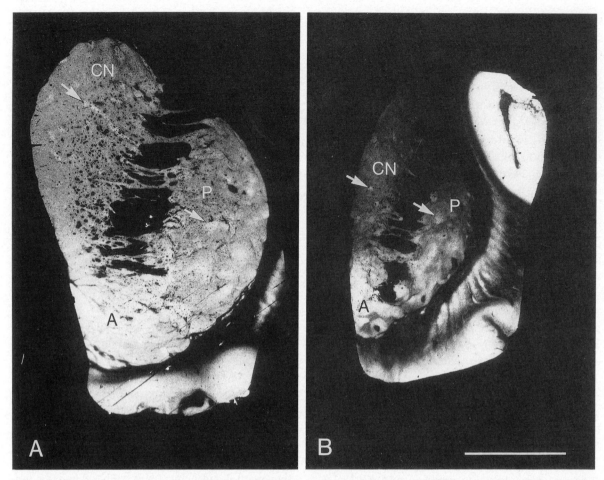

Fig. 1. Autoradiographic distribution of GABA$_A$-benzodiazepine receptors in the striatum of the normal and Huntington's disease brain. Autoradiograms showing the distribution of GABA$_A$-benzodiazepine receptors in transverse sections of the human striatum (comprised of the caudate nucleus, putamen, and nucleus accumbens) from *A,* a neurologically normal case, H8 (female, aged 43 years, 18 h post-mortem delay), and *B,* case HC13 (female, aged 57 years, 19 h post-mortem delay) who died with a clinical diagnosis of Huntington's disease. Neuropathological analysis of sections from case HC13 revealed advanced neuronal degeneration which was designated grade 3 using the five point (0 – 4) neuropathological grading scale of Vonsattel et al. (1985) (see text for further details). Sections *A* and *B* were incubated under identical conditions with 1 nM [^{3}H]flunitrazepam (a ligand with a high affinity for both Type I and Type II GABA$_A$-benzodiazepine receptors). The arrows in *A* and *B* indicate patches of high receptor density in the caudate nucleus and putamen. A, nucleus accumbens; CN, caudate nucleus; P, putamen. Scale bar, 1 cm.

changes is present in the basal ganglia of the quinolinic acid-lesioned animal model of Huntington's disease. In both the human and animal studies, the distribution of GABA$_A$-benzodiazepine receptors was investigated using autoradiography following in vitro labelling of cryostat sections with a tritiated ligand ([^{3}H]flunitrazepam) and immunohistochemical techniques with a monoclonal antibody (bd-17)

to the $\beta_{2,3}$ subunits of the GABA$_A$-benzodiazepine receptor complex.

The distribution of GABA$_A$-benzodiazepine receptors in the striatum and globus pallidus of the normal human brain

Striatum. The autoradiograms demonstrated

moderate to high concentrations of GABA$_A$-benzodiazepine receptors throughout all subdivisions of the normal striatum; namely the caudate nucleus, putamen and nucleus accumbens (Figs. 1*A*, 3*A*). The highest concentration of receptors in the striatum was consistently seen in the most ventral region, the nucleus accumbens (Fig. 1*A*). In the striatum the receptors were distributed in an uneven, complex, mosaic fashion where irregularly shaped patches of high densities of receptors were set

against a background matrix of lower receptor density (Figs. 1*A*, 3*A*).

The high-density patches of receptors were most clearly marked in the caudate nucleus where the edges of the patches were easily delineated from the background matrix region (Fig. 1*A*). The patches in the caudate nucleus showed considerable variation in size and shape; they varied from small, round and oblong shapes to slender, narrow (0.2 – 0.4 mm in width), elongated profiles measuring up to 7.0 mm

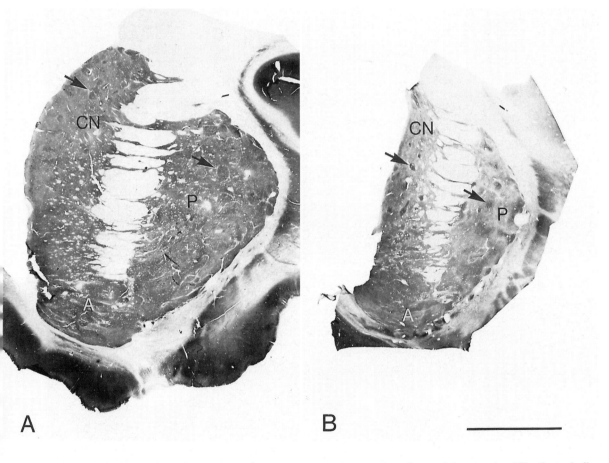

A

B

Fig. 2. Immunohistochemical distribution of GABA$_A$-benzodiazepine receptors in the striatum of the normal and Huntington's disease brain. Photomicrographs showing the distribution of GABA$_A$-benzodiazepine receptors in transverse sections of the human striatum (comprised of the caudate nucleus, putamen, and nucleus accumbens) from *A*, a neurologically normal case, H115 (male, aged 73 years, 13.3 h post-mortem delay) and *B*, case HC48 (male, aged 62 years, 20 h post-mortem delay) who died with a clinical diagnosis of Huntington's disease. Neuropathological analysis of sections from case HC48 revealed advanced neuronal degeneration which was designated grade 3 using the five point (0 – 4) neuropathological grading scale of Vonsattel et al. (1985) (see text for further details). Sections *A* and *B* were immunohistochemically processed following identical procedures using the monoclonal antibody bd-17 specific for the $\beta_{2,3}$ subunits of the GABA$_A$-benzodiazepine receptor complex. The arrows in *A* and *B* indicate patches of increased receptor immunoreactivity in the caudate nucleus and putamen. A, nucleus accumbens; CN, caudate nucleus; P, putamen. Scale bar, 1 cm.

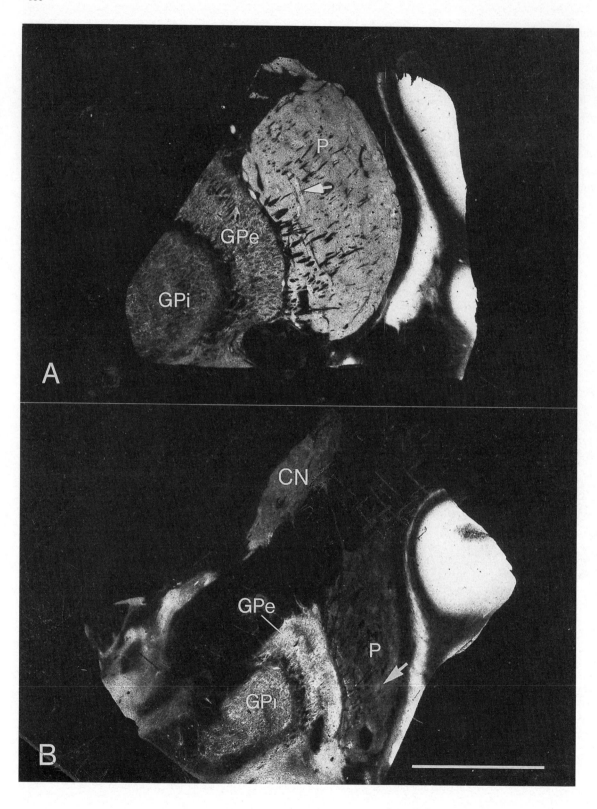

in length (Fig. 1A). In the putamen the autoradiograms showed that the patches were not so clearly distinguished as those in the caudate nucleus (Figs. 1A, 3A). In the putamen the patches generally appeared as rather poorly defined regions of higher densities of receptors which merged imperceptibly with the surrounding background matrix region of lower receptor densities. In anterior regions of the putamen (Fig. 1A) the patches appeared as rather diffuse regions of high receptor densities while at posterior levels, in the region of the lenticular nucleus (Fig. 3A), the patches were not easily distinguished in the autoradiograms and appeared considerably smaller and in the form of round or elongated profiles. In the nucleus accumbens the dense patches of receptors were especially conspicuous and occupied most of the region (Fig. 1A); here, the patches appeared as large, continuous, diffuse regions of very high receptor densities with minimal intervening matrix of lower receptor densities.

A very similar pattern of receptor distribution was seen in the striatum sections processed using immunohistochemical techniques and a monoclonal antibody to the $\beta_{2,3}$ subunits of the GABA$_A$-benzodiazepine receptor complex. GABA$_A$-benzodiazepine receptor immunoreactivity was distributed throughout all regions of the normal human striatum. In the caudate nucleus, small round to oval patches of dense immunoreactivity were set against a background matrix of less dense receptor immunoreactivity (Fig. 2A). In the putamen the patches of higher receptor immunoreactivity were less conspicuous (Fig. 2A) and not as easily distinguished as in the autoradiograms (Fig. 1A). In fact, at caudal levels of the putamen (Fig. 4A), receptor immunoreactivity appeared to be uniformly distributed with no clear evidence of the patches which were seen in the autoradiograms (Fig. 3A). In the

nucleus accumbens the density of receptor immunoreactivity was generally greater than that in the caudate nucleus and putamen although the difference in the intensity of staining was not as great as that seen in the autoradiograms.

Comparison of the localization of the GABA$_A$-benzodiazepine receptor patches in the caudate nucleus and putamen which were seen in the autoradiograms and the immunohistochemical sections with the pattern of AChE staining in adjacent sections showed that the high-density patches of receptors corresponded with the AChE-poor regions in the striatum.

Comparison of the density of autoradiographic labelling in adjacent sections of the striatum which had been incubated with [³H]flunitrazepam in the presence and absence of CL218,872 indicated that the striatum contained both Type I and Type II GABA$_A$-benzodiazepine receptors.

Globus pallidus. The pattern of distribution and density of GABA$_A$-benzodiazepine receptors in the normal human globus pallidus was virtually identical in both the autoradiograms (Fig. 3A) and in the sections processed for immunohistochemistry (Fig. 4A). In all cases (Figs. 3A, 4A), moderate to low concentrations of GABA$_A$-benzodiazepine receptors were present in both subdivisions of the globus pallidus. As demonstrated in both Fig. 3A and Fig. 4A, the concentration of receptors in the globus pallidus was markedly less than that in the adjacent putamen. Moderate densities of receptors were present in the external segment of the globus pallidus (GPe, Figs. 3A, 4A), while lower levels of receptors were present in the internal segment (GPi, Figs. 3A, 4A). By contrast with the patchy pattern of distibution of receptors in the striatum, the receptor labelling in the globus pallidus in both the autoradi-

Fig. 3. Autoradiographic distribution of GABA$_A$-benzodiazepine receptors in the lenticular nucleus of the normal and Huntington's disease brain. Autoradiograms showing the distribution of GABA$_A$-benzodiazepine receptors in transverse sections of the human lenticular nucleus (comprised of the putamen, globus pallidus externus and globus pallidus internus) from *A*, a neurologically normal case, H8, and *B*, case HC13 who died with a clinical diagnosis of Huntington's disease. Sections *A* and *B* were incubated under identical conditions with 1 nM [³H]flunitrazepam. See legend to Fig. 1 for further details. The arrows in *A* and *B* indicate patches of high receptor density in the putamen. GPe, globus pallidus externus; GPi, globus pallidus internus; P, putamen. Scale bar, 1 cm.

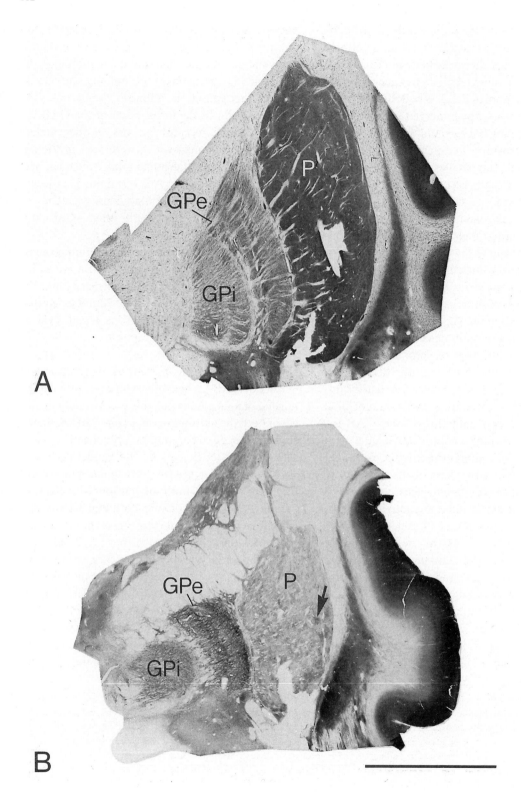

A

B

ograms (Fig. 3A) and in the immunohistochemical sections (Fig. 4A) appeared to be distributed in a honeycomb-like pattern; this pattern was especially evident in the more heavily labelled globus pallidus externus (Figs. 3A, 4A). Comparison of the autoradiograms with the original slide-mounted cryostat sections counterstained for myelin and cells showed that this pattern of labelling was due to the dispersed nature of the pallidal neuropil resulting from the presence of fascicles of heavily myelinated fibres traversing the globus pallidus.

Comparison of the density of labelling in adjacent sections of the globus pallidus which had been incubated with [^{3}H]flunitrazepam in the presence and absence of CL218,872 indicated that only Type I GABA$_A$-benzodiazepine receptors are present in the normal human globus pallidus.

The distribution of GABA$_A$-benzodiazepine receptors in the striatum and globus pallidus of the Huntington's disease human brain

The 23 cases of Huntington's disease which were examined in this study showed a variable extent of degeneration and atrophy of the striatum. The cases were graded using the grading scale of Vonsattel, Myers and colleagues (Vonsattel et al., 1985; Myers et al., 1991) who designated five grades (0 – 4) in ascending order of severity of neuropathological change in the basal ganglia: viz, grade 0 cases show no discernible loss of striatal neurons (Vonsattel et al., 1985) but an increased number of oligodendrocytes (Myers et al., 1991) while grade 4 cases show advanced macroscopical and microscopical neuropathological changes in the basal ganglia (Vonsattel et al., 1985; Myers et al., 1991). The 23 cases were graded as follows: three cases were designated grade 0; two cases showed minimum neuropathological

changes and were designated grade 1; seven cases showing moderate neuronal loss were grade 2; nine cases showed major neuronal loss and striatal atrophy and were designated grade 3; and two cases with very advanced neuropathology were graded stage 4.

In order to describe and illustrate the pattern of GABA$_A$-benzodiazepine receptors in Huntington's disease, the results in two representative grade 3 cases (case HC13, female, aged 57 years, 19 h post-mortem delay, Figs. 1B, 3B; and case HC48, male, aged 62 years, 20 h post-mortem delay, Figs. 2B, 4B) have been selected for detailed presentation.

The changes in the density and distribution of GABA$_A$-benzodiazepine receptors in Huntington's disease are best illustrated by comparison with the results from neurologically normal cases. In order to validate the comparison in each group of experiments, the sections from both the control and diseased tissue were normally processed together for receptor autoradiography or for receptor immunohistochemistry in an identical fashion using exactly the same procedures and incubation solutions. Also, control cases were selected which were matched as closely as possible for sex, age and post-mortem delay to the Huntington's cases.

Striatum. A comparison of the sections from the normal (Figs. 1A, 2A, 3A, 4A) and Huntington's disease (Figs. 1B, 2B, 3B, 4B) cases showed a dramatic loss of GABA$_A$-benzodiazepine receptors in the striatum in Huntington's disease. The overall pattern of receptor loss in the Huntington's cases was remarkably similar in the sections processed for receptor autoradiography (Figs. 1B, 3B) and receptor immunohistochemistry (Figs. 2B, 4B). The autoradiograms and the immunohistochemical sec-

Fig. 4. Immunohistochemical distribution of GABA$_A$-benzodiazepine receptors in the lenticular nucleus of the normal and Huntington's disease brain. Photomicrographs showing the distribution of GABA$_A$-benzodiazepine receptors in transverse sections of the human lenticular nucleus (comprised of the putamen, globus pallidus externus and globus pallidus internus) from A, a neurologically normal case H58 (male, aged 29 years, 4.5 h post-mortem delay) and B, case HC48 (male, aged 62 years, 20 h post-mortem delay) who died with a clinical diagnosis of Huntington's disease (see legend to Fig. 2 for further details). Sections A and B were immunohistochemically processed following identical procedures using the monoclonal antibody bd-17 specific for the $\beta_{2,3}$ subunits of the GABA$_A$-benzodiazepine receptor complex. The arrow in B indicates a patch of increased receptor immunoreactivity in the putamen. GPe, globus pallidus externus; GPi, globus pallidus internus; P, putamen. Scale bar, 1 cm.

tions both showed a major loss of receptors in the caudate nucleus and putamen. In the autoradiograms, the loss of receptors was especially marked in the caudate nucleus, the dorsal half of the rostral putamen and throughout the full extent of the caudal putamen (Figs. 1B, 3B). A similar regional pattern of receptor loss was seen in the sections processed for immunohistochemistry (Figs. 2B, 4B) except that the loss of receptor staining was less extensive being mainly localized to the dorsal half of the caudate nucleus (Fig. 2B). The extent of receptor loss in the putamen was virtually identical in the autoradiograms and immunohistochemical sections; viz, a major loss in the dorsal half of the rostral putamen (Figs. 1B, 2B) and an almost total loss in all regions of the caudal putamen (Figs. 3B, 4B).

Comparison of the regional pattern of receptor loss in representative cases of the various neuropathological gradings of the disease (i.e., from grade 0 to grade 4) showed that the pattern and extent of receptor loss closely followed the regional pattern of neuronal cell death which characterises the degenerative process in Huntington's disease (Vonsattel et al., 1985; Ferrante et al., 1987). Thus, the loss of receptors progressed from periventricular dorsomedial to ventral regions of the caudate nucleus and from dorsal to ventral regions of the putamen. In particular, at the very earliest stages of the disease, that is, in grade 0 cases which showed no detectable loss of striatal neurons, there was already a marked loss of receptors in the dorsal regions of · the caudate nucleus and putamen.

Of particular interest is the demonstration that in both the autoradiograms and immunohistochemical sections the pattern of receptor loss in the caudate nucleus and putamen occurred in a conspicuous heterogeneous fashion. This was especially evident in the caudate nucleus and rostral putamen where the remaining receptors were mainly concentrated into small patches surrounded by a background matrix of markedly reduced receptor staining (Figs. 1B, 2B). In the caudate nucleus the patches of receptors were well delineated with sharp boundaries and mainly small to round in shape (0.2 – 0.5 mm in diameter) (Figs. 1B, 2B). In the rostral putamen, however, the islands of receptor staining appeared less well defined with poorly delineated edges (Figs. 1B, 2B). Although the heterogeneous pattern of receptor loss was especially apparent in the caudate nucleus and rostral putamen, there was also evidence of a similar pattern of loss in the caudal putamen. This was especially apparent in the sections processed for immunohistochemistry (Fig. 4B) where a number of patches of receptors were evident against a background matrix showing virtually no receptor staining. These islands of receptor staining in the caudal putamen were not as conspicuous in the autoradiograms (Fig. 3B).

Comparison of this heterogeneous distribution of receptors with adjacent sections stained for AChE showed that the remaining patches of $GABA_A$-benzodiazepine receptors in the caudate nucleus and putamen corresponded with the AChE-poor striosomes.

By contrast with the major loss of receptors in the caudate nucleus and putamen of the dorsal striatum, the nucleus accumbens of the ventral striatum appeared to be relatively spared showing only minimal losses of receptors in the autoradiograms (Fig. 1B) and no clearly detectable loss of staining in the immunohistochemical sections (Fig. 2B).

Comparison of the density of autoradiographic labelling in adjacent sections of the striatum which had been incubated with [^{3}H]flunitrazepam in the presence and absence of CL218,872 showed that the receptor population remaining in the striatum in Huntington's disease contained both Type I and Type II $GABA_A$-benzodiazepine receptors.

An essentially similar pattern of receptor loss in the striatum was seen in the other Huntington's cases, with the extent of the receptor changes paralleling the grade of neuropathological degeneration in the striatum.

Globus pallidus. By contrast with the loss of receptors in the striatum, the globus pallidus showed a dramatic increase in $GABA_A$-benzodiazepine receptors in Huntington's disease (Figs. 3B, 4B). The increase in receptor staining was clearly evident in both the autoradiograms (Fig. 3B) and in the sections processed for receptor immuno-histochemistry (Fig. 4B). The increase in the receptor staining was especially conspicuous in the external segment of the globus pallidus; this increase was most obvious in the autoradiograms (Fig. 3B) but was also clearly evident with immunohistochemistry (Fig. 4B). The globus pallidus internus also consistently showed increased $GABA_A$-benzodiazepine receptor staining in Huntington's disease but the increase in staining was not as clearly marked as that in the external segment (Figs. 3A, 4A). As with the external segment receptor changes, the increase in receptors in the internal segment was more pronounced in the autoradiograms (Fig. 3B) than in the sections processed for immunohistochemistry (Fig. 4B).

Comparison of the density of autoradiographic labelling in adjacent sections of the globus pallidus which had been incubated with [³H]flunitrazepam in the presence and absence of the subtype discriminating ligand CL218,872 clearly showed that the increased number of receptors in the globus pallidus externus were mainly of the Type I $GABA_A$-benzodiazepine receptor variety.

This overall pattern of increased receptor staining in the globus pallidus was seen consistently in all cases of Huntington's disease using both receptor autoradiography and receptor immunohistochemistry. The extent of the increase in receptor staining closely followed the neuropathological grading with a progressively more intense pattern of staining in cases of more advanced neuropathology. Of special interest is the observation that the increased receptor staining was already clearly evident in the very earliest stages of the disease, i.e., in the grade 0 cases where neuropathological changes could not be detected.

The distribution of GABA_A-benzodiazepine receptors in the striatum and globus pallidus of the rat brain following unilateral quinolinic acid lesions in the striatum

Striatum. On the normal, unoperated side of the brain, $GABA_A$-benzodiazepine receptors were homogeneously distributed throughout the striatum (Fig. 5A). The extent of the quinolinic acid lesion on the operated right side of the striatum was clearly delineated in the autoradiograms by the region of receptor loss (Fig. 5A). At all survival times (1 – 32 weeks) there was virtually a total loss of receptors in the region of the lesion. The region of receptor loss on the lesioned side correlated exactly with the region of neuronal cell loss as verified by Nissl staining of the sections used to generate the autoradiograms.

Comparison of the density of autoradiographic labelling in adjacent sections which had been incubated with [³H]flunitrazepam in the presence and absence of CL218,872 showed that the receptor population in the rat striatum contained both Type I and II receptors, and that both types of receptors were lost in the region of the quinolinic acid lesion.

Globus pallidus. On the normal side, moderate densities of $GABA_A$-benzodiazepine receptors were distributed throughout the globus pallidus. On the lesioned side of the brain, there was a clearly delineated region of increased density of receptors in the globus pallidus which was evident as early as one week following the placement of the lesion and was detectable in autoradiograms at all subsequent survival times up to 32 weeks (Fig. 5B). This region of increase in receptor staining was also clearly evident in sections processed for receptor immuno-histochemistry (Fig. 6). The size and topography of the region of increased receptor staining in the globus pallidus varied with the size and topography of the striatal lesion. Most of the quinolinic acid lesions were placed in the dorsolateral two-thirds of the striatal complex (Fig. 5A) and the resulting region of increased receptor staining in the globus pallidus was localized in the lateral region of the ipsilateral globus pallidus (Figs. 5B, 6).

Autoradiographic studies on the subtype composition of the pallidal receptors showed that as in the Huntington's disease cases, the binding of 1 nM [³H]flunitrazepam in the rat globus pallidus was completely displaced by 200 nM CL218,872 on both the normal and lesioned sides indicating that the rat

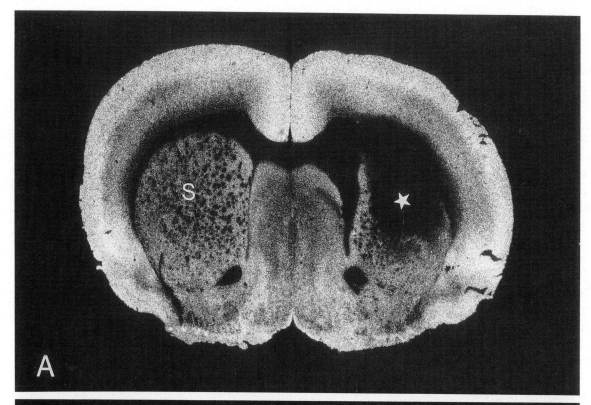

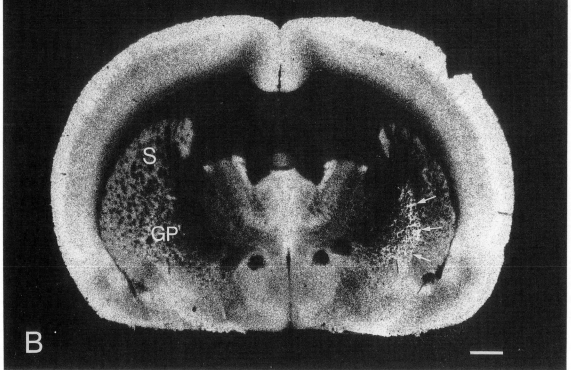

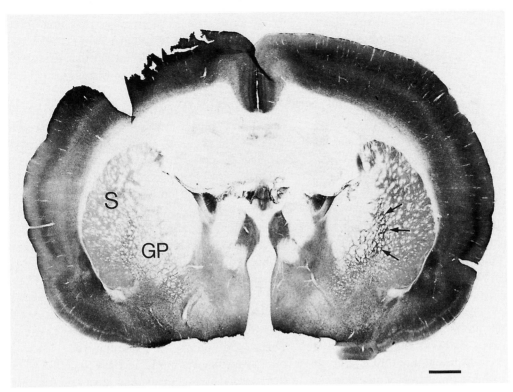

Fig. 6. Immunohistochemical distribution of GABA$_A$-benzodiazepine receptors in the globus pallidus of the rat following a quinolinic acid lesion in the striatum. Photomicrograph showing the distribution of GABA$_A$-benzodiazepine receptors in the globus pallidus following an injection of quinolinic acid in the right striatum of the rat in experiment QA86. The animal was killed 32 weeks following the injection and the section was immunohistochemically processed using the monoclonal antibody bd-17 specific for the $\beta_{2,3}$ subunits of the GABA$_A$-benzodiazepine receptor complex. The arrows indicate the region of increased receptor immunoreactivity in the right globus pallidus. GP, globus pallidus; S, striatum. Scale bar, 1 mm.

pallidal GABA$_A$-benzodiazepine receptors were of the Type I variety.

Discussion

This study provides a detailed analysis of the distribution of GABA$_A$-benzodiazepine receptors in the basal ganglia of the normal and Huntington's disease human brain and in the quinolinic acid-lesioned

rat model of Huntington's disease. The overall objective of this study was first to detail the major GABA$_A$-benzodiazepine receptor changes in Huntington's disease by comparison with the findings in the normal human brain and then to investigate whether the same pattern of receptor changes was present in the basal ganglia of the quinolinic acid-lesioned rat model of the disease. Here the separate findings on the normal and Huntington's disease

Fig. 5. Autoradiographic distribution of GABA$_A$-benzodiazepine receptors in the basal ganglia of the rat following a quinolinic acid lesion in the striatum. Autoradiograms showing the distribution of GABA$_A$-benzodiazepine receptors in A, the striatum and B, the globus pallidus following an injection of quinolinic acid in the right striatum of the rat in experiment QA15. The animal was killed two weeks following the injection and the sections incubated with 1 nM [^{3}H]flunitrazepam. The star in A indicates the region of the quinolinic acid lesion which is clearly delineated by the absence of GABA$_A$-benzodiazepine receptors. The arrows in B indicate the region of increased receptor density in the right globus pallidus. GP, globus pallidus; S, striatum. Scale bar, 1 mm.

human brain and on the animal model are first discussed before comparing and contrasting the results of these studies.

The distribution of GABA$_A$-benzodiazepine receptors in the striatum and globus pallidus of the normal human brain

The first aim of this study was to document the anatomical distribution of GABA$_A$-benzodiazepine receptors in the normal human basal ganglia using both receptor autoradiography and receptor immunohistochemistry. Previous studies on the distribution of GABA$_A$-benzodiazepine receptors in the human basal ganglia have only used receptor autoradiography following in vitro labelling of cryostat sections with tritiated ligands (Penney and Young, 1982; Walker et al., 1984; Whitehouse et al., 1985; Faull and Villiger, 1986, 1988; Penney and Pan, 1986). The additional use of immunohistochemistry in this study not only provides the opportunity to verify the receptor autoradiographic findings but by using subunit-specific monoclonal antibodies, important additional information can also be gained on the subunit composition of the receptors in the basal ganglia. Also, apart from our earlier quantitative autoradiographic studies (Faull and Villiger, 1986, 1988), the previous autoradiographic studies on GABA$_A$-benzodiazepine receptors in the human basal ganglia have been primarily directed towards receptor changes in Huntington's disease and have reported only briefly on the distribution of receptors in the basal ganglia of the normal human brain (Penney and Young, 1982; Walker et al., 1984; Whitehouse et al., 1985; Penney and Pan, 1986).

Striatum. The autoradiographic and immunohistochemical results show a similar regional pattern in the distribution of GABA$_A$-benzodiazepine receptors in the normal human striatum. That is, receptors are distributed throughout all subdivisions of the striatum with the highest density of receptors in the ventral striatum (Figs. 1*A*, 2*A*, 3*A*, 4*A*). In agreement with previous studies in the human (Penney and Young, 1982; Walker et al., 1984;

Whitehouse et al., 1985; Penney and Pan, 1986; Faull and Villiger, 1988), our findings showed that the density of receptors in the normal striatum is markedly higher than those in the globus pallidus (Figs. 3*A*, 4*A*).

Confirming our previous studies in the human (Faull and Villiger, 1986, 1988), one of the most striking features concerning the distribution of GABA$_A$-benzodiazepine receptors in the human striatum is the patchy distribution of receptors. This heterogeneous distribution of receptors is evident in both the autoradiograms (Figs. 1*A*, 3*A*) and immunohistochemical sections (Fig. 2*A*) and is most clearly delineated in autoradiograms of the dorsal striatum (i.e., caudate nucleus and putamen, Figs. 1*A*, 3*A*). As detailed and previously described (Faull and Villiger, 1986, 1988), the high-density patches of GABA$_A$-benzodiazepine receptors in the dorsal striatum align with the AChE-poor striosomes. Thus, the patchy distribution of GABA$_A$-benzodiazepine receptors appears to fit the same striosome/matrix compartmental mosaic organisation which has been demonstrated for other neurochemical markers in the striatum of the human and other mammalian brains (see Faull and Villiger, 1986, 1988; Faull et al., 1989; Graybiel, 1990).

Globus pallidus. As detailed in previous autoradiographic studies in the human (Penney and Young, 1982; Walker et al., 1984; Whitehouse et al., 1985; Penney and Pan, 1986; Faull and Villiger, 1988), our autoradiographic (Fig. 3*A*) and immunohistochemical (Fig. 4*A*) results clearly demonstrate that the globus pallidus in the normal human brain contains a much lower density of GABA$_A$-benzodiazepine receptors than the striatum, with the density of receptors in the internal segment of the globus pallidus being considerably lower than that in the external segment. Furthermore, in agreement with our earlier studies in the human (Faull and Villiger, 1988) and other studies in the rat (Young et al., 1981; Penney and Pan, 1986; Richards et al., 1987a), the GABA$_A$-benzodiazepine receptors in the globus pallidus are predominantly of the Type I variety. This is in contrast to the subtype composition of the receptors in the striatum, which comprise a mixture of Type I and Type II GABA$_A$-benzodiazepine receptors (Faull and Villiger, 1988).

The distribution of GABA$_A$-benzodiazepine receptors in the striatum and globus pallidus of the Huntington's disease human brain

Comparison of the distribution of GABA$_A$-benzodiazepine receptors in the basal ganglia in Huntington's disease with the results in normal cases clearly demonstrated that the Huntington's disease brains were distinguished by quite striking receptor changes which showed a consistent pattern in both the autoradiographic and immuno-histochemical studies (Figs. 1 – 4).

Striatum. The caudate nucleus and putamen consistently showed a marked loss of receptors; the extent of receptor loss reflected the degree of neuron degeneration as measured by the neuropathological grading. These findings confirm the results of previous autoradiographic studies (Penney and Young, 1982; Walker et al., 1984; Whitehouse et al., 1985; Penney and Pan, 1986) showing a reduction in caudate and putamen receptor binding sites without changes in affinity (Walker et al., 1984; Whitehouse et al., 1985; Penney and Pan, 1986).

The most novel and interesting finding in our studies is the demonstration that in Huntington's disease GABA$_A$-benzodiazepine receptors are not uniformly lost from both the matrix and striosome compartments of the striatum. Instead, our findings clearly demonstrate that receptors are selectively lost from the matrix compartment of the caudate nucleus and putamen (Figs. 1B, 2B) resulting in a relatively more intense receptor labelling of the patches which align with the AChE-poor zones in the striatum. This pattern of a selective GABA$_A$-benzodiazepine receptor loss in the striatal matrix in Huntington's disease is especially evident with immunohistochemistry (Fig. 2B).

The selective compartmental loss of GABA$_A$-benzodiazepine receptors observed in our studies is in agreement with other studies on Huntington's disease showing a marked loss of calbindin im-

munoreactivity in the striatal matrix zone (Seto-Ohshima et al., 1988), a selective reduction of the striatal AChE-rich matrix (Ferrante et al., 1987), and the results of a preliminary report indicating that dopamine, cholinergic and benzodiazepine receptors are enriched in AChE-poor regions of the striatum in Huntington's disease (Olsen et al., 1986). Taken together with our present results, these findings all suggest that it is the matrix compartment of the striatum that is primarily affected in Huntington's disease. However, in a recent study on the pattern of NADPH-diaphorase staining in the striatum in Huntington's disease, we have shown that in the very early stages of the disease (grade 0), there is a selective loss of NADPH staining in the regions of the neuropil which correspond with the AChE-poor striosomes and that at later stages of the disease both the striosome and matrix compartments are affected (Morton et al., 1993). These collective findings demonstrate that Huntington's disease is not simply a matrix compartment disease but rather is a much more complex neurodegenerative process that variably affects both the matrix and striosome compartments depending on the neurochemical parameter under study. Clearly, the significance of the compartmental pattern of chemical anatomical changes in the striatum in Huntington's disease will not be elucidated until we have a better understanding of the pathogenesis of the disease and of the neuronal and compartmental localization of the various neurotransmitters and receptors in the normal striatum.

Globus pallidus. The most dramatic change in GABA$_A$-benzodiazepine receptors in Huntington's disease was seen in the globus pallidus. The autoradiographic (Fig. 3B) and immunohistochemical (Fig. 4B) studies consistently showed a marked increase in receptor staining in the globus pallidus. The increase in staining was especially pronounced in the globus palidus externus which contrasted with the virtual total loss of receptors in the immediately adjacent putamen (Figs. 3B, 4B). Previous autoradiographic studies have also demonstrated an increase in pallidal receptors in Huntington's disease (Penney and Young, 1982; Walker et al., 1984; Whitehouse et al., 1985; Penney and Pan, 1986) showing that the increase in receptor staining is due to an increase in receptor numbers without changes in affinity. This dramatic increase in $GABA_A$-benzodiazepine receptors in the globus pallidus was evident in the very earliest stages of the disease (i.e., grade 0 cases) where it was not possible to detect neurodegenerative changes in the striatum.

Our autoradiographic studies have shown that the $GABA_A$-benzodiazepine receptors in the globus pallidus in the normal and Huntington's disease human brain and in the rat brain are predominantly of the Type I variety. Since the localization of receptors in the globus pallidus can also be demonstrated using immunohistochemistry and subunit-specific monoclonal antibodies, then clearly, these findings can be used to indicate the subunit configuration of the Type I receptor. Molecular biological cloning studies have identified that the $GABA_A$ receptor complex is comprised of four different classes of subunits designated α, β, γ and δ (for review, see Möhler et al., 1991) and that there are at least six α-subunits (α_{1-6}), three β-subunits (β_{1-3}), two γ-subunits ($\gamma_{1,2}$) and one δ-subunit (Möhler et al., 1990 and Olsen and Tobin, 1990). Furthermore, recent in situ hybridization studies (Wisden et al., 1989) and pharmacological studies (Pritchett et al., 1989; Lüddens and Wisden, 1991) suggest that the Type I $GABA_A$-benzodiazepine receptor has the $\alpha_1 \beta_x \gamma_2$ (where β_x is any β subunit) subunit configuration. Our immunohistochemical findings suggest that the $\beta_{2,3}$ subunits are components of the Type I $GABA_A$-benzodiazepine receptor complex in the globus pallidus. Clearly, in situ hybridization studies using the subunit-specific oligonucleotide probes and/or further immunohistochemical studies using additional subunit-specific monoclonal antibodies are necessary in order to precisely specify the overall subunit composition of the $GABA_A$ pallidal receptors in the human and rat brain.

Our autoradiographic and immunohistochemical studies on $GABA_A$-benzodiazepine receptors in the basal ganglia in Huntington's disease clearly demonstrate that there is a *contrasting pattern of receptor changes in the striatum and globus pallidus in Huntington's disease* and that this pattern of receptor change is present from the very earliest stages of the disease before there is any detectable striatal neuronal loss (i.e., grade 0). The change in the striatum is characterized by a major loss of receptors from the caudate-putamen which selectively affects the matrix compartment. By contrast, there is a dramatic increase of $GABA_A$-benzodiazepine receptors in the globus pallidus. Our studies therefore suggest that Huntington's disease is characterised by a reversal in the striato-pallidal ratio of $GABA_A$-benzodiazepine receptors. Since these findings have been consistent in all 23 cases of Huntington's disease included in this study, we suggest that this pattern of $GABA_A$-benzodiazepine receptor changes in the basal ganglia is pathognomonic for Huntington's disease and therefore may serve as a reliable criterion for the post-mortem diagnosis of Huntington's disease and for distinguishing it from other neurological diseases.

The distribution of $GABA_A$-benzodiazepine receptors in the striatum and globus pallidus of the quinolinic acid-lesioned rat model of Huntington's disease

In order to investigate whether the pattern of $GABA_A$-benzodiazepine receptor changes in the basal ganglia in Huntington's disease is replicated in the basal ganglia of the quinolinic acid-lesioned rat model of Huntington's disease, receptor autoradiographic and receptor immunohistochemical studies were undertaken following unilateral quinolinic lesions of the striatum in the rat. The results showed that there was virtually a total loss of $GABA_A$-benzodiazepine receptors in the region of the quinolinic acid lesion and that at all survival times studied (1–32 weeks) the lesion resulted in an increase of Type I $GABA_A$-benzodiazepine receptors in the ipsilateral globus pallidus (the homologue of the globus pallidus externus in the human brain).

Thus, there is a remarkable similarity in the general pattern of $GABA_A$-benzodiazepine receptor changes in Huntington's disease and in the quinolinic acid-lesioned rat. Both the human and rat basal ganglia show a loss of receptors in the striatum and an increase of Type I GABA$_A$-benzodiazepine receptors in the ipsilateral globus pallidus. The only major difference between the two species is that in the human striatum the receptor loss occurs in the matrix compartment, whereas in the rat the loss occurs throughout the full extent of the striatal lesion area and does not differentiate between the matrix and striosome compartments. It is interesting that Pan and colleagues (Pan et al., 1984; Penney and Pan, 1986) have shown that striatal lesions in the rat induced by another excitotoxin, kainic acid, similarly resulted in an increase of GABA$_A$-benzodiazepine receptors in the globus pallidus. However, in contrast to our finding of an increase in Type I receptors in the globus pallidus one week after placement of a quinolinic acid lesion, Pan et al. (Pan et al., 1984; Penney and Pan, 1986) showed that kainic acid lesions in the striatum resulted in an increase of Type II GABA$_A$-benzodiazepine receptors in the globus pallidus 2 – 3 months after placement of the lesion. It is difficult to reconcile the differences in the time course and the receptor subtype resulting from the two different excitotoxic lesions since presumably in both cases the increase in the GABA$_A$-benzodiazepine receptors is the result of denervation supersensitivity of receptors in the globus pallidus following the loss of GABAergic afferents from the striatum.

Irrespective of these differences, it is clear from our results that the quinolinic acid-lesioned rat is a useful experimental model for studying the possible mechanisms that may be involved in the receptor changes that occur in the basal ganglia of the human brain in Huntington's disease. In particular, it would be of enormous benefit to our understanding of GABA$_A$ receptors to identify the intracellular events which provide the link between GABAergic denervation of the globus pallidus and the activation of the appropriate GABA$_A$ subunit genes in pallidal neurons to effect the increase in the production of Type I GABA$_A$-benzodiazepine receptors. These questions cannot be readily answered from human studies, but can be addressed using the quinolinic acid-lesioned rat. Such studies using the animal model should provide vital new information on the neuronal mechanisms involved in the monitoring and control of GABA$_A$ receptors in the mammalian brain and thus enable a better understanding of the neurochemical changes in Huntington's disease.

Acknowledgements

This study was supported by grants from the Health Research Council of New Zealand, the New Zealand Neurological Foundation and the New Zealand Lottery Board.

References

Beal, M.F., Kowall, N.W., Ellison, D.W., Mazurek, M.F., Swartz, K.J. and Martin, J.B. (1986) Replication of the neurochemical characteristics of Huntington's disease by quinolinic acid. *Nature,* 321: 168 – 171.

Beal, M.F., Kowall, N.W., Swartz, K.J., Ferrante, R.J. and Martin, J.B. (1989) Differential sparing of somatostatin-neuropeptide Y and cholinergic neurons following striatal excitotoxin lesions. *Synapse,* 3: 38 – 47.

Boegman, R.J., Smith, Y. and Parent, A. (1987) Quinolinic acid does not spare striatal neuropeptide Y-immunoreactive neurons. *Brain Res.,* 415: 178 – 182.

Davies, S.W. and Roberts, P.J. (1987) No evidence for preservation of somatostatin-containing neurons after intrastriatal injections of quinolinic acid. *Nature,* 327: 326 – 329.

Dawbarn, D., De Quidt, M.E. and Emson, P.C. (1985) Survival of basal ganglia neuropeptide Y-somatostatin neurones in Huntington's disease. *Brain Res.,* 340: 251 – 260.

DiFiglia, M. (1990) Excitotoxic injury of the neostriatum: a model for Huntington's disease. *Trends Neurosci.,* 13: 286 – 289.

Ellison, D.W., Beal, M.F., Mazurek, M.F., Malloy, J.R., Bird, E.D. and Martin, J.B. (1987) Amino acid neurotransmitter abnormalities in Huntington's disease and the quinolinic acid animal model of Huntington's disease. *Brain,* 110: 1657 – 1673.

Faull, R.L.M. and Villiger, J.W. (1986) Heterogeneous distribution of benzodiazepine receptors in the human striatum: a quantitative autoradiographic study comparing the pattern of receptor labelling with the distribution of acetylcholinesterase staining. *Brain Res.,* 381: 153 – 158.

Faull, R.L.M. and Villiger, J.W. (1988) Multiple benzodiazepine receptors in the human basal ganglia: a detailed pharmacological and anatomical study. *Neuroscience,* 24: 433 – 451.

Faull, R.L.M., Dragunow, M. and Villiger, J.W. (1989) The distribution of neurotensin receptors and acetylcholinesterase in the human caudate nucleus: evidence for the existence of a third neurochemical compartment. *Brain Res., 488*: 381 – 386.

Ferrante, R.J., Kowall, N.W., Beal, M.F., Richardson, E.P., Bird, E.D. and Martin, J.B. (1985) Selective sparing of a class of striatal neurons in Huntington's disease. *Science, 230*: 561 – 563.

Ferrante, R.J., Kowall, N.W., Beal, M.F., Martin, J.B., Bird, E.D. and Richardson, E.P. (1987) Morphologic and histochemical characteristics of a spared subset of striatal neurons in Huntington's disease. *J. Neuropathol. Exp. Neurol., 46*: 12 – 27.

Graveland, G.A., Williams, R.S. and DiFiglia, M. (1985) Evidence for degenerative and regenerative changes in neostriatal spiny neurons in Huntington's disease. *Science, 227*: 770 – 773.

Graybiel, A.M. (1990) Neurotransmitters and neuromodulators in the basal ganglia. *Trends Neurosci., 13*: 244 – 254.

Gusella, J.F., Wexler, N.S., Conneally, P.M., Naylor, S.L., Anderson, M.A., Tanzi, R.E., Watkins, P.C., Ottina, K., Wallace, M.R., Sakaguchi, A.Y., Young, A.B., Shoulson, I., Bonilla, E. and Martin, J.B. (1983) A polymorphic DNA marker genetically linked to Huntington's disease. *Nature, 306*: 234 – 238.

Häring, P., Stähli, C., Schoch, P., Takács, B., Staehelin, T. and Möhler, H. (1985) Monoclonal antibodies reveal structural homogeneity of γ-aminobutyric acid/benzodiazepine receptors in different brain areas. *Proc. Natl. Acad. Sci. U.S.A., 82*: 4837 – 4841.

Hayden, M.R. (1981) *Huntington's Chorea,* Springer, New York, 192 pp.

Houser, C.R., Olsen, R.W., Richards, J.G. and Möhler, H. (1988) Immunohistochemical localization of benzodiazepine/GABA$_A$ receptors in the human hippocampal formation. *J. Neurosci., 8*: 1370 – 1383.

Klepner, C.A., Lippa, A., Benson, D.I., Sano, M.C. and Beer, B. (1979) Resolution of two biochemically and pharmacologically distinct benzodiazepine receptors. *Pharmacol. Biochem. Behav., 11*: 457 – 462.

Kowall, N.W., Ferrante, R.J. and Martin, J.B. (1987) Patterns of cell loss in Huntington's disease. *Trends Neurosci., 10*: 24 – 29.

Lo, M.M., Strittmatter, S.M. and Snyder, S.H. (1982) Physical separation and characterization of two types of benzodiazepine receptors. *Proc. Natl. Acad. Sci. U.S.A., 79*: 680 – 684.

Lüddens, H. and Wisden, W. (1991) Function and pharmacology of multiple GABA$_A$ receptor subunits. *Trends Pharmacol Sci., 12*: 49 – 51.

Martin, J.B. and Gusella, J.F. (1986) Huntington's disease. Pathogenesis and management. *N. Engl. J. Med., 315*: 1267 – 1276.

Möhler, H., Malherbe, P., Draguhn, A. and Richards, J.G. (1990) GABA$_A$-receptors: structural requirements and sites of gene expression in mammalian brain. *Neurochem. Res., 15*: 199 – 207.

Möhler, H., Malherbe, P., Richards, J.G., Persohn, E., Benke, D., Barth, M., Rhyner, T. and Sigel, E. (1991) GABA$_A$-receptor gene expression and regulation. In: E. Coata (Ed.), *Neurotransmitter Regulation of Gene Transcription – Fidia Research Foundation Series, Vol. 7,* Thieme, New York, pp. 111 – 124.

Morton, A.J., Nicholson, L.F.B. and Faull, R.L.M. (1993) Compartmental loss of NADPH diaphorase in the neuropil of the human striatum in Huntington's disease. *Neuroscience, 53*: 159 – 168.

Myers, R.H., Vonsattel, J.P., Paskevich, P.A., Kiely, D.K., Stevens, T.J., Cupples, L.A., Richardson, E.P. and Bird, E.D. (1991) Decreased neuronal and increased oligodendroglial densities in Huntington's disease caudate nucleus. *J. Neuropathol. Exp. Neurol., 50*: 729 – 742.

Olsen, J.M.M., Penney, J.B., Shoulson, I. and Young, A.B. (1986) Inhomogeneities of striatal receptor binding in Huntington's disease. *Neurology, 36*: 342.

Olson, R.W. and Tobin, A.J. (1990) Molecular biology of GABA$_A$-receptors. *FASEB J., 4*: 1469 – 1480.

Pan, H.S., Penney, J.B. and Young, A.B. (1984) Characterization of benzodiazepine receptor changes in substantia nigra, globus pallidus and entopeduncular nucleus after striatal lesions. *J. Pharmacol. Exp. Ther., 230*: 768 – 775.

Penney, J.B. and Pan, H.S. (1986) Quantitative autoradiography of GABA and benzodiazepine binding in studies of mammalian and human basal ganglia function. In: C.A. Boast, E.W. Snowhill and C.A. Altar (Eds.), *Quantitative Receptor Autoradiography,* Alan R. Liss, New York, pp. 29 – 52.

Penney, J.B. and Young, A.B. (1982) Quantitative autoradiography of neurotransmitter receptors in Huntington disease. *Neurology, 32*: 1391 – 1395.

Pritchett, D.B., Lüddens, H. and Seeburg, P.H. (1989) Type I and Type II GABA$_A$ benzodiazepine receptors produced in transfected cells. *Science, 245*: 1389 – 1392.

Reisine, T.D., Wastek, G.J., Speth, R.C., Bird, E.D. and Yamamura, H.I. (1979) Alterations in the benzodiazepine receptor of Huntington's diseased human brain. *Brain Res., 165*: 183 – 187.

Reisine, T.D., Overstreet, D., Gale, K., Rossor, M., Iversen, L. and Yamamura, H.I. (1980) Benzodiazepine receptors: the effect of GABA on their characteristics in human brain and their alteration in Huntington's disease. *Brain Res., 199*: 79 – 88.

Richards, J.G., Möhler, H. and Haefely, W. (1986) Mapping benzodiazepine receptors in the CNS by radiohistochemistry and immunohistochemistry. In: P. Panula, H. Paivarinta and S. Soinila (Eds.), *Neurohistochemistry: Modern Methods and Applications,* Alan R. Liss, New York, pp. 629 – 677.

Richards, J.G., Möhler, H. and Haefely, W. (1987a) Benzodiazepine receptors and their ligands. In: G.N. Woodruff (Ed.), *Mechanisms of Drug Action,* Macmillan, London, pp. 131 – 176.

Richards, J.G., Schoch, P., Häring, P., Takacs, B. and Möhler, H. (1987b) Resolving GABA$_A$/benzodiazepine receptors: cellular and subcellular localization in the CNS with monoclonal antibodies. *J. Neurosci.,* 7: 1866–1886.

Schoch, P., Richards, J.G., Häring, P., Takacs, B., Stähli, C., Staehelin, T., Haefely, W. and Möhler, H. (1985) Co-localization of GABA$_A$ receptors and benzodiazepine receptors in the brain shown by monoclonal antibodies. *Nature,* 314: 168–171.

Schwarcz, R., Whetsell, W.O. and Mangano, R.M. (1983) Quinolinic acid: an endogenous metabolite that produces axon-sparing lesions in rat brain. *Science,* 219: 316–318.

Seto-Ohshima, A., Emson, P.C., Lawson, E., Mountjoy, C.Q. and Carrasco, L.H. (1988) Loss of matrix calcium-binding protein-containing neurons in Huntington's disease. *Lancet,* ii: 1252–1255.

Vonsattel, J-P., Myers, R.H., Stevens, T.J., Ferrante, R.J., Bird, E.D. and Richardson, E.P. (1985) Neuropathological classification of Huntington's disease. *J. Neuropathol. Exp.*

Neurol., 44: 559–577.

Walker, F.O., Young, A.B., Penney, J.B., Dovorini-Zis, K. and Shoulson, I. (1984) Benzodiazepine and GABA receptors in early Huntington's disease. *Neurology,* 34: 1237–1240.

Whitehouse, P.J., Trifiletti, R.R., Jones, B.E., Folstein, S., Price, D.L., Snyder, S.H. and Kuhar, M.J. (1985) Neurotransmitter receptor alterations in Huntington's disease: autoradiographic and homogenate studies with special reference to benzodiazepine receptor complexes. *Ann. Neurol.,* 18: 202–210.

Wisden, W., Morris, B.J., Darlison, M.G., Hunt, S.P. and Barnard, E.A. (1989) Localization of GABA$_A$ receptor α subunit mRNAs in relation to receptor subtypes. *Mol. Brain Res.,* 5: 305–310.

Young, W., Niehoff, D.L., Kuhar, M.J., Beer, B. and Lippa, A.S. (1981) Multiple benzodiazepine receptor localization by light microscopic radiohistochemistry. *J. Pharmacol. Exp. Ther.,* 216: 425–430.

G.W. Arbuthnott and P.C. Emson (Eds.)
Progress in Brain Research, Vol. 99
© 1993 Elsevier Science Publishers B.V. All rights reserved.

CHAPTER 8

Chemical signalling in the globus pallidus in parkinsonism

Jonathan Brotchie, Alan Crossman, Ian Mitchell, Susan Duty, Camille Carroll, Alison
Cooper, Brian Henry, Neill Hughes and Yannick Maneuf

*Experimental Neurology and Myology Group, Department of Cell and Structural Biology, Medical School, University of
Manchester, Manchester M13 9PT, U.K.*

Introduction

Dysfunction of the basal ganglia results in a wide range of movement disorders ranging from those characterised by reductions in voluntary movement, e.g., Parkinson's disease, through to those characterised by increased, or inappropriate, movements, e.g., chorea, hemiballism. The last five years have witnessed remarkable progress in our understanding of the neural signalling underlying the symptomatology of such diseases, especially parkinsonism. This work has led to a greater appreciation of the neural mechanisms underlying both physiological and pathophysiological motor control. Additionally, several approaches that might provide novel means of therapeutic intervention in these basal ganglia-related disorders have been proposed. The current chapter will present some of our more recent data, taking chemical signalling by excitatory amino acids, neuropeptides and ATP-sensitive potassium channels as examples, to illustrate this point with regard to Parkinson's disease.

Background

It has become widely accepted that the basal ganglia represent one of the major centres involved in the control of movement in the mammalian brain.

The role of the basal ganglia in this respect might be described as being: (i) the collation of information from diverse regions of the brain to provide a representation of the environment, including current motor state; and (ii) the processing of information to provide an output to the cortex (via the thalamus) and other motor centres such as the pedunculopontine nucleus, that can coordinate motor programmes.

The neural mechanisms required for such control of voluntary movement must undoubtedly be of great complexity given the many degrees of freedom in which the body must move and maintain posture (Jordan, 1989; Nguyen and Widrow, 1989). Given the relatively slow speed of neuronal processing, it might be anticipated that the biological correlate of such a computationally intensive task would be reflected in a high level of neuroanatomical sophistication within the basal ganglia. Indeed, basal ganglia structure does appear to reflect this requirement. At one level this is seen in the organisation of connections between and within constituent nuclei, e.g., many recurrent connections, overlap of "receptive fields". An additional level of structural complexity is imparted by the use of multiple chemical signals. Such molecules interact with each other in complex ways to enrich neurotransmission. These neuromodulators represent a diverse range of molecules including the "classical" transmitters (e.g., dopamine, GABA and the excitatory amino acids (EAAs)), peptides (enkephalins and substance P) and intracellular messengers (e.g., cAMP and

ATP). A small selection of the chemical signals used within the basal ganglia will form the focus of this chapter.

Parkinson's disease is characterised classically by a triad of symptoms, namely hypokinesia, rigidity and tremor. The primary pathology underlying these symptoms is widely recognised as being degeneration of dopaminergic cells in the substantia nigra pars compacta which project to the striatum. Most current therapies for parkinsonism rely on replacement of this decreased dopamine transmission in the striatum. However, whilst such therapies can provide remarkable improvements in symptomatology, especially in the short term, they are not without their problems (Marsden, 1977). Parkinsonian patients chronically treated with dopaminergic agents invariably develop dyskinetic side effects such as dystonia or chorea. Such iatrogenic side effects can eventually become more debilitating than the underlying Parkinson's disease. We have therefore become interested in developing ideas that might lead to alternative treatment strategies for parkinsonism which are not based on the direct manipulation of striatal dopamine systems. The approach we have taken is to investigate the abnormalities of neuronal signalling within the basal ganglia that result from the initial pathology in the dopaminergic nigrostriatal system.

Neural mechanisms underlying parkinsonism

Functional anatomy

A detailed theoretical model of the neural mechanisms mediating parkinsonian symptoms has been constructed on the basis of data from several laboratories utilising techniques including 2-deoxyglucose metabolic tracing, electrophysiology, in situ mRNA hybridization, behavioural pharmacology and neurochemical receptor studies (Penney and Young, 1986; Mitchell et al., 1989). The work described below comes from an increasing body of data acquired from the MPTP-treated primate, the 6-hydroxydopamine-treated rat and the reserpine-treated rat models of parkinsonism.

In terms of functional anatomy it has become in-creasingly useful to describe the basal ganglia as a series of sequential connections of constituent nuclei. As already alluded to, the dopaminergic substantia nigra pars compacta projects to the striatum. The striatum projects to the lateral segment of the globus pallidus (globus pallidus in the rat). This pathway uses GABA and a peptide, enkephalin, as its neurotransmitters. The lateral segment of the globus pallidus influences the subthalamic nucleus with a GABAergic pathway. The subthalamic nucleus projects massively to the output regions of the basal ganglia, that is the medial segment of the globus pallidus (entopeduncular nucleus in the rat) and the substantia nigra pars reticulata. These subthalamic efferents are thought to use an excitatory amino acid (EAA) as their transmitter (Brotchie and Crossman, 1991). The medial pallidal segment and the substantia nigra pars reticulata also receive direct projections from the striatum. These pathways utilise GABA and the peptides substance P and dynorphin as their transmitters. Recently, the lateral pallidal segment has been shown to send a large GABAergic projection to both the medial pallidal segment and the substantia nigra pars reticulata; this pathway may be of great functional significance (Hazrati et al., 1990).

Striatum. In the simplest form of the model of the neural mechanisms underlying parkinsonism, a sequence of events is initiated by loss of the dopaminergic cells of the substantia nigra pars compacta. Dopamine is thought to have functionally opposite effects on those striatal cells that project to the lateral pallidal segment compared to those projecting to the medial pallidal segment and substantia nigra (Pan et al., 1985). Dopamine is thought to inhibit striatal neurons projecting to the lateral pallidal segment but excite those neurons projecting directly to the medial segment and substantia nigra. The degeneration of the dopaminergic input to the striatum therefore leads to two distinct effects:

(i) Disinhibition of GABA/enkephalin striatal cells that project to the lateral segment of the globus pallidus. The striato-lateral-pallidal projection is therefore rendered overactive.

(ii) Inhibition of GABA/substance P/dynorphin projections to the medial pallidal segment and substantia nigra.

Lateral segment of the globus pallidus. The suggestion of increased activity in the striato-lateral-pallidal pathway is supported by several lines of evidence. Hence, in the MPTP-treated primate, increased terminal activity, assessed by 2-deoxyglucose metabolic tracing, is observed in the lateral segment of the globus pallidus (Mitchell et al., 1989). Increases in GABA release are also implied by findings that GABA and benzodiazepine receptor numbers are down-regulated in the parkinsonian lateral pallidal segment in the MPTP-treated primate and in the globus pallidus of 6-hydroxydopamine-treated rat models of parkinsonism (Pan et al., 1985). Evidence of increased enkephalinergic transmission in the striatopallidal projection has also been provided. In the 6-hydroxydopamine-induced model of parkinsonism in the rat, increased enkephalin is found in the globus pallidus (Engber et al., 1991). In the parkinsonian striatum increased mRNA for pre-proenkephalin has been demonstrated using in situ hybridisation techniques in both MPTP-treated primates and 6-hydroxydopamine-treated rats (Augood et al., 1989; Gerfen et al., 1990; Frayne et al., 1991).

The consequence of this overactivity in the striatopallidal projection is excessive inhibition of the lateral segment of the globus pallidus which thus becomes abnormally underactive in the parkinsonian state. Two consequences arise from the resulting underactivity of the GABAergic efferents from lateral pallidal segment:

(i) Reduced inhibition of the subthalamic nucleus. The subthalamic nucleus is therefore overactive.

(ii) Reduced inhibition of the medial pallidal segment and substantia nigra pars reticulata.

Subthalamic nucleus. The proposition that the subthalamic nucleus is overactive in parkinsonism due to decreased inhibition from the lateral pallidal segment is supported by behavioural, electrophysiological and metabolic tracing experiments. 2-

Deoxyglucose tracing studies suggest that in parkinsonism there is decreased terminal activity in the area of the subthalamic nucleus receiving input from the lateral pallidal segment (Mitchell et al., 1989). Electrophysiological recording in the MPTP-treated primate shows a marked increase in the mean firing rate of neurons of the subthalamic nucleus (Wichmann et al., 1990). However, perhaps the most exciting finding relating to this point are the reports that lesion of the subthalamic nucleus can alleviate parkinsonian symptoms (Bergman et al., 1990; Aziz et al., 1991). These findings may have great clinical relevance especially in the light of reports that marked bilateral anti-parkinsonian effects are seen following unilateral lesion of the subthalamic nucleus with radiofrequency lesion generators of a type used routinely in neurosurgical clinics (Aziz et al., 1991).

The subthalamic nucleus is thought to use an excitatory amino acid, probably glutamate, as its neurotransmitter (Brotchie and Crossman, 1991). We therefore suppose that the regions of the basal ganglia receiving input from the subthalamic nucleus, the medial pallidal segment and substantia nigra pars reticulata receive excessive excitation in parkinsonism.

Medial pallidal segment and substantia nigra pars reticulata. As has been described above, in parkinsonism the output regions of the basal ganglia receive abnormal inputs from three sources: (i) overactive EAA input from the subthalamic nucleus; (ii) underactive GABA/substance P/dynorphin input from the striatum; and (iii) underactive GABA input from the lateral segment of the globus pallidus. All of these abnormal afferents tend to have the same effect, that is to increase the activity of the output neurons of the medial pallidal segment and substantia nigra pars reticulata. Such increased activity is found electrophysiologically in MPTP-treated primates (Miller and Delong, 1987; Filion et al., 1988).

The abnormalities in the inputs from the subthalamic nucleus and lateral pallidal segment have been discussed in the relevant sections above. The evidence for parkinsonism being characterised by decreased activity of the striatal neurons projecting to the medial pallidal segment and substantia nigra pars reticulata comes from two sources. Firstly, in both the MPTP-treated primate and the 6-hydroxydopamine-treated rat there is an up-regulation of GABA receptors and the allosterically linked benzodiazepine receptors suggesting decreased GABA transmission (Pan et al., 1985). Secondly, both in situ mRNA hybridisation and immunocytochemistry report significant decreases in the synthesis and levels of substance P by striatal outputs to these regions (Gerfen et al., 1990; Engber et al., 1991). Smaller decreases are also seen in the synthesis and levels of dynorphin.

Summary. It is now generally considered that the major changes in neural activity that accompany parkinsonian symptoms are:

(i) Decreased activity in the dopaminergic nigro-striatal pathway.

(ii) Increased activity in the GABA/enkephalin striato-lateral-pallidal pathway.

(iii) Increased activity of the subthalamic nucleus.

(iv) Increased activity of the regions of the basal ganglia that project to non-basal ganglia motor regions, i.e., the medial pallidal segment and the substantia nigra pars reticulata.

This theoretical model, though very simple, appears to describe the neural mechanisms underlying parkinsonism remarkably well. Basal ganglia manipulations that reverse the neural dysfunction proposed by the scheme are surprisingly successful in alleviating parkinsonian symptoms. For instance, injections of the GABA antagonist bicuculline directly into the globus pallidus of the reserpine-induced rat model of parkinsonism provide dose-dependent reversal of parkinsonian symptoms (Fig. 4). The mechanism underlying this effect is presumed to be blockade of the overactive GABA input from the striatum suggested by the model.

In order to enrich the representation of basal ganglia function by the theoretical model described above we have recently begun to investigate the way in which the diversity of chemical signals used by each of the given connections might interact both with each other and at the molecular level within the neuron. In our work to date we have concentrated on three aspects on basal ganglia function:

(i) The receptor pharmacology employed by the EAA-utilising projection from the subthalamic nucleus to the medial pallidal segment.

(ii) The role of peptide neuromodulators in striatofugal pathways.

(iii) The role of ATP-sensitive potassium channels in modulating neurotransmitter release.

EAA transmission in subthalamic nucleus efferents

Throughout the last decade, considerable basic pharmacological research has elucidated several receptor subtypes involved in EAA transmission. At least four receptor subtypes have been proposed (NMDA, AMPA, kainate and ACPD). Additionally, several other possible receptors have been proposed (e.g., APB), and many sites that modulate transmission at the NMDA receptor have been described (e.g., glycine and PCP site) (Collingridge and Lester, 1989). In addition to the main subtypes of EAA receptors a further tier of organisation probably exists. Several distinct molecular forms of both NMDA and non-NMDA receptors have been proposed on the basis of sequence data from molecular cloning experiments (Kutsuwada et al., 1992). In the case of the NMDA receptors there is also evidence from pharmacological studies that subtypes of NMDA receptors exist (Thomson et al., 1985; Monaghan et al., 1988; Monaghan, 1991; Monaghan and Beaton, 1991).

Given the proposal that the outputs of the subthalamic nucleus to the medial pallidal segment are overactive in parkinsonism we hypothesised that antagonism of EAA transmission in the medial pallidal segment would have anti-parkinsonian actions. Local blockade of EAA transmission by intracerebral injections of the broad spectrum EAA receptor antagonist kynurenate in the medial pallidal segment of the MPTP-treated macaque and marmoset were found to reverse parkinsonian symptoms (Graham et al., 1990; Brotchie et al., 1991). Similar anti-parkinsonian effects are also seen following injections of kynurenate in the entopeduncular nucleus of the rat in the 6-hydroxydopamine and reserpine-induced models of parkinsonism (Brotchie et al., 1990, 1991). Klockgether and colleagues have shown anti-parkinsonian effects of single doses of the NMDA receptor-specific compound CPP (Klockgether and Turski, 1990) and the AMPA-specific compound NBQX (Klockgether et al., 1991) in the reserpine-treated rat.

The subtype of EAA receptor utilised by a given pathway has enormous bearing on the mode of neural processing in which any synapse can participate. For instance, the activated NMDA receptor causes excitatory post-synaptic potentials (EPSPs) of very long duration, which are sensitive to the membrane potential, and signal via an influx of Ca^{2+}. In contrast, the AMPA receptor, when activated, causes fast, non-voltage-sensitive, excitatory currents carried almost solely by Na^+ and K^+. If our model of basal ganglia function is to progress to an appreciation of the means by which different chemical messengers might interact, the starting point must surely include an understanding of the signalling mecha-

nisms employed by each of the separate transmitters.

The aim of the experiments presented in this section was to define which EAA receptor subtype(s) is (are) involved in the anti-parkinsonian effects of EAA antagonism in the medial pallidal segment/entopeduncular nucleus of the MPTP-treated marmoset and the reserpinised rat.

In the rodent experiments, rats were rendered parkinsonian by subcutaneous injection of reserpine (5 mg/kg). After 18 h a parkinsonian syndrome was seen that was stable for at least 6 h. During this time injections were made into the entopeduncular nucleus via previously implanted cannulae. The pharmacological selectivity of the different antagonists used is shown in Table I. A total of 279 injections were made within the entopeduncular nucleus. A wide variety of the compounds active at EAA-mediated synapses were capable of alleviating reserpine-induced akinesia following unilateral injection in the entopeduncular nucleus (see Table II). The list of compounds having anti-parkinsonian actions included agents acting selectively at both the NMDA receptor-ionophore complex (CPP, AP7, MK-801, 7-chlorokynurenate and HA-966) and non-NMDA receptors (CNQX). Surprisingly, the

TABLE I

Pharmacological specificity of EAA antagonists injected into the medial pallidal segment

	"NMDA"			AMPA	Kainate
	NMDA	PCP	glycine		
Kynurenate	***	–	***	***	***
CPP	****	–	–	–	–
CNQX	–	–	*	****	****
MK-801	–	****	–	–	–
APV	****	–	–	–	–
7-Cl-KYN	–	–	****	–	–
HA-966	–	–	***	–	–

The table illustrates the approximate potency and selectivity of each of the EAA antagonists injected into the medial pallidal segment of the MPTP-treated marmoset and the reserpinised rat. The number of asterisks represents the approximate potency of a compound as an antagonist at a particular receptor; –, denotes little significant effect. Abbreviations: 7-Cl-KYN, 7-chlorokynurenate; APV, 2-amino-5-phosphonovaleric acid; CNQX, 6-cyano-7-nitroquinoxaline-2,3-dione; CPP, 3-(carboxypiperazin-4-yl)-propyl-1-phosphonic acid.

130

TABLE II

Pharmacological profile of EAA antagonism in alleviating reserpine-induced akinesia

Compound	EC$_{50}$ (mM)	Threshold (mM)
CPP	21.4	2.0
MK-801	21.6	2.7
D-AP7	53.5	7.2
7-Cl-KYN	59.0	3.7
HA-966	87.6	11.7
Kynurenate	106.2	10.9
CNQX	117.9	11.1
D-APV	NE	NE
L-APV	NE	NE

Compounds are displayed in order of potency (as estimated by EC$_{50}$) in alleviating akinesia following unilateral injection in the entopeduncular nucleus of the reserpine-treated rat model of parkinsonism. Drugs that had no anti-akinetic effect are denoted by NE. Anti-parkinsonian effects were assessed as described in Brotchie et al. (1991)

prototypical NMDA receptor antagonist APV had no anti-parkinsonian effects (Fig. 1).

In all cases the anti-parkinsonian effects were very similar to those described previously with kynurenate (Brotchie et al., 1991). The anti-parkinsonian effects were dose-dependent and reversible. For some compounds the dose – response curves for the anti-parkinsonian effects were bell-shaped (Fig. 1). Compounds that produced bell-shaped dose – response curves were either NMDA receptor antagonists, e.g., CPP, or NMDA channel blockers, e.g., MK-801. Compounds acting at non-NMDA receptors, e.g., CNQX, or at the NMDA receptor-associated glycine site, e.g., 7-chlorokynurenate, did not exhibit this phenomenon.

Similar findings were also seen following injections of subtype-specific EAA antagonists in the medial pallidal segment of MPTP-treated marmoset. In this study eleven adult marmosets (*Callithrix jacchus*) were rendered parkinsonian by administration of MPTP (6 mg/kg, Brotchie et al., 1991; Close and Elliot, 1991). Bilateral intracerebral injections of EAA antagonists were made into the

medial pallidal segment. Injections of the NMDA receptor antagonist CPP, the NMDA receptor-associated glycine site antagonist 7-chloro-kynurenate, and the non-NMDA antagonist CNQX all alleviated parkinsonian symptoms (Fig. 2). As in the rodent study, these effects were dose-dependent. Again the NMDA receptor antagonist CPP ex-

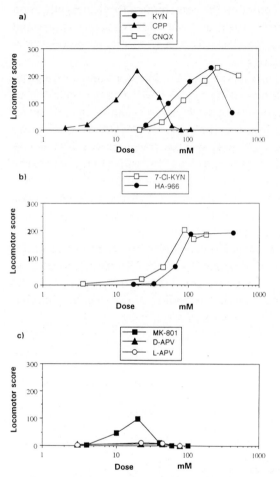

Fig. 1. Pharmacology of reversal of reserpine-induced parkinsonism by EAA antagonist injections in the entopeduncular nucleus. The figure shows the dose – response curves for the effects of EAA antagonists injected unilaterally into the entopeduncular nucleus in reserpine-treated parkinsonian rats. Locomotor scores, measured in arbitrary locomotor units (ALUs) per 15 min, are shown following each injection (Brotchie et al., 1991). Each point represents the median of three injections at different sites. Compounds shown are:- (*a*) KYN, CPP and CNQX; (*b*) the glycine site antagonists 7-Cl-KYN and HA-966; (*c*) MK-801, D-APV and L-APV. Abbreviations as in Table I.

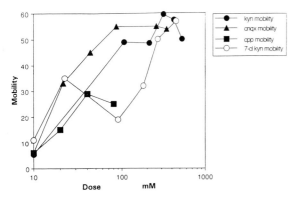

Fig. 2. Pharmacology of reversal of MPTP-induced parkinsonism by EAA antagonist injections in the medial pallidal segment in the marmoset. This figure shows the dose–response curves for the anti-parkinsonian effects of injections into the medial pallidal segment of antagonists with different specificity profiles for EAA receptor subtypes. Dose is plotted against a measure of mobility as determined by a clinical rating scale (Brotchie et al., 1991).

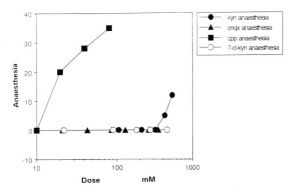

Fig. 3. Pharmacology of anaesthetic side effects in the MPTP-treated marmoset following EAA antagonist injections in the medial pallidal segment. This figure shows dose–response curves for the anaesthetic effects of injections of antagonists with different specificity profiles for EAA receptor subtypes into the medial pallidal segment of the MPTP-treated marmoset. Dose is plotted against anaesthesia score. The anaesthesia score represents the number of minutes during which anaesthesia was observed in the 40 min period immediately post-injection.

hibited a bell-shaped dose–response curve with regard to its anti-parkinsonian action.

Given the propensity of some NMDA antagonists to cause anaesthesia, e.g., ketamine (Thomson et al., 1985), we also assessed the presence of anaesthesia in MPTP-treated marmosets following the in-

tracerebral injections. Neither 7-chlorokynurenate nor CNQX produced any anaesthetic-like symptoms. However, CPP injections were followed by symptoms characteristic of dissociative anaesthesia (Fig. 3). These anaesthetic effects were dose-dependent. We propose that the bell-shape and lower maximal value of the dose–response curve for the anti-parkinsonian effects of CPP are due at least in part to the appearance of anaesthesia which impairs the mobility of the animal. We also suggest that similar mechanisms may underlie the bell-shaped dose–response curves for the anti-parkinsonian effects of some NMDA antagonists in the reserpinised rat.

From both sets of experiments we conclude that in the medial segment of the pallidal complex, both the NMDA channel and associated receptors, and non-NMDA receptors are involved in the mechanisms underlying parkinsonian symptoms. Antagonism of any of these receptors in the medial pallidal segment can alleviate parkinsonian symptoms. EAA antagonists acting at the NMDA or PCP receptors also induce dissociative anaesthesia. However, glycine site or non-NMDA antagonists

TABLE III

Pharmacological profile of EAA antagonism in alleviating MPTP-induced parkinsonism and inducing dissociative anaesthesia

Compound	EC$_{50}$ (mM)	
	Anti-parkinsonian effects	Anaesthetic effects
CPP	18	17
CNQX	20	> 300
Kynurenate	44	> 300
7-Cl-KYN	108	> 300

Compounds are displayed in order of potency (as estimated by EC$_{50}$) in increasing mobility following bilateral injection in the medial pallidal segment of the MPTP-treated marmoset model of parkinsonism. Mobility and anaesthesia were assessed as defined in Figs. 2 and 3 and by Brotchie et al. (1991) and Close et al. (1992).

only have anti-parkinsonian effects in the medial pallidal segment.

The anaesthetic effects of CPP in the marmoset highlight a potential problem with the idea of using EAA antagonists as a systemic treatment for Parkinson's disease. Indeed, the appearance of anaesthetic side effects may be responsible for the inability of MK 801 to alleviate parkinsonian symptoms when injected systemically in the MPTP-treated macaque (Crossman et al., 1989). However, as it does appear possible to dissociate the anti-parkinsonian effects of EAA antagonism from the anaesthetic effects several potential therapeutic approaches to parkinsonism using EAA antagonists do become apparent. Either non-NMDA receptors or the NMDA receptors-associated glycine site might be useful targets for EAA antagonist therapies in parkinsonism as these receptors do not appear to be involved in the mediation of anaesthesia.

We propose that of these two possibilities, glycine site manipulation is potentially the most fruitful with regard to novel therapies. Glycine site antagonism would allow transmission at non-NMDA systems. This would thus allow the vast majority of excitatory transmission to proceed normally. A further advantage of glycine site manipulation is the current availability of partial agonists which act to attenuate NMDA transmission without abolishing it altogether (Pullan et al., 1991). Partial glycine site agonists may alleviate parkinsonian symptoms whilst permitting NMDA transmission to occur at a level which would avoid compromising other NMDA-associated processes such as memory and other important cognitive processes (Morris et al., 1986). Various forms of experimentally induced dyskinesia are thought to be mediated via abnormally low levels of EAA transmission in the medial pallidal segment (e.g., Robertson et al., 1989). Partial agonists at the glycine site might be less likely to lead to dyskinetic side effects than would be the case if EAA transmission was abolished altogether.

A further potential approach to selectively alleviating parkinsonism without eliciting anaesthesia may also be suggested by the lack of anti-parkinsonian effects seen with APV. This is in ap-

parent contradiction to the potent anti-akinetic effects of several other antagonists at the NMDA channel complex. APV has been shown to have NMDA antagonist action in a variety of in vivo preparations in other areas of the brain (Morris et al., 1986; Salt, 1986). This paradox may be resolved by the suggestion that separate subtypes of the NMDA receptor-ionophore complex are involved in the anti-parkinsonian effects as opposed to the anaesthetic effects of EAA antagonism. The presence of multiple subtypes of NMDA receptors has gained increasing credence recently (Monaghan et al., 1988; Stone and Burton, 1988; Monaghan, 1991; Monaghan and Beaton, 1991; Kutsuwada et al., 1992). The NMDA complex is now thought to represent a heterodimeric complex of two protein subunits. An active NMDA receptor-ionophore complex is assembled from a NR1 subunit and an NR2 subunit. At present, there are thought to be four subtypes of the NR2 subunit which are expressed in different anatomical regions. The identity of the NR2 subunit appears to determine to a large extent the pharmacological characteristics of the channel when expressed in *Xenopus* oocytes (Kutsuwada et al., 1992). The apparent efficacy of glycine antagonists, e.g., 7-chlorokynurenate, and ineffectiveness of APV in alleviating parkinsonian symptoms is very similar to the pharmacological profile of the NMDA receptors composed of NR1/NR2c or NR1/NR2b NMDA subunits. If this is the case it may become possible, with the development of novel antagonists, to alleviate parkinsonism with EAA antagonists selective for specific subtypes of NMDA receptors without affecting EAA transmission in areas where other subtypes of NMDA receptors are concentrated.

Peptides in striatal outputs

The basal ganglia appear to be one of the major areas of the vertebrate brain which take advantage of peptide co-transmission.

These peptidergic systems are most obvious in the striatum. In the striatum a wide variety of peptides are expressed. Individual peptide transmitters are localised in distinct populations of striatal output cells. These striatal output neurons use GABA and a peptide, normally thought to subserve a modulatory role, as their transmitters. The peptides used by striatal outputs for this role are the opioids met-enkephalin and dynorphin, and the neurokinin substance P.

In rat striatum, three quarters of the substance P-positive neurons contain dynorphin and vice versa. However, enkephalin is found in very few (< 5%) of the substance P neurons and in virtually none of the dynorphin neurons (Anderson and Reiner, 1990). This split between substance P/dynorphin and enkephalin-utilising cells appears to have been conserved throughout evolution and may be of great functional significance. Hence, similar patterns of distribution are seen in the striata of the primate, cat, bird and reptile (Anderson and Reiner, 1990; Besson et al., 1990).

An additional level of organisation in the partitioning of striatal peptides is seen when considering the basal ganglia region to which a striatal output

neuron projects. Met-enkephalin is co-localised with GABA in the striatal neurons projecting to the lateral pallidal segment (rodent globus pallidus). In contrast, substance P and dynorphin are used by the striatal neurons projecting to the medial pallidal segment (rodent entopeduncular nucleus) and the substantia nigra. Given this well-defined neurochemical dichotomy the striatal output system has hence been suggested as a ideal system in which to study peptide modulation of neurotransmission. The functional properties provided by partitioning populations of striatal output cells in terms of their peptide transmitters remain to be elucidated. We have begun to address this issue by investigating the role of enkephalin in modulating GABA transmission in the striatal projection to the rat globus pallidus.

Using behavioural pharmacology strategies in catecholamine-depleted rats (reserpine, 5 mg/kg, s.c.) we have shown that the behavioural effects of GABAergic transmission in the globus pallidus are modulated by manipulations of opioid transmission. Local GABA antagonism by bicuculline injection in the globus pallidus increases locomotor activity in rats rendered parkinsonian by systemic injection of reserpine (Fig. 4). These anti-akinetic effects are thought to be due to blockade of the GABAergic input from the striatum which is suggested as being overactive in parkinsonism. These anti-parkinsonian effects are dose-dependent. The EC_{50} for the effects is 0.78 μM. Injections of the opioid antagonist naloxone (0.005 – 0.1 M), to antagonise the effects of endogenous enkephalin, have no effect on parkinsonian symptoms. However, when a dose – response curve for the anti-parkinsonian effect of bicuculline is constructed in the presence of co-injected 0.1 M naloxone the EC_{50} of the parkinsonian effects of bicuculline is increased to 1.40 μM. These data are illustrated in Fig. 4. From this experiment we concluded that enkephalin antagonists reduce the behavioural effects of GABA antagonists. This finding suggests functionally opposing roles for the amino acid and peptide in controlling the activity of the globus pallidus. We suggested that enkephalin co-transmission

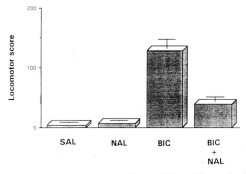

Fig. 4. Anti-parkinsonian effects of bicuculline and naloxone injections in the globus pallidus of the reserpine-treated rat. This figure illustrates the effects of unilateral intracerebral injections in the globus pallidus in the reserpine-treated rat model of parkinsonism. Following injection of bicuculline (0.8 μM) marked locomotor activity was observed. Following injection of saline or naloxone (0.1 M) no anti-parkinsonian action was observed. Following co-injection of bicuculline (0.8 μM) and naloxone (0.1 M) increased locomotor activity was observed but this was significantly different from that seen in the presence of bicuculline alone ($P < 0.05$, ANOVA, THSD). Locomotor activity is measured in arbitrary locomotor units per 15 min as described elsewhere (Brotchie et al., 1991). Abbreviations: BIC, 0.8 μM bicuculline; SAL, saline; NAL, 0.1 M naloxone.

134

with GABA in striatopallidal neurons attenuates the effects of GABA.

In the homologous region of the ventral portion of the basal ganglia, the ventral pallidum, a similar situation is found (Austin and Kalivas, 1990). Both GABA antagonists or mu-opioid agonists increase locomotor activity. These results again suggest opposing actions of the two transmitter systems. Again, evidence of functional interactions between the two systems at the behavioural level was also seen. However, neither behavioural study described above proffered evidence of direct interactions between the transmitter systems.

In the globus pallidus, mu-opioid receptors thought to interact with transmitter enkephalin are localised, at least in part, on the terminals of affer-

ents from the striatum (Abou-Khalil et al., 1984). We proposed that these receptors may provide a site for direct interaction between GABA and opioids. We have begun to elucidate in vitro the mechanisms by which such interactions might occur. An assay was developed to measure release of GABA from terminals in the globus pallidus.

Briefly, slices of globus pallidus were incubated in artificial cerebrospinal fluid (aCSF, 30°C, pH 7.4, aerated with 95% O_2/5% CO_2) containing 1 μM [^{3}H]GABA, in the presence of the GABA transaminase inhibitor amino-oxyacetic acid, to load terminals of striatopallidal fibres with labelled GABA. The pallidal slice was washed and the release of loaded transmitter measured. Release of [^{3}H] labelled GABA was measured every 5 min. Release was expressed as a fractional release rate (percentage of that present at the start of each time interval). For the purpose of this experiment, neurotransmitter release was defined as the Ca^{2+}-dependent release evoked by the addition of 5 min pulses of 40 mM K^+ to the aCSF. The Ca^{2+} dependency of the release was demonstrated by replacing $CaCl_2$ in the aCSF with $CoCl_2$.

Met-enkephalin caused marked reductions in Ca^{2+}-dependent K^+-evoked GABA release from slices of globus pallidus pre-loaded with [^{3}H] GABA (Fig. 5). This effect was dose-dependent, the IC_{50} being 0.53 μM (Fig. 6). This attenuation of GABA release by enkephalin was itself antagonised by the opiate antagonist naloxone (5 mM). On the

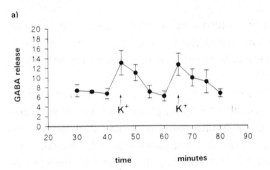

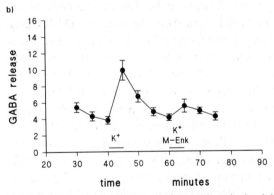

Fig. 5. Effect of met-enkephalin on GABA release in the globus pallidus. This figure shows GABA release from 400 μm slices of globus pallidus pre-loaded with [^{3}H]GABA (method as described in text and Amoroso et al., 1990). GABA release is expressed as percentage fractional release. (*a*) Pulses of K^+ (40 mM) evoke reproducible peaks of GABA release. (*b*) Met-enkephalin (M-Enk, 10 nM) added to the second K^+ pulse inhibits GABA release to 23% of the control value observed in the presence of vehicle ($P < 0.05$, $n = 6$, ANOVA).

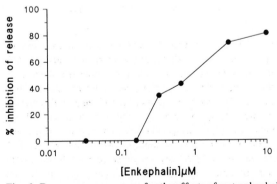

Fig. 6. Dose – response curves for the effects of met-enkephalin in attenuating GABA release in the globus pallidus. This figure shows the dose dependency of met-enkephalin inhibition of K^+-evoked [^{3}H]GABA release in the globus pallidus.

basis of these in vitro data we propose that the modulation of GABAergic transmission by opioids in the globus pallidus, described in behavioural experiments, may result, at least in part, from a presynaptic mechanism causing decreased GABA release.

These conclusions from both the in vivo and in vitro experiments presented here lead to interesting speculations regarding the functional roles of GABA and enkephalin in parkinsonism. Both neurotransmitters appear to be released in abnormally high levels in the lateral pallidal segment in parkinsonism (see above). However, as they have apparently opposing actions we have been led to speculate that, in simple terms at least, the role of increased enkephalinergic transmission in parkinsonism is to compensate for excessive GABAergic transmission. In this way it is suggested that increases in enkephalin synthesis in parkinsonism are not part of the neural mechanisms responsible for the symptomatology, but actually serve to limit the symptoms to some extent. Compensatory mechanisms such as this may help explain why very large reductions in dopaminergic transmission in the striatum ($>$ 90%) are required before parkinsonian symptoms are observed.

ATP-sensitive potassium channels

In the past decade, complex ionophores have become de rigueur in neurobiology. The ability of an ion channel to integrate signals from several sources has been shown to have great functional significance, e.g., the voltage-sensitive nature of EAA-induced opening of the NMDA ionophore has important consequences for learning and memory, as well as giving insight into the pathophysiology of epilepsy and stroke.

The ATP-sensitive potassium channel (K_{ATP}) is another example of a complex ionophore capable of integrating numerous and disparate chemical signals. In the pancreas, K_{ATP}s have been known to perform a vital role in the regulation of insulin release. The major class of non-insulin therapies for diabetes mellitus are the sulphonylureas, e.g., tol-butamide and glibenclamide. Sulphonylureas exert their actions by blockade of K_{ATP}s. However, it is only recently that clues have begun to emerge which describe the role K_{ATP}s might play in modulating neurotransmission in the CNS, particularly in the output regions of the basal ganglia.

A neural K_{ATP} would confer important properties on neurons that would enrich their processing ability. These properties would result from the diversity of regulatory signals which are known to modulate this channel in the pancreas, e.g., intracellular ATP and Ca^{2+} levels, sulphonylureas, peptides such as somatostatin and galanin. Chemical signals within the neuron derived from distinct signalling systems, e.g., ions, second messengers and metabolic status, could thus be integrated by neurons possessing K_{ATP}s. These integrative functions of the K_{ATP} impart the pancreas with the ability to control insulin secretion tightly in response not only to blood glucose levels (and hence intracellular ATP) but also in relationship to the levels of other insulin-controlling factors, e.g., levels of somatostatin. In a similar way it might be speculated that the K_{ATP} along with other highly regulated ionophores would provide the molecular basis for the complex neuronal hardware undoubtedly required to perform computationally intensive tasks of which the control of movement is a prime example. The sensitivity of the channel to ATP levels might allow the neuron to represent a temporal aspect of information. As the length of time for which a neuron was firing increased, the intracellular ATP levels would fall, so blocking the K_{ATP}. Such temporal representation by a chemical signal would be required for computational problems such as motor control which undoubtedly involve the recognition and generation of sequential information.

A sulphonylurea binding site has recently been identified in homogenate preparations from whole pig brain using [^{3}H]glibenclamide binding assays. The pharmacology of the CNS effects of sulphonylureas and the results from $^{86}Rb^+$ efflux experiments are indicative that this sulphonylurea binding site is indeed an ATP-sensitive potassium channel similar to that found in the periphery

(Amoroso, 1990). The regional distribution of this sulphonylurea binding site within the rat brain has been studied using [3H]glibenclamide (Mourre, 1990; Treherne and Ashford, 1991) and [125I]glyburide (Gehlert, 1991) receptor autoradiography. Interestingly, in these studies, the sulphonylurea binding sites were found to be selectively concentrated in the basal ganglia, specifically in the globus pallidus, entopeduncular nucleus and substantia nigra pars reticulata. We have conducted experiments to define the cellular location of these K_{ATP}s in the basal ganglia.

Unilateral quinolinic acid lesions (5 μg) were made in the striatum to lesion the terminals of the striatal projection to the globus pallidus, entopeduncular nucleus and substantia nigra pars reticulata. After a survival period of 14 days, which has been found to maximise terminal degeneration, the animals were sacrificed and the brains removed and snap frozen. [3H]glibenclamide was used to quantify K_{ATP} channel numbers using a standard autoradiographic binding assay (20 μm cryostat cut sections incubated in [3H]glibenclamide (2.5 nM, in 40 mM Hepes · NaOH (pH 7.5) at 4°C for 60 min)). Lesions were located and quantified using PK 11195 autoradiography (Benavides et al., 1990).

Following lesion of the striatum significant reductions in the numbers of sulphonylurea binding sites were seen in the globus pallidus, entopeduncular nucleus and substantia nigra pars reticulata (decreases of 40%, 11% and 24%, respectively, $P < 0.05$, paired t-test with Bonferroni correction, $n = 6$). No significant changes were seen in other brain regions. We interpret these data as suggesting that K_{ATP}s in the globus pallidus, entopeduncular nucleus and substantia nigra are localised, at least in part, pre-synaptically on terminals of axons originating in the striatum. Such a location would place the K_{ATP} in an ideal location to "monitor" terminal activity in striatal efferents and regulate the release of GABA from such terminals.

In the globus pallidus and substantia nigra pars reticulata we and others investigated the effects of sulphonylureas in modulating GABA release. The techniques used were essentially those described

above for investigating the modulation of GABA release by enkephalin. A range of sulphonylureas have been shown to have potent actions in evoking release of GABA from pallidal and nigral slices pre-loaded with [3H]GABA (e.g., Fig. 7, Amoroso et al., 1990). Conversely, diazoxide, a K_{ATP} opener in the periphery, causes reductions in the K^+-evoked release of [3H]GABA from slices of the globus pallidus pre-loaded with [3H]GABA (Fig. 8). The mechanism by which K_{ATP} blockade increases GABA release is suggested as being the same as that proposed for the similar increases in insulin release in the pancreas. Blockade of a potassium conductance limits hyperpolarisation, leading to some depolarisation of the membrane potential. This depolarisation causes a rise in intracellular Ca^{2+} levels which, in turn, leads to increased transmitter release by Ca^{2+}-dependent exocytosis.

Further evidence for a role of K_{ATP}s in modulating GABA transmission involved in the control of movement is proffered by behavioural data. It has previously been reported that injections of a range of sulphonylureas into the substantia nigra pars reticulata of rats result in circling behaviour (Levesque and Greenfield, 1991). Furthermore, intracerebral injection of the K_{ATP} opener diazoxide in the globus pallidus in the reserpine-treated rat alleviates parkinsonian symptoms (Fig. 9). As parkin-

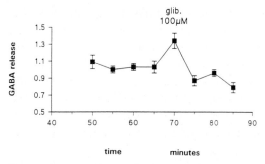

Fig. 7. Effect of glibenclamide on GABA release in the globus pallidus. This figure shows GABA release from 400 μm slices of globus pallidus pre-loaded with [3H]GABA (method as described in text and Amoroso et al., 1990). GABA release is expressed as percentage fractional release. Glibenclamide (100 μM) added to the superperfusion medium caused a significant increase in the release of GABA compared to baseline levels ($P < 0.05$, $n = 6$, paired t-test).

sonism is thought to be characterised by increased GABA release in the globus pallidus these effects are in keeping with our in vitro [³H]GABA release studies described above showing that diazoxide reduces GABA release in the globus pallidus.

Additionally, injections of the sulphonylurea tolbutamide in the entopeduncular nucleus and substantia nigra pars reticulata of the parkinsonian rat alleviate akinesia (Fig. 10). This finding may have important clinical implications. The neural activity in both these regions is thought to be abnormally increased in parkinsonism. To date all manipulations

in primates that act to decrease this overactivity have led to a reversal of parkinsonian symptoms. From our in vitro [³H]GABA release study we suppose that the anti-parkinsonian effects of tolbutamide are due to an increase in GABA release in these basal ganglia output regions. Such increased GABA release would serve to reverse the abnormal overactivity of basal ganglia projections to other motor centres. The selective concentration of K_{ATP} channels in the basal ganglia, compared to other regions of the brain, may allow selective targeting of GABA release in the basal ganglia. Such anatomical targeting may allow alleviation of parkinsonian symptoms without compromising other important brain functions.

In 1960 Gates and Hyman reported "a considerable reduction of tremor or rigidity or both" in eleven out of fifteen patients suffering from Parkinson's disease following treatment with tolbutamide (Gates and Hyman, 1960). They were unable to provide any explanation of the mechanisms that might underlie these effects and "indicate(d) the need for further research on man and animals". We would like to suggest that the data presented here begin to

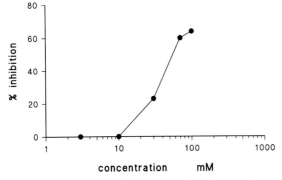

Fig. 8. Effect of diazoxide on GABA release in the globus pallidus. This figure shows the dose − response curve for the effects of diazoxide in decreasing K^+-evoked GABA release from 400 μm slices of globus pallidus pre-loaded with [³H]GABA (method as described in text and Amoroso et al., 1990).

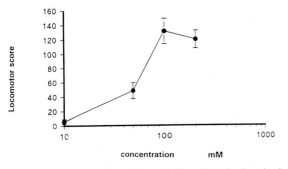

Fig. 9. Anti-parkinsonian effects of diazoxide injections in the globus pallidus of the reserpine-treated rat model of parkinsonism. The figure shows the dose − response curve for the effects of diazoxide injected unilaterally into the globus pallidus in reserpine-treated parkinsonian rats. Locomotor scores, measured in arbitrary locomotor units (ALUs) per 15 min, are shown following each injection. Each point represents the mean ± S.E.M. of five injections at different sites.

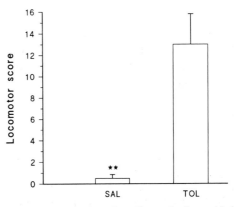

Fig. 10. Anti-parkinsonian effects of tolbutamide injections in the entopeduncular nucleus of the reserpine-treated rat. This figure illustrates the effects of unilateral intracerebral injections in the entopeduncular nucleus in the reserpine-treated rat model of parkinsonism. Following injection of saline (SAL) no anti-parkinsonian effects were seen. Following injection of tolbutamide (TOL, 5 mM) significant increases in locomotor activity were observed ($P < 0.05$, $n = 6$, t-test). Locomotor activity is measured in arbitrary locomotor units per 15 min as described elsewhere.

reconcile the findings of this interesting clinical report with our current model of the pathophysiology of parkinsonism.

Conclusion

The data discussed in this chapter begin to address some aspects of neuron-neuron and intraneuronal signalling in the basal ganglia. Many important questions remain to be answered concerning the mechanisms by which signalling mechanisms interact, and the molecular mechanisms by which such interactions occur. A fuller understanding of the control of movement by the basal ganglia at the molecular level will provide exciting insights into how the brain addresses the difficult computational problems involved in the control of movement. Progress in this area will also suggest potential avenues for novel therapeutic approaches to parkinsonism. Such innovations might reduce our reliance on dopamine-agonist replacement therapies as the primary symptomatic treatment for Parkinson's disease.

Acknowledgements

The experiments reported in this paper have been supported by the Medical Research Council, the Wellcome Trust, the Royal Society and the Parkinson's Disease Society.

References

Abou-Khalil, B., Young, A.B. and Penny, J.B. (1984) Evidence for the presynaptic localisation of opiate binding sites on striatal efferent fibres. *Brain Res.*, 323: 21 – 29.

Amoroso, S., Schmid-Antomarchi, H., Fosset, M. and Lazdunski, M. (1990) Glucose, sulfonylureas and neurotransmitter release: role of ATP-sensitive K^+ channels. *Science*, 247: 852 – 854.

Anderson, K.D. and Reiner, A. (1990) Extensive co-occurrence of substance P and dynorphin in striatal projection neurons: an evolutionarily conserved feature of basal ganglia organization. *J. Comp. Neurol.*, 295: 339 – 369.

Augood, S.J., Emson, P.C., Mitchell, I.J., Boyce, S., Clarke, C.E. and Crossman, A.R. (1989) Cellular localisation of enkephalin gene expression in MPTP-treated cynomolgus monkeys. *Mol. Brain Res.*, 6: 85 – 92.

Austin, M.C. and Kalivas, P.W. (1990) Dopaminergic involvement in locomotion elicited from the ventral pallidum/substantia innominata. *Brain Res.*, 542: 123 – 131.

Aziz, T., Peggs, D., Sambrook, M.A. and Crossman, A.R. (1991) Lesions of the subthalamic nucleus in the alleviation of parkinsonism in the MPTP-exposed primate. *Movement Dis.*, 6: 288 – 292.

Benavides, J., Capdeville, C., Dauphin, F., Dubois, A., Duverger, D., Fage, D., Gotti, B., Mackenzie, E.T. and Scatton, B. (1990) The quantification of brain lesions with an omega3 site ligand: a critical analysis of animal models of cerebral ischemia and neurodegeneration. *Brain Res.*, 522: 275 – 289.

Bergman, H., Wichmann, T. and Delong, M.R. (1990) Amelioration of parkinsonian symptoms by inactivation of the subthalamic nucleus in MPTP-treated monkeys. *Science*, 249: 1436 – 1438.

Besson, M.J., Graybiel, A.M. and Quinn, B. (1990) Co-expression of neuropeptides in the cat's striatum: an immunohistochemical study of substance P, dynorphin B and enkephalin. *Neuroscience*, 39: 33 – 58.

Brotchie, J.M. and Crossman, A.R. (1991) D-[^{3}H]-Aspartate and [^{14}C]-GABA uptake in the basal ganglia of rats following lesions in the subthalamic region suggests a role for excitatory amino acid but not GABA-mediated transmission in subthalamic nucleus efferents. *Exp. Neurol.*, 113: 171 – 181.

Brotchie, J.M., McGuire, S.G., Mitchell, I.J. and Crossman, A.R. (1990) Alleviation of akinesia by intracerebral injections of EAA antagonists in the 6-OHDA model of parkinsonism. *Neurosci. Lett.* (Suppl.), 38: S76.

Brotchie, J.M., Mitchell, I.J., Sambrook, M.A. and Crossman, A.R. (1991) Alleviation of parkinsonism by antagonism of excitatory amino acid transmission in the medial segment of the globus pallidus in rat and primate. *Movement Dis.*, 6: 133 – 138.

Close, S.P. and Elliott, P.J. (1991) Procedure for assessing the behavioral effects of novel anti-parkinsonian drugs in normal and MPTP-treated marmosets following central microinfusions. *J. Pharmacol. Methods,* 25: 123 – 131.

Collingridge, G.L. and Lester, R.A.J. (1989) Excitatory amino acids receptors in the vertebrate central nervous system. *Pharmacol. Rev.*, 40: 143 – 210.

Crossman, A.R., Peggs, D., Boyce, S., Luquin, M.R. and Sambrook, M.A. (1989) Effect of the NMDA antagonist MK-801 on MPTP-induced parkinsonism in the monkey. *Neuropharmacology*, 28: 1271 – 1273.

Engber, T.M., Susel, Z., Kuo, S., Gerfen, C.R. and Chase, T.N. (1991) Levodopa replacement therapy alters enzyme activities in the striatum and neuropeptide content in striatal output regions of 6-hydroxydopamine-lesioned rats. *Brain Res.*, 552: 113 – 118.

Filion, M., Tremblay, L. and Bedard, P.J. (1988) Abnormal influences of passive limb movement on the activity of globus pallidus neurons in parkinsonian monkeys. *Brain Res.*, 444:

165 – 176.

Frayne, S., Mitchell, I.J., Sharpe, P.T., Sambrook, M.A. and Crossman, A.R. (1991) Distribution of enkephalin gene expression in the striatum of the parkinsonian primate: implications for dopamine agonist-induced dystonia. *Mol. Neuropharmacol.*, 1: 53 – 58.

Gates, E.W. and Hyman, I. (1960) Use of tolbutamide in paralysis agitans. *JAMA*, 172: 1351 – 1354.

Gehlert, D.R., Gackenheimer, S.L., Mais, D.E. and Robertson, D.W. (1991) Quantitative autoradiography of the binding sites for [^{125}I] iodoglyburide, a novel high-affinity ligand for ATP-sensitive potassium channels in rat brain. *J. Pharmacol. Exp. Ther.*, 257: 901 – 907.

Gerfen, C.R., Engber, T.M., Mahan, L.C., Susel, Z., Chase, T.N., Monsma Jr., F.J. and Sibley, D.R. (1990) D1 and D2 dopamine receptor-regulated gene expression of striatonigral and striatopallidal neurons. *Science*, 250: 1429 – 1432.

Graham, W.G., Robertson, R.G., Sambrook, M.A. and Crossman, A.R. (1990) Injection of excitatory amino acid antagonists into the medial pallidal segment of a MPTP-treated primate reverses motor symptoms of parkinsonism. *Life Sci.*, 47: 91 – 97.

Hazrati, L.N., Parent, A., Mitchell, S. and Haber, S.N. (1990) Evidence for interconnections between the two segments of the globus pallidus in primates: a PHA-L anterograde tracing study. *Brain Res.*, 533: 171 – 176.

Jordan, M.I. (1989) Generic constraints on underspecified target trajectories. In: *Proceedings of the International Joint Conference on Neural Networks*, IEEE Press, New York, pp. 217 – 225.

Klockgether, T. and Turski, L. (1990) NMDA antagonists potentiate anti-parkinsonian actions of L-dopa in monoamine-depleted rats. *Ann. Neurol.*, 28: 539 – 546.

Klockgether, T., Turski, L., Honore, T., Zhang, Z., Gask, G.M., Kurlan, R. and Greenamyre, J.T. (1991) The AMPA receptor antagonist NBQX has antiparkinsonian effects in monoamine-depleted rats and MPTP-treated monkeys. *Ann. Neurol.*, 30(5): 715 – 723.

Kutsuwada, T., Kashiwabuchi N., Mori, H., Sakimura, K., Kushiya, E., Araki, K., Meguro, H., Masaki, H., Kumanishi, T., Arakawa, M. and Mishina, M. (1992) Molecular diversity of the NMDA receptor channel. *Nature*, 358: 36 – 41.

Levesque, D. and Greenfield, S.A. (1991) Psychopharmacological evidence for a role of the ATP-sensitive potassium channel in the substantia nigra of the rat. *Neuropharmacology*, 30: 359 – 365.

Marsden, C.D. and Parkes, J.D. (1977) Success and problems of long term therapy in Parkinson's disease. *Lancet*, i: 345 – 349.

Miller, W.C. and Delong, M.R. (1987) Altered tonic activity of neurons in the globus pallidus and subthalamic nucleus in the primate MPTP model of parkinsonism. In: M.B. Carpenter and A. Jayaraman (Eds.), *Advances in Behavioral Biology, Vol. 32: The Basal Ganglia, II. Structure and Function — Current Concepts*, Plenum, New York, pp. 395 – 403.

Mitchell, I.J., Clarke, C.E., Boyce, S., Robertson, R.G., Peggs, D., Sambrook, M.A. and Crossman, A.R. (1989) Neural

mechanisms underlying parkinsonian symptoms based upon regional uptake of 2-deoxyglucose in monkeys exposed to 1-methyl-4-phenyl-1,2,3,6-tetrahydropyridine (MPTP). *Neuroscience*, 32: 213 – 226.

Monaghan, D.T. (1991) Differential stimulation of [^{3}H]-MK-801 binding to subpopulations of NMDA receptors. *Neurosci. Lett.*, 122: 21 – 24.

Monaghan, D.T. and Beaton, J.A. (1991) Quinolinate differentiates between forebrain and cerebellar NMDA receptors. *Eur. J. Pharmacol.*, 194: 123 – 125.

Monaghan, D.T., Olverman, H.J., Nguyen, L., Watkins, J.C. and Cotman, C.W. (1988) Two classes of N-methyl-D-aspartate recognition sites: differential distribution and differential regulation by glycine. *Proc. Natl. Acad. Sci. U.S.A.*, 85: 9836 – 9840.

Morris, R.G.M., Anderson, E., Lynch, G.S. and Baudry, M. (1986) Selective impairment of learning and blockade of long-term potentiation of an N-methyl-D-aspartate receptor antagonist, APV. *Nature*, 319: 774 – 776.

Mourre, C., Widmann, C. and Lazdunski, M. (1990) Sulfonylurea binding sites associated with ATP-regulated K$^+$ channels in the central nervous system: autoradiographic analysis of their distribution and ontogenesis, and of their localization in mutant mice cerebellum. *Brain Res.*, 519: 29 – 43.

Nguyen, D. and Widrow, B. (1989) The truck backer-upper: an example of self learning in neural networks. In: *Proceedings of the International Joint Conference on Neural Networks, 2*, IEEE Press, New York, pp. 357 – 363.

Pan, H.S., Penney, J.B. and Young, A.B. (1985) GABA and benzodiazepine receptor changes induced by unilateral 6-hydroxydopamine lesions of the medial forebrain bundle. *J. Neurochem.*, 45: 1396 – 1404.

Penney, J.B. and Young, A.B. (1986) Striatal inhomogeneities and basal ganglia function. *Movement Dis.*, 1: 3 – 15.

Pullan, L.M., Verticelli, A.M. and Paschetto, K.A. (1991) Agonist-like character of the (R)-enantiomer of 1-hydroxy-3-aminopyrrolid-2-one (HA-966). *Eur. J. Pharmacol.*, 208: 25 – 29.

Robertson, R.G., Farmery, S.M., Sambrook, M.A. and Crossman, A.R. (1989) Dyskinesia in the primate following injection of an excitatory amino acid antagonist into the medial segment of the globus pallidus. *Brain Res.*, 476: 317 – 322.

Salt, T.E. (1986) Mediation of thalamic sensory input by both NMDA and non-NMDA receptors. *Nature*, 322: 263 – 265.

Stone, T.W. and Burton, N.R. (1988) NMDA receptors and ligands in the vertebrate CNS. *Prog. Neurobiol.*, 30: 333 – 368.

Thomson, A.M., West, D.C. and Lodge, D. (1985) An NMDA receptor mediated synapse in rat cerebral cortex: a site of action of ketamine. *Nature*, 313: 479 – 481.

Treherne, J.M. and Ashford, M.L. (1991) The regional distribution of sulphonylurea binding sites in rat brain. *Neuroscience*, 40: 523 – 531.

Wichmann, T., Bergman, H. and Delong, M.R. (1990) Increased neural activity in the subthalamic nucleus (STN) of MPTP-treated monkeys. *Movement Dis.*, 5: (Suppl. 1): 283.

SECTION II

The Genetic Control of Signalling

G.W. Arbuthnott and P.C. Emson (Eds.)
Progress in Brain Research, Vol. 99
© 1993 Elsevier Science Publishers B.V. All rights reserved.

CHAPTER 9

Regulation of glutamic acid decarboxylase gene expression in efferent neurons of the basal ganglia

Marie-Françoise Chesselet, Marianne Mercugliano, Jean-Jacques Soghomonian, Pascal Salin, Ying Qin and Cathleen Gonzales

Department of Pharmacology, University of Pennsylvania, Philadelphia, PA 19104, U.S.A.

Introduction

The majority of efferent neurons of the striatum and of its main target areas, the pallidum and substantia nigra pars reticulata, are GABA-ergic (Ribak, 1981; Mugnaini and Oertel, 1985; Pasik et al., 1988). Therefore, GABA-ergic neurons constitute the backbone of the output system of the basal ganglia, and regulation of GABA synthesis is likely to play a critical role in the adaptation of basal ganglia neurons to physiological and pathological challenges. The limiting step in GABA synthesis is catalyzed by glutamic acid decarboxylase (GAD), an enzyme detected with immunohistochemical techniques in brain GABA-ergic neurons (Ribak, 1981; Bolam et al., 1985; Mugnaini and Oertel, 1985). In recent years, we have examined the changes in steady-state levels of GAD and its mRNA occurring in the basal ganglia in response to lesions of neuronal inputs and pharmacological treatments. The ultimate goal of this research is to provide new insights into the plasticity of GAD gene expression in the basal ganglia and its functional significance in neurodegenerative diseases and chronic drug therapy.

Distribution of GAD and GAD mRNA in neurons of the basal ganglia in adult rats

Earlier studies with a radiolabeled RNA probe complementary to the mRNA encoding GAD M_r 67000 (GAD67; Kaufman et al., 1986) have revealed the presence of this mRNA in neurons previously identified as GABA-ergic on the basis of immunohistochemical studies (Chesselet et al., 1987). Specifically, numerous densely labeled neurons with the morphology of efferent cells were observed in both pallidal segments and in the substantia nigra pars reticulata. The striatum contained both numerous weakly labeled medium-sized neurons and much fewer very densely labeled medium-to-large cells (Fig. 1*B*). Both weakly and densely labeled cells were present in the striosomal and extrastriosomal compartments of the striatum (Chesselet and Robbins, 1989b). There were no observable differences in the level of labeling for GAD67 mRNA in the two compartments, in contrast to previous observations (Chesselet and Robbins, 1989a) of the levels of mRNA encoding tachykinins, neuropeptides colocalized with GAD in a subpopulation of GABA-ergic neurons (Reiner and Anderson, 1991).

Morphological analysis revealed that the densely labeled cells had indented nuclei, suggesting that they may correspond to those striatal interneurons exhibiting dense immunoreactivity to GAD and GABA (Bolam et al., 1985; Kita and Kitai, 1988; Pasik et al., 1988). This hypothesis was recently confirmed by the observation (Qin et al., 1992b) that the majority of neurons densely labeled for GAD67 mRNA in rat striatum also contain the mRNA encoding parvalbumin, a calcium-binding protein

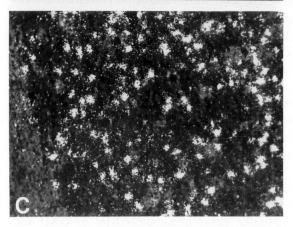

present in striatal GABA-ergic interneurons (Cowan et al., 1990; Kita et al., 1990). Like other striatal interneurons (Beal et al., 1986; Chesselet et al., 1990; Qin et al., 1992a), these GABA-ergic interneurons are relatively resistant to transient global ischemia in gerbils (Gonzales et al., 1992) and to local injections of quinolinic acid in the striatum of rats (Qin et al., 1992a).

Biochemical evidence indicates that several isoforms of GAD exist in brain (for review, see Erlander and Tobin, 1991). It has recently been shown that GAD M_r 65000 (GAD65) and GAD67 are encoded by separate genes (Erlander et al., 1991). We have compared the distributions of mRNAs encoding GAD65 and GAD67 in neurons of the basal ganglia, and found that both mRNAs were expressed in the same GABA-ergic neurons of striatum, pallidum and substantia nigra pars reticulata, but at different levels (Table I) (Mercugliano et al., 1992b). In the striatum, medium-sized efferent neurons express higher levels of GAD65 than GAD67 mRNA (Fig. 2), whereas the opposite is true for the interneurons. In the globus pallidus (external pallidal segment), the two mRNAs were expressed at similar levels. In contrast, neurons of the entopeduncular nucleus (internal pallidal segment) expressed higher levels of GAD65 than GAD67. As a result, the ratio of labeling in EP versus GP was greater for GAD65 than for GAD67 (Fig. 3). GAD67 mRNA was significantly higher in the lateral than in the medial part of the substantia nigra pars reticulata (Fig. 4). In the lateral part, GAD67 was slightly higher than GAD65, but the two mRNAs were expressed at similar levels in the medial part.

Thus, higher levels of GAD65 than GAD67 were found in two distinct populations of output neurons, the efferent neurons of the striatum and of the entopeduncular nucleus, which differ in their func-

Fig. 1. Darkfield photomicrographs of sections of rat striatum hybridized with antisense ^{35}S-radiolabeled RNA probes complementary to mRNAs encoding preproenkephalin (*A*), GAD67 (*B*) and preprotachykinin (*C*). (For experimental details, see Chesselet et al., 1987.) Exposure times were much longer for the tachykinin probe (40 days) than for the enkephalin (five days) and GAD67 probe (seven days). Note the dense labeling of numerous medium-sized neurons for enkephalin and tachykinin mRNAs. With the GAD67 RNA probe, dense labeling in a small population of medium-sized neurons (arrows) contrasts with weak labeling of the majority of striatal neurons.

tion and rate of activity, whereas neurons with similar patterns of activity such as those of the entopeduncular nucleus and substantia nigra pars reticulata had very different ratios of labeling for the two mRNAs. This argues against the hypothesis

that patterns of firing activity determine the relative level of expression of the two GAD mRNAs. The functional significance of the high level of expression of GAD65 in the entopeduncular nucleus is unknown, and experiments are in progress to deter-

TABLE I

Schematic diagram of the relative levels of labeling for GAD67 and GAD65 mRNA in neurons of the basal ganglia in rats, ranging from low (+) to very dense (+ + + +)

	GAD67 mRNA	GAD 65 mRNA
Striatum efferents	+	+ +
interneurons	+ + + +	+ +
Globus pallidus	+ + +	+ + +
Entopeduncular nucleus	+ +	+ + + + +
Substantia nigra pars reticulata	+ + +	+ + +

For detailed quantitative data, see Mercugliano et al. (1992b).

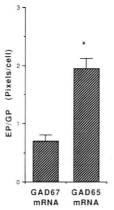

Fig. 3. Comparison of levels of labeling for GAD67 and GAD65 mRNAs in the two pallidal segments of rats. Sections were processed as described for Fig. 2. Ratios of labeling in entopeduncular nucleus (EP) to labeling in the globus pallidus (GP) in sections processed in parallel were calculated for each probe in individual rats and averaged. Data are mean ± S.E.M. (n = 4). * P < 0.05 when the corresponding means are compared with a Mann-Whitney U-test.

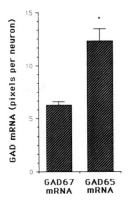

Fig. 2. Levels of labeling for GAD67 and GAD65 mRNA in rat striatum. Serially adjacent sections from five different rats were processed in parallel with ^{35}S-radiolabeled RNA probes of identical specific activity complementary to GAD67 and GAD65 mRNA, respectively. Levels of labeling for each mRNA were measured in a random sample (50 cells per rat) of labeled neurons with an image analysis system (for details, see Mercugliano et al., 1992b). The data are mean ± S.E.M. of the medians of frequency distributions of levels of labeling determined in individual rats (n = 5). Medians were compared rather than means because the frequency distributions for GAD67 mRNA are markedly asymmetrical in striatum due to the presence of the very densely labeled cells (see Fig. 1 and Soghomonian et al., 1992). * P < 0.005 when compared to GAD67 mRNA (Mann-Whitney U-test).

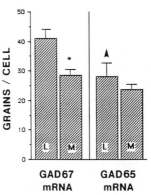

Fig. 4. Levels of labeling for GAD67 and GAD65 mRNAs in the substantia nigra pars reticulata of rats. Levels of labeling for each mRNA were measured with the image analysis system in serially adjacent sections from five different rats. Sections were processed as for Fig. 2. Data are mean ± S.E.M. of level of labeling (grains per neuron) in individual rats. * P < 0.05 when labeling in medial (M) and lateral (L) parts of substantia pars reticulata were compared; P < 0.05 when compared to labeling for GAD67 mRNA in corresponding regions (Mann-Whitney U-test).

mine whether the same ratio between the two mRNAs also exists in the internal pallidal segment of primates.

Most previous immunohistochemical work on the localization of GAD in brain has been accomplished with non-selective antibodies recognizing both GAD67 and, to a larger extent, GAD65 (Kaufman et al., 1991). Thanks to the cloning of the mRNA encoding GAD67 and its expression in bacteria, it has been possible to generate a polyclonal antibody specific for GAD67 (Kaufman et al., 1991). In an effort to determine whether all neurons previously identified as GAD-positive in the basal ganglia express GAD67, we have mapped the distribution of this GAD isoform in the rat by immunohistochemistry with the selective polyclonal antibody (Gonzales et al., 1991). In the striatum, both intensely stained and numerous weakly labeled neurons were observed, in agreement with the distribution of GAD67 mRNA. Double labeling studies with the GAD antibody and an antibody against parvalbumin (Celio and Heizmann, 1981) showed that most of the intensely labeled cells expressed immunoreactivity to parvalbumin (Soghomonian et al., 1992), confirming that they are interneurons (Cowan et al., 1990; Kita et al., 1990). In contrast to previous studies, however, neuronal cell bodies in pallidum and substantia nigra pars reticulata were intensely stained with the GAD67-specific antibody. A strong immunolabeling of axon terminals, as observed with the non-selective antibodies, was only seen in sections processed in the presence of triton-X 100 to increase the sensitivity of the immunostaining. Thus the results suggest that GAD67 is present in all neuronal types previously identified as GABA-ergic in the basal ganglia, but GAD67 may be more abundant or more accessible than GAD65 in neuronal cell bodies (see also Kaufman et al., 1991).

Lesions of dopaminergic inputs to the striatum differentially regulate levels of GAD mRNA in efferent neurons and interneurons

Several groups have reported that lesions of the nigro-striatal pathway by a unilateral injection of 6-hydroxydopamine in the substantia nigra increased GAD mRNA levels in the striatum ipsilateral to the lesion (Vernier et al., 1988; Lindefors et al., 1989; Segovia et al., 1990). We have confirmed this finding, and showed that immunoreactivity to GAD67 also increased in the dopamine-depleted striatum three weeks after the lesion, suggesting that the increase in mRNA levels leads to increased synthesis of new enzyme molecules (Soghomonian et al., 1992). Single cell analysis in emulsion-coated sections, however, revealed that the increase in GAD67 mRNA levels was restricted to the population of striatal neurons normally expressing low levels of GAD67 mRNA and corresponding to striatal efferent neurons. In contrast, the levels of GAD67-mRNA were decreased in the very densely labeled cells corresponding to GABA-ergic interneurons (Soghomonian et al., 1992). These results suggest that dopamine exerts opposite effects on GAD gene expression in these two distinct populations of GABA-ergic neurons in the striatum (Table II).

It has been shown previously that dopamine depletion increases the firing and bursting activity of striatal efferent neurons, as well as GABA release in the striatum and the pallidum (Arbuthnott, 1974; Orr et al., 1986; Tossman et al., 1986; Calabresi et al., 1988; Lindefors et al., 1989). Therefore, increased levels of GAD67 mRNA in striatal efferent neurons represent an adaptive response to increased

TABLE II

Summary of changes in levels of GAD67 mRNA observed in the striatum, the globus pallidus (GP) and the entopeduncular nucleus (EP) three weeks after a unilateral nigro-striatal lesion by injection of 6-hydroxydopamine in the substantia nigra

	Ipsilateral	Contralateral
Striatum	↑ (1) ↓ (2)	0
GP	↑	0
EP	0	↓

Arrows indicate direction of changes; 0 indicates no effect; (1): efferent neurons; (2): interneurons.

GABA-ergic transmission in these neurons. Conversely, decreased levels of GAD mRNA in striatal GABA-ergic interneurons could result from a decreased activity of these cells in the dopamine-depleted striatum. This hypothesis is of particular interest in view of recent evidence suggesting that striatal GABA-ergic interneurons may play a critical role in the generation of inhibitory potentials in striatal efferent neurons (Wilson et al., 1989). Accordingly, a decreased activity of GABA-ergic interneurons could contribute significantly to the functional consequences of dopamine depletion (Albin et al., 1989). Recent double labeling studies indicate that at least a subpopulation of striatal GABA-ergic interneurons expresses a mRNA encoding D2 dopamine receptors, but no detectable level of D1 dopamine receptor mRNA (Qin et al., 1992b). Thus dopamine may exert its effects on these interneurons through a D2 receptor-mediated mechanism. The effects of selective D1 and D2 antagonists on the level of expression of GAD67 mRNA in striatal interneurons are currently under investigation.

It is still unclear whether all GABA-ergic efferent neurons of the striatum exhibit increased levels of GAD67 mRNA after unilateral 6-hydroxydopamine lesions. There is evidence to suggest a dual regulation of striatal efferent neurons by dopamine (Albin et al., 1989). In particular, nigro-striatal lesions result in opposite changes in the levels of mRNAs encoding enkephalin and tachykinin, neuropeptides present in neurons projecting to the external and internal pallidum, respectively (for review, see Graybiel, 1990). In our experiments, exposure times for the emulsion autoradiograms were chosen so that about half of striatal efferent neurons expressed detectable levels of GAD67 mRNA in controls. Whereas a global increase in mRNA would be expected to result in an increased proportion of labeled neurons, we observed the same number of labeled neurons in lesioned and control striata, suggesting that the increase in GAD67 mRNA levels was restricted to a subpopulation of striatal efferent neurons. Confirmation of this hypothesis awaits the results of quantitative double-labeling studies which are in progress.

In spite of the robust changes in GAD67 mRNA levels observed by us and others in the striatum of rats with unilateral 6-hydroxydopamine lesions, we did not observe any concomitant changes in the levels of GAD65 mRNA in the same animals (Soghomonian et al., 1992). This is compatible with evidence that GAD65 is only partially saturated with its cofactor, pyridoxal phosphate, and is more likely to be principally regulated at the level of its enzymatic activity (Erlander and Tobin, 1991). The GAD67, in contrast, is present as a holoenzyme in brain and synthesis of new enzyme molecules may play a more critical role in its upregulation.

Effects of 6-hydroxydopamine lesions on GAD mRNA levels in the pallidum

One important characteristic of GAD mRNA in brain neurons is that it is localized to the cell bodies of GABA-ergic neurons, but it is not detectable in their axon terminals. In the pallidum, for example, GAD mRNA can be detected specifically in pallidal neuronal cell bodies unlike GAD and GABA which are also present in axon terminals of striato-pallidal neurons (Chesselet et al., 1987). This provides a unique opportunity to obtain information on pallidal efferent neurons, which are difficult to study with biochemical methods because homogenates of pallidum contain GAD and GABA originating from afferents as well as from intrinsic neurons. Therefore, we examined the effects of nigro-striatal lesions on the levels of GAD67 and GAD65 mRNAs in the globus pallidus and entopeduncular nucleus.

In the globus pallidus, GAD67, but not GAD65 mRNA levels were increased on the side ipsilateral to the lesion, three weeks after surgery (Table II) (Soghomonian and Chesselet, 1990; Soghomonian and Chesselet, 1992). This result was at first surprising, in view of evidence indicating that the inhibitory input from the striatum onto the external pallidum is increased after nigro-striatal lesions, resulting in inhibition of firing of pallidal efferent neurons (Pan and Walters, 1988). Electrophysiological experiments, however, also revealed an increased bursting pattern of pallidal neurons after nigro-striatal lesions (Miller and DeLong, 1987; Pan and Walters, 1988; Filion and Tremblay, 1991). It is unclear whether this change in firing pattern results in increased GABA release from axon terminals of these neurons, but our results suggest that it may play a role in the regulation of GAD67 gene expression. These results have recently been confirmed by Kincaid et al. (1991), who showed that the increase in GAD mRNA occurred in globus pallidus neurons projecting to the substantia nigra pars reticulata.

There was a marked asymmetry between the levels of GAD67 mRNA in the ipsi- and contralateral entopeduncular nuclei of rats after unilateral nigro-striatal lesions (Soghomonian and Chesselet, 1990). However, no detectable changes in GAD67 or GAD65 mRNA were found in the entopeduncular nucleus ipsilateral to the lesion when compared to unlesioned controls (Soghomonian and Chesselet, 1992). Indeed, the asymmetry resulted from a decreased level of the mRNA on the side contralateral to the lesion, further indicating that unilateral nigro-striatal lesions affect the contralateral basal ganglia (Table II). Interestingly, the levels of GAD65 mRNA, which are particularly high in the entopeduncular nucleus (see above) were also decreased in the contralateral entopeduncular nucleus of rats with a unilateral lesion of the nigro-striatal pathway, whereas it remained unchanged in the striatum and globus pallidus where GAD67 mRNA was affected by the lesion (Soghomonian and Chesselet, 1992).

In conclusion, unilateral nigro-striatal lesions induce an asymmetry in the levels of GAD67 mRNA in both pallidal segments. Compared to the contralateral side, the level of mRNA is higher on the side of the lesion both in the globus pallidus and in the entopeduncular nucleus, but the neuronal mechanisms responsible for this asymmetry appear different in the case of each pallidal segment: levels in globus pallidus are increased compared to controls in the ipsilateral globus pallidus and decreased in the contralateral entopeduncular nucleus. This contralateral effect may reflect compensatory changes in the activity of GABA-ergic neurons of the internal pallidum on the side contralateral to

dopamine depletion which may play a role in maintaining symmetrical movements in unilaterally lesioned rats.

Expression of GAD67 and GAD67 mRNA in striatal efferent neurons after unilateral cortical lesions

In addition to the nigro-striatal pathway, the striatum receives a massive input from the cerebral cortex (Selemon and Goldman-Rakic, 1985; McGeorges and Faull, 1989). Corticostriatal neurons are glutamatergic and synapse on the dendritic spines of striatal efferent neurons (Somogyi et al., 1981; Hassler et al., 1982). They are therefore likely to provide a driving force to the striatal output pathways. In an effort to determine the long-term consequences of unilateral cortical lesions on GAD gene expression in striatal output neurons, we have measured GAD67 mRNA in the striatum, as well as GAD67 immunoreactivity in striatum, pallidum and substantia nigra of rats with extensive lesions of the fronto-parietal cortex by thermocoagulation of pial vessels (Errami and Nieoullon, 1986). This procedure results in complete loss of cortical tissue under the thermocoagulated area within a few days. In order to obtain quantitative data, immunodetection of GAD67 was performed with the selective polyclonal antibody (Kaufman et al., 1991), an ^{125}I-radiolabeled secondary antibody, and densitometric analysis of film autoradiograms (Mc Lean et al., 1985).

The levels of GAD mRNA were increased in the dorsolateral part of the striatum ipsilateral to the cortical lesion five, 21 and even 90 days after surgery (Salin and Chesselet, 1993). At the 21 day time point, the increase in labeling was more pronounced, and also observed on the contralateral side (Fig. 5). The increase in mRNA levels was observed on emulsion-coated slides at all time points, confirming that the effect was due to an increased level of labeling per individual neuron. Single cell analysis also indicated that the increase occurred in those striatal cells normally exhibiting low levels of GAD mRNA (efferent neurons). In contrast, no de-

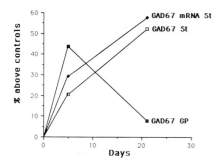

Fig. 5. Time course of changes in GAD67 immunoreactivity in the striatum (St) and globus pallidus (GP), and of GAD67 mRNA in the striatum of rats sacrificed five and 21 days after unilateral thermocoagulation of pial vessels supplying the frontoparietal cortex. Immunolabeling was performed with a radiolabeled secondary antibody and the signal quantified by measuring optical densities of film autoradiograms. In situ hybridization was performed with a ^{35}S-radiolabeled RNA probe. Levels of mRNA were measured at the single cell level in emulsion-coated slides with an image analysis system as described in Salin et al. (1990). Data are means of level of labeling in 5 – 7 rats expressed as percent of corresponding controls. S.E.M. were < 3% of the means.

tectable changes in GAD67 mRNA levels were observed in the densely labeled cells (interneurons).

Levels of GAD67 immunoreactivity were measured in the striatum and its target areas in animals sacrificed five and 21 days after surgery. The increase in levels of GAD67 mRNA observed in the striatum was accompanied by an increase in immunoreactive GAD67 in the striatum and in the axon terminals of striatal efferent neurons in the pallidum and the substantia nigra. The time course of these changes, however, was dramatically different in the striatum and in its target areas (Fig. 5). In the striatum, the increase in GAD67 immunoreactivity followed closely the changes in mRNA on the ipsilateral side at the two time points examined. In both pallidal segments and in the substantia nigra, GAD67 immunoreactivity was markedly increased five days after surgery, but except for a small ipsilateral increase in entopeduncular nucleus, was unchanged compared to controls at 21 days. These results suggest that unilateral lesions of the cortex by thermocoagulation induce long-lasting increases in GAD mRNA in the region of the striatum that receives most inputs from the lesioned cortex

(McGeorge and Faull, 1989). The increase in GAD mRNA appears to lead to synthesis of new GAD molecules. Whereas the level of GAD protein increases in axon terminals of striatal efferent neurons shortly after the lesion, at a later time the increase in GAD is restricted to the striatum, suggesting an impairment of transport of newly synthesized enzyme molecules to the terminal fields of striatal neurons.

It is likely that the experimental protocol used to generate the cortical lesions plays a critical role in the effects observed. This is suggested by the fact that we have observed different effects on peptide mRNAs in rats with similar lesions than those previously reported after acute decortication by aspiration. Whereas levels of enkephalin and tachykinin mRNAs were increased in the striatum after thermocoagulatory lesions (Chesselet and Salin, 1990), they were decreased after lesions by aspiration (Uhl et al., 1988; Sommers and Beckstead, 1990). One obvious difference between the two procedures is that, in the case of thermocoagulation, the loss of cortical neurons is progressive over a period of several days, and is secondary to the interruption of blood flow to the affected cortical area. The effects of this local ischemic lesion are likely to be different from those of acute cortical ablation. Therefore, rather than being the direct result of the loss of cortical inputs to the dorsolateral striatum, the increase in GAD synthesis observed after thermocoagulatory lesions of the cortex in rats may be triggered by excitatory amino acids released from dying cortical neurons (Benveniste et al., 1984) followed by plastic changes of the denervated striatal neurons (Chen and Hillman, 1990). Whatever their mechanisms, the long-lasting changes in GAD mRNA observed after thermocoagulatory lesions of the cortex further support the hypothesis that regulation of GAD gene expression plays a role in the long-term adaptation of GABA-ergic neurons to loss of inputs and are relevant to the understanding of the consequences of cortical strokes in humans.

GAD mRNA and antipsychotic treatment

Classical antipsychotics such as haloperidol cause

extrapyramidal symptoms in humans and induce catalepsy in laboratory rats. In contrast to classical neuroleptics, antipsychotics such as clozapine are devoid of both early and delayed extrapyramidal side effects (Matz et al., 1974; Tarsy and Baldessarini, 1986). Therefore, comparison of the effects induced by these drugs provides a useful tool to determine the neuronal mechanisms underlying extrapyramidal movement disorders. Whereas the effects of these two prototypical drugs on a variety of neurochemical markers have been examined over the years, there is still little information on the effects of prolonged treatments with haloperidol and clozapine on efferent neurons of the pallidum that are directly involved in the generation of extrapyramidal symptoms (DeLong, 1990).

We have examined the effects of four weeks of daily intraperitoneal injections of either haloperidol (1 mg/kg) or clozapine (20 mg/kg) on the levels of GAD67 mRNA in neurons of the globus pallidus and entopeduncular nucleus in rats (Mercugliano et al., 1992a). Under these experimental conditions, treatment with clozapine resulted in a 37% increase in GAD67 mRNA levels in the globus pallidus, whereas haloperidol increased GAD67 mRNA in the entopeduncular nucleus (Fig. 6). No significant

changes in GAD67 mRNA levels were observed in the striatum with either treatment at this time point (Mercugliano et al., 1992a).

In an effort to determine whether the increase in GAD mRNA induced by clozapine in the globus pallidus resulted from an action of this drug on striatopallidal neurons, we have measured the levels of mRNA encoding enkephalin, a neuropeptide present in striatal neurons projecting to the globus pallidus (Reiner and Anderson, 1990). We found that after four weeks of daily intraperitoneal injections, haloperidol did not modify enkephalin mRNA levels in the striatum, whereas enkephalin mRNA levels were decreased in the clozapine-treated animals at this time point (Mercugliano and Chesselet, 1992). The results suggest that long-term treatment with clozapine and haloperidol differentially affect striatal efferent neurons projecting to the globus pallidus, which may lead to the differential effects of the two drugs on GAD mRNA expression in this brain region.

The observation of differential effects of haloperidol and clozapine on the expression of GAD67 mRNA in the two pallidal segments is of interest in view of their different ability to induce motor side effects. The main target of efferent GABAergic neurons of the globus pallidus is the ipsilateral subthalamic nucleus (Alexander and Crutcher, 1990). If, as in other neuronal systems (Vernier et al., 1988; Litwak et al., 1990), GAD mRNA increased in response to an increased GABA production and release from the corresponding neurons, one may speculate that clozapine treatment results in an increased inhibition of the subthalamic nucleus by the globus pallidus (Fig. 7). Because lesions of the subthalamic nucleus have recently been shown to ameliorate parkinsonian symptoms in MPTP-treated monkeys (Bergman et al., 1990), inhibition of the subthalamic nucleus could play a critical role in the absence of extrapyramidal symptoms in patients treated with clozapine. Conversely, haloperidol-induced increase in GAD mRNA in the entopeduncular nucleus is compatible with evidence that the neuronal firing rate increases in the internal pallidum of monkeys with MPTP-induced parkin-

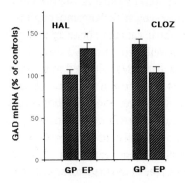

Fig. 6. Levels of labeling for GAD67 mRNA in the globus pallidus (GP) and entopeduncular nucleus (EP) of rats treated daily for 28 days with haloperidol (HAL: 1 mg/kg, i.p.) or clozapine (CLOZ: 20 mg/kg, i.p.). Data are mean ± S.E.M. of average levels of labeling calculated for each rat and expressed as percent of values in vehicle injected controls. * $P < 0.05$ when absolute values were compared to control animals (Mann-Whitney U-test). $n = 8$ (EP) and 12 (GP).

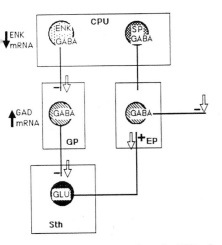

Fig. 7. Schematic representation of mRNA changes (black arrows) observed in clozapine-treated animals (20 mg/kg, i.p., daily, 28 days). Open arrows indicate hypothetical consequences of these effects on neuronal interactions in the basal ganglia. CPU, caudate-putamen (striatum); GP, globus pallidus; EP, entopeduncular nucleus; Sth, subthalamic nucleus; ENK, enkephalin; SP, tachykinins; GLU, glutamate (for references on connections, see Alexander and Crutcher, 1990).

sonism (Miller and DeLong, 1986; Filion and Tremblay, 1991).

Significance of changes in GAD mRNA in the basal ganglia

The results summarized here clearly indicate that a variety of experimental situations results in long term-changes in the steady state levels of GAD mRNA in neurons of the basal ganglia. In most cases, changes were restricted to the mRNA encoding GAD67, suggesting that different mechanisms are involved in the regulation of these two GAD isoforms in response to altered activity of GABA-ergic neurons. When changes in immunoreactive GAD67 were examined, they paralleled changes in GAD67 mRNA in the striatum, suggesting that the increase in mRNA levels leads to an increased synthesis of the enzyme.

In some instances, it has been possible to correlate increases in GAD67 gene expression with an increase in GAD activity and in the firing or bursting

activity of the corresponding GABA-ergic neurons (Vernier et al., 1988; Litwak et al., 1990). Whereas the relationship between neuronal activity and mRNA regulation is likely to be complex (see Weiss-Wunder and Chesselet, 1992), it is reasonable to speculate that increases in GAD mRNA most likely occur when neurons are challenged to produce more GABA in response to increased release of this neurotransmitter. Because they can be detected after prolonged pharmacological treatments and experimental lesions mimicking neuropathological conditions, levels of GAD67 mRNA provide a novel index of long-term alterations in GABA-ergic neurons.

Conclusion

The ability to measure GAD mRNA levels in single neurons allows for a detailed analysis of the topography and cell types involved. This is particularly useful in a region like the striatum which contains several distinct populations of GABA-ergic neurons, and in the pallidum and substantia nigra pars reticulata in which efferent GABA-ergic neurons are difficult to study at the molecular level with biochemical methods. Application of this method to the study of long-term effects of lesions of striatal inputs revealed opposite changes in GAD67 gene expression in efferent neurons and in interneurons of the striatum after lesions of the nigro-striatal pathway. In addition, the results indicated that these lesions result in asymmetric levels of GAD mRNA in globus pallidus and entopeduncular nucleus in the two hemispheres. Different changes in GAD67 mRNA levels were also observed in the two pallidal segments after chronic treatment with either haloperidol or clozapine, suggesting a novel mechanism for the absence of extrapyramidal side effects during treatment with atypical neuroleptics. Finally, the prolonged alterations in GAD gene expression in the striatum after thermocoagulation of pial vessels provide evidence of lasting transsynaptic changes in subcortical GABA-ergic neurons after ischemic lesions of the cerebral cortex.

152

Acknowledgements

This work has been supported by Public Health Service grants BNS86-16841, MH 44894 and NS 29230, Training Grant MH 14654, the Pharmaceutical Manufacturers Association Foundation, the Hereditary Disease Foundation, the Tourette Syndrome Association and ICI Pharmaceuticals Group. We are grateful to Dr. A.J. Tobin, UCLA, for his invaluable contribution to this work through helpful discussions and the gift of cDNAs and antibodies.

References

Albin, R.L., Young, A.B. and Penney, J.B. (1989) The functional anatomy of basal ganglia disorders. *Trends Neurosci.*, 12: 366 – 375.

Alexander, G.E. and Crutcher, M.D. (1990) Functional architecture of basal ganglia circuits: neural substrates of parallel processing. *Trends Neurosci.*, 13: 266 – 271.

Arbuthnott, G.W. (1974) Spontaneous activity of single units in the striatum after unilateral destruction of the dopamine input. *J. Physiol. (Lond.)*, 239: 121 – 122.

Beal, M.F., Kowall, N.W., Ellison, D.W., Mazurek, M.F., Swartz, K.J. and Martin, J.B. (1986) Replication of the neurochemical characteristics of Huntington's disease by quinolinic acid. *Nature,* 321: 168 – 171.

Benveniste, H., Drejer, A., Shousboe, A. and Diemer, N.H. (1984) Elevation of the extracellular concentrations of glutamate and aspartate in rat hippocampus during transient cerebral ischemia monitored by intracerebral microdialysis. *J. Neurochem.*, 43: 1369 – 1374.

Bergman, H., Wichmann, T. and DeLong, M.R. (1990) Reversal of experimental parkinsonism by lesions of the subthalamic nucleus. *Science,* 249: 1436 – 1438.

Bolam, J.P., Powell, J.F, Wu, J.-Y. and Smith, A.D. (1985) Glutamate decarboxylase-immunoreactive neurons in the rat neostriatum: a correlated light and electronmicroscopic study including a combination of Golgi impregnation with immunohistochemistry. *J. Comp. Neurol.*, 237: 1 – 20.

Calabresi, P., Benedetti, M., Mercuri, N.B. and Bernardi, G. (1988) Endogenous dopamine and dopaminergic agonists modulate synaptic excitation in striatum: intracellular studies from naive and catecholamine-depleted rats. *Neuroscience,* 27: 145 – 157.

Celio, M.R. and Heizmann, C.W. (1981) Calcium-binding protein parvalbumin as a neuronal marker. *Nature,* 293: 300 – 302.

Chen, S. and Hillman, D.E. (1990) Robust synaptic plasticity of striatal cells following partial deafferentation. *Brain Res.,*

520: 103 – 114.

Chesselet, M.-F. and Robbins, E.(1989a) Regional differences in substance P-like immunoreactivity in the striatum correlate with levels of pre-protachykinin mRNA. *Neurosci. Lett.,* 96: 47 – 53.

Chesselet, M.-F. and Robbins, E. (1989b) Characterization of striatal neurons expressing high levels of glutamic acid decarboxylase messenger RNA. *Brain Res.,* 492: 237 – 244.

Chesselet, M.-F. and Salin, P. (1990) Effects of cortical lesion on striatal gene expression in the rat: I. Efferent neurons. *Soc. Neurosci. Abstr.,* 16: 1232.

Chesselet, M.-F., Weiss, L., Wuenschell, C., Tobin, A.J. and Affolter, H.-U. (1987) Comparative distribution of mRNAs for glutamic acid decarboxylase, tyrosine hydroxylase, and tachykinins in the basal ganglia: an in situ hybridization study in the rodent brain. *J. Comp. Neurol.,* 262: 125 – 140.

Chesselet, M.-F., Gonzales, C., Lin, C.-S., Polsky, K. and Jin, B.-K. (1990) Ischemic damage in the gerbil striatum: relative sparing of somatostatinergic and cholinergic interneurons contrasts with loss of efferent neurons. *J. Exp. Neurol.,* 110: 209 – 218.

Cowan, R.L., Wilson, C.J., Emson, P.C. and Heizmann, C.W. (1990) Parvalbumin-containing GABAergic interneurons in the rat neostriatum. *J. Comp. Neurol.,* 302: 197 – 205.

DeLong, M. (1990) Primate models of movement disorders of basal ganglia origin. *Trends Neurosci.,* 13: 281 – 285.

Erlander, M.G. and Tobin, A.J. (1991) The structural and functional heterogeneity of glutamic acid decarboxylase: a review. *Neurochem. Res.,* 16: 215 – 226.

Erlander, M.G., Tillakaratne, N.J.K., Feldblum, S., Patel, N. and Tobin, A.J. (1991) Two genes encode distinct glutamate decarboxylases. *Neuron,* 7: 91 – 100.

Errami, M. and Nieoullon, A. (1986) Development of a micromethod to study the Na^+-independent L-^{3}H glutamic acid binding to rat striatal membranes, II. Effects of selective striatal lesions and deafferentations. *Brain Res.,* 366: 178 – 186.

Fillion, M. and Tremblay, L. (1991) Abnormal spontaneous activity of globus pallidus neurons in monkeys with MPTP-induced parkinsonism. *Brain Res.,* 547: 142 – 151.

Gonzales, C., Kaufman, D., Tobin, A. and Chesselet, M.-F. (1991) Distribution of GAD 67 in the basal ganglia of the rat: an immunohistochemical study with a selective cDNA-generated polyclonal antibody. *J. Neurocytol.,* 20: 953 – 961.

Gonzales, C., Lin, R.C.-S. and Chesselet, M.-F. (1992) Relative sparing of GABA-ergic interneurons in the striatum of gerbils with ischemia-induced lesions. *Neurosci. Lett.,* 135: 53 – 58.

Graybiel, A.M. (1990) Neurotransmitters and neuromodulators in the basal ganglia. *Trends Neurosci.,* 13: 244 – 254.

Hassler, R., Haug, P., Nitsch, C., Kim, J.S. and Paik, K. (1992) Effect of motor and premotor cortex ablation on concentration of amino acids, monoamines and acetylcholine and on the ultrastructure in rat striatum. A confirmation of glutamate as the specific cortico-striatal transmitter. *J. Neurochem.,* 38:

1087 – 1098.

Kaufman, D.L., McGinnis, J.F., Krieger, N.R. and Tobin, A.J. (1986) Brain glutamate decarboxylase cloned in lambda gt11: fusion protein produces gamma-aminobutyric acid. *Science*, 232: 1138 – 1140.

Kaufman, D.L., Houser, C.R. and Tobin, A.J. (1991) Two forms of the GABA synthetic enzyme glutamate decarboxylase have distinct intraneuronal distributions. *J. Neurochem.*, 56: 720 – 723.

Kincaid, A.E., Albin, R.L., Newman, S.W., Penney, J.B. and Young, A.B. (1991) Dopaminergic regulation of glutamic acid decarboxylase mRNA in pallidal projection neurons. *Soc. Neurosci. Abstr.*, 17: 854.

Kita, H. and Kitai, S.T. (1988) Glutamate decarboxylase immunoreactive neurons in rat neostriatum: their morphological types and populations. *Brain Res.*, 447: 346 – 352.

Kita, H., Kosaka, T. and Heizmann, C.W. (1990) Parvalbumin-immunoreactive neurons in the rat neostriatum: a light and electron microscopic study. *Brain Res.*, 536: 1 – 15.

Lindefors, N., Brene, S., Herrera-Marschitz, M. and Persson, H. (1989) Region specific regulation of glutamic acid decarboxylase mRNA expression by dopamine neurons in rat brain. *Exp. Brain Res.*, 77: 611 – 620.

Litwak, J., Mercugliano, M., Chesselet, M.-F. and Oltmans, G.A. (1990) Increased glutamic acid decarboxylase (GAD) mRNA and GAD activity in cerebellar Purkinje cells following lesion-induced increases in cell firing. *Neurosci. Lett.*, 116: 179 – 183.

Matz, R., Rick, W., Oh, D., Thompson, H. and Gershon, S. (1974) Clozapine – a potential antipsychotic agent without extrapyramidal manifestations. *Curr. Ther. Res.*, 16: 687 – 695.

McGeorge, A.J. and Faull, R.L.M. (1989) The organization of the projection from the cerebral cortex to the striatum in the rat. *Neuroscience*, 29: 503 – 537.

McLean, S., Skirboll, L.R. and Pert, C.B. (1985) Comparison of substance P and enkephalin distribution in rat brain: an overview using radioimmunocytochemistry. *Neuroscience*, 14: 837 – 852.

Mercugliano, M. and Chesselet, M.-F. (1992) Clozapine decreases enkephalin mRNA in rat striatum. *Neurosci. Lett.*, 136: 10 – 14.

Mercugliano, M., Saller, A., Salama, A., U'Prichard, D. and Chesselet, M.-F. (1992a) Haloperidol and clozapine have differential effects on glutamic acid decarboxylase mRNA in the pallidal nuclei of the rat. *Neuropsychopharmacology*, 6: 179 – 187.

Mercugliano, M., Soghomonian, J.-J., Qin, Y., Nguyen, H.Q., Feldblum, S., Erlander, M.G., Tobin, A.J. and Chesselet, M.-F. (1992b) Comparative distribution of messenger RNAs encoding glutamic acid decarboxylases (M_r 65,000 and M_r 67,000) in the basal ganglia of the rat. *J. Comp. Neurol.*, 318: 245 – 254.

Miller, C.W. and DeLong, M.R. (1986) Altered tonic activity of neurons in the globus pallidus and subthalamic nucleus in the primate MPTP model of parkinsonism. In: M.B. Carpenter and A. Jayaraman (Eds.), *The Basal Ganglia II. Structure and Function – Current Concepts – Advances in Behavioral Biology, Vol. 32,* Plenum, New York, pp. 415 – 427.

Mugnaini, E. and Oertel, W.H. (1985) An atlas of the distribution of GABAergic neurons and terminals in the CNS as revealed by GAD immunohistochemistry. In: A. Björklund and T. Hökfelt (Eds.), *Handbook of Neuroanatomy, Vol. 4, Part 1,* Elsevier, Amsterdam, pp. 436 – 608.

Orr, W.B., Gardiner, T.W., Stricker, E.M., Zigmond, M.J. and Berger, T.W. (1986) Short-term effects of dopamine-depleting lesions on spontaneous activity of striatal neurons: relation to local dopamine concentration and behavior. *Brain Res.*, 376: 20 – 28.

Pan, H.S. and Walters, J.R. (1988) Unilateral lesion of the nigrostriatal pathway decreases the firing rate and alters the firing pattern of globus pallidus neurons in the rat. *Synapse*, 2: 560 – 565.

Pasik, P., Pasik, T., Holstein, G. and Hamori, J. (1988) GABAergic elements in the neuronal circuits of the monkey neostriatum: a light and electronmicroscopic immunocytochemical study. *J. Comp. Neurol.*, 270: 157 – 170.

Qin, Y., Soghomonian, J.-J. and Chesselet, M.-F. (1992a) Effects of quinolinic acid on messenger RNAs encoding somatostatin and glutamic acid decarboxylase in the striatum of adult rats. *Exp. Neurol.*, 115: 200 – 211.

Qin, Y., Robbins, E., Baldino, F. and Chesselet, M.-F. (1992b) GABA-ergic interneurons of the striatum express D2 receptor mRNA: a double-labelling study with digoxigenin- and radiolabeled-RNA probes. *Soc. Neurosci. Abstr.*, 18: 1044.

Reiner, A. and Anderson, K.D. (1990) The patterns of neurotransmitter and neuropeptide co-occurrence among striatal projection neurons: conclusions based on recent findings. *Brain Res. Rev.*, 15: 251 – 265.

Ribak, C.E. (1981) The GABA-ergic neurons of the extrapyramidal system as revealed by immunohistochemistry. *Adv. Biochem. Psychopharmacol.*, 30: 23 – 36.

Salin, P. and Chesselet, M.-F. (1993) Expression of GAD (Mr 67,000) and its mRNA in basal ganglia and cerebral cortex after ischemic cortical lesions in rats. *Exp. Neurol.*, 119: 291 – 301.

Salin, P., Mercugliano, M. and Chesselet, M.-F. (1990) Differential effects of chronic treatment with haloperidol and clozapine on the level of preprosomatostatin mRNA in the striatum, nucleus accumbens, and frontal cortex of the rat. *Cell. Mol. Neurobiol.*, 10: 127 – 144.

Segovia, J., Tillakaratne, N.J.K., Whelan, K., Tobin, A.J. and Gale, K. (1990) Parallel increases in striatal glutamic acid decarboxylase activity and mRNA levels in rats with lesions in the nigrostriatal pathway. *Brain Res.*, 529: 345 – 348.

Selemon, L.D. and Goldman-Rakic, P.S. (1985) Longitudinal topography and interdigitation of corticostriatal projections in the rhesus monkey. *J. Neurosci.*, 5: 776 – 794.

Soghomonian, J.-J. and Chesselet, M.-F. (1990) Effect of 6-

154

hydroxydopamine lesions of the substantia nigra on the levels of glutamic acid decarboxylase and preprosomatostatin mRNAs in the rat pallidum. *Soc. Neurosci. Abstr.,* 16: 1232.

Soghomonian, J.-J. and Chesselet, M.-F. (1992) Effects of nigrostriatal lesions on the levels of messenger RNAs encoding two isoforms of glutamate decarboxylase in the globus pallidus and entopeduncular nucleus of the rat. *Synapse,* 11: 124 – 133.

Soghomonian, J.-J., Gonzales, C. and Chesselet, M.-F. (1991) Nigrostriatal lesions differentially affect mRNAs encoding glutamate-decarboxylases (GADs) in subpopulations of striatal neurons. *Soc. Neurosci. Abstr.,* 17: 856.

Soghomonian, J.-J., Gonzales, C. and Chesselet, M.-F. (1992) Messenger RNAs encoding glutamate decarboxylases are differentially affected by nigrostriatal lesions in subpopulations of striatal neurons. *Brain Res.,* 576: 68 – 79.

Sommers, D.L. and Beckstead, R.M. (1990) Striatal preprotachykinin and preproenkephalin mRNA levels and the levels of nigral substance P and pallidal metenkephalin depend on corticostriatal axons that use the excitatory amino acid neurotransmitters aspartate and glutamate: quantitative radioimmunocytochemical and in situ hybridization evidence. *Mol. Brain Res.,* 8: 143 – 158.

Somogyi, P., Bolam, J.P. and Smith, A.D. (1981) Monosynaptic cortical input and local axon collaterals of identified striatonigral neurons. A microscopic study using the Golgi-peroxidase transport degeneration procedure. *J. Comp. Neurol.,* 195: 567 – 584.

Tarsy, D. and Baldessarini, R.J. (1986) Movement disorders induced by psychotherapeutic agents. In: N.S. Shah and A.G. Donald (Eds.), *Movement Disorders,* Plenum, New York, pp. 365 – 389.

Tossman, U., Segovia, J. and Ungerstedt, U. (1986) Extracellular levels of amino acids in striatum and globus pallidus of 6-hydroxydopamine-lesioned rats measured with microdialysis. *Acta Physiol. Scand.,* 127: 547 – 551.

Uhl, G.R., Navia, B. and Douglas, J. (1988) Differential expression of preproenkephalin and preprodynorphin mRNAs in striatal neurons: high levels of preproenkephalin expression depend on cerebral cortical afferents. *J. Neurosci.,* 8: 4755 – 4764.

Vernier, P., Julien, J.-F., Rataboul, P., Fourrier, O., Feuerstein, C. and Mallet, J. (1988) Similar time course changes in striatal levels of glutamic acid decarboxylase and proenkephalin mRNA following dopaminergic deafferentation in the rat. *J. Neurochem.,* 51: 1375 – 1380.

Weiss-Wunder, L.T. and Chesselet, M.-F. (1992) Acute and repeated administration of fluphenazine-N-mustard alter levels of tyrosine hydroxylase messenger RNA in subsets of mesencephalic dopaminergic neurons. *Neuroscience,* 49: 297 – 305.

Wilson, C.J., Kita, H. and Kawaguchi, Y. (1989) GABA-ergic interneurons rather than spiny cell axon collaterals are responsible for the IPSP responses to afferent stimulation in neostriatal spiny neurons. *Soc. Neurosci. Abstr.,* 15: 907.

G.W. Arbuthnott and P.C. Emson (Eds.)
Progress in Brain Research, Vol. 99
© 1993 Elsevier Science Publishers B.V. All rights reserved.

CHAPTER 10

Chemical signalling and striatal interneurones

P.C. Emson, S.J. Augood, R. Señaris, R. Guevara Guzman*, J. Kishimoto,
K. Kadowaki, P.J. Norris and K.M. Kendrick*

*MRC Molecular Neuroscience Group and * Department of Neurobiology, AFRC, Institute of Animal Physiology and Genetics Research, Babraham, Cambridge, CB2 4AT, U.K.*

Introduction

The majority of neostriatal neurones are medium-sized spiny neurones which have diameters between 10 and 20 μm (Wilson, 1990). These cells were originally believed to be interneurones (Kemp et al., 1971; Fox et al., 1972); however, retrograde transport studies established them as projection neurones (Sorimachi and Kataoka, 1974; Bunney and Aghajanian, 1976; Faull et al., 1976; Kocsis et al., 1977; Bak et al., 1978; Graybiel et al., 1979; Szabo, 1979; Wilson and Groves, 1980; Preston et al., 1980). Parallel studies showed that GABA inhibition (or more strictly disinhibition) controls the majority of functional activity in the basal ganglia (Precht and Yoshida, 1971; Yoshida and Precht, 1971; Yoshida et al., 1979; Wilson, 1990; Kita, this volume). In addition to the medium-sized spiny cells, the larger aspiny cells, 20 – 60 μm diameter, constitute some 4 – 5% of all striatal neurones and these are now known to be short axoned interneurones, although there are occasional reports of aspiny projection neurones (Bolam et al., 1981b). These interneurones integrate activity between output pathways through the striatum providing feed forward and feedback loops (Kita, this volume). In addition, interneurones may represent relatively specific targets for cortical or thalamic inputs (Lapper and Bolam, 1992). In this article we discuss some of our recent work exploring the phenotypes of striatal interneurones and present evidence indicating

that nitric oxide may be a novel intercellular messenger in the striatum modulating the effects of glutamate on N-methyl-D-aspartate (NMDA) receptors expressed by striatal neurones. Stimulation of NMDA receptors in vivo activates local acetylcholine (ACh) release as does local application of substance P and substance P agonists. The exquisite sensitivity of cholinergic neurones to substance P and NMDA suggests that these neurones represent an important target both for local striatal axon collaterals containing substance P, and thalamic excitatory inputs releasing glutamate (Lapper and Bolam, 1992).

Phenotypes of neurones

The original anatomical and pathway tracing studies (Kemp et al., 1971; Fox et al., 1972; Bunney et al., 1976; Faull et al., 1976; Kocsis et al., 1977; Bak et al., 1978; Graybiel et al., 1979; Somogyi et al., 1979; Szabo, 1979; Preston et al., 1980) did not provide any evidence for the neurotransmitter phenotypes of striatal neurones and evidence for the involvement of γ-aminobutyric acid (GABA), ACh, amino acids and later neuropeptides as striatal transmitters was originally based on biochemical measurements (for review, see Graybiel and Ragsdale, 1983). Subsequently the development of immunohistochemical techniques revealed, in particular, two principal populations of medium-sized spiny neurones, the GABA-substance P-dynorphin cells, projecting particularly to the substantia nigra (Kanazawa et al., 1977; Jessell et al., 1978) and the GABA-enkephalin cells projecting to the globus pallidus (Cuello and Paxinos, 1978; Penny et al., 1986). More recently, in situ hybridization combined with the use of retrograde tracers has confirmed this phenotypic classification (Young et al., 1986; Gerfen et al., 1991). Thus substance P mRNA was particularly associated with cells labelled by fluorogold from nigra injections, while enkephalin mRNA was found in another population of medium-sized cells (projecting to the globus pallidus) (Gerfen and Young, 1988). Co-expression studies using combinations of isotopic and non-isotopic probes carried out by Bloch and colleagues (Le Moine et al., 1990a,b) and Augood et al. (this volume) also confirmed the presence of distinct and generally non-overlapping populations of enkephalin and substance P neurones. In situ hybridization has also confirmed that most medium-sized cells contain glutamic acid decarboxylase (GAD) mRNA (Chesselet et al., 1987, this volume). This was important as immunohistochemical studies with existing anti-GAD antibodies had given variable percentages of positive cells (estimates varying from 4 to 80% of striatal cells) (Ribak et al., 1979; Chesselet et al., this volume; Kita, this volume). In this respect, in situ hybridization is likely to be more specific and we can say that the majority of output cells contain GAD mRNA, which is of course consistent with the extensive evidence for the inhibitory nature of striato-pallidal/striato-nigral projections (Yoshida et al., 1971, 1979).

The GABA-ergic enkephalin and substance P neurones therefore constitute the majority of striatal output cells. However, the medium to large aspiny cells which seem to constitute the interneurone types are perhaps of more interest as they must provide the links between the phenotypically distinct "substance P" and "enkephalin" pathways through the striatum.

Cholinergic neurones

Early biochemical studies had shown that ACh was present in large amounts in the striatum along with the biosynthetic enzyme choline acetyltransferase (ChAT) and the degradative enzyme acetylcholinesterase (AChE) (McGeer et al., 1971; Cheney et al., 1975) and that lesions of projection pathways did not influence striatal content of ChAT or ACh (McGeer et al., 1974). Retrograde tracing studies also failed to label AChE-positive large cells when injections were placed in pallidum or nigra indicating that cholinergic cells were likely to be interneurones (Bak et al., 1978; Henderson, 1981; Woolf and Butcher, 1981; Parent et al., 1981). These observations were subsequently confirmed by immunohistochemistry when large aspiny ChAT immunoreactive cells were shown to comprise $2-3\%$ of striatal cells. These large cells had widespread processes which distributed throughout the striatum (Wainer et al., 1984; Bolam et al., 1984a,b). More recent work using in situ hybridization with ChAT mRNA-specific in situ probes have also confirmed that it is expressed in $2-3\%$ of medium to large striatal cells (Fig. 1). The role of these neurones in striatal functioning has recently been clarified by Lapper and Bolam (1992) who have shown that they receive a prominent thalamic input but little cortical input. This observation would suggest that the cholinergic cells may provide a means of "coding" thalamic information throughout the striatum. Consistent with this suggestion is the finding that cholinergic terminals innervate medium-sized neurones, including striato-nigral neurones (Izzo and Bolam, 1988), and that ACh influences enkephalin release. Both enkephalin- and substance P-containing output neurones are known to express muscarinic receptor mRNAs (Bernard et al., 1992), as do the cholinergic neurones themselves, allowing ACh neurones to influence their own activity.

Cholinergic neurones are also known to be under the control of dopaminergic nigro-striatal neurones acting on dopamine receptors expressed on these cells (Dawson et al., 1990; Weiner et al., 1990; Le Moine et al., 1990b). ACh and dopamine interact in a complex manner (Lehmann and Langer, 1983; Stoof et al., 1992) which may depend on patch/matrix organisation (Kemel et al., 1989; Gauchy et al., 1991).

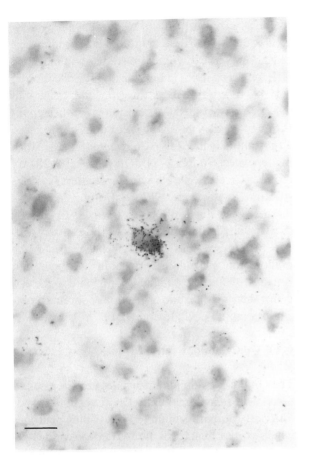

Fig. 1. Localisation of choline acetyltransferase (ChAT) mRNA in a large neurone of the rat striatum. The ChAT mRNA signal was detected using a ^{35}S labelled specific ChAT antisense probe and the sites of hybridization detected by emulsion autoradiography. Scale bar, 40 μm.

In contrast to the interest in dopamine-acetylcholine interactions less has been done to consider how excitatory amino acids (glutamate) and neuropeptides (substance P and enkephalin) influence cholinergic cells. The influence of substance P on cholinergic cells is of particular interest as these cells are known to express the majority of striatal tachykinin receptors which are of the neurokinin-1 type (Gerfen, 1991) and substance P-containing terminals have been reported to synapse on the somatodendritic tree of cholinergic neurones (Bolam et al., 1983b, 1986). Similarly, although the cholinergic cells are known to be sensitive to the excitatory amino acid agonist NMDA (Scatton and Lehmann,

1982) this had not been re-examined with recent techniques of in vivo microdialysis which can measure endogenous transmitter release, rather than the release of [3H]ACh in in vitro preparations. We therefore undertook studies of the effects of substance P and NMDA on ACh release in vivo using microdialysis.

The effects of local infusion of substance P by retrodialysis on ACh release in urethane anaesthe-

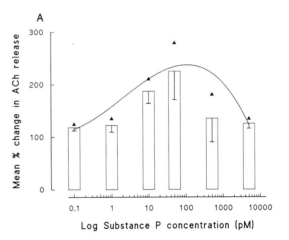

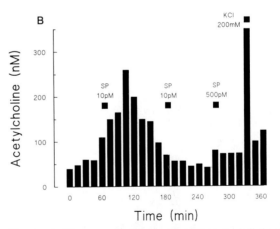

Fig. 2. *A.* Histogram and curve illustrating the bell-shaped dose – response effect of substance P on acetylcholine release in the anaesthetized rat. Values are means ± S.E.M. from 4 – 8 experiments for each dose of substance P. *B.* Graph showing ACh release in response to successive doses of substance P (10 pM). Note the marked release of ACh at the first application of substance P; subsequent application of substance P (SP) at 10 pM or 500 pM doses fails to elicit a response although depolarization with potassium chloride (KCl, 200 mM) readily produces a response.

tized rats is shown in Fig. 2*A*. Substance P elicited a dose-dependent increase in ACh release at low concentrations of substance P (1 – 50 pM); however, at higher concentrations (between 500 pM and 5 nM) the response declined giving a bell-shaped dose – response curve. The response to substance P also rapidly desensitized, with further application of substance P over the next few hours failing to elicit ACh release (Fig. 2*B*). These observations indicate that whatever substance P does in the striatum it does not do it very often! Parallel measurements of dopamine release indicated that it was not influenced by the substance P-evoked ACh release. As expected from the observations of Gerfen (1991) this response seems to be mediated by a neurokinin-1 receptor as the Pfizer NK-1 antagonist CP-96,345 (100 pM) and the Rhone Poulenc NK-1 antagonist RP67580 (500 pM) blocked the ACh release produced by application of substance P (50 pM) (Guevara-Guzman et al., 1993).

The localization of a tachykinin receptor on the cholinergic cells together with the presence of substance P-immunoreactive terminals on cholinergic cells (Bolam et al., 1986) suggests that the cholinergic cells are an important target for substance P af-

ferents. In contrast, in situ studies have not so far localized NMDA receptors to the large cholinergic cells; however, earlier in vitro studies had indicated [^{3}H]ACh release could be evoked by application of NMDA to striatal slices (Scatton and Lehmann, 1982). We confirmed this result in vivo when application of NMDA (50 μM) by retrodialysis produced a substantial increase in ACh release (Fig. 3). Much higher concentrations of NMDA (250 – 500 μM) are required to release amino acid transmitters from the striatum (Bustos et al., 1992) confirming the relative increased sensitivity of cholinergic cells to NMDA (Scatton and Lehmann, 1982). As the excitatory input to these cells is now believed to be predominantly from the thalamus (Lapper and Bolam, 1992), these data may contribute to the evidence that the thalamic projections contain the excitatory amino acid glutamate.

GABA-parvalbumin interneurones

The GABA-parvalbumin neurones are discussed in detail by Kita in this volume. They constitute an additional group of medium to large aspiny neurones which express high levels of GAD mRNA and GAD immunoreactivity (Bolam et al., 1983a; Kita and Kitai, 1988; Chesselet and Robbins, 1989; Cowan et al., 1990). The most important feature of these cells is that they provide a feed forward inhibitory circuit in which they receive excitatory inputs (mostly from cortex) and inhibit both spiny output cells and interneurones including those containing somatostatin (Kita, this volume). The parvalbumin cells also ignore patch-matrix boundaries allowing them to influence activity in areas associated with both limbic and motor cortex inputs (Cowan et al., 1990). Little is yet known of the receptor phenotype of these cells, although given their cortical glutamatergic input we would expect them to express excitatory amino acid receptors. They are known to express the inhibitory dopamine (D$_2$) but not the excitatory (D$_1$) dopamine receptor indicating that functionally they will respond to dopamine inputs as do the GABA-enkephalin-containing cells of the striato-pallidal pathway (Chesselet et al., this volume).

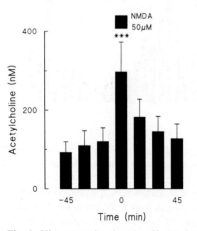

Fig. 3. Histogram showing the effects of N-methyl-D-aspartate (NMDA) (50 μM) on acetylcholine release from the striatum of the anaesthetized rat (*n* = 8 rats; *** *P* < 0.01 compared to control concentrations, paired *t*-test).

Somatostatin-neuropeptide Y-nitric oxide synthase interneurones

These medium-sized aspiny interneurones were originally identified by Pearse and colleagues (Thomas and Pearse, 1964) who identified a group of solitary active cells by their high content of "diaphorase" activity that could be observed by tetrazolium salt histochemistry. Pearse and colleagues also noted that these neurones were resistant to anoxia. Subsequent work by Vincent and colleagues (Vincent and Johansson, 1983; Vincent et al., 1983) showed that in the striatum these cells also contained the neuropeptides, neuropeptide Y and somatostatin (Fig. 4). However, it is only recently that the work of Vincent and colleagues (Hope et al., 1990, 1991) and Snyder and colleagues (Bredt and Snyder, 1989, 1990) has identified the brain NADPH-diaphorase activity as being primarily due to a calcium/calmodulin-activated enzyme, nitric oxide synthase (NOS). The idea that nitric oxide (NO), a soluble gas, might be an intercellular messenger has attracted a lot of interest (Snyder and Bredt 1991, 1992) and the physiological role(s) of NO in the central nervous system (CNS) are currently of considerable interest. In this context these

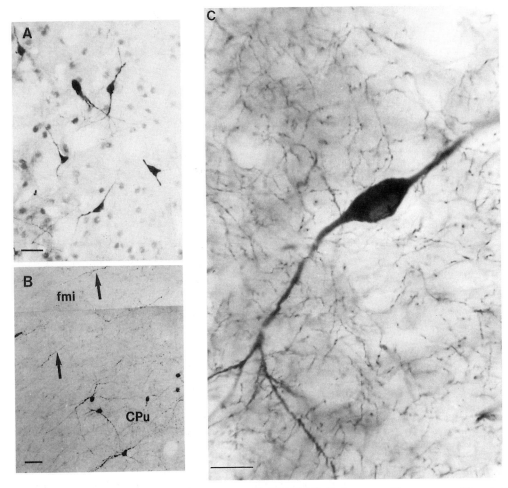

Fig. 4. Histochemical characterization of the neuropeptide Y/NADPH-diaphorase-positive neurones of the rat striatum. *A* and *B* show neuropeptide Y-immunoreactive neurones which are morphologically identical to those visualized by NADPH-diaphorase staining (*C*). These neurones are medium to large size neurones. Scale bars: *A*, 60 μm; *B*, 100 μm; and *C*, 20 μm.

cells, whose processes may bridge patch-matrix boundaries (Takagi et al., 1983) and receive prominent cortical (excitatory) and pallidal (inhibitory) inputs (Staines and Hincke, 1991), are well placed to influence activity throughout the striatum. It is therefore of considerable interest to understand what role local striatal release of NO gas may have. One possibility (and perhaps the most likely) is as a local vasodilator. The established role of NO is as endothelium-derived relaxing factor (EDRF) (Knowles and Moncada, 1992); however, local NO release will certainly influence guanylate cyclase and cGMP formation and the freely moving gas "NO"

would be ideally suited to integrate activity in local circuits or in a functional pathway. The striatum is one of the richest sites in the CNS for guanylate cyclase and cGMP content and NO released from NOS/somatostatin cells will activate guanylate cyclase in surrounding medium-sized spiny neurones (Ariano and Matus, 1981; Ariano et al., 1982; Ariano, 1983, 1984; Matsuoka et al., 1992). It is not known how increased cGMP formation would influence local neurones and activation of cGMP kinase may phosphorylate and influence the activity of a number of protein targets including ion channels and other kinases in a second messenger cas-

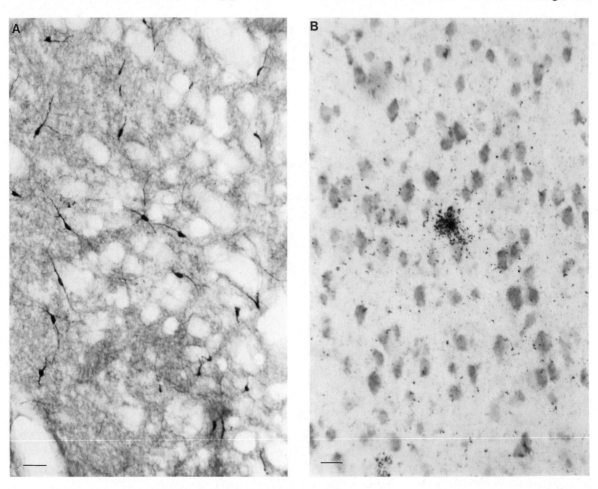

Fig. 5. Demonstration of nitric oxide synthase (NOS)-immunoreactive neurones (*A*) and NOS mRNA signal (*B*) in the rat striatum. The strongly stained NOS-immunoreactive neurones are identical in appearance to those stained with neuropeptide Y antibodies or NADPH-diaphorase histochemistry (Fig. 4). A similarly sized population of neurones also contains NOS mRNA signal (*B*). Scale bar: *A*, 100 μm; *B*, 40 μm.

cade. We might therefore expect cGMP increases to influence neuronal excitability and transmitter release.

To localize NO producing neurones, and study the expression of NOS in the CNS, we have recently cloned and isolated fragments of rat and human brain-specific NOS cDNA (Kishimoto et al., 1992), using primers based on Bredt et al. (1991) and used these cDNA fragments to express NOS and raise antibodies to the N-terminal portions of NOS (the portion with NOS activity, rather than the electron transferring oxido-reductase C-terminus). Antibodies and in situ probes confirm that the NOS cells correspond to somatostatin/neuropeptide Y cells (Fig. 5) and co-existence studies show that NOS and somatostatin in situ signals are co-localized (Fig. 6). These medium-sized NOS-somatostatin-neuropeptide Y cells are presumably the medium-sized aspiny cells which do not contain GAD mRNA (Chesselet and Robbins, 1989b).

To consider what effect local release of NO might have on striatal neurone activity we used Fura-2-loaded foetal striatal neurones in culture and investigated the effects of local NO releasers on the response of these cells to glutamate agonists (NMDA and kainate). Application of NMDA to cultured neurones produced a large intracellular Ca^{2+} pulse (Fig. 7) consistent with opening the NMDA receptor Ca^{2+} channel. Application of NO

releasers such as isosorbide and S-nitrosoacetyl penicillamine (SNAP) did not influence the response of the neurones to application of kainate or to potassium chloride (opening the voltage-sensitive calcium channels) (Fig. 7A); however, the response of these neurones to NMDA was reduced in a dose-dependent fashion (Fig. 7B). These data would suggest that local release of NO in the striatum would tend to reduce the excitatory effects of cortical or thalamic excitatory inputs on striatal neurones providing a feed back inhibitory mechanism which may be neuroprotective. The mechanism of this effect of NO on the NMDA receptor itself is not understood. It may involve modification of the oxidation-reduction site but is certainly directly on the NMDA receptor, rather than through cGMP and the guanylate cyclase pathway, as the effect can be observed in isolated membrane patches (Manzoni et al., 1992).

Conclusion

The striatal interneurones discussed here provide feed forward and feed back control between the phenotypically distinct output pathways of the striatum and link between patch and matrix compartments. In this regard they receive relatively selective inputs from cortex, thalamus and pallidum which

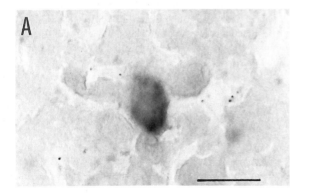
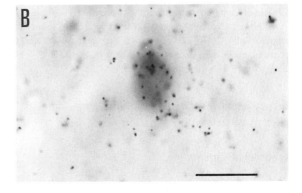

Fig. 6. Demonstration of the co-expression of somatostatin mRNA signal (*A*) and nitric oxide synthase mRNA (*B*) in the same striatal neurone. Note the non-isotopic in situ signal for somatostatin mRNA (*A*) is localized in the same neurones as the NOS-mRNA signal (isotopic probe). The autoradiographic emulsion coats the tissue section so that the silver grains (*B*) overlie the somatostatin-positive neurone (*A*) demonstrating the co-expression of the two target mRNAs in the same cell. Scale bar, 20 μm.

162

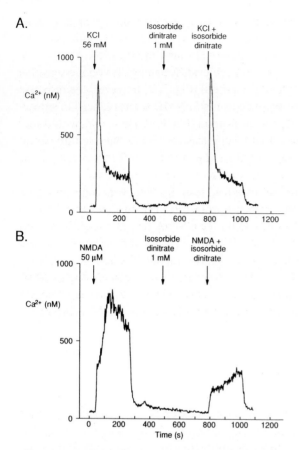

A.

B.

Fig. 7. Video imaging of a Fura-2-loaded cultured striatal neurone. (*A*) The response of the neurone to the application of a
depolarizing pulse of KCl (56 mM) is not influenced by the
presence of the nitric oxide releaser isosorbide dinitrate. The
response to KCl indicates that NO does not influence the opening
of voltage-sensitive Ca^{2+} channels in the neurone. (*B*) The
response of the same striatal neurone imaged in (*A*) to application of NMDA. The application of NMDA produces a rapid rise
in intracellular Ca^{2+}. The response is, however, substantially
reduced (and in some neurones abolished) when NMDA is applied together with isosorbide.

will presumably serve to distinguish these "inputs"
in terms of striatal information processing.

Acknowledgements

We are grateful to the MRC for their continued support. PJN is supported by Bayer, Germany, RS by
the Government of Galicia and JK by Shiseido Inc.,
Yokohoma, Japan. SJA acknowledges the financial
support of the Tourette Syndrome Association
(U.S.A.).

References

Ariano, M.A. (1983) Distribution of components of the guano-
sine 3′,5′-phosphate system in rat caudate-putamen. *Neuroscience*, 10: 707 – 723.

Ariano, M.A. (1984) Rat striatal cyclic nucleotide-reactive cells
and acetylcholinesterase-reactive interneurons are separate
populations. *Brain Res.*, 296: 160 – 163.

Ariano, M.A. and Matus, A.I. (1981) Ultrastructural localization of cyclic GMP and cyclic AMP in rat striatum. *J. Cell
Biol.*, 91: 287 – 292.

Ariano, M.A., Lewicki, J.A., Branswein, H.J. and Murad, F.
(1982) Immunohistochemical localization of guanylate cyclase
within neurons of rat brain. *Proc. Natl. Acad. Sci. U.S.A.*, 79:
1316 – 1320.

Bak, I.J., Markham, C.H., Cook, M.L. and Stevens, J.G. (1978)
Ultrastructural and immunoperoxidase study of striatonigral
neurons by means of retrograde axonal transport of herpes
simplex virus. *Brain Res.*, 143: 361 – 368.

Bernard, V., Normand, E. and Bloch, B. (1992) Phenotypical
characterization of the rat striatal neurons expressing muscarinic receptor genes. *J. Neurosci.*, 12: 3591 – 3600.

Bolam, J.P., Powell, J.F., Totterdell, S. and Smith, A.D.
(1981a) The proportion of neurons in the rat neostriatum that
project to the substantia nigra demonstrated using horseradish
peroxidase conjugated with wheatgerm agglutin. *Brain Res.*,
220: 339 – 343.

Bolam, J.P., Somogyi, P., Totterdell, S. and Smith, A.D.
(1981b) A second type of striatonigral neuron: a comparison
between retrogradely labelled and Golgi-stained neurons at the
light and electron microscopic levels. *Neuroscience*, 6:
2141 – 2157.

Bolam, J.P., Clark, D.J., Smith, A.D. and Somogyi, P. (1983a)
A type of aspiny neuron in the rat neostriatum accumulates
[^{3}H]γ-aminobutyric acid; combination of Golgi-staining, autoradiography and electron microscopy. *J. Comp. Neurol.*,
213: 121 – 134.

Bolam, J.P., Somogyi, P., Takagi, H., Fodor, I. and Smith A.D.
(1983b) Localization of substance P-like immunoreactivity in
neurons and nerve terminals in the neostriatum of the rat: a
correlated light and electron microscopic study. *J. Neurocytol.*, 12: 325 – 344.

Bolam, J.P., Ingham, C.A. and Smith, A.D. (1984a) The section
Golgi impregnation procedure, III. Combination of Golgi-
impregnation with enzyme histochemistry and electron
microscopy to characterize acetylcholinesterase-containing
neurons in the rat neostriatum. *Neuroscience*, 12: 687 – 718.

Bolam, J.P., Wainer, B.H. and Smith, A.D. (1984b) Characterization of cholinergic neurons in the rat neostriatum. A combination of choline acetyltransferase immunocytochemistry,

Golgi impregnation and electron microscopy. *Neuroscience,* 12: 711 – 718.

Bolam, J.P., Ingham, C.A., Izzo, P.M., Levey, A.I., Rye, D.B., Smith, A.D. and Wainer, B.H. (1986) Substance P-containing terminals in synaptic contact with cholinergic neurons in the neostriatum and basal forebrain: a double immunocytochemical study in the rat. *Brain Res.,* 397: 279 – 289.

Bredt, D.S. and Snyder, S.H. (1989) Nitric oxide mediates glutamate-linked enhancement of cGMP levels in the cerebellum. *Proc. Natl. Acad. Sci. U.S.A.,* 86: 9030 – 9033.

Bredt, D.S. and Snyder, S.H. (1990) Isolation of nitric oxide synthase, a calmodulin-requiring enzyme. *Proc. Natl. Acad. Sci. U.S.A.,* 87: 682 – 685.

Bredt, D.S., Hwang, P.M., Glatt, C.E., Lowenstein, C.L., Reed, R.R. and Snyder, S.H. (1991) Cloned and expressed nitric oxide synthase structurally resembles cytochrome P-450 reductase. *Nature,* 351: 714 – 719.

Bunney, B.S. and Aghajanian, G.K. (1976) The precise localization of nigral afferents in the rat as determined by a retrograde tracing technique. *Brain Res.,* 117: 423 – 436.

Bustos, G., Abarca, J., Forray, M.I., Gysling, K., Bradberry, C.W. and Roth, R.H. (1992) Regulation of excitatory amino acid release by *N*-methyl-D-asparate receptors in rat striatum: in vivo microdialysis studies. *Brain Res.,* 585: 105 – 115.

Cheney, D.L., LeFevre, H.F. and Racagni, G. (1975) Choline acetyltransferase activity and mass fragmentographic measurement of acetylcholine in specific nuclei and tracts of rat brain. *Neuropharmacology,* 14: 801 – 809.

Chesselet, M.-F. and Robbins, E. (1989) Characterization of striatal neurons expressing high levels of glutamic acid decarboxylase messenger RNA. *Brain Res.,* 492: 237 – 244.

Chesselet, M.-F., Weiss, L., Wuenschell, C., Tobin, A.J. and Affolter, H.-U. (1987) Comparative distribution of mRNAs for glutamic acid decarboxylase, tyrosine hydroxylase, and tachykinins in the basal ganglia: in situ hybridization study in the rodent brain. *J. Comp. Neurol.,* 262: 125 – 140.

Cowan, R.L., Wilson, C.J., Emson, P.C. and Heizmann, C.W. (1990) Parvalbumin-containing GABAergic interneurons in the rat neostriatum. *J. Comp. Neurol.,* 302: 197 – 205.

Cuello, A.C. and Paxinos, G. (1978) Evidence for a long Leu-enkephalin striopallidal pathway in rat brain. *Nature,* 271: 178 – 180.

Dawson, V.L., Dawson, T.M. and Wamsley, J.K. (1990) Muscarinic and dopaminergic receptor subtypes on striatal cholinergic interneurons. *Brain Res. Bull.,* 25: 903 – 912.

Faull, R.L.M. and Mehler, W.R. (1976) Studies of the fiber connections of the substantia nigra in the rat using the method of retrograde transport of horseradish peroxidase. *Soc. Neurosci. Abstr.,* 2: 62.

Fox, C.A., Andrade, A., Hillman, D.E. and Schwyn, R.C. (1972) The spiny neurons in the primate striatum: a Golgi and electron microscopic study. *J. Hirnforsch.,* 13: 181 – 201.

Gauchy, C., Desban, M., Krebs, M.O., Glowinski, J. and Kemel, M.L. (1991) Role of dynorphin-containing neurons in the presynaptic inhibitory control of the acetylcholine-evoked release of dopamine in the striosomes and the matrix of the cat caudate nucleus. *Neuroscience,* 41: 449 – 458.

Gerfen, C.R. (1991) Substance P (neurokinin-1) receptor mRNA is selectively expressed in cholinergic neurons in the striatum and basal forebrain. *Brain Res.,* 556: 165 – 170.

Gerfen, C.R. and Young III, W.S. (1988) Distribution of striatonigral and striatopallidal peptidergic neurons in both patch and matrix compartments: an in situ hybridization histochemistry and fluorescent retrograde tracing study. *Brain Res.,* 460: 161 – 167.

Graybiel, A.M., and Ragsdale Jr., C.W. (1983) Biochemical anatomy of the striatum. In: P.C. Emson (Ed.), *Chemical Neuroanatomy,* Raven Press, New York, pp. 427 – 504.

Graybiel, A.M., Ragsdale, C.W. and Moon Edley, S. (1979) Compartments in the striatum of the cat observed by retrograde cell-labeling. *Exp. Brain Res.,* 34: 189 – 195.

Guevara Guzman, R., Kendrick, K.M. and Emson, P.C. (1993) Effect of substance P on acetylcholine and dopamine release in the rat striatum: a microdialysis study. *Brain Res.,* in press.

Henderson, Z. (1981) Ultrastructure and acetylcholinesterase content of neurones forming connections between the striatum and substantia nigra of rat. *J. Comp. Neurol.,* 197: 185 – 196.

Hope, B.T., Michael, G.J., Knigge, K.M. and Vincent, S.R. (1990) NADPH-diaphorase synthesizes a second messenger; yes or no. *Soc. Neurosci. Abstr.,* 16: 538.

Hope, B.T., Michael, G.J., Knigge, K.M. and Vincent, S.R. (1991) Neuronal NADPH-diaphorase is a nitric oxide synthase. *Proc. Natl. Acad. Sci. U.S.A.,* 88: 2811 – 2814.

Izzo, P.N. and Bolam, J.P. (1988) Cholinergic synaptic input to different parts of spiny striatonigral neurons in the rat. *J. Comp. Neurol.,* 269: 219 – 234.

Jessell, T.M., Emson, P.C., Paxinos, G. and Cuello, A.C. (1978) Topographic projection of substance P and GABA pathways in the striato- and pallido-nigral system: a biochemical and immunohistochemical study. *Brain Res.,* 152: 487 – 498.

Kanazawa, I., Emson, P.C. and Cuello, A.C. (1977) Evidence for the existence of substance P-containing fibres in striato-nigral and pallido-nigral pathways in rat brain. *Brain Res.,* 119: 447 – 453.

Kemel, M.L., Desban, M., Glowinski, J. and Gauchy, C. (1989) Distinct presynaptic control of dopamine release in striosomal and matrix areas of the cat caudate nucleus. *Proc. Natl. Acad. Sci. U.S.A.,* 86: 9006 – 9010.

Kemp, J.M. and Powell, T.P.S. (1971) The structure of the caudate nucleus of the cat: light and electron microscopy. *Phil. Trans. R. Soc. Lond. (Biol.),* 262: 383 – 401.

Kishimoto, J., Spurr, N., Emson, P.C. and Xu, W. (1992) Localization of brain nitric oxide synthase to human chromosome 12. *Genomics,* 14: 802 – 804.

Kita, H. and Kitai, S.T. (1988) Glutamate decarboxylase immunoreactive neurons in rat neostriatum: their morphological types and populations. *Brain Res.,* 447: 346 – 352.

Knowles, R.G. and Moncada, S. (1992) Nitric oxide as a signal in blood vessels. *Trends Biochem. Sci.,* 17: 399–402.

Kocsis, J.D., Sugimori, M. and Kitai, S.T. (1977) Convergence of excitatory synaptic inputs to caudate spiny neurons. *Brain Res.,* 124: 403–413.

Lapper, S.R. and Bolam, J.P. (1992) Input from the frontal cortex and the parafascicular nucleus to cholinergic interneurons in the dorsal striatum of the rat. *Neuroscience,* 51: 533–545.

Lehmann, J. and Langer, S.Z. (1983) The striatal cholinergic interneuron: synaptic target of dopaminergic terminals? *Neuroscience,* 10: 1105–1120.

Le Moine, C., Normand, E., Guitteny, A.F., Fouque, B., Teoule, R. and Bloch, B. (1990a) Dopamine receptor gene expression by enkephalin neurons in rat forebrain. *Proc. Natl. Acad. Sci. U.S.A.,* 87: 230–234.

Le Moine, C., Tison, F. and Bloch, B. (1990b) D2 dopamine receptor gene expression by cholinergic neurons in the rat striatum. *Neurosci. Lett.,* 117: 248–252.

Manzoni, O., Prezeau, L., Marin, P., Deshager, S., Bockaert, J. and Fagni, L. (1992) Nitric oxide-induced blockade of NMDA receptors. *Neuron,* 8: 653–662.

Matsuoka, I., Giuili, G., Poyard, M., Stengel, D., Parma, J., Guellaen, G. and Hanoune, J. (1992) Localization of adenylyl and guanylyl cyclase in rat brain by in situ hybridization: comparison with calmodulin mRNA distribution. *J. Neurosci.,* 12: 3350–3360.

McGeer, P.L., McGeer, E.G., Fibiger, H.C. and Wickson, V. (1971) Neostriatal choline acetylase and cholinesterase following selective brain lesions. *Brain Res.,* 35: 308–314.

McGeer, P.L., McGeer, E.G., Singh, V.K. and Chase, W.H. (1974) Choline acetyltransferase localization in the central nervous system by immunohistochemistry. *Brain Res.,* 81: 373–379.

Parent, A., Boucher, R. and O'Reilly-Fromentin, J. (1981) Acetylcholinesterase-containing neurons in cat pallidal complex: morphological characteristics and projection towards the neocortex. *Brain Res.,* 230: 356–361.

Penny, G.R., Afsharpour, S. and Kitai, S.T. (1986) The glutamate decarboxylase-, leucine enkephalin-, methionine enkephalin- and substance P-immunoreactive neurons in the neostriatum of the rat and cat: evidence for partial population overlap. *Neuroscience,* 17: 1011–1045.

Precht, W. and Yoshida, M. (1971) Blockage of caudate-evoked inhibition of neurons in the substantia nigra by picrotoxin. *Brain Res.,* 32: 229–233.

Preston, R.J., Bishop, G.A. and Kitai, S.T. (1980) Medium spiny neuron projection from the rat striatum: an intracellular horseradish peroxidase study. *Brain Res.,* 183: 253–263.

Ribak, C.E., Vaughn, J.E. and Roberts, E. (1979) The GABA neurons and their axon terminals in rat corpus striatum as demonstrated by GAD immunocytochemistry. *J. Comp. Neurol.,* 187: 261–283.

Scatton, B. and Lehmann, J. (1982) N-methyl-D-aspartate type receptor mediates striatal ^{3}H-acetylcholine release evoked by excitatory amino acids. *Nature,* 297: 422–424.

Somogyi, P. and Smith, A.D. (1979) Projection of neostriatal spiny neurons to the substantia nigra. Application of a combined Golgi-staining and horseradish peroxidase transport procedure at both light and electron microscopic levels. *Brain Res.,* 178: 3–15.

Sorimachi, M. and Kataoka, K. (1974) Choline uptake by nerve terminals: a sensitive and a specific marker of cholinergic innervation. *Brain Res.,* 72: 350–353.

Staines, W.A. and Hincke, M.T.C. (1991) Substantial alterations in neurochemical and metabolic indices in select basal ganglia neurons follow lesions of globus pallidus neurons in rats. *Soc. Neurosci. Abstr.,* 17 (1): 456.

Stoof, J.C., Drukarch, B., De Boer, P., Westerink, B.H.C. and Groenewegen, H.J. (1992) Regulation of the activity of striatal cholinergic neurons by dopamine. *Neuroscience,* 47: 755–770.

Snyder, S.H. and Bredt, D.S. (1991) Nitric oxide as a neuronal messenger. *Trends Pharmacol. Sci.,* 12: 125–128.

Snyder, S.H. and Bredt, D.S. (1992) Biological roles of nitric oxide. *Sci. Am.,* May 1992: 28–35.

Szabo, J. (1979) Strionigral and nigrostriatal connections. *Appl. Neurophysiol.,* 42: 9–12.

Takagi, H., Somogyi, P., Somogyi, J. and Smith, A.D. (1983) Fine structural studies on a type of somatostatin-immunoreactive neuron and its synaptic connections in the rat neostriatum: a correlated light and electron microscopic study. *J. Comp. Neurol.,* 214: 1–16.

Thomas, E. and Pearse, A.G.E. (1964) The solitary active cells. Histochemical demonstration of damage-resistant nerve cells with a TPN-diaphorase reaction. *Acta Neuropathol. (Berl.),* 3: 238–249.

Vincent, S.R. and Johansson, O. (1983) Striatal neurons containing both somatostatin- and avian pancreatic polypeptide (APP)-like immunoreactivities and NADPH-diaphorase activity: a light and electron microscopic study. *J. Comp. Neurol.,* 217: 264–270.

Vincent, S.R., Johansson, O., Hökfelt, T., Skirboll, L., Elde, R.P., Terenius, L., Kimmel, J. and Goldstein, M. (1983) NADPH-diaphorase: a selective histochemical marker for striatal neurons containing both somatostatin- and avian pancreatic polypeptide (APP)-like immunoreactivities. *J. Comp. Neurol.,* 217: 252–263.

Wainer, B.H., Bolam, J.P., Freund, T.F., Henderson, Z., Totterdell, S. and Smith, A.D. (1984) Cholinergic synapses in the rat brain: a correlated light and electron microscopic immunohistochemical study employing a monoclonal antibody against choline acetyltransferase. *Brain Res.,* 308: 69–76.

Weiner, D.M., Levey, A.I. and Brann, M.R. (1990) Expression of muscarinic acetylcholine and dopamine receptor mRNAs in rat basal ganglia. *Proc. Natl. Acad. Sci. U.S.A.,* 87: 7050–7054.

Wilson, C.J. (1990) Basal ganglia. In: G.M. Shepherd (Ed.), *The Synaptic Organisation of the Brain,* Oxford University Press, Oxford, pp. 279–317.

Wilson, C.J. and Groves, P.M. (1980) Fine structure and synaptic connections of the common spiny neuron of the rat neostriatum: a study employing intracellular injection of horseradish peroxidase. *J. Comp. Neurol.,* 194: 599 – 615.

Woolf, N.J. and Butcher, L.L. (1981) Cholinergic neurons of the caudate-putamen complex proper are intrinsically organized: a combined Evans blue and acetylcholinesterase analysis. *Brain Res. Bull.,* 7: 487 – 507.

Yoshida, M. and Omata, S. (1979) Blocking by picrotoxin of nigra-evoked inhibition of neurons of ventromedial nucleus of the thalamus. *Experimentia,* 35: 794.

Yoshida, M. and Precht, W. (1971) Monosynaptic inhibition of neurons in the substantia nigra by caudate-nigral fibers. *Brain Res.,* 32: 225 – 228.

Young III, W.S., Bonner, T.I. and Brann, M.R. (1986) Mesencephalic dopamine neurons regulate the expression of neuropeptide mRNAs in the rat forebrain. *Proc. Natl. Acad. Sci. U.S.A.,* 83: 9827 – 9831.

G.W. Arbuthnott and P.C. Emson (Eds.)
Progress in Brain Research, Vol. 99
© 1993 Elsevier Science Publishers B.V. All rights reserved.

CHAPTER 11

Dopamine receptors: structure and function

Philip G. Strange

Biological Laboratory, The University, Canterbury, Kent, CT2 7NJ, U.K.

Introduction

Receptors for the neurotransmitter dopamine have been studied intensively over the past 30 years and something of a consensus was reached in the late 1970s from biochemical and pharmacological studies that there were two subtypes of dopamine receptor (D_1, D_2) (Kebabian and Calne, 1979) (Table I). This relatively simple picture has been transformed with the application of molecular biology techniques to the study of dopamine receptors in the recent years. These studies have shown that there are at least six dopamine receptor isoforms defined on the basis of cloned DNA sequences and the corresponding amino acid sequences (summarised in Table II). Although this seems very complex, the different receptor isoforms may be grouped in to sub-families that resemble the D_1 (cloned D_1, D_5) and D_2 (cloned $D_{2(short)}$, $D_{2(long)}$, D_3, D_4) receptors proposed previously. Below I shall show how this grouping in to sub-families can be justified on structural and functional grounds and refer to the sub-families as D_1-like and D_2-like receptors.

The nomenclature for dopamine receptors has become rather cumbersome and confusing. Indeed it has been suggested that a new nomenclature should be used based on the D_1-like and D_2-like sub-families (Sibley and Monsma, 1992). Thus D_1 and D_5 would become D_{1A} and D_{1B} and D_2, D_3 and D_4 would become D_{2A}, D_{2B} and D_{2C}. Although this has some rational basis, it may be prudent to retain older nomenclatures until it is known that all the dopamine receptor subtypes have been cloned.

In the subsequent sections of this chapter I shall describe the common features of the different dopamine receptor isoforms, then their individual features and finally offer some speculations on the functional implications of the findings.

Features common to the dopamine receptor isoforms

Each isoform contains about 400 amino acids corresponding to a protein mass of about 50000 daltons. This will then be glycosylated with oligosaccharide chains whose mass is likely to be in the region of 20000 daltons. It is not possible to be more precise about this as estimates of molecular weights (from SDS-PAGE analysis) are at present subject to uncertainty (see, for example, Clagett Dame and McKelvy, 1989).

When the amino acid sequences are subjected to hydropathy analysis in all cases seven sequences of hydrophobic amino acids long enough to form transmembrane α-helices are recognised. Thus each isoform conforms to the, now classical, model for G-protein-linked receptors of seven putative transmembrane α-helices linked by extracellular and intracellular loops with an extracellular amino terminal section and an intracellular carboxyterminal tail. This places the dopamine receptors as members of the super-family of G-protein-linked receptors (see Strange, 1991c, for a review).

When the layout of the sequences with respect to the membrane is examined some differences can be seen. The D_1-like receptors (D_1, D_5) have relatively

168

TABLE I

Dopamine receptor subtypes defined on the basis of pharmacological and biochemical studies

	D_1	D_2
Pharmacological profile		
Selective agonists	SKF 38393, fenoldopam	N-O437, quinpirole
Selective antagonists	SCH 23390, SKF 83566	Domperidone, sulpiride, YM 091512
Effector responses		
		Adenylyl cyclase ↓
	Adenylylcyclase ↑	K^+ channel ↑
	Phospholipase C ↑	Ca^{2+} channel ↓

The pharmacologically and biochemically defined D_1 and D_2 receptors, originally defined by Kebabian and Calne (1979), correspond to D_1-like and D_2-like sub-families of cloned receptor isoforms (Table II).

short third intracellular loops and long carboxyterminal tails. The D_2-like receptors (D_2, D_3, D_4) have relatively long third intracellular loops and short carboxyterminal tails. This presumably in some way reflects their function, the former arrangement being similar to other receptors that signal via the G-protein G_s and the latter being similar to some receptors that signal via G_o/G_i.

There is no firm information on the functional regions of the receptors but it is assumed that oligosaccharides are placed on the extracellular part of the receptors and consensus sequences for glycosylation are found in the amino terminal section (D_{1-5}) and second extracellular loop (D_1, D_5). By analogy with other G-protein-linked receptors a major site of interaction with the G-protein is likely to be on the third intracellular loop. There is a cysteine in the carboxyterminal section of each isoform that is probably palmitoylated and this may lead to the formation of an additional intracellular loop (O'Dowd et al., 1989). The ligand-binding site of the receptors is thought to be formed by the bundling together of the transmembrane spanning α-helices generating a cavity in to which ligands bind via inter-

actions with certain amino acid side chains (see below).

Comparison of the amino acid sequences of the different isoforms supports the D_1-like, D_2-like sub-grouping. Between isoforms within a sub-group, e.g., D_1, D_5, there is considerable homology especially in the transmembrane spanning regions. Between isoforms in different sub-groups, e.g., D_1, D_2, the homology is less and about the same as that with other G-protein-linked receptors.

Within the amino acid sequences certain conserved residues can be recognised and it is then presumed that these play important functional roles. For example, aspartic acid residues within the second and third transmembrane spanning regions can be seen in each isoform. The former is about two thirds in to the membrane, is conserved in a wide range of G-protein-linked receptors in addition to the dopamine receptors and is likely to play a rather general role in G-protein-linked receptor function, perhaps in maintaining the conformation of the protein (see below for more discussion). The aspartic acid in the third transmembrane region (about a third in to the membrane) is conserved only in receptors that bind cationic amine ligands and is thought to be important for providing the counterion for the cationic amine head group in binding to the receptor.

Two serine residues in the fifth transmembrane α-helix are also conserved in each dopamine receptor and are thought to be important for interaction with the catechol hydroxyl groups of dopamine. Within the sub-group of D_2-like receptors (D_2, D_3, D_4) a histidine and a tyrosine in the sixth and seventh transmembrane spanning regions can be seen. These may also be important for receptor function as will be explored below.

Individual features of the dopamine receptor isoforms

D_1-like receptor isoforms

When D_1 and D_5 receptors are expressed in animal cells they all show the pharmacological profile for D_1-like receptors (high affinity for SCH

23390, low affinity for spiperone). The principal differences in pharmacological properties are that D_5 shows a higher affinity (ten-fold) for dopamine and a lower affinity (nine-fold) for $(+)$-butaclamol compared to D_1. A dopamine receptor subtype has been cloned from rat and termed D_{1B} (Tiberi et al., 1991). This appears, however, to be the rat homologue of the D_5 receptor originally cloned from a human source.

When expressed from their cloned genes, D_1 and D_5 receptors lead to stimulation of adenylyl cyclase, the classical second messenger response linked to D_1-like receptors. There are, however, reports of D_1-like receptor stimulation of phospholipase C in some tissues (Andersen et al., 1990) so that additional D_1-like receptor isoforms may yet be cloned.

The polymerase chain reaction (PCR) and in situ hybridisation have been used to determine the localisation of mRNA for D_1 and D_5 receptor isoforms (Table II). This showed that mRNA for D_1 receptors is found at high levels in the neostriatum (caudate nucleus/putamen) and the nucleus accumbens and olfactory tubercle as expected from ligand-binding studies. mRNA for D_5 receptors is present at lower levels in several brain regions. In the earlier work on D_1 receptors no mRNA could be detected

TABLE II

Dopamine receptor isoforms from gene cloning

	"D_1-like"		"D_2-like"		
	D_1	D_5	D_2	D_3	D_4
Amino acids	446(h,r)	477(h) 475(r)	414/443(h) 415/444(r)	400(h) 446(r)	387(h) 368(r)
Pharmacological specificity	SCH 23390 (0.35), dopamine (2340)	SCH 23390 (0.30), dopamine (228)	Spiperone (0.05), raclopride (1.8), clozapine (56), dopamine (1705)	Spiperone (0.61), raclopride (3.5), clozapine (180), dopamine (27)	Spiperone (0.05), raclopride (237), clozapine (9), dopamine (450)
Localisation	Caudate/putamen, nucleus accumbens, olfactory tubercle, frontal cortex	Caudate/putamen, nucleus accumbens, olfactory tubercle, hippocampus, hypothalamus, frontal cortex (all low)	Caudate/putamen, nucleus accumbens, olfactory tubercle, cerebral cortex (low)	Nucleus accumbens, olfactory tubercle, islands of Calleja, cerebral cortex (low)	Frontal cortex, amygdala, medulla (all low), cardiovascular system, retina
Effector response	cAMP ↑	cAMP ↑	cAMP ↓	?	?
References	See, for example, Dearry et al. (1990)	Sunahara et al. (1991); Tiberi et al. (1991)	See, for example, Dal Toso et al. (1989)	Sokoloff et al. (1990); Giros et al. (1990); Bouthenet et al. (1991)	Van Tol et al. (1991); O'Malley et al. (1992)

The properties of the principal dopamine receptor isoforms identified by gene cloning are shown. They are divided up into "D_1-like" and "D_2-like" groups to reflect amino acid homology, functional similarity and similar pharmacological properties. This grouping also conforms with previous classifications based only on pharmacological and biochemical properties (see Table I; Kebabian and Calne, 1979). Under amino acids, h and r refer to human and rat sequences respectively. Under the D_2 isoform two sizes are shown referring to the $D_{2(short)}$ and $D_{2(long)}$ isoforms. These isoforms differ by a 29 amino acid insertion in the $D_{2(long)}$ form and are derived by alternative splicing of a common genomic sequence (Strange, 1990b). Under pharmacological specificity the figures are the dissociation constants (nM) for selected ligands taken from the published data and some are for rat, some human. The figures for dopamine are in the presence of Gpp(NH)p. The localisations shown are the principal ones known at present which in some cases have not been examined exhaustively. For general reviews, see Strange (1990b, 1991a,c).

in peripheral tissues such as the kidney or heart where it is known that D_1-like receptors are present from functional studies. A recent report has, however, described the localisation of mRNA for D_1 dopamine receptors in rat kidney (Meister et al., 1991).

D₂-like dopamine receptor isoforms

In this sub-group of dopamine receptors the D_2 isoform was the first to be cloned at the end of 1988 (Bunzow et al., 1988). It soon became apparent that there were two forms of the D_2 receptor which have been termed $D_{2(short)}$ and $D_{2(long)}$ (see, for example, Dal Toso et al., 1989; reviewed in Strange, 1990b). These are derived by alternative splicing of a common genomic sequence. The two splice variants code for proteins that are identical except for a 29 amino acid insertion in the third intracellular loop of the receptor, hence $D_{2(short)}$ and $D_{2(long)}$. The insertion is contained on a single exon and the gene for the D_2 dopamine receptor contains multiple exons and introns (Gandelman et al., 1991). This is unusual for G-protein-linked receptors as these are mostly expressed as single exons.

Subsequently the D_3 and D_4 isoforms were identified by gene cloning (Sokoloff et al., 1990; Van Tol et al., 1991; reviewed in Strange, 1991a,b). In both cases the genes contain multiple exons and introns so the D_2-like sub-group can be identified by the complexity of the genomic structure. It is not known at present whether "short" and "long" variants of D_3 and D_4 receptors exist.

When D_2, D_3 and D_4 receptors were expressed in animal cells, although each isoform was found to bind classical dopamine antagonists, e.g., haloperidol and spiperone with high affinity, there were also significant differences for certain ligands. $D_{2(short)}$ and $D_{2(long)}$ when expressed did not show any differences in antagonist affinities although there were some minor differences in the behaviour of agonists in binding to these isoforms (Giros et al., 1989). An exhaustive study of the differences between the two isoforms has not been carried out but the behaviour is consistent with the structural difference between the two. The 29 amino acid insertion

in $D_{2(long)}$ is in the third intracellular loop, a region of the receptor thought not to be important for ligand binding but thought to be important for interaction with G-proteins (Lefkowitz and Caron, 1988). This difference between $D_{2(short)}$ and $D_{2(long)}$ ought therefore to influence agonist but not antagonist binding. More recent studies outlined below tend to question this interpretation.

If a comparison of the affinities of some key representative ligands for D_2, D_3 and D_4 receptors is made then some trends can be discerned (Table II). D_3 is distinguished from D_2 by its lower affinity for binding typical dopamine antagonists, e.g., spiperone, but a relatively similar ability to bind certain antagonists including the substituted benzamides, e.g., raclopride. Agonist, e.g., dopamine affinities are notably higher at D_3 than at D_2. D_4 binds some typical dopamine antagonists with similar affinity to D_2 but has a rather lower affinity for others including some substituted benzamide antagonists and a relatively higher affinity for ligands such as clozapine. Although certain trends can be discerned for groups of compounds each of the isoforms has its own particular pharmacological profile.

Functionally the D_2 isoforms ($D_{2(short)}$ and $D_{2(long)}$) are the only ones to which functions may be attached. The D_2 isoforms both inhibit adenylyl cyclase when expressed in CHO cells. $D_{2(short)}$ appears to couple more effectively to inhibition of adenylyl cyclase than does $D_{2(long)}$ (Dal Toso et al., 1989; Montmayeur and Borelli, 1991) supporting the idea that there is a difference between the two isoforms in coupling to G-proteins (see above).

The D_3 receptor when expressed in CHO cells neither affects adenylyl cyclase nor shows coupling to the endogenous G-proteins (Sokoloff et al., 1990). This may reflect the lack of suitable G-proteins in this cell line and requires expression of the D_3 receptor in another cell line containing a different complement of G-proteins. The D_4 receptor when expressed in COS-7 cells does couple to G-proteins but there is no report at present about coupling to second messenger systems (Van Tol et al., 1991).

The tissue distributions of the different isoforms have been determined in greater or lesser detail and the principal localisations are given in Table II. These distributions have been determined at the mRNA level (in situ hybridisation, polymerase chain reaction, solution hybridisation/protection) (for example, Mansour et al., 1990; O'Malley et al., 1990; Gandelman et al., 1991; Snyder et al., 1991) and may not reflect precisely the distributions at the protein level. For the D_2 receptor isoforms the highest mRNA concentrations are found in the ventral tegmental area and the substantia nigra pars compacta where the cell bodies of mesocortical and mesostriatal dopamine neurones are found and in the neostriatum (caudate nucleus/putamen) and certain limbic regions (olfactory tubercle, nucleus accumbens) which are the areas of termination of these neurones. Detailed distribution studies have been performed (O'Malley et al., 1990; Mansour et al., 1990; Fremeau et al., 1991; Gandelman et al., 1991). The relative abundances of $D_{2(short)}$ and $D_{2(long)}$ have been examined and there is some inter-experimenter and inter-species variation in the data (Giros et al., 1989; O'Malley et al., 1990; Gandelman et al., 1991; Neve et al., 1991b; Snyder et al., 1991).

Generally, the D_3 receptor seems to be concentrated in limbic regions of the brain with very low levels in the neostriatum whereas the D_4 receptor has a distribution that is different again. In terms of understanding the functions of the different receptor subtypes it will be very important to determine the distributions in detail. This will also need to be determined at the level of expressed protein and may require the raising of antibodies specific for the receptor isoforms (Chazot et al., 1991) as the currently available radioligands distinguish only D_1-like or D_2-like receptors and not the individual isoforms. Equally important will be the relative abundances of the different isoforms. This information is not very clear at present and is only available at the mRNA level. For D_4 receptors it seems that these are present in the brain at much lower levels (10–100-fold less) than D_2 receptors (Van Tol et al., 1991). High levels of D_4 receptors may be

present in the cardiovascular system so that the D_4 receptor may be predominantly a peripheral dopamine receptor (O'Malley et al., 1992). Some previous pharmacological studies of peripheral D_2-like receptors may, therefore, have been examining D_4 receptors. For D_3 receptors the information is rather confusing. Sokoloff et al. (1990) imply that in some brain regions D_3 receptor mRNA is more abundant than that for D_2 receptors whereas in the study by Van Tol et al. (1991) the abundance of D_3 and D_4 receptors is said to be similar and low. It may be that generally D_3 receptor mRNA is found at low levels but there are certain brain regions, e.g., limbic, where it is more abundant than that for the D_2 receptor. More recent studies also indicate that although some brain regions do express both D_2 and D_3 receptors, in some limbic regions the distributions are complementary and non-overlapping (Bouthenet et al., 1991).

Multiple dopamine receptor isoforms: implications for dopamine function and drug action

By considering the distributions of the receptor isoforms in more detail some ideas may be obtained about how dopamine controls brain function. The principal isoforms in the neostriatum are D_1 and D_2. Since the neostriatum is a brain region important for motor control, it seems that the binding of dopamine to D_1 and D_2 receptors may be important for controlling motor function. This will be considered in more detail later.

In individual limbic and cortical brain regions there are varying mixtures of D_1, D_2, D_3, D_4 and D_5 receptors, with D_1 and D_2 generally predominating. The control of behaviour, emotion and motivation by dopamine in these brain regions will therefore be dependent on dopamine interacting with various combinations of receptor isoforms. The localisation of the D_3 receptor may be particularly interesting, found as it is in certain limbic brain regions (nucleus accumbens, olfactory tubercle) and at lower levels in cortical regions. These are brain regions important for regulation of behaviour, mood and emotion, functions which are disturbed when patients suffer from psychosis. Therefore the D_3 receptor may be of particular interest as a site of action for dopamine in controlling the activities of these brain regions and their associated functions. D_1 and D_2 receptors are, however, also found in these brain regions and the relative importance of D_1, D_2 and D_3 actions of dopamine are unclear.

These considerations show that the drugs used to treat Parkinson's disease such as L-Dopa (generating dopamine) are interacting with D_1 and D_2 receptors in the neostriatum to control motor function (see below). Where there are psychotomimetic side effects some of these may be due to interaction with D_3 (or D_4, D_5) receptors in limbic or cortical regions. A selective D_1/D_2 receptor agonist might therefore control motor function but have reduced psychotomimetic side effects.

Antipsychotic drugs were thought previously to achieve their effects mainly via interaction with D_2-like dopamine receptors (Strange, 1991b). It is now clear that this could include actions at D_2, D_3 and D_4 receptors which all have related pharmacological profiles with high affinities for antipsychotic drugs. Blockade of D_1 and D_2 receptors in the neostriatum is likely to be responsible for the extrapyramidal motor side effects of the drugs. The selective localisation of D_3 dopamine receptors in limbic brain regions implicates this isoform in the control of certain aspects of behaviour, emotion and motivation. Since the psychotic symptoms of schizophrenia represent disturbances of these functions, a drug that selectively blocked D_3 receptors might be a selective antipsychotic drug without extrapyramidal effects. It is not known, however, whether blockade of D_2 receptors in limbic and cortical brain regions is also important for achieving an antipsychotic effect.

When the D_3 and D_4 receptors were cloned it was suggested that these might be specific sites of action of particular drugs. It was noted that the "atypical" antipsychotic drugs (showing reduced extrapyramidal side effects) had quite similar affinities for D_2 and D_3 receptors whereas the "typical" antipsychotic drugs (which do show extrapyramidal side ef-

fects) had higher affinities for the D_2 isoform than the D_3 isoform. The interaction of "atypical" antipsychotics with D_3 receptors then might be important for their particular therapeutic profile (Sokoloff et al., 1990). The ability of D_4 receptors to bind drugs such as clozapine which have a selective ability to treat the negative symptoms of schizophrenia (Kane et al., 1988) was proposed as evidence that the D_4 receptor was the site of action of clozapine (Van Tol et al., 1991). All these drugs, however, have actions at a number of receptor subtypes (receptors for dopamine and other neurotransmitters) and it is more likely that the particular spectrum of interactions at different receptors generates the profile of action of the drug.

D_1/D_2 receptor localisation in the neostriatum, implications for striatal function

The localisation of the principal dopamine receptor isoforms in the neostriatum (D_1/D_2) has begun to be defined at the cellular level using in situ hybridisation. This localisation in turn allows speculation about the function of the receptor isoforms.

The neostriatum is important for motor function and dopamine plays a key role in controlling striatal neurone activity. The clearest illustration of this comes from Parkinson's disease where the motor disorder is due to loss of dopamine neurones innervating the striatum (reviewed in Strange, 1992). The neostriatum contains one major cell type as defined morphologically. This is the medium spiny neurone which constitutes 95% of the striatal neuronal population (Gerfen, 1988). Medium spiny neurones are the output cells of the striatum using GABA as neurotransmitter. Subpopulations of medium spiny neurone exist defined by a coexisting neuropeptide (enkephalin or substance P, see below) (Albin et al., 1989). Other neuronal types in the neostriatum include cholinergic interneurones.

Medium spiny neurones receive their principal input from excitatory glutamatergic projections from the cerebral cortex. The medium spiny cells project to the two output nuclei of the basal ganglia, the globus pallidus (internal segment) (GP_i) and the pars reticulata of the substantia nigra (SN_r). These output nuclei project to the thalamus which in turn projects to specific regions of the cerebral cortex so that cortico-striato-pallido/nigro-thalamo-cortical loops are set up (Fig. 1) (Alexander et al., 1986, 1990). Several of these loops exist based on different cortical and striatal regions. For the discussion of motor function a loop based on motor and premotor regions of the cerebral cortex and the putamen within the neostriatum is important, termed the motor circuit. Another important input to the medium spiny neurones is from the pars compacta of the substantia nigra. These are the mesostriatal dopamine neurones lost in Parkinson's disease.

From ligand binding studies (which do not differentiate the cloned receptor isoforms) it is known that D_1-like and D_2-like receptors are present on medium spiny neurones (Filloux et al., 1988a; De Keyser and Ebinger, 1990), D_2-like receptors are found on cholinergic interneurones (Dawson et al., 1988) and on the terminals of mesostriatal dopamine neurones (Wolf and Roth, 1987).

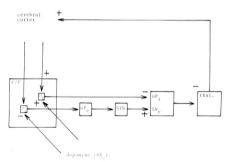

Fig. 1. Localisation of D_1 and D_2 dopamine receptor isoforms on medium spiny neostriatal neurones in relation to cortico-striato-pallido/nigro-thalamo-cortical loops. The diagram shows input from the cerebral cortex to the neostriatum (caudate nucleus/putamen, C/P). The "direct" pathway linking the C/P to the globus pallidus (internal segment)/substantia nigra pars reticulata (GP_i/SN_r) and "indirect" pathway via the globus pallidus (external segment) (GP_e) and subthalamic nucleus (STN) are shown. The output of the GP_i/SN_r is to the thalamus (thal). Dopamine neurones from the substantia nigra pars compacta (SN_c) are shown. D_1 receptors at which dopamine facilitates activity in the "direct" pathway and D_2 receptors at which dopamine inhibits activity in the "indirect" pathway are shown. For more details, see Albin et al. (1989) and Alexander and Crutcher (1990).

In some but not all studies D_2-like receptors have been described on terminals of the cortico-striatal glutamate neurones (see references cited in Trugman et al., 1986; Joyce and Marshall, 1987; Filloux et al., 1988b; De Keyser and Ebinger, 1990; Strange, 1990a).

Recent studies at the mRNA level have shown that the distribution of D_1 and D_2 receptors on medium spiny neurones partly parallels their chemical differentiation (Gerfen et al., 1990; Le Moine et al., 1991). It seems that the medium spiny neurones form two distinct pathways linking the neostriatum to the GP_i/SN_r (Albin et al., 1989). The "direct" pathway is a direct neuronal link formed by GABA-containing medium spiny neurones. The "indirect" link is via the external segment of the globus pallidus (GPe) and the subthalamic nucleus (STN) (Fig. 1). The medium spiny neurones participating in the "direct" pathway contain GABA and substance P, dopamine facilitates their activity and these neurones contain D_1 receptors preferentially. The medium spiny neurones participating in the "indirect" pathway contain GABA and enkephalin, dopamine inhibits the activity of these neurones and the neurones contain preferentially D_2 receptors. Mechanisms for facilitation and inhibition by dopamine have been considered elsewhere (Strange, 1990a). Although there is a preferential localisation of D_1 and D_2 dopamine receptors on different populations of medium spiny neurones, examples have been described of medium spiny neurones expressing both D_1 and D_2 receptor mRNA (Meador-Woodruff et al., 1991). There may also be facilitatory effects of dopamine on D_1 receptors located on terminals of the striato-nigral neurones (Robertson, 1992).

This preferential localisation of dopamine receptor subtypes has important implications for understanding how neostriatal neurone activity controls motor function. The medium spiny neurones of the neostriatum receive information from several regions of the cerebral cortex via excitatory glutamatergic neurones. Medium spiny neurones project to the GP_i/SN_r and for the "direct" projection the effects will be inhibitory (GABA is the neurotransmitter). Projections from GP_i/SN_r to the thalamus are also inhibitory so that activity in the "direct" neostriatal output pathway will tend to dis-inhibit the thalamus which may drive the cerebral cortex and enable motor function to occur. This motor function derives from cerebral cortical neuronal activity but it seems that the thalamocortical signals are important for enabling the cerebral cortical activity to generate motor function. The cortico-striato-pallido/nigro-thalamo-cortical motor loop then acts to allow motor function to be driven by inputs from several cerebral cortical regions (for further discussion, see Alexander and Crutcher, 1990; De Long, 1990). In the "indirect" pathway the neurotransmitters are such that activity in neostriatal neurones of the "indirect" pathway results in inhibition of the thalamus so that the effects of the "indirect" pathway are to oppose those of the "direct" pathway (Albin et al., 1989). It is therefore likely that normal motor function may depend on setting a balance between the "direct" and "indirect" pathways with activity in the former being in excess in order to allow motor function to occur. Dopamine facilitates activity in the "direct" pathway via D_1 receptors and inhibits activity in the "indirect" pathway via D_2 receptors. Dopamine therefore facilitates motor function and at least part of the function of dopamine may be to act as a gain-setting device so that the activities of medium spiny striatal neurones in "direct" and "indirect" pathways are balanced correctly. A facilitation of motor activity may also result from the small increase in dopamine neuronal activity that precedes a movement (Strange, 1990c). These ideas also provide some explanation for the need in experimental animals for D_1 and D_2 receptor stimulation to generate motor activity (Waddington and O'Boyle, 1987). If both receptor subtypes are not stimulated then the appropriate balanced neostriatal neuronal action will not occur.

In Parkinson's disease, the classical hypokinetic motor disorder, there is a loss of the dopamine neuronal control of the neostriatum. This will lead to a shift in the balance of neostriatal neuronal activity in a favour of the "indirect" pathway and hence a reduction in motor function. In early Huntington's disease, which is a typical hyperkinetic disorder, there is a selective loss of the neostriatal neurones from the "indirect" pathway (Albin et al., 1989). This will result in a shift in the balance of neostriatal neuronal activity towards the "direct" pathway. Since the "direct" pathway facilitates motor function, this emphasis on the actions of the "direct" pathway unchecked by the counterbalance of the "indirect" pathway may lead to excessive movements. The cerebral cortex may receive too strong a facilitatory signal. Other hyperkinetic disorders such as tardive dyskinesia (in schizophrenic patients) and L-Dopa-induced dyskinesias (in parkinsonian patients) may also reflect disturbances in the balance of neostriatal neuronal activity in favour of the "direct" pathway.

It should be apparent that a knowledge of the locations of dopamine receptor isoforms on individual neostriatal neurones has significant implications for understanding the functions of the isoforms.

The structure of the ligand-binding site of D_2 dopamine and related D_2-like dopamine receptors

There is now much interest in designing compounds with selective actions at the different dopamine receptor subtypes for use as selective therapeutic agents. The design of such compounds should be aided by understanding the mechanism of ligand-binding to the receptors and this section considers the mechanisms that may be involved for D_2 dopamine receptors.

The overall binding energy that drives the interaction of ligands (agonists and antagonists) with receptors will be contributed to by electrostatic, hydrophobic, hydrogen-bond and Van der Waals interactions. This energy will be realised from the interactions of the ligand with the side chains of amino acids lining the cavity formed from the bundling of the seven transmembrane spanning α-helices. Dopamine agonists and antagonists contain cationic amine groups so one interaction is likely to be electrostatic with a negatively charged group on the receptor. An aspartic acid residue in the third transmembrane α-helix (Asp 114 in the D_2 sequence) is conserved in the G-protein-linked receptors that bind cationic amines and so is a prime candidate for this residue. Indeed, Dixon et al. (1988) have shown that mutation of the corresponding residue in the β-adrenergic receptor reduces agonist and antagonist affinities by a factor of 10^4. In the case of the D_2 dopamine receptor chemical modification with dicyclohexylcarbodiimide has provided evidence for the importance of a carboxyl group (presumably Asp 114) in the binding of the antagonist [3H]spiperone (Williamson and Strange, 1990).

It is of interest, however, that for the nicotinic acetylcholine receptor no evidence has been obtained so far for the participation of carboxyl groups in the binding of the cationic ligand acetylcholine (Galzi et al., 1991). Interactions with the side chains of other amino acids, e.g., tyrosine, may be important and the interactions may be via hydrogen-bond and hydrophobic forces (Lehn, 1985). Although this is not a G-protein-linked receptor these observations suggest that interactions with amino acid side chains other than those containing carboxyl groups should be considered for the interaction of the cationic head groups of ligands with G-protein-linked receptors.

In the case of the β-adrenergic receptor even after mutation of the important aspartic acid residue in the third transmembrane region the receptor still binds ligands with the correct specificity albeit with a much lower affinity (Dixon et al., 1988). This shows that other interactions between the receptor and other parts of the ligand are essential for binding. For agonists further important interactions are likely to be hydrogen bonds between the catechol hydroxyl groups and two conserved serine residues in α-helix 5. Interactions between the catechol ring and adjacent phenylalanine residues in α-helix 6 may also be important. These interactions are likely to be found for D_2 dopamine receptors as well and the combination of interactions must then provoke a conformational change in the receptor that leads to signalling across the membrane. For antagonists other interactions again are likely and hydrophobic

interactions should be important reflecting the nature of the antagonist molecules. Although agonist and antagonist interactions with the receptor must be competitive, the basis of binding of the two classes of ligand may be quite different.

Further circumstantial support for these ideas comes from modelling studies. A three-dimensional model of the D_2 dopamine receptor has been constructed based on the coordinates of bacteriorhodopsin (Livingstone et al., 1992). In this model it was possible to show that dopamine and other agonists could bind via electrostatic interaction with Asp 114 and hydrogen-bond interaction with serine residues in α-helix 5. The model also suggested that stacking interactions might be important between aromatic amino acid side chains and aromatic moieties of ligands. Of particular interest was the proximity of a histidine (365) and tyrosine (388, $D_{2(short)}$) residue to the agonist-binding region. The agonist-binding region seems to be within the membrane spanning pocket about a third of the way in from the outside (Strange, 1991c). His 365 and Tyr 388 are both in this region. His 365 is found only in D_2-like dopamine receptors and provides a potential ionisable group in the ligand-binding pocket. Tyr 388 is a residue that is conserved in G-protein-linked receptors that bind cationic amines and has been highlighted as potentially important in transmembrane signalling (Hulme et al., 1990). Chemical modification studies using reagents selective for histidine and tyrosine residues have provided some evidence for their participation in ligand-binding but the evidence is not unequivocal and requires extension (Williamson and Strange, 1990; Srivastava and Mishra, 1990).

Further information on the amino acid residues that contribute to ligand-binding can be obtained by determining the pH dependence of ligand-binding to the receptors. Ligand-binding is generally of lower affinity when the pH is reduced and apparent pKa values may be assigned to the receptor in its interaction with ligands. This pKa value should reflect the nature of the group that undergoes protonation as the pH is reduced, the protonation then affecting receptor-ligand interaction. For D_2 dopamine receptors, dopamine antagonists may be divided into two groups when subjected to such an analysis. For the binding of standard antagonists, e.g., haloperidol and spiperone, D_2 dopamine receptors show pKa values of about six whereas for the binding of antagonists of the substituted benzamide class, e.g., sulpiride, the receptors show pKa values closer to seven (Williamson and Strange, 1990; Presland and Strange, 1991; D'Souza and Strange, 1992). These data show that the two classes of antagonist bind to D_2 dopamine receptors differently and the substituted benzamide drugs are particularly sensitive to changes of pH. Substituted benzamide drugs were already known to be unusual in their binding to D_2-like dopamine receptors in that their binding was dependent on Na^+ ions unlike other antagonists (Theodorou et al., 1980).

It is not possible as yet to assign these pKa values to the ionisation of particular amino acid residues on the receptor although this is an important goal. It seems likely, however, that the amino acid residue of pKa about six is Asp 114 whose protonation interferes with electrostatic interaction with the ligands. The group of pKa about seven could be a histidine residue and His 365 within the sixth α-helix is a possible candidate residue. Mutagenesis studies on these residues will be required for unambiguous assignment.

One mutagenesis study has been published concerning D_2 dopamine receptors. Neve et al. (1991a) mutated Asp 80 (in α-helix 2) to Ala-80. This aspartic acid residue is conserved in almost every G-protein-linked receptor and so is likely to play an important role in maintaining the conformation of such proteins and perhaps is important to the signalling process. This makes it a very interesting residue to study but also means that its mutagenesis may have multiple effects via altered conformational states.

Although in the Ala-80 mutant the binding of [^{3}H]spiperone is unaltered so that the gross receptor conformation is unchanged, several other effects are seen. The binding of the substituted benzamide drugs is of lower affinity in the mutant and these drugs also lose their sensitivity to Na^+. The pH de-

pendency of substituted benzamide binding is altered but these ligands retain a greater sensitivity to the effects of pH. The mutant receptor can also no longer signal inhibition of adenylyl cyclase.

Interpretation of these effects is rather difficult. The elimination of Na^+ dependence of substituted benzamide binding may be a specific effect of the Ala-80 mutation and the reduction in the affinity of substituted benzamide binding may simply reflect this. A plausible explanation is that the receptor exists in two conformations with higher (R') and lower (R'') affinities for substituted benzamide drugs but equal affinities for other antagonists. Na^+ ions are required to form R'. Mutation of Asp 80 to Ala 80 renders R' unattainable. This could be due to a direct interaction of Na^+ and Asp 80 in R'. This conclusion is reinforced by the finding that for α_2 adrenergic receptors mutation of the corresponding aspartic acid residue also eliminates the regulation of ligand-binding by Na^+ (Horstman et al., 1990).

The pH dependency data of Neve et al. (1991a) are not developed fully enough to be interpreted in any detail. In the Ala-80 mutant the binding of substituted benzamide drugs is still more pH dependent than other antagonists. This suggests that Asp 80 is not responsible for the greater pH dependency of substituted benzamide binding and some other residue may be important. That the pH dependency is altered in the mutant is not surprising as the conformation of the receptor will be altered and it seems that generally the binding of the substituted benzamide drugs is very conformation-dependent and the conformation can be affected by Na^+, pH and the Ala 80 mutation. As for the effects on the receptor-mediated inhibition of adenylyl cyclase in the Ala 80 mutant these are also unlikely to be direct effects of the mutation. It seems more likely that in the mutant the conformation of the receptor is altered so that it cannot effect transmembrane signalling.

Further evidence for the conformational sensitivity and the binding of substituted benzamide drugs comes from recent studies on $D_{2(short)}$ and $D_{2(long)}$ receptors expressed from cloned genes in animal cells (Castro and Strange, 1992). Whereas the binding of most antagonists to $D_{2(short)}$ and $D_{2(long)}$ was essentially identical, the binding of the substituted benzamide antagonists showed a 2 – 5-fold higher affinity to $D_{2(short)}$. These receptor isoforms differ only by the 29 amino acid insertion in the third intracellular loop and this part of the receptor is not normally considered important for forming the ligand-binding site. The 29 amino acid insertion may, however, alter the conformation of the third intracellular loop which in turn may alter the conformation of the receptor. If the binding of the substituted benzamide drugs is very conformation-dependent then their binding may differ to the two forms of receptor.

In conclusion, these kinds of biophysical/biochemical approaches are beginning to give insights into the mechanism of ligand-binding. Nevertheless there is much more to be done in terms of mutagenesis and chemical approaches in order to understand how ligands bind to these receptors.

Acknowledgement

I thank Sue Davies for excellent manuscript preparation.

References

Albin, R.L., Young, A.B. and Penney, J.B. (1989) The functional anatomy of basal ganglia disorders. *Trends Neurosci.*, 12: 366 – 375.

Alexander, G.E. and Crutcher, M.D. (1990) Functional architecture of basal ganglia circuits: neural substrates of parallel processing. *Trends Neurosci.*, 13: 266 – 271.

Alexander, G.E., De Long, M.R. and Strick, P.L. (1986) Parallel organisation of functionally segregated circuits linking basal ganglia and cortex. *Annu. Rev. Neurosci.*, 9: 357 – 381.

Alexander, G.E., Crutcher, M.D. and De Long, M.R. (1990) Basal ganglia-thalamocortical circuits: parallel substrates for motor, oculomotor, prefrontal, and limbic functions. *Prog. Brain Res.*, 85: 119 – 146.

Andersen, P.H., Gingrich, J.A., Bates, M.D., Dearry, A., Falardeau, P., Senogles, S.E. and Caron, M.G. (1990) Dopamine receptor subtypes: beyond the D_1/D_2 classification. *Trends Pharmacol. Sci.*, 11: 231 – 236.

Bouthenet, M.L., Souil, E., Martres, M.P., Sokoloff, P., Giros, B. and Schwartz, J.C. (1991) Localisation of dopamine D_3 receptor mRNA in the rat brain using in situ hybridization to histochemistry: comparison with dopamine D_2 receptor mRNA. *Brain Res.*, 564: 203 – 219.

Bunzow, J.R., Van Tol, H.H.M., Grandy, D.K., Albert, P., Salon, J., Christie, M., Machida, C.A., Neve, K.A. and Civelli, O. (1988) Cloning and expression of a rat D_2 dopamine receptor cDNA. *Nature*, 336: 783 – 787.

Castro, S. and Strange, P.G. (1992) Characterisation of the two forms of the D_2 dopamine receptor expressed in mammalian cell lines. *Br. J. Pharmacol.*, 106: 55.

Chazot, P.L., Wilkins, M. and Strange, P.G. (1991) Site specific antibodies as probes of the structure and function of the brain D_2 dopamine receptor. *Biochem. Soc. Trans.*, 19: 143S.

Clagett-Dame, M. and McKelvy, J.F. (1989) N-linked oligosaccharides are responsible for rat striatal dopamine D2 receptor heterogeneity. *Arch. Biochem. Biophys.*, 274: 145 – 154.

De Long, M.R. (1990) Primate models of movement disorders of basal ganglia origin. *Trends Neurosci.*, 13: 281 – 286.

Dal Toso, R., Sommer, B., Ewert, M., Herb, A., Pritchett, D.B., Bach, A., Shivers, B.D. and Seeburg, P.H. (1989) The dopamine D_2 receptor: two molecular forms generated by alternative splicing. *EMBO J.*, 8: 4025 – 4034.

Dawson, V.L., Dawson, T.M., Filloux, F.M. and Wamsley, J.K. (1988) Evidence for dopamine D-2 receptors on cholinergic interneurons in the rat caudate-putamen. *Life Sci.*, 42: 1933 – 1939.

Dearry, A., Gingrich, J.A., Falardeau, P., Fremeau, R.T., Bates, M.D. and Caron, M.G. (1990) Molecular cloning and expression of the gene for a human D_1 dopamine receptor. *Nature*, 347: 72 – 76.

De Keyser, J. and Ebinger, G. (1990) Neostriatal dopamine receptors. *Trends Neurosci.*, 13: 324.

Dixon, R.A.F., Sigal, I.S. and Strader, C.D. (1988) Structure function analysis of the β-adrenergic receptor. *Cold Spring Harbor Symp. Quant. Biol.*, 53: 487 – 497.

D'Souza, U. and Strange, P.G. (1992) Structural analysis of the D_2 dopamine receptor. *Biochem. Soc. Trans.*, 20: 146S.

Filloux, F., Dawson, T.M. and Wamsley, J.K. (1988a) Localisation of nigrostriatal dopamine receptor subtypes and adenylate cyclase. *Brain Res. Bull.*, 20: 447 – 459.

Filloux, F., Liu, T.H., Hsu, C.Y., Hunt, M.A. and Wamsley, J.K. (1988b) Selective cortical infarction reduces [³H]sulpiride binding in rat caudate-putamen: autoradiographic evidence for presynaptic D_2 receptors on corticostriate terminals. *Synapse*, 2: 521 – 531.

Fremeau, R.T., Duncan, G.E., Fornaretto, M.G., Dearry, A., Gingrich, J.A., Breese, G.R. and Caron, M.G. (1991) Localisation of D_1 dopamine receptor mRNA in brain supports a role in cognitive, affective and neuroendocrine aspects of dopaminergic neurotransmission. *Proc. Natl. Acad. Sci. U.S.A.*, 88: 3727 – 3736.

Galzi, J.L., Revah, F., Bessis, A. and Changeux, J.P. (1991) Functional architecture of the nicotinic acetylcholine receptor. *Annu. Rev. Pharmacol. Toxicol.*, 31: 37 – 72.

Gandelman, K.Y., Harmon, S., Todd, R.D. and O'Malley, K.L. (1991) Analysis of the structure and expression of the human dopamine D_{2A} receptor gene. *J. Neurochem.*, 56:

178

1024 – 1029.

Gerfen, C.R. (1988) Synaptic organisation of the striatum. *J. Electron Microsc.,* 10: 265 – 281.

Gerfen, C.R., Engber, T.M., Mahan, L.C., Susel, Z., Chase, T.N., Monsma, F.J. and Sibley, D.R. (1990) D_1 and D_2 dopamine receptor regulated gene expression of striatonigral and striatopallidal neurones. *Science,* 250: 1429 – 1432.

Giros, B., Sokoloff, P., Martres, M.P., Riou, J.F., Emorine, L.J. and Schwartz, J.C. (1989) Alternative splicing directs the expression of two dopamine receptor isoforms. *Nature,* 342: 923 – 926.

Giros, B., Martres, M.P., Sokoloff, P. and Schwartz, J.L. (1990) cDNA cloning of the human dopaminergic D_3 receptor and chromosome identification. *C.R. Acad. Sci. Paris, Serie III:* 501 – 508.

Horstman, D.A., Brandon, S., Wilson, A.L., Guyer, C.A., Cragoe, E.J. and Limbird, L.E. (1990) An aspartate conserved among G-protein linked receptors confers allosteric regulation of α_2-adrenergic receptors by sodium. *J. Biol. Chem.,* 265: 21590 – 21595.

Hulme, E.C., Birdsall, N.J.M. and Buckley, N.J. (1990) Muscarinic receptor subtypes. *Annu. Rev. Pharmacol. Toxicol.,* 30: 633 – 673.

Joyce, J.N. and Marshall, J.F. (1987) Quantitative autoradiography of dopamine D_2 sites in rat caudate-putamen. Localisation to intrinsic neurones and not to neocortical afferents. *Neuroscience,* 20: 773 – 795.

Kane, J.M., Honigfeld, G., Singer, J., Meltzer, H.Y. and the Clozaril collaborative study group (1988) Clozapine for the treatment resistant schizophrenic. *Arch. Gen. Psych.,* 45: 789 – 796.

Kebabian, J.W. and Calne, D.B. (1979) Multiple receptors for dopamine. *Nature,* 277: 93 – 96.

Le Moine, C., Normand, E. and Block, B. (1991) Phenotypical characterisation of the rat striatal neurons expressing the D_1 dopamine receptor gene. *Proc. Natl. Acad. Sci. U.S.A.,* 8: 4205 – 4209.

Lefkowitz, R.J. and Caron, M.G. (1988) Adrenergic receptors. *J. Biol. Chem.,* 263: 4993 – 4996.

Lehn, J.M. (1985) Supramolecular chemistry: receptors, catalysts and carriers. *Science,* 227: 849 – 856.

Livingstone, C.D., Strange, P.G. and Naylor, L.H. (1992) Molecular modelling of D_2-like dopamine receptors. *Biochem. J.,* 287: 277 – 282.

Mansour, A., Meador-Woodruff, J.H., Bunzow, J.R., Civelli, O., Akil, H. and Watson, S.J. (1990) Localisation of dopamine D_2 receptor mRNA and D_1 and D_2 receptor binding in rat brain and pituitary: an in situ hybridisation-receptor autoradiography analysis. *J. Neurosci.,* 10: 2587 – 2600.

Meador-Woodruff, S.H., Mansour, A., Healy, D.J., Kuehn, R., Zhou, Q., Bunzow, J.R., Akil, H., Civelli, O. and Watson, S.J. (1991) Comparison of the distributions of D_1 and D_2 dopamine receptor mRNAs in rat brain. *Neuropsychopharmacology,* 5: 231 – 242.

Meister, B., Holgert, H., Aperia, A. and Hökfelt, T. (1991) Dopamine D_1 receptor mRNA in rat kidney: localisation by in situ hybridisation. *Acta Physiol. Scand.,* 143: 447 – 449.

Montmayeur, J.P. and Borrelli, E. (1991) Transcription mediated by a cAMP responsive promoter element is reduced upon activation of dopamine D_2 receptors. *Proc. Natl. Acad. Sci. U.S.A.,* 88: 3135 – 3139.

Neve, K.A., Cox, B.A., Henningsen, R.A., Spanoyannis, A. and Neve, R.L. (1991a) Pivotal role for aspartate-80 in the regulation of dopamine D_2 receptor affinity for drugs and inhibition of adenylate cyclase. *Mol. Pharmacol.,* 39: 733 – 739.

Neve, K.A., Neve, R.L., Fidel, S., Janowsky, A. and Higgins, G.A. (1991b) Increased abundance of alternatively spliced forms of D_2 dopamine receptor mRNA after denervation. *Proc. Natl. Acad. Sci. U.S.A.,* 88: 2802 – 2806.

O'Dowd, B.F., Hnatowich, M., Caron, M.G., Lefkowitz, R.J. and Bouvier, M. (1989) Palmitoylation of the human β_2-adrenergic receptor. *J. Biol. Chem.,* 264: 7564 – 7569.

O'Malley, K.L., Mack, K., Gandelman, K. and Todd, R.D. (1990) Organisation and expression of the rat D_{2A} receptor gene: identification of alternative transcripts and a variant splice donor site. *Biochemistry,* 29: 1367 – 1371.

O'Malley, K.L., Harmon, S., Tang, L. and Todd, R.D. (1992) The rat dopamine D_4 receptor: sequence, gene structure and demonstration of expression in the cardiovascular system. *New Biologist,* 4: 137 – 146.

Presland, J.R. and Strange, P.G. (1991) pH dependence of sulpiride binding to D_2 dopamine receptors in bovine brain. *Biochem. Pharmacol.,* 41: R9 – R12.

Robertson, H.A. (1992) Synergistic interations of D-1 and D-2 selective dopamine agonists. Animal models for Parkinson's disease: sites of action and implications for the pathogenesis of dyskinesias. *Can. J. Neurol. Sci.,* 19: 147 – 152.

Sibley, D.R. and Monsma, F.J. (1992) Molecular biology of dopamine receptors. *Trends Pharmacol. Sci.,* 13: 61 – 69.

Snyder, L.A., Roberts, J.L. and Sealfon, S.C. (1991) Distribution of dopamine D_2 receptor mRNA splice variants in the rat by solution hybridisation/protection assay. *Neurosci. Lett.,* 122: 37 – 40.

Sokoloff, P., Martres, M.P., Delandre, M., Redouane, K. and Schwartz, J.C. (1984) [^{3}H]domperidone binding sites differ in rat striatum and pituitary. *Naunyn Schmiedeberg's Arch. Pharmacol.,* 327: 221 – 227.

Sokoloff, P., Giros, B., Martres, M.P., Bouthenet, M.L. and Schwartz, J.C. (1990) Molecular cloning and characterisation of a novel dopamine receptor (D_3) as a target for neuroleptics. *Nature,* 347: 146 – 151.

Srivastava, L.K. and Mishra, R.K. (1990) Chemical modification reveals involvement of tyrosine in ligand binding to dopamine D_1 and D_2 receptors. *Biochem. Int.,* 21: 705 – 714.

Strange, P.G. (1990a) Neostriatal dopamine receptors. *Trends Neurosci.,* 13: 324 – 325.

Strange, P.G. (1990b) Aspects of the structure of the D_2 dopamine receptor. *Trends Neurosci.,* 13: 373 – 378.

Strange, P.G. (1990c) Role of the mesostriatal dopamine pathway. *Trends Neurosci.*, 13: 93 – 94.

Strange, P.G. (1991a) Interesting times for dopamine receptors. *Trends Neurosci.*, 14: 43 – 45.

Strange, P.G. (1991b) Neuroleptic drugs and dopamine receptors. *Am. J. Psychiatry*, 148: 1101.

Strange, P.G. (1991c) Receptors for neurotransmitters and related substances. *Curr. Opinion Biotechnol.*, 2: 269 – 277.

Strange, P.G. (1992) *Brain Biochemistry and Brain Disorders*, Oxford University Press, Oxford.

Sunahara, R.K., Guan, H.C., O'Dowd, B.F., Seeman, P., Laurier, L.G., Ng, G., George, S.R., Torchia, J., Van Tol., H.H.M. and Niznik, H.B. (1991) Cloning of the gene for a human dopamine D_5 receptor with higher affinity for dopamine than D_1. *Nature,* 350: 614 – 619.

Theodorou, A.E., Hall, M.D., Jenner, P. and Marsden, C.D. (1980) Cation regulation differentiates specific binding of [^{3}H]sulpiride and [^{3}H]spiperone to rat striatal preparations. *J. Pharm. Pharmacol.*, 32: 441 – 444.

Tiberi, M., Jarvie, K.R., Silvia, C., Falardeau, P., Gingrich, J.A., Godinot, N., Bertrand, L., Yang Feng, T.L., Fremeau, R.T. and Caron, M.G. (1991) Cloning, molecular characterisation and chromosomal assignment of a gene encoding a second D_1 dopamine receptor subtype: differential expression patterns in rat brain compared with the D1A subtype. *Proc. Natl. Acad. Sci. U.S.A.*, 88: 7491 – 7495.

Trugman, J.M., Geary, W.A. and Wooten, G.F. (1986) Localisation of D-2 dopamine receptors to intrinsic striatal neurones by quantitative autoradiography. *Nature,* 323: 267 – 269.

Van Tol, H.H.M., Bunzow, J.R., Guan, H.C., Sunahara, R.K., Seeman, P., Niznik, H.B and Civelli, O. (1991) Cloning of the gene for a human dopamine D_4 receptor with high affinity for the antipsychotic clozapine. *Nature,* 350: 610 – 614.

Waddington, J.L. and O'Boyle, K.M. (1987) The D-1 dopamine receptor and the search for its functional role: from neurochemistry to behaviour. *Rev. Neurosci.*, 1: 157 – 184.

Williamson, R.A. and Strange, P.G. (1990) Evidence for the importance of a carboxyl group in the binding of ligands to the D_2 dopamine receptor. *J. Neurochem.*, 55: 1357 – 1365.

Wolf, M.E. and Roth, R.H. (1987) Dopamine autoreceptors. I. Creese and C.M. Fraser (Eds.), *Dopamine Receptors,* A.R. Liss, New York, pp. 45 – 96.

G.W. Arbuthnott and P.C. Emson (Eds.)
Progress in Brain Research, Vol. 99
© 1993 Elsevier Science Publishers B.V. All rights reserved.

CHAPTER 12

Neuroleptics and striatal neuropeptide gene expression

S.J. Augood[1], K. Westmore[1], R.L.M. Faull[2] and P.C. Emson

[1]*MRC Group, Department of Neurobiology, AFRC Babraham Institute, Babraham, Cambridge, CB2 4AT, U.K. and*
[2]*Department of Anatomy, School of Medicine, University of Auckland, Private Bag, Auckland, New Zealand*

Introduction

Neuroleptics (nerve seizing) are a broad spectrum of agents which, historically, were introduced into clinical medicine due to their ability to potentiate the effects of anaesthetics. Administered alone these compounds result in a diminished state of arousal and a tendency to sleep without loss of consciousness. Thus it was not long before the beneficial "soothing" ability of these compounds was recognized by clinical psychiatrists in the treatment of psychosis. Whilst treatment of psychotic patients with neuroleptics may not necessarily be an effective "cure", they may be effective in controlling/suppressing the socially unacceptable behaviour patterns exhibited by these patients. Consequently, chlorpromazine, the archetypal neuroleptic, was introduced into clinical psychiatry in the 1950s as an effective treatment for psychosis. Subsequent biochemical studies in experimental animals demonstrated that the sedated behaviour induced by these compounds could be mimicked by drugs that blocked dopamine (DA) neurotransmission, for example, these agents could inhibit stereotypic behaviour induced by amphetamine, a non-selective DA agonist, or as in the case of reserpine, isolated from *Rauwolfia serpentina* and used in the 1930s in the treatment of insanity and hypertension, deplete catecholamine stores rendering experimental subjects rigid and bradykinetic. Consequently, interest in the physiology and neurobiology of catechola-

mines and the diversity of their roles in mediating cognition and locomotion has exploded over the past three decades and progressed rapidly. Neuroleptics, DA receptor antagonists, are now widely used in clinical medicine, for treating both psychiatric and neurodegenerative disorders where a dysfunction in DA transmission has been implicated; haloperidol (a typical neuroleptic) is used in the treatment of Gilles de la Tourette's Syndrome, clozapine (an atypical neuroleptic) is used in the treatment of schizophrenia while L-Dopa (DA precursor) is used successfully in the treatment of Parkinson's disease.

The effects of endogenous DA in vivo are manifested through interaction with selective DA receptors. To date, five main mammalian DA receptors subtypes, termed $D_1 - D_5$, have been isolated and sequenced (Bunzow et al., 1988; Dearry et al., 1990; Sokoloff et al., 1990; Sunahara et al., 1990; Zhou et al., 1990; Van Tol et al., 1991). The D_2 and D_3 subtypes are the main target receptors for the action of typical neuroleptics, the D_4 subtype displays high affinity for the atypical anti-psychotic clozapine and the D_5 subtype has greater affinity for DA than the D_1 subtype. As these cDNA sequences are now available it is possible to study in detail the precise cellular localizations of these various receptor subtypes within the CNS using the technique of in situ hybridization. Therefore the sites of action of DAergic drugs can be more clearly defined.

There exists a wealth of experimental data consistent with the suggestion that it is the D_2 receptor which is the dominant DA receptor mediating the effects of typical neuroleptics (and the extrapyramidal side effects associated with long-term neuroleptic treatment). Numerous ligand-binding and in situ hybridization studies have shown that the mammalian striatum is particularly enriched with both D_1 and D_2 receptors (Joyce and Marshall, 1987; Leslie and Bennett, 1987); D_1 receptors being localized to postsynaptic striatal cells and their associated processes whilst D_2 receptors are localized on both presynaptic nigro-striatal DA nerve terminals and on post-synaptic striatal cells and their processes. Data from combined retrograde tracing and in situ hybridization studies have shown also that most striatal cells expressing the D_1 receptor subtype comprise a sub-population of GABAergic medium-sized spiny cells which preferentially project to the substantia nigra (SN) and contain the neuropeptides substance P (SP) and dynorphin; conversely GABAergic striatal cells which project preferentially to the globus pallidus (external segment in primates) express the D_2 receptor subtype and contain mRNA encoding the opioid peptide enkephalin (ENK: Gerfen et al., 1990). The expression of these neuropeptides in separate cells is illustrated in Fig. 1.

Thus, from the studies of Gerfen and colleagues (1990) it appears that the two major GABAergic striatal output pathways may be chemically differentiated by expression of DA receptor subtype and co-expressed neuropeptides; such revelations provide a neurochemical tool by which the regulation/activity of these two major output pathways may be differentially assessed. Given the enrichment of DA receptors in the striatum, its extensive DAergic innervation by the nigro-striatal pathway and the behavioural manifestations associated with DA receptor blockade (e.g., akinesia) it seems likely that the main targets for the action of typical neuroleptics are striatal DA receptors, blockade of which may result in a cascade of changes in downstream pallidal and nigral signalling and thus may influence the activity of colliculo-spinal neurones and motor activity.

The basal ganglia nuclei principally function through a series of inhibitory and disinhibitory pathways consequently affecting locomotion. It is well established that GABA is the principal neurotransmitter in striatal efferent fibres, whilst intrinsic striatal signalling is mediated by a small percentage (<10%) of interneurones including cholinergic cells which have extensive dendritic arborizations in addition to GABA/parvalbumin cells (Cowan et al., 1990), somatostatin (SRIF)-/neuropeptide Y-/NADPH-diaphorase-positive

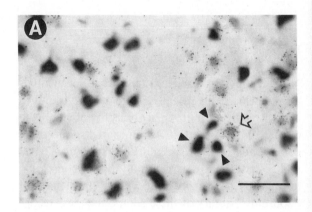

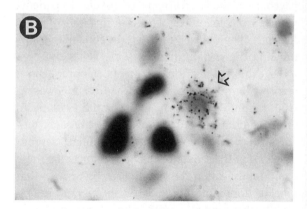

Fig. 1. A. Photomicrograph of a coronal section of dorsal striatum simultaneously hybridized with an AP-ENK oligonucleotide (darkly stained cells) and a ^{35}S-labelled SP oligonucleotide (silver grains). Essentially the two gene transcripts are expressed by different cell populations. Examples of ENK mRNA-containing cells are illustrated by filled arrow heads, SP mRNA-containing cells by an open arrow head. Scale bar, 40 μm. B. High-power photomicrograph of the cells illustrated in A; three ENK-positive cells and one SP-positive cell (open arrow head) can be seen.

cells (Takagi et al., 1983; Vincent and Johansson, 1983; Smith and Parent, 1986) and possibly the recently described population of medium-sized calretinin-immunoreactive interneurones (Bennett et al., 1992). Given the prevalence of neuroleptic treatment in clinical neurology/psychiatry we will describe in this article how we have used the techniques of in situ hybridization to study the effects of acute neuroleptic treatment in the rat on striatal neurochemical signalling; particular emphasis is placed on the association of D_2 receptors with the GABA/ENK striato-pallidal pathway and the association of D_1 receptors with the GABA/SP striato-nigral pathway. In addition, the effects of these treatments on striatal neurotensin- (NT) and SRIF-containing cells is presented as there are extensive biochemical data pertaining to an interaction of DA with these neuropeptide-containing striatal cell types.

Enkephalin

It is well established from neuroanatomical tracing techniques, lesion studies and electron microscopy that the activity of striatal GABA/ENK cells can be influenced by the activity of the DAergic cells in the ipsilateral SN pars compacta (Young et al., 1986; Normand et al., 1988). As predominantly symmetrical synaptic specializations have been demonstrated between tyrosine hydroxylase (TH)-immunoreactive axonal boutons and ENK-immunoreactive proximal dendrites and cell soma (Kubota et al., 1986a) the interaction between these two systems is thought to be direct.

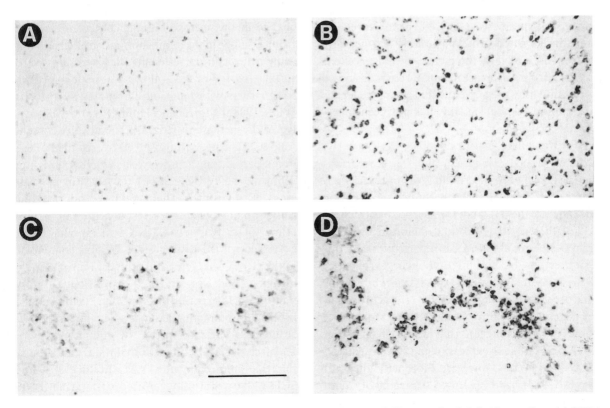

Fig. 2. Illustration of the induction in ENK gene expression in the dorsal striatum and olfactory tubercle following a unilateral 6-OHDA lesion. Sections hybridized with the AP-ENK probe; cells containing ENK mRNA are visualized by the concentration of AP reaction product within the cell cytoplasm. *B* and *D*, ipsilateral 6-OHDA-lesioned side; *A* and *C*, contralateral unlesioned side. Scale bar, 250 μm.

Numerous in situ hybridization and Northern analysis studies have shown that removal of the DA input to the striatum (by either electrolytically lesioning or chemically lesioning the nigro-striatal pathway with the neurotoxins 6-OHDA or MPTP) results in a significant increase in ENK gene expression in the ipsilateral DA denervated striatum (Angulo et al., 1986; Shivers et al., 1986; Young et al., 1986; Normand et al., 1988; Augood et al., 1989; Morris et al., 1989), as illustrated in Fig. 2. Reducing striatal DA content with reserpine, predominantly a catecholamine depletor, similarly increases striatal ENK gene expression in a dose-dependent manner (Zheng et al., 1988). Increases in the tissue content of met-ENK immunoreactivity have been reported in both the ipsilateral striatum and globus pallidus (the principal target nucleus of GABA/ENK striatal efferents) of 6-OHDA-lesioned rats (Voorn et al., 1987; Ingham et al., 1991; Manier et al., 1991) suggesting that the increase in ENK gene expression results in increased protein synthesis and possibly release. Alternatively, the increased tissue content may arise from a decrease in peptide degradation or an accumulation of peptide within the nerve terminal (reduced release) but this has not been investigated.

To differentiate, where possible, D_1- from D_2-mediated events selective D_1 and D_2 receptor antagonists have been used in an attempt to manipulate striatal neuropeptide gene expression. *Chronic* blockade of the D_1 and D_2 subtypes with SCH 23390 (Iorio et al., 1983) and raclopride, respectively (Köhler et al., 1985), is reported to have opposing effects on striatal ENK gene expression; SCH 23390 attenuates ENK expression while raclopride potentiates it, paralleling the effects of striatal DA denervation (Morris et al., 1988b; Morris and Hunt, 1991). This suggests that the dominant action of DA on ENK gene expression in vivo is mediated via D_2 receptors. However, Mocchetti and colleagues (1987) have presented contradictory data from Northern analysis studies whilst Bannon and colleagues (1989) have reported a potentiation in ENK expression following electrical stimulation of the medial forebrain bundle and acute administra-

tion of quinpirole, a D_2 agonist. Again this is in contrast to in situ data demonstrating that a 6-OHDA-induced increase in striatal ENK expression may be reversed by subsequent continuous treatment with this D_2 agonist (Gerfen et al., 1990). Thus there is still controversy about the effects of DA receptor antagonists on striatal GABA/ENK cells. To address the problem of the effects of endogenous DA on post-synaptic ENK cells we have examined the effects of acute raclopride (D_2 antagonist; 5 mg/kg i.p.) and SCH 23390 (D_1 antagonist; 0.25 mg/kg i.p.) treatment on ENK gene expression using non-radioactive in situ hybridization (Augood et al., 1992). One advantage of non-radioactive oligonucleotides, to which the enzyme alkaline phosphatase (AP) is directly conjugated, is the clarity and exceptional cellular resolution of the cytoplasmic hybridization signal. This approach, therefore, allows one to differentiate between a change in the average cellular content of mRNA from a change in the number of positive cells. In our acute neuroleptic experiments, rats were allowed to survive for 1, 3 or 9 h following a single injection. In agreement with data from chronic studies (Morris et al., 1988b; Morris and Hunt, 1991) we also detected an increase in striatal ENK mRNA content following acute raclopride (D_2) treatment, but noted only a transient decrease in ENK expression following acute SCH 23390 (D_1) treatment (Augood et al., 1992). These data corroborate our earlier findings where the effect of acute haloperidol (4 mg/kg i.p.) on striatal ENK gene expression was examined; in these studies the cellular content of ENK mRNA was increased within 30 min of a single injection, and this increased expression was sustained for a long period (> 24 h; Fig. 3; data unpublished). Radioimmunoassay studies have reported an increase in striatal met-ENK immunoreactivity 1 h after a single i.p. injection of the D_2 antagonist sulpiride, but treatment of rats with SKF 38393 or SCH 23390 were without effect on striatal met-ENK tissue concentrations (Taylor et al., 1991). Thus, as both our results and those of Morris and colleagues used in situ hybridization to study the effects of neuroleptic treatment whilst Mocchetti and co-workers

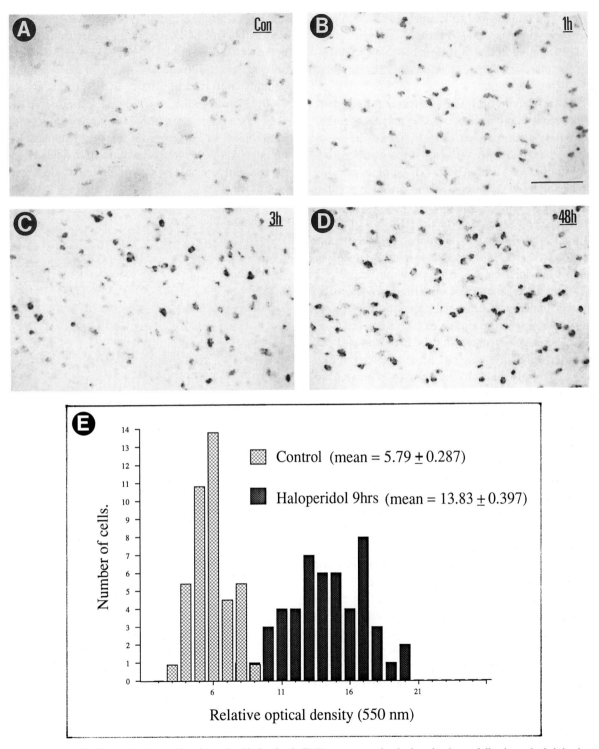

Fig. 3. Time profile illustrating the rapid and sustained induction in ENK gene expression in dorsal striatum following a single injection of haloperidol (4 mg/kg i.p.). *A*, control; *B*, 1 h; *C*, 3 h; *D*, 48 h following the injection. Note the increase in intensity of AP reaction product concentrated within the cytoplasm of cells indicating an increase in the cellular content of ENK mRNA. As can be seen in *E* an increase in the cellular content of ENK mRNA is reflected by a shift to the right of the distribution profile. Scale bar, 100 μm.

(1987) and Bannon and colleagues (1987,1989) used Northern analysis (and DA receptor agonists as opposed to antagonists), it is possible that the difference in analytical approach may partly explain these conflicting results.

How can these contrasting effects on ENK gene expression by blockade of the D_1 and D_2 receptor subtypes be interpreted? Firstly, there is the possibility that there are at least two distinct subpopulations of striatal ENK cells; one expressing predominantly D_1 receptors and another population expressing predominantly D_2 receptors. If this is the case, by comparing the distributions of populations of ENK cells from vehicle-treated striatal sections (SCH 23388) with those from SCH 23390- and raclopride-treated sections one may expect the D_1- and D_2-treated ENK distributions to be bimodal, indicative of two cell populations responding differently to the antagonist. This is a very simplistic idea as it assumes that the two proposed cell populations do not overlap. As can be seen in Fig. 4 Gaussian distributions are actually observed, indicative of a single cell population responding to both drug treatments.

One of the most likely explanations for these data is that the D_2 response is via the direct interaction of raclopride with D_2 receptors expressed by ENK cells (Le Moine et al., 1990b), whilst the D_1 response is indirect, mediated via interactions with other neurochemically defined striatal cells expressing the D_1 subtype (such as the GABA/SP cells). D_1 mRNA-positive cells may then influence ENK gene expression via interaction with striatal interneurones, for example cholinergic cells express SP (NK-1) receptor mRNA (Gerfen, 1991). Blockade of D_1 receptors on GABA/SP striato-nigral cells may also influence the activity of post-synaptic nigral DA cells which in turn innervate striatal ENK cells. In support of this latter hypothesis, a SCH 23390-mediated inhibition of forskolin-stimulated [3H] GABA efflux from slices of rat SN has been reported (Starr, 1987), local application of a D_1 agonist has been shown to increase [3H]GABA release in the dorsal striatum whilst local application of a D_2 agonist similarly decreases [3H]GABA

release (Girault et al., 1986). In vitro studies confirm that activation of D_1 receptors located on striatal nerve terminals stimulates [3H] GABA release from SN pars reticulata, entopeduncular nucleus, globus pallidus and striatal tissue slices (Floran et al., 1990). Therefore the D_1-mediated decrease in ENK gene expression may be through binding of SCH 23390 to D_1 receptors (expressed by striato-nigral GABA/SP cells) resulting in a decrease in nigral GABA release, which in turn results in a con-

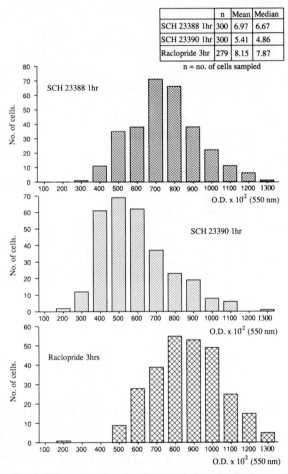

	n	Mean	Median
SCH 23388 1hr	300	6.97	6.67
SCH 23390 1hr	300	5.41	4.86
Raclopride 3hr	279	8.15	7.87

n = no. of cells sampled

Fig. 4. Histograms showing the population distributions and parameters of individual optical density readings of ENK mRNA-containing cells sampled after SCH 23388 (1 h), SCH 23390 (1 h) and raclopride (3 h) survival times following a single i.p. injection. Figure reproduced from Augood and colleagues (1992) with permission from Oxford University Press.

comitant increase in nigral DA cell activity and possibly an increase in the inhibitory action of DA on post-synaptic striatal ENK cells mediated via D_2 receptors. Thus, it could be predicted that acute SCH 23390 treatment may result in an increase in DA concentrations in the striatum. We have previously reported a slight increase in striatal DA concentrations (Augood et al., 1992) 3 h after SCH 23390 administration; however, this increase was not found to be significantly different from vehicle-treated values suggesting that the D_1 attenuation in ENK gene expression may be mediated via intrinsic signalling pathways. The role of the cholinergic interneurones in mediating the raclopride-induced increase in ENK gene expression has recently been addressed by Pollack and Wooten (1992) who have shown that scopolamine (a muscarinic antagonist) can attenuate the eticlopride- and 6-OHDA-induced increase in ENK gene expression. Administration of scopolamine alone was without effect on expression. Possible signal transduction mechanisms involved in mediating the effects of acute DA receptor blockade of ENK gene expression are discussed later in the chapter.

Neurotensin

In addition to GABA/ENK and GABA/SP striatal efferents, populations of NT-immunoreactive medium-sized projection cells have been described, which in the cat suggest that in contrast to the ENK and SP projections only 20% of NT cells co-exist with the classical transmitter GABA suggesting that there may be several sub-populations of striatal NT cells (Sugimoto and Mizuno, 1987). This is in contrast to rat studies which suggest that most striatal projection neurones are GABAergic (Kita and Kitai, 1988).

Since the suggestion of Nemeroff (1980) that NT may be acting as an endogenous neuroleptic, numerous studies have been carried out in an attempt to characterize further the possible neuroleptic-like effects of exogenously administered NT. The striatum is particularly enriched in DA and NT receptor binding sites (Goedert et al., 1984b; Moyse et al., 1987)

and there exists an inverse relationship between the compartmental localization of NT receptors and NT-LI in the cat (Goedert et al., 1983,1984a) where NT receptors are localized within the striatal matrix compartment while NT-LI is concentrated within the striatal patch compartment.

There is an increasing body of evidence consistent with a functional interaction between the DA and NT systems in the rat basal ganglia. Indeed, NT receptor mRNA is found concentrated in the SN and ventral tegmental area (Sato et al., 1992) consistent with the localization of NT receptors on DA cells and associated processes (Palacios and Kuhar, 1981). Recent studies by Castel and colleagues (1990, 1991) provide further data in support of a direct interaction between these two systems by demonstrating that monoiodo-Tyr[3] NT (8–13) injected into the rat striatum is retrogradely transported, intact (as assessed by HPLC), to the SN pars compacta resulting in a potentiation in TH gene expression within these retrogradely labelled nigral cells (Burgevin et al., 1992). The authors suggest that this retrograde transport involves binding of the labelled NT to NT receptors on DAergic nerve terminals which are then internalized and transported back to the nerve cell soma.

As with most biochemical studies the role of neuroactive substances in vivo are inferred from denervation studies, this is particularly true in the case of striatal NT, the content of which has been measured following DA denervation or DA receptor blockade (Goedert et al., 1984b; Letter et al., 1987; Merchant et al., 1989; Zahm and Johnson, 1989).

In contrast to the striatal ENK system, there is concordance amongst authors about the effects of DA denervation on striatal NT gene expression; a rapid induction in NT gene expression is observed following DA denervation and both chronic and acute D_2 receptor blockade (Augood et al., 1991b). Indeed a rapid and sustained potentiation in NT gene expression is detected following a single injection of haloperidol (1 mg/kg i.p.; Merchant et al., 1992). In contrast, no induction is detected following acute D_1 receptor blockade with SCH 23390 (Augood et al., 1991b). A potentiation in NT gene expression is also observed 6 h after reserpine treatment (Bean and Hökfelt, 1992) and 3 h following administration of BMY 14802, a potential antipsychotic sigma receptor antagonist (Levant and Nemeroff, 1990; Levant et al., 1992) indicating that striatal NT cells, like GABA/ENK striatal cells, are under the influence of the DAergic nigro-striatal pathway. In all cases reported, the induction in NT mRNA is relatively restricted to the dorso-lateral subcallosal rim, an area of striatum particularly enriched in D_2 receptor binding sites and D_2 receptor mRNA (Weiner and Brann, 1989; Mansour et al., 1990). Acute treatment of rats with the atypical neuroleptic clozapine (20 mg/kg i.p.) is reported to be without effect on striatal NT gene expression; at more toxic doses (40 mg/kg) an induction was detected in the dorso-lateral rim, however, not all animals survived the injection. In contrast, an induction in expression was detected in the nucleus accumbens at the lower dose (Merchant et al., 1992) consistent with the suggestion that the main target sites for the action of clozapine are DA D_4 receptors located in limbic-related structures.

These in situ data may be interpreted as extending the pharmacological findings of Frey and co-workers (1986, 1988) who detected an increase in the tissue content of NT peptide, measured by radioimmunoassay, in rat striatum after D_2 antagonist treatment and a decrease in peptide concentrations following D_1 blockade. They suggest that the increased peptide concentration detected after D_2 blockade may be due to an accumulation of the peptide in nerve terminals; however, such an increase may also arise from enhanced peptide synthesis which, assuming that an increase in transcription is paralleled by an increase in post-transcriptional processing, would account for the increased peptide content.

In view of this and other data a theoretical synaptic arrangement which may underlie DA-NT interactions has been proposed (Bean et al., 1989), with D_2 receptor-mediated alterations in NT peptide content being associated with D_2 receptors located on cortico-striate processes. However, from D_2 receptor in situ hybridization studies localizing sites of D_2 receptor gene expression (Weiner and Brann, 1989) it is clear that the majority of striatal D_2 receptors are located on intrinsic neurones and/or their processes and not on cortico-striate processes (Joyce and Marshall, 1987) suggesting that a considerable proportion of NT-DA interactions in the striatum occurs locally. While the mechanism of NT induction following acute D_2 receptor blockade and DA denervation remains to be established, it is of interest to note that the differential effects of acute D_1 and D_2 receptor antagonism on striatal NT content parallel those observed for striatal ENK, suggesting that endogenous DA may influence the expression of this gene through similar signal transduction pathways. An insight into the possible pathways and gene transcription factors involved are discussed later in this article.

Substance P

The tachykinin undecapeptide substance P (SP) is generated by differential RNA splicing of three preprotachykinin (PPT) mRNAs termed α, β and γ (Krause et al., 1987) all of which are derived from a single PPT gene which also encodes neurokinin A (substance K). As mentioned earlier, SP mRNA is expressed by a population of striatal GABA medium-sized spiny cells (Young et al., 1986; Chesselet and Affolter, 1987) which preferentially project to the SN resulting in a dense plexus of SP-immunoreactive nerve fibres and terminals localized in both the pars compacta and pars reticulata (Kanazawa and Jessell, 1976; Brownstein et al., 1977; Kanazawa et al., 1977). Whilst the majority of striatal SP cells have spiny processes, aspiny immunoreactive cells have been reported in the rat and cat (Bolam et al., 1983; Penney et al., 1986). Nevertheless, it is the spiny nerve cells which are believed to be the source of the GABA/SP-containing striato-nigral pathway.

Electron microscopy studies have shown that SP-immunoreactive terminals (presumably arising from GABA/SP striatal cells) form synaptic specializations with TH-immunoreactive dendrites and cell bodies in the rat SN (Somogyi et al., 1982;

Kawai et al., 1987) suggesting that the GABA/SP striato-nigral pathway can directly influence the DAergic nigro-striatal pathway. Terminals from DAergic pars compacta cells have also been shown to monosynaptically influence striato-nigral GABA/SP cells (Kubota et al., 1986b). However, the search for a functional/physiological role for SP in the nigra is compounded by the paradox of an anatomical mismatch between regions enriched in SP binding sites and regions enriched in SP peptide. Despite the high concentration of immunoreactive peptide localized in nerve terminals in the nigra and the absence, to date, of SP binding sites/receptors (NK-1 receptors) there is a wealth of pharmacological, electrophysiological and biochemical data consistent with an interaction between the SP and DA systems. SP applied electrophoretically into the SN of rats and cats in vivo has been found to significantly increase the activity of the majority of nigral cells tested (Davis and Dray, 1976), and potentiate the release of DA in the ipsilateral striatum (Cheramy et al., 1977; Reid et al., 1990) resulting in turning behaviour (James and Starr, 1977), suggesting activation of the DAergic nigro-striatal pathway. Furthermore, administration of Spantide II (0.7 nmol), a modified SP peptide analogue lacking histamine-releasing activity but effective as a tachykinin antagonist (Folkers et al., 1990), into the pars reticulata of anaesthetized rats has been found to block SP stimulation (0.07 nmol) of striatal DA release and, when administered alone, transiently decrease extracellular levels of DA in the ipsilateral striatum (Reid et al., 1990). As NK-1 receptor mRNA in the striatum is expressed exclusively by cholinergic interneurones (Gerfen, 1991), it is possible that these cells mediate the release of DA from pre-synaptic nerve terminals.

To investigate in more detail interactions between the SP- and DA-containing systems in the rat basal ganglia, neurotoxins, such as 6-OHDA, and selective DA receptors agonists and antagonists have been used. It has been reported that striatal SP gene expression is significantly decreased following DA denervation (Young et al., 1986) or chronic haloperidol and sulpiride treatment (Bannon et al.,

1987; Angulo et al., 1990). A concomitant decrease in nigral SP content (Oblin et al., 1984; Bannon et al., 1987; Cruz and Beckstead, 1988; Sivam, 1989) and ventral striatal immunostaining is detected following such treatments (Voorn et al., 1987), suggesting that the attenuation in gene expression may be paralleled by a decrease in peptide synthesis. In contrast to this, chronic treatment of rats with SCH 23390 results in a significant increase in SP immunoreactivity in the ipsilateral SN (Cruz and Beckstead, 1988). Our preliminary radioactive in situ data suggest that acute SCH 23390 results in a transient potentiation in striatal SP gene expression whilst administration of raclopride attenuates the expression of this gene when compared to uninjected control animals. This again indicates that blockade of the D_1 and D_2 receptor subtypes can differentially modulate the expression of this gene. Chronic treatment of rats with low doses of the D_4 receptor antagonist clozapine (2 mg/kg s.c.) is reported to be without effect on SP gene expression (Angulo et al., 1990).

Possibly the most surprising and potentially interesting finding from our preliminary in situ study was a rapid and sustained increase in SP gene expression following injection of SCH 23388, the biologically inactive S-enantiomer of SCH 23390. From previous acute studies using this compound (Augood et al., 1991a,b, 1992) it is clear that SCH 23388 has no effect on ENK, NT or SRIF gene expression, indicating a specific interaction of SCH 23388 with the striatal tachykinin system. One interpretation of this rapid and sustained increase in SP expression is an interaction of SCH 23388 with the serotonin (5-HT) system, as subchronic p-chloro-phenylalanine treatment of rats, which results in a depletion of striatal 5-HT levels, significantly decreases striatal SP mRNA content. Conversely administration of zimelidine (a 5-HT uptake inhibitor) or DOI (a 5-HT_2 agonist) significantly increases both SP gene expression and SP immunoreactivity in striatum (Walker et al., 1991). These data suggest that SCH 23388 may act to increase 5-HT transmission. Destruction of the 5-HT dorsal raphe-striatal pathway similarly results in a reduction in prodynorphin gene expression (co-expressed by most striatal GABA/SP cells) without affecting striatal ENK gene expression (Morris et al., 1988a). It is clear from these studies that striatal SP gene expression is influenced by both the DAergic nigro-striatal pathway and the 5-HT raphe-striatal pathway, which have opposing effects.

Somatostatin

Unlike the three striatal neuropeptide systems discussed above, striatal SRIF cells belong to a relatively small population of medium-sized interneurones with aspiny dendrites and indented nuclei as demonstrated by immunocytochemical studies (Takagi et al., 1983; Chesselet and Graybiel, 1986; Smith and Parent, 1986) which do not contain GABA (Chesselet and Robbins, 1989). Examples of SRIF neurones, visualized using in situ hybridization and immunocytochemistry, are shown in Fig. 5.

Although it is not clear which other striatal cells SRIF interneurones interact with, it has been suggested on the basis of their anatomical localization, lining the chemically demarcated patch/matrix boundaries, that they may relay information between these two striatal compartments (Gerfen, 1984). In addition to SRIF, these interneurones are reported, in the cat, rat and squirrel, to contain NPY and have NADPH-diaphorase activity (Vincent and Johansson, 1983; Smith and Parent, 1986). As with most neurochemically defined striatal cell types an interaction between the DA system and SRIF interneurones has been suggested. As indeed symmetrical synaptic specializations have been demonstrated between TH-immunoreactive axon terminals, presumed to originate from the SN, and approximately 50% of striatal NPY-immunoreactive perikarya and proximal dendrites (Kubota et al., 1988), a direct interaction of DA with this interneuronal cell population is likely.

The majority of radioimmunoassay, immunocytochemical and in situ hybridization data are con-

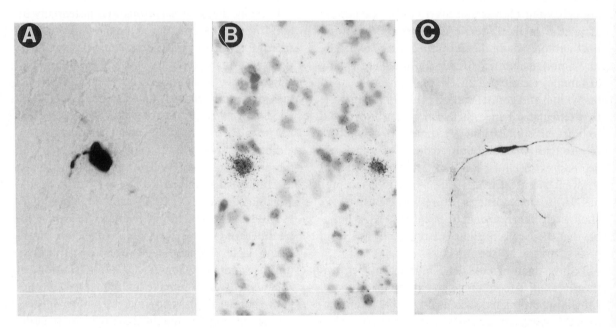

Fig. 5. Examples of striatal SRIF mRNA-containing (A and B) and SRIF-immunoreactive cells (C). A. Cryostat section (15 μm) hybridized with an AP-SRIF probe. B. Cryostat section (15 μm) hybridized with a ^{35}S-labelled SRIF probe and then counterstained to visualize cell bodies. Two SRIF-positive cells can be seen (clustering of silver grains over the cell soma). C. Microtome section (40 μm) processed to visualize SRIF immunoreactivity (illustration kindly provided by Dr. A. Herbison, Department of Neurobiology, AFRC Babraham Institute, Babraham, Cambridge).

sistent with such an interaction (Beal and Martin, 1984; Martin-Iverson et al., 1986; Radke et al., 1988; Weiss and Chesselet, 1989; Soghomonian and Chesselet, 1989; Salin et al., 1990); more recent findings have, however, questioned the role of DA in influencing SRIF cell activity (Salin et al., 1990). The majority of studies have investigated a possible DA-SRIF interaction by disrupting the DA innervation to the striatum with 6-OHDA (Beal and Martin, 1984; Salin et al., 1990), or by chronically treating rats with typical (usually haloperidol) or atypical neuroleptics and measuring the effect of DA denervation on the tissue content of SRIF immunoreactivity. In general a significant reduction in both SRIF mRNA and SRIF immunoreactivity is detected following subchronic D_2 receptor blockade (Beal and Martin, 1984; Radke et al., 1988; Weiss and Chesselet, 1989); in contrast to this, despite a reduction in SRIF gene expression following DA denervation (Soghomonian and Chesselet, 1991) no detectable change in peptide content has been measured (Vuillet et al., 1989). Using an acute drug regime we have shown that D_1 and D_2 receptor blockade results in a decrease in SRIF gene expression; no change in the density of SRIF mRNA-containing cells was detected (Augood et al., 1991a). These data are supportive of a DA-SRIF interaction, as the cellular reduction in SRIF mRNA content occurred within 60 min of a single injection of SCH 23390. In contrast, the cellular reduction in SRIF mRNA content was not detected until 3 h after an injection of raclopride and this decrease was still apparent 9 h later.

To date there are no data describing the effects of chronic D_1 receptor blockade on striatal SRIF gene expression. The differential effects of chronic D_2 receptor blockade versus total DA denervation on striatal SRIF levels may indicate either the importance of the D_1 receptor in modulating SRIF levels (as striatal cells expressing this receptor would still be activated by endogenous DA following D_2 receptor blockade) and/or that the striatal SRIF system possesses a high degree of plasticity and has recovered from the primary effects of the 6-OHDA lesion during the 2 – 3 weeks post-operative period. Possi-

ble explanations for the regulation of the SRIF gene through activation of DA D_1 receptors are discussed below with emphasis on the likely signal transduction pathways which may be mediating these complex responses.

Studies of the effect of chronic clozapine administration report an increase in SRIF gene expression in the nucleus accumbens with no change in expression in the striatum (Salin et al., 1990). As no change in either D_1 and D_2 receptor binding is detected in rat membrane homogenates following chronic clozapine treatment this suggests that the principal action of clozapine is not blockade of either D_1 and D_2 receptors (Riva and Creese, 1990) but rather interaction with D_4 receptors localized within limbic-related structures, particularly in the nucleus accumbens (Van Tol et al., 1991). In light of the suggestion that D_4 receptors, like striatal D_2 receptors, may couple to the inhibitory adenylate cyclase-linked GTP-binding protein (Gi) when activated, it is possible that the increase in SRIF gene expression detected following chronic clozapine treatment may be explained partly by alterations in intracellular cAMP levels. This concept is discussed in more detail later in this chapter.

Selectivity of SCH 23390 and raclopride for DA D_1 and D_2 receptors

Detailed studies of the localization of DA D_1 and D_2 receptor binding sites as visualized using [³H]SCH 23390 and [³H]raclopride have shown that both ligands interact with a single population of binding sites with high affinity (Kd = 1.5 and 2.2 nM, respectively). In addition, approximately four times as many D_1 than D_2 sites are detected as reflected by the B_{max} values of 86.0 fmol/mg (D_1) and 20.0 fmol/mg (D_2) of tissue (Köhler et al., 1985; Mansour et al., 1990). A similar high-affinity Kd value has been reported for [³H]raclopride binding to human putamen membranes (3.9 nM; Hall et al., 1990).

As with all exogenously administered agents the degree of pharmacological selectivity of a compound for a particular class of receptors is relative and highly dose-dependent. This is expecially true for SCH 23390 which possesses some degree of affinity for receptors other than those belonging to the DA D_1 subtype. In particular while SCH 23390 is reported to have low affinity for alpha-1, alpha-2 adrenergic, muscarinic, histamine and serotonin 5-HT_1 receptors it has been found to have a nanomolar affinity for 5-HT_2 receptors in forebrain (Bischoff et al., 1986) and 5-HT_{1c} receptors in the choroid plexus (Nicklaus et al., 1988) as determined by in vitro binding studies. However, in vivo doses of approximately 0.1 mg/kg are sufficient to inhibit DA-dependent behaviours, such as contralateral turning and locomotion, elicited by stimulation of D_1 receptors (by SKF 38393) in the 6-OHDA-lesioned rat but much larger doses are required to inhibit [³H]spiperone binding to 5-HT_2 receptors in frontal cortex (doses of > 1.5 mg/kg required for 50% inhibition; see review by Clark and White, 1987). It would appear that blockade of 5-HT_2 receptors by SCH 23390 is not responsible for the behavioural effects observed suggesting that the primary sites of action of this compound are D_1 receptors. Nevertheless, the nanomolar affinity of [³H]SCH 23390 for 5-HT_2 receptors in vitro is noteworthy.

DA receptors and involvement of transcription factors

One pharmacological characteristic distinguishing striatal D_1 and D_2 receptors is their opposing effects on adenylate cyclase activity and second messenger, cAMP, formation. In vitro striatal D_1 and D_2 receptors have been shown to have either a stimulatory or inhibitory effect respectively on adenylate cyclase activity (Kebabian and Calne, 1979; Stoof and Kebabian, 1981) when stimulated by selective agonists. In view of this, the wealth of literature pertaining to the regulation of expression of ENK, NT and SRIF genes by cAMP and cAMP analogues and the demonstration of (putative) cAMP-responsive elements (termed CREs) located within the 5' untranslated promoter regions of these genes, upstream of the initiation codon, it is feasible that the

effects of DA receptor blockade discussed here may be explained, in part, by (transient) changes in intracellular cAMP concentrations.

Consistent with this suggestion, data obtained from PC 12 phaeochromocytoma cells transfected with the SRIF gene have shown a four-fold increase in SRIF gene expression within 4 h following the addition of 10 μM forskolin (a direct activator of adenylate cyclase) to the culture medium (Montminy et al., 1986). In addition SRIF secretion is increased by agents that stimulate adenylate cyclase activity (Chihara et al., 1979; Shimatsu et al., 1982; Tapia-Arancibia and Reichlin, 1985). The content of ENK mRNA and its translational products, met- and leu-ENK, have been shown to be significantly elevated in vitro by forskolin and cAMP analogues (Eiden et al., 1984; Quach et al., 1984; Folkesson et al., 1989; Wan et al., 1991). Activation of a transfected ENK fusion gene by membrane depolarisation in PC 12 and C6 glioma cells is proportional to extracellular Ca^{2+} concentrations and is inhibited by verapamil (a Ca^{2+} channel blocker; Nguyen et al., 1990).

Studies on the regulation of SRIF gene expression by cAMP by Montminy and colleagues (1986) have shown by selective base pair deletions of parts of the 5'-region of the SRIF gene promotor, that the nucleotide sequence important for conferring cAMP responsiveness to the SRIF gene sequence, termed the CRE consensus sequence, is an eight nucleotide palindrome: 5'-TGACGTCA-3' located at position − 41 relative to the initiation codon. Subsequently, the human ENK gene has also been found to contain two functionally distinct CREs, termed ENKCRE-1 at position − 104 and ENKCRE-2 at position − 92 (Comb et al., 1988). In contrast to the SRIF CRE, neither ENKCRE-1 nor ENKCRE-2 is palindromic; the consensus sequences being 5'-TGGCGTA-3' and 5'-TGCGTCA-3', respectively. These elements have been shown to act synergistically, as activation of ENKCRE-1 in the absence of a funtionally active ENKCRE-2 is not sufficient to activate ENK gene transcription. Further, the base pair spacing between these two elements appears to be critical for activation of gene transcription. It has also been noted that the promoter sequence of the rat NT/NN gene contains a base pair sequence, 5'-TGACATCA-3', at position −155 which closely resembles the SRIF CRE consensus sequence whilst the human sequence contains two putative CRE's (Bean et al., 1992). In support of the NT/NN gene containing a CRE, the tissue content of NT peptide and NT mRNA are reported to be significantly increased in response to activators of adenylate cyclase (Kislauskis et al., 1988). Further, data from in vitro studies suggest that D_2 receptors mediate the inhibition of intracellular cAMP formation by DA in striatal primary neuronal cultures, and that this process is pertussis toxin-sensitive suggesting interaction with the inhibitory G protein, Gi (Weiss et al., 1985).

Given the opposing effects of D_1 and D_2 activation on adenylate cyclase activity it is feasible that the significant reductions in the cellular content of ENK and SRIF mRNAs, expressed by striatal cells, following D_1 receptor blockade may be associated with a reduction in intracellular cAMP formation and thus a reduction in the activation of CREs contained within the promoter region of these neuropeptide genes. In contrast, blockade of D_2 receptors is associated with a potentiation of second messenger cAMP formation and thus an increase in activation of CREs. While a significant increase in ENK and NT gene expression is observed following raclopride treatment, SRIF gene expression is attenuated suggesting an indirect effect of raclopride on SRIF interneurones but perhaps a direct effect on striatal ENK and NT mRNA-containing cells.

Implications for striatal signalling

The suggestions detailed above for the regulation of ENK, NT and SRIF gene expression in the rat striatum by DA D_1 and D_2 receptors are partly corroborated by recent data demonstrating the cellular co-expression of PPE A and D_2 mRNA within individual striatal neurones (Le Moine et al., 1990b). Furthermore Le Moine notes that striatal SRIF cells do not appear to express D_2 receptor mRNA. This is consistent with an indirect polysynaptic effect of raclopride on SRIF gene expression as opposed to a direct effect. If this is the case, one may speculate that the D_2 effect may be mediated via an interaction of raclopride with presynaptic D_2 receptors on DAergic nerve terminals, or/and ENK striatal neurones which may contact aspiny striatal cells or/and striatal cholinergic interneurones which also express D_2 receptor mRNA (Le Moine et al., 1990a) and form symmetrical synaptic contacts with NPY-immunoreactive somata and proximal dendrites (Vuillet et al., 1992). It has been suggested that the activities of these two interneuronal cell populations may be functionally linked as reciprocal NPY-ChAT interactions have been described (Vuillet et al., 1992).

Explanations for the contrasting effects of neuroleptics on SP expression are likely to be equally complex, however, the increase in expression following acute SCH 23390 treatment is likely to be direct as these striatal GABAergic cells express D_1 receptor mRNA (Le Moine et al., 1991). Explanations for the D_2-mediated effect are more complex, as there is still much controversy concerning the localization of D_2 receptors on GABA/SP striatonigral neurones (Meador-Woodruff et al., 1991; Ariano et al., 1992).

To date, little is known about the localization of DA receptors on striatal NT cells. One possible explanation for the significant induction in NT gene expression following raclopride treatment is analogous to that of striatal ENK cells, namely striatal NT cells also express D_2 receptors, blockade of which would be predicted to result in a potentiation in cAMP formation and thus an increase in the activation of the putative CRE resulting in an increase in NT gene transcription. However, the exact mechanism for the complex regulation needs to be established.

Consideration of all the data raises the question of the cellular co-expression of D_1 and D_2 receptors by individual striatal cells, particularly those expressing ENK mRNA. While there are some electrophysiological data consistent with the co-localization of D_1 and D_2 receptors (Ohno et al., 1987) and various biochemical and pharmacological studies have suggested that such a cellular co-expression may exist (Stoof and Kebabian 1981; Weiner et al., 1991), there is no unequivocal evidence demonstrating the cellular co-expression of D_1 and D_2 receptors in vivo (but see also Surmeier and Kitai, this volume). By combining retrograde tracing experiments with in situ hybridization studies, Gerfen and colleagues (1990) have reported that only a small percentage of striatal projection cells express both receptor subtypes. Data from our combined radioactive and non-radioactive in situ hybridization studies in control naive rats are in good agreement; striatal ENK cells express mainly D_2 mRNA (Fig. 6A) and not D_1 mRNA (Fig. 6B,

data unpublished) when detected by in situ hybridization.

However, recent in situ hybridization data, using ^{35}S-labelled riboprobes on semi-thin serial sections, report that approximately 33% of striatal cells express both receptor mRNAs (Meador-Woodruff et al., 1991). From these contradictory findings it is apparent that the balance between D_1 and D_2-mediated effects may be of major importance in the normal functioning of the mammalian basal ganglia. Understanding this balance is likely to be important for therapeutic intervention in basal ganglia-associated disorders.

Acknowledgements

The authors would like to thank the MRC, the Tourette Syndrome Association (U.S.A.) and SmithKline (1982) Foundation for financial support. The contribution of Eileen McGowan is gratefully acknowledged.

References

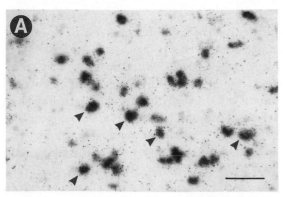
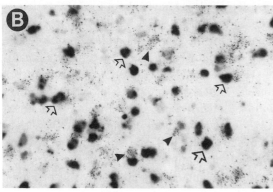

Fig. 6. Cryostat sections of rat dorsal striatum simultaneously hybridized with AP-ENK oligo + ^{35}S-D$_2$ oligo (A), and AP-ENK oligo + ^{35}S-D$_1$ oligo (B). Note that the two hybridization signals (coloured AP reaction product and silver grains) may be clearly resolved. A. Both hybridization signals are seen concentrated in the same cell illustrating that ENK cells contain D_2 mRNA. B. The two hybridization signals are found concentrated in different cells, illustrating that in control naive rats ENK (filled arrows) and D_1 (open arrows) transcripts are not extensively co-expressed. Scale bar, 50 μm.

Angulo, A., Davis, L., Buckhart, B. and Cristoph, G. (1986) Reduction of striatal dopaminergic transmission elevates proenkephalin mRNA. *Eur. J. Pharmacol.*, 130: 341 – 343.

Angulo, J.A., Cadet, J.L. and McEwen, B.S. (1990) Effect of typical and atypical neuroleptic treatment on protachykinin mRNA levels in the striatum of the rat. *Neurosci. Lett.*, 113: 217 – 221.

Ariano, M.A., Stromski, C.J., Smyk-Randall, E.M. and Sibley, D.R. (1992) D_2 dopamine receptor localization on striatonigral neurons. *Neurosci. Lett.*, 144: 215 – 220.

Augood, S.J., Emson, P.C., Mitchell, I.J., Boyce, S., Clarke, C.E. and Crossman, A.R. (1989) Cellular localization of enkephalin gene expression in MPTP-treated cynomolgus monkeys. *Mol. Brain Res.*, 6: 85 – 92.

Augood, S.J., Kiyama, H., Faull, R.L.M. and Emson, P.C. (1991a) Dopaminergic D_1 and D_2 receptor antagonists decrease prosomatostatin mRNA expression in rat striatum. *Neuroscience*, 44: 35 – 44.

Augood, S.J., Kiyama, H., Faull, R.L.M. and Emson, P.C. (1991b) Differential effects of acute dopaminergic D_1 and D_2 receptor antagonists on proneurotensin mRNA expression in rat striatum. *Mol. Brain Res.*, 9: 341 – 346.

Augood, S.J., Faull, R.L.M. and Emson, P.C. (1992) Contrasting effects of raclopride and SCH 23390 on the cellular content of proenkephalin A mRNA in rat striatum; a quantitative non-radioactive in situ hybridization study. *Eur. J., Neurosci.,* 4: 102 – 112.

Bannon, M.J., Elliot, P.J. and Bunney, E.B. (1987) Striatal tachykinin biosynthesis; regulation of mRNA and peptide levels by dopamine agonists and antagonists. *Mol. Brain Res.,* 3: 31 – 37.

Bannon, M.J., Kelland, M. and Chido, L.A. (1989) Medial forebrain bundle stimulation or D-2 dopamine receptor activation increases proenkephalin mRNA in rat striatum. *J. Neurochem.,* 52: 859 – 862.

Beal, M.F. and Martin, J.B. (1984) Effects of neuroleptic drugs on brain somatostatin-like immunoreactivity. *Neurosci. Lett.,* 47: 125 – 130.

Bean, A.J. and Hökfelt, T. (1992) Reserpine increases striatal neurotensin mRNA levels. *Mol. Brain Res.,* 12: 345 – 348.

Bean, A.J., During, M.J., Deutch, A.Y. and Roth, R.H. (1989) Effects of dopamine depletion on striatal neurotensin: biochemical and immunohistochemical studies. *J. Neurosci.,* 9: 4430 – 4438.

Bean, A.J., Dagerlind, A., Hökfelt, T. and Dobner, P.R. (1992) Cloning of human neurotensin/ neuromedin N genomic sequences and expression in the ventral mesencephalon of schizophrenics and age/ sex matched controls. *Neuroscience,* 50: 259 – 268.

Bennett, B., Lapper, S.R., Francis, C.M., Rogers, J., Celio, M.R. and Bolam, J.P. (1992) Characterization of striatal neurones that display immunoreactivity for calcium binding proteins. *Neurosci. Lett. (Suppl.),* 42: S36.

Bischoff, S., Heinrich, M., Sonntag, J.M. and Krauss, J. (1986) The D_1 dopamine receptor antagonist SCH 23390 also interacts potently with brain serotonin (5-HT$_2$) receptors. *Eur. J. Pharmacol.,* 129: 367 – 370.

Bolam, J.P., Somogyi, P., Takagi, H., Fodor, I. and Smith, A.D. (1983) Localisation of substance P-like immunoreactivity in neurons and nerve terminals in the neostriatum of the rat; a correlated light and electron micrscopic study. *J. Neurocytol.,* 12: 325 – 344.

Brownstein, M.J., Mroz, E.A., Tappaz, M.L. and Leeman, S.E. (1977) On the origin of substance P and glutamic acid decarboxylase (GAD) in the substantia nigra. *Brain Res.,* 135: 315 – 323.

Bunzow, J.R., Van Tol, H.H.M., Grandy, D.K., Albert, P., Salon, J., Christie, M., Machida, C.A., Neve, K.A. and Civelli, O. (1988) Cloning and expression of a rat D$_2$ dopamine receptor cDNA. *Nature,* 336: 783 – 787.

Burgevin, M.-C., Castel, M.-N., Quarteronet, D., Chevet, T. and Laduron, P.M. (1992) Neurotensin increases tyrosine hydroxylase messenger RNA-positive neurons in substantia nigra after retrograde axonal transport. *Neuroscience,* 49: 627 – 633.

Castel, M.-N., Malgouris, C., Blanchard, J.-C. and Laduron, P.M. (1990) Retrograde axonal transport of neurotensin in the dopaminergic nigrostriatal pathway in the rat. *Neuroscience,* 36: 425 – 430.

Castel, M.N., Faucher, D., Cuiné, F., Dubédat, P., Boireau, A. and Laduron, P.M. (1991) Identification of intact neurotensin in the substantia nigra after its retrograde axonal transport in dopaminergic neurons. *J. Neurochem.,* 56: 1816 – 1818.

Cheramy, A., Nieoullon, A., Michelot, R. and Glowinski, J. (1977) Effects of intranigral application of dopamine and substance P on the in vivo release of newly sythesized ^{3}H-dopamine in the ipsilateral caudate nucleus of the cat. *Neurosci. Lett.,* 4: 105 – 109.

Chesselet, M.-F. and Affolter, H.-U. (1987) Preprotachykinin messenger RNA detected by in situ hybridization in striatal neurons of the human brain. *Brain Res.,* 410: 83 – 88.

Chesselet, M.-F. and Graybiel, A.M. (1986) Striatal neurons expressing somatostatin-like immunoreactivity: evidence for a peptidergic interneuronal system in the cat. *Neuroscience,* 17: 547 – 571.

Chesselet, M.-F. and Robbins, E. (1989) Characterization of striatal neurons expressing high levels of glutamic acid decarboxylase messenger RNA. *Brain Res.,* 492: 237 – 244.

Chihara, K., Arimura, A. and Schally, A. (1979) Effect of intraventricular injection of dopamine, norepinephrine, acetylcholine and 5-hydroxytryptamine on immunoreactive somatostatin release into rat hypophyseal portal blood. *Endocrinology,* 104: 1656 – 1682.

Clark, D. and White, F.J. (1987) Review: D-1 dopamine receptor – the search for a function. *Synapse,* 1: 347 – 388.

Comb, M., Mermod, H., Hyman, S.E., Pearlberg, J., Ross, M.E. and Goodman, H.M. (1988) Proteins bound at adjacent DNA elements act synergistically to regulate human proenkephalin cAMP inducible transcription. *EMBO J.,* 7: 3793 – 3805.

Cowan, R.L., Wilson, C.J., Emson, P.C. and Heizmann, C.W. (1990) Parvalbumin-containing GABAergic interneurons in the rat neostriatum. *J. Comp. Neurol.,* 302: 197 – 205.

Cruz, C.J. and Beckstead, R.M. (1988) Quantitative radioimmunocytochemical evidence that haloperidol and SCH 23390 induce opposite changes in substance P levels of rat substantia nigra. *Brain Res.,* 457: 29 – 43.

Davis, J. and Dray, A. (1976) Substance P in the substantia nigra. *Brain Res.,* 107: 623 – 627.

Dearry, A., Gingrich, J.A., Falardeau, P., Fremeau, R.T., Bates, M.D. and Caron, M.G. (1990) Molecular cloning and expression of the gene for a human D$_1$ dopamine receptor. *Nature,* 347: 72 – 76.

Eiden, L.E., Giraud, P., Affolter, H-U., Herbert, E. and Hotchkiss, A.J. (1984) Alternative modes of enkephalin biosynthesis regulation by reserpine and cyclic AMP in cultured chromaffin cells. *Proc. Natl. Acad. Sci. U.S.A.,* 81: 3949 – 3953.

Floran, B., Aceves, J., Sierra, A. and Martinez-Fong, D. (1990) Activation of D-1 dopamine receptors stimnulates the release of GABA in the basal ganglia of the rat. *Neurosci. Lett.,* 116: 136 – 140.

Folkers, K., Feng, D.M., Asano, N., Håkanson, R., Wiesenfeld-Hallin, Z. and Leanders, S. (1990) Spantide II, an effective tachykinin antagonist having high potency and negligible neurotoxicity. *Proc. Natl. Acad. Sci. U.S.A.*, 87: 4833 – 4835.

Folkesson, R., Monstein, H.-J., Geijer, T. and Terenius, L. (1989) Modulation of proenkephalin A gene expression by cyclic AMP. *Mol. Brain Res.*, 5: 211 – 217.

Frey, P., Fuxe, K., Eneroth, P. and Agnatis, L.F. (1986) Effects of acute and long term treatment with neuroleptics on regional telencephalic neurotensin levels in the male rat. *Neurochem. Int.*, 8: 429 – 434.

Frey, P., Lis, M. and Coward, D.M. (1988) Neurotensin concentrations in rat striatum and nucleus accumbens: further studies of their regulation. *Neurochem. Int.*, 12: 39 – 45.

Gerfen, C.R. (1984) The neostriatal mosaic; compartmentalization of corticostriatal input and striatonigral output systems. *Nature*, 311: 461 – 464.

Gerfen, C.R. (1991) Substance P (neurokinin-1) receptor mRNA is selectively expressed in cholinergic neurons in the rat striatum and basal forebrain. *Brain Res.*, 556: 165 – 170.

Gerfen, C.R., Engber, T.M., Mahan, L.C., Susel, Z., Chase, T.N., Monsma, F.J. and Sibley, D.R. (1990) D_1 and D_2 receptor-regulated gene expression of striatonigral and striatopallidal neurons. *Science*, 250: 1429 – 1432.

Girault, J.A., Spampinato, U., Savaki, H.E., Glowinski, J. and Besson, M.J. (1986) In vivo release of [^{3}H]-aminobutyric acid in the rat neostriatum, I. Characterization and topographical heterogeneity of the effects of dopaminergic and cholinergic agents. *Neuroscience*, 19: 1101 – 1108.

Goedert, M., Mantyh, P.W., Hunt, S.P. and Emson, P.C. (1983) Mosaic distribution of neurotensin-like immunoreactivity in the cat striatum. *Brain Res.*, 274: 176 – 179.

Goedert, M., Mantyh, P.W., Emson, P.C. and Hunt, S.P. (1984a) Inverse relationship between neurotensin receptors and neurotensin-like immunoreactivity in cat striatum. *Nature*, 307: 543 – 546.

Goedert, M., Pittaway, K. and Emson, P.C. (1984b) Neurotensin receptors in the rat striatum: lesion studies. *Brain Res.*, 299: 164 – 168.

Hall, H., Wedel, I., Halldim, C., Kopp, J. and Farde, L. (1990) Comparison of the in vitro receptor binding properties of N-[^{3}H] methyl spiperone and [^{3}H] raclopride to rat and human membranes. *J. Neurochem.*, 55: 2048 – 2057.

Ingham, C.A., Hood, S.H. and Arbuthnott, G.W. (1991) A light and electron microscopy study of enkephalin-immunoreactive structures in the rat neostriatum after removal of the nigrostriatal dopaminergic pathway. *Neuroscience*, 42: 715 – 730.

Iorio, L.C., Barnett, A., Leitz, F.H., Houser, V.P. and Korduba, C.A. (1983) SCH 23390, a potential benzazepine antipsychotic with unique interactions on dopaminergic systems. *J. Pharmacol. Exp. Ther.*, 226: 462 – 468.

James, T.A. and Starr, M.S. (1977) Behavioural and biochemical effects of substance P injected into the substantia nigra of the rat. *J. Pharm. Pharmacol.*, 29: 181 – 182.

Joyce, J.N. and Marshall, J.F. (1987) Quantitative autoradiography of dopamine D_2 sites in rat caudate-putamen: localisa-

tion to intrinsic neurons and not to neocortical afferents. *Neuroscience*, 20: 773 – 795.

Kanazawa, I. and Jessell, T. (1976) Post mortem changes and regional distribution of substance P in the rat and mouse nervous system. *Brain Res.*, 117: 362 – 367.

Kanazawa, I., Emson, P.C. and Cuello, A.C. (1977) Evidence for the existence of substance P containing fibres in striatonigral and pallido-nigral pathways in rat brain. *Brain Res.*, 119: 447 – 453.

Kawai, Y., Takagi, H., Kumoi, Y., Shiosaka, S. and Tohyama, M. (1987) Nigrostriatal dopamine neurons receive synaptic substance P-ergic inputs in the substantia nigra: application of the immunoelectron microscopic mirror technique to fluorescent double-staining for transmitter specific projections. *Brain Res.*, 401: 371 – 376.

Kebabian, J.W. (1978) Multiple classes of dopamine receptors in mammalian central nervous system: the involvement of dopamine-sensitive adenylyl cyclase. *Life Sci.*, 23: 479 – 484.

Kebabian, J.W. and Calne, D.B. (1979) Multiple receptors for dopamine. *Nature*, 277: 93 – 96.

Kebabian, J.W., Petzold, G.L. and Greengard, P. (1972) Dopamine-sensitive adenylate cyclase in caudate nucleus of rat brain, and its similarity to the "Dopamine Receptor". *Proc. Natl. Acad. Sci. U.S.A.*, 69: 2145 – 2149.

Kislauskis, E., Bullock, B., McNeil, S. and Dobner, P.R. (1988) The rat gene encoding neurotensin and neuromedin N. *J. Biol. Chem.*, 263: 4963 – 4968.

Kita, H. and Kitai, S.T. (1988) Glutamate decarboxylase immunoreactive neurons in rat neostriatum: their morphological types and populations. *Brain Res.*, 447: 346 – 352.

Köhler, C., Hall, H., Ogren, S.-O. and Gawell, L. (1985) Specific in vitro binding of ^{3}H-raclopride. A potent substituted benzamide drug with high affinity for dopamine D_2 receptors in rat brain. *Biochem. Pharmacol.*, 34: 2251 – 2259.

Krause, J.E., Chirqwin, J.M., Carter, M.S., Xu, Z.S. and Hershey, A.D. (1987) Three rat preprotachykinin mRNAs encode the neuropeptides substance P and neurokinin A. *Proc. Natl. Acad. Sci. U.S.A.*, 84: 881 – 885.

Kubota, Y., Inagaki, S., Kito, S., Takagi, H. and Smith, A.D. (1986a) Ultrastructural evidence of dopaminergic input to enkephalinergic neurons in rat neostriatum. *Brain Res.*, 367: 374 – 378.

Kubota, Y., Inagaki, S. and Kito, S. (1986b) Innervation of substance P neurons by catecholaminergic terminals in the neostriatum. *Brain Res.*, 375: 163 – 167.

Kubota, Y., Inagaki, S., Kito, S., Schimada, S., Okayama, T., Hatanaka, H., Pelletier, G., Takagi, H. and Tohyama, M. (1988) Neuropeptide Y-immunoreactive neurons receive synaptic inputs from dopaminergic axon terminals in the rat neostriatum. *Brain Res.*, 458: 389 – 393.

Le Moine, C., Normand, E., Guitteny, A.F., Fouque, B., Teoule, R. and Bloch, B. (1990b) Dopamine receptor gene expression by enkephalin neurons in rat forebrain. *Proc. Natl. Acad. Sci. U.S.A.*, 87: 230 – 234.

Le Moine, C., Tison, F. and Bloch, B. (1990a) D_2 dopamine receptor gene expression by cholinergic neurons in the rat striatum. *Neurosci. Lett.*, 117: 248 – 252.

Le Moine, C., Normand, E. and Bloch, B. (1991) Phenotypical characterization of the rat striatal neurons expressing the D_1 dopamine receptor gene. *Proc. Natl. Acad. Sci. U.S.A.*, 88: 4205 – 4209.

Leslie, C.A. and Bennett, J.P. (1987) Striatal D_1 and D_2 dopamine receptor sites are separately detectable in vivo. *Brain Res.*, 415: 90 – 97.

Letter, A.A., Matsuda, L.A., Merchant, K.M., Gibb, J.W. and Hanson, G.R. (1987) Characterisation of dopaminergic influence on striato-nigral neurotensin systems. *Brain Res.*, 422: 200 – 203.

Levant, B. and Nemeroff, C.B. (1990) Sigma receptor "antagonist" BMY 14802 increases neurotensin concentrations in the rat nucleus accumbens and caudate. *J. Pharmacol. Exp. Ther.*, 254: 330 – 335.

Levant, B., Merchant, K.M., Dorsa, D.M. and Nemeroff, C.B. (1992) BMY 14802, a potential antipsychotic drug, increases expression of proneurotensin mRNA in the rat striatum. *Mol. Brain Res.*, 12: 279 – 284.

Manier, M., Abrous, D.N., Feuerstein, C., Le Moal, M. and Herman, J.P. (1991) Increase of striatal methionine enkephalin content following lesion of the nigrostriatal dopaminergic pathway in adult rats and reversal following the implantation of embryonic dopaminergic neurons. *Neuroscience*, 42: 427 – 439.

Mansour, A., Meador-Woodruff, J.H., Bunzow, J.R., Civelli, O., Akil, H. and Watson, S.J. (1990) Localisation of dopamine D-2 receptor mRNA and D-1 and D-2 receptor binding in the rat brain and pituitary: an in situ hybridization-receptor autoradiographic analysis. *J. Neurosci.*, 10: 2587 – 2600.

Martin-Iverson, M.T., Radke, J.M. and Vincent, S.R. (1986) The effects of cysteamine on dopamine-mediated behaviours: evidence for dopamine-somatostatin interactions in the striatum. *Pharmacol. Biochem. Behav.*, 24: 1707 – 1714.

Meador-Woodruff, J.H., Mansour, A., Healy, D.J., Kuehn, R., Zhou, Q.-Y., Bunzow, J.R., Akil, H., Civelli, O. and Watson, S.J. (1991) Comparison of the distributions of D_1 and D_2 dopamine receptor mRNAs in rat brain. *Neuropsychopharmacology*, 5: 231 – 242.

Merchant, K.M., Bush, L.G., Gibb, J.W. and Hanson, G.R. (1989) Dopamine D-2 receptors exert tonic regulation over discrete neurotensin systems of the rat brain. *Brain Res.*, 500: 21 – 29.

Merchant, K.M., Dobner, P.R. and Dorsa, D.M. (1992) Differential effects of haloperidol and clozapine on neurotensin gene transcription in rat neostriatum. *J. Neurosci.*, 12: 652 – 663.

Mocchetti, I., Naranjo, J.R. and Costa, E. (1987) Regulation of striatal enkephalin turnover in rats receiving antagonists of specific receptor subtypes. *J. Pharmacol. Exp. Ther.*, 241: 1120 – 1124.

Montminy, M.R., Sevarino, K.A., Wagner, J.A., Mandel, G. and Goodman, R.H. (1986) Identification of a cyclic-AMP responsive element within the rat somatostatin gene. *Proc. Natl. Acad. Sci. U.S.A.*, 83: 6682 – 6686.

Morris, B.J. and Hunt, S.P. (1991) Proenkephalin mRNA levels in rat striatum are increased and decreased, respectively, by selective D_2 and D_1 dopamine receptor antagonists. *Neurosci. Lett.*, 125: 201 – 204.

Morris, B.J., Reimer, S., Höllt, V. and Herz, A. (1988a) Regulation of striatal prodynorphin mRNA levels by the raphe-striatal pathway. *Mol. Brain Res.*, 4: 15 – 22.

Morris, B.J., Höllt, V. and Herz, A. (1988b) Dopaminergic regulation of striatal proenkephalin mRNA and prodynorphin mRNA: contrasting effects of D1 and D2 antagonists. *Neuroscience*, 25: 525 – 532.

Morris, B.J., Herz, A. and Höllt, V. (1989) Localization of striatal opioid gene expression and its modulation by the mesostriatal dopamine pathway: an in situ hybridization study. *J. Mol. Neurosci.*, 1: 9 – 18.

Moyse, E., Rostene, W., Vial, M., Leonard, K., Mazella, J., Kitabgi, P., Vincent, J.P. and Beaudet, A. (1987) Distribution of neurotensin binding sites in rat brain: a light microscopic radioautographic study using monoiodo $[^{125}I]$ Tyr^3-neurotensin. *Neuroscience*, 22: 525 – 536.

Nemeroff, C.B. (1980) Neurotensin: per chance an endogenous neuroleptic? *Biol. Psychiatry*, 15: 283 – 301.

Nguyen, T.V., Kobierski, L., Comb, M. and Hyman, S.E. (1990) The effect of depolarization on expression of the human proenkephalin gene is synergistic with cAMP and dependent upon a cAMP-inducible enhancer. *J. Neurosci.*, 10: 2826 – 2831.

Nicklaus, K.J., McGonogle, P. and Molinoff, P.B. (1988) $[^3H]$-SCH 23390 labels both dopamine-1 and 5-hydroxytryptamine$_{1c}$ receptors in the choroid plexus. *J. Pharmacol. Exp. Ther.*, 247: 343 – 347.

Normand, E., Popovici, T., Onteniente, B., Fellman, D., Piatier-Tonneau, D., Auffray, C. and Bloch, B. (1988) Dopaminergic neurons of the substantia nigra modulate preproenkephalin A gene expression in rat striatal neurons. *Brain Res.*, 439: 39 – 46.

Oblin, A., Zivkovic, B. and Bartholini, G. (1984) Involvement of the D_2 dopamine receptor in the neuroleptic-induced decrease in nigral substance P. *Eur. J. Pharmacol.*, 105: 175 – 177.

Ohno, Y., Sasa, M. and Takaori, S. (1987) Coexistence of inhibitory dopamine D-1 and excitatory D-2 receptors on the same caudate nucleus neurones. *Life Sci.*, 40: 1937 – 1945.

Palacios, J.M. and Kuhar, M.J. (1981) Neurotensin receptors are located on dopamine-containing neurones in rat midbrain. *Nature*, 294: 587 – 589.

Penney, G.R., Afsharpour, S. and Kitai, S.T. (1986) The glutamate decarboxylase-, leucine enkephalin-, methionine enkephalin- and substance P-immunoreactive neurons in the neostriatum of the rat and cat: evidence for partial population overlap. *Neuroscience*, 17: 1011 – 1045.

Pollack, A.E. and Wooten, G.F. (1992) D_2 dopaminergic regulation of striatal preproenkephalin mRNA levels is mediated at least in part through cholinergic interneurons. *Mol. Brain Res.*, 13: 35–41.

Quach, T.T., Tang, F., Kegeyama, H., Mocchetti, I., Guidotti, A., Meek, J.L., Costa, E. and Schwartz, J.P. (1984) Enkephalin biosynthesis in adrenal medulla; modulation of proenkephalin mRNA content of cultured chromaffin cells by 8-bromo-adenosine 3′,5′-monophosphate. *Mol. Pharmacol.*, 26: 255–260.

Quirion, R., Chieueh, C.C., Everist, H.D. and Pert, A. (1985) Comparative localisation of neurotensin receptors on nigrostriatal and mesolimbic dopaminergic terminals. *Brain Res.*, 327: 385–389.

Radke, J.M., MacLennan, A.J., Vincent, S.R. and Fibiger, H.C. (1988) Comparison between short- and long-term haloperidol administration on somatostatin and substance P concentrations in the rat brain. *Brain Res.*, 445: 55–60.

Reid, M.S., Hökfelt, T., Herrera-Marschitz, M., Håkanson, R., Feng, D.M., Folkers, K., Goldstein, M. and Ungerstedt, U. (1990) Intranigral substance P stimulation of striatal dopamine release is inhibited by Spantide II: a new tachykinin antagonist without apparent neurotoxicity. *Brain Res.*, 532: 175–181.

Riva, M.A. and Creese, I. (1990) Effect of chronic administration of dopamine receptor antagonists on D-1 and D-2 dopamine receptors and sigma/haloperidol binding sites in rat brain. *Mol. Neuropharmacol.*, 1: 17–22.

Salin, P., Mercugliano, M. and Chesselet, M.-F. (1990) Differential effects of chronic treatment with haloperidol and clozapine on the level of preprosomatostatin mRNA in the striatum, nucleus accumbens and frontal cortex of the rat. *Cell. Mol. Neurobiol.*, 10: 127–143.

Sato, M., Kiyama, H. and Tohyama, M. (1992) Different postnatal expression of cells expressing mRNA encoding neurotensin receptor. *Neuroscience*, 48: 137–149.

Schmidt, M.J. and Hill, L.E. (1977) Effects of ergots on adenylate cyclase activity in the corpus striatum and pituitary. *Life Sci.*, 20: 789–798.

Shimatsu, A., Kato, Y., Matsushita, N., Katami, H., Yanihara, N. and Imura, H. (1982) Effects of glucagon, neurotensin and vasoactive intestinal polypeptide on somatostatin release from perifused rat hypothalamus. *Endocrinology*, 110: 2113–2117.

Shivers, B.B., Harlan, R.E., Roamo, G.J., Howells, R.D. and Pfaff, D.W. (1986) Cellular location and regulation of proenkephalin mRNA in rat brain. In: G.R. Uhl (Ed.), *In Situ Hybridization in Brain*, Plenum Press, New York, pp. 3–20.

Sivam, S.P. (1989) D$_1$ dopamine receptor-mediated substance P depletion in the striatonigral neurons of rats subjected to neonatal dopaminergic denervation: implications for self-injurious behaviour. *Brain Res.*, 500: 119–129.

Smith, Y. and Parent, A. (1986) Neuropeptide Y-immunoreactive neurons in the striatum of cat and monkey: morphological characteristics, intrinsic organization and co-localization with

somatostatin. *Brain Res.*, 372: 241–252.

Soghomonian, J.J. and Chesselet, M.-F. (1989) 6-Hydroxydopamine (6-OHDA)-induced changes in levels of striatal mRNAs encoding somatostatin (SOM) and glutamic acid decarboxylase (GAD) as detected by in situ hybridization histochemistry (ISHH). *Soc. Neurosci. Abstr.*, 359.2.

Sokoloff, P., Giros, B., Martres, M-P., Bouthenet, M-L. and Schwartz, J-C. (1990) Molecular cloning and characterization of a novel dopamine receptor (D$_3$) as a target for neuroleptics. *Nature*, 347: 146–151.

Somogyi, P., Priestly, J.V., Cuello, A.C., Smith, A.D. and Bolam, J.P. (1982) Synaptic connections of substance P immunoreactive nerve terminals in the substantia nigra of the rat. *Cell Tissue Res.*, 223: 469–486.

Starr, M. (1987) Opposing roles of dopamine D1 and D2 receptors in nigral gamma-[^{3}H] aminobutyric acid release? *J. Neurochem.*, 49: 1042–1049.

Stoof, J.C. and Kebabian, J.W. (1981) Opposing roles for D-1 and D-2 dopamine receptors in efflux of cyclic AMP from rat neostriatum. *Nature*, 294: 366–368.

Sugimoto, T. and Mizuno, N. (1987) Neurotensin in projection neurons of the striatum and nucleus accumbens, with reference to coexistence with enkephalin and GABA: an immunohistochemical study in the cat. *J. Comp. Neurol.*, 257: 383–395.

Sunahara, R.K., Guan, H-C., O'Dowd, B.F., Seeman, P., Laurier, L.G., Ng, G., George, S.R., Torchia, J., Van Tol, H.H.M. and Niznik, H.B. (1990) Cloning of the gene for a human dopamine D$_5$ receptor with higher affinity for dopamine than D$_1$. *Nature*, 350: 614–619.

Takagi, H., Somogyi, P., Somogyi, J. and Smith, A.D. (1983) Fine structural studies on a type of somatostatin-immunoreactive neuron and its synaptic connections in the rat neostriatum. *J. Comp. Neurol.*, 214: 1–16.

Tapia-Arancibia, L. and Reichlin, S. (1985) Vasoactive intestinal peptide and PHI stimulate somatostatin release from rat cerebral cortical and diencephalic cells in dispersed cell culture. *Brain Res.*, 336: 67–72.

Taylor, M.D., De Ceballos, M.L., Jenner, P. and Marsden, C.D. (1991) Acute effects of D$_1$ and D$_2$ dopamine receptor agonist and antagonist drugs on basal ganglia (met^5)- and (leu^5)-enkephalin and neurotensin content in the rat. *Biochem. Pharmacol.*, 41: 1385–1391.

Van Tol, H.H.M., Bunzow, J.R., Guan, H.-C., Sunahara, R.K., Seeman, P., Niznik, H.B. and Civelli, O. (1991) Cloning of the gene for a human dopamine D$_4$ receptor with high affinity for the antipsychotic clozapine. *Nature*, 350: 610–614.

Vincent, S.R. and Johansson, O. (1983) Striatal neurons containing both somatostatin- and avian pancreatic polypeptide (APP)-like immunoreactivities and NADPH-diaphorase activity: a light and electron microscopic study. *J. Comp. Neurol.*, 217: 264–270.

Voorn, P., Roest, G. and Groenewegen, H.J. (1987) Increase of enkephalin and decrease of substance P immunoreactivity in the dorsal and ventral striatum of the rat after midbrain 6-hydroxydopamine lesions. *Brain Res.,* 412: 391 – 396.

Vuillet, J., Kerkerian, L., Salin, P. and Nieoullon, A. (1989) Ultrastructural features of NPY-containing neurons in the rat striatum. *Brain Res.,* 477: 241 – 251.

Vuillet, J., Dimova, R., Nieoullon, A. and Kerkerian-Le-Goff, L. (1992) Ultrastructural relationships between choline acetyltransferase- and neuropeptide Y-containing neurons in the rat striatum. *Neuroscience,* 46: 351 – 360.

Walker, P.D., Riley, L.A., Hart, R.P. and Jonakait, G.M. (1991) Serotonin regulation of tachykinin biosynthesis in the rat neostriatum. *Brain Res.,* 546: 33 – 39.

Wan, D.C.C., Marley, P.D. and Livett, B.G. (1991) Coordinate and differential regulation of proenkephalin A and PNMT mRNA expression in cultured bovine adrenal chromaffin cells: responses to cAMP elevation and phorbol esters. *Mol. Brain Res.,* 9: 135 – 142.

Weiner, D.M. and Brann, M.R. (1989) The distribution of a dopamine D_2 receptor mRNA in rat brain. *FEBS Lett.,* 253: 201 – 213.

Weiner, D.M., Levey, A.I., Sunahara, R.K., Niznik, H.B., O'Dowd, B.F., Seeman, P. and Brann, M.R. (1991) D-1 and D-2 dopamine receptor mRNA in rat brain. *Proc. Natl. Acad. Sci. U.S.A.,* 88: 1859 – 1863.

Weiss, L.T. and Chesselet, M.-F. (1989) Regional distribution and regulation of preprosomatostatin messenger RNA in the striatum as revealed by in situ hybridization histochemistry. *Mol. Brain Res.,* 5: 121 – 130.

Weiss, S., Sebben, M., Garcia-Sainz, J.A. and Bockaert, J. (1985) D_2-dopamine receptor-mediated inhibition of cyclic AMP formation in striatal neurons in primary culture. *Mol. Pharmacol.,* 27: 595 – 599.

Young, W.S., Bonner, T.I. and Brann, M.R. (1986) Mesencephalic dopamine neurons regulate the expression of neuropeptide mRNAs in the rat forebrain. *Proc. Natl. Acad. Sci. U.S.A.,* 83: 9827 – 9831.

Zahm, D.S. and Johnson, S.N. (1989) Asymmetrical distribution of neurotensin immunoreactivity following unilateral injection of 6-hydroxydopamine in rat ventral tegmental area (VTA). *Brain Res.,* 483: 301 – 311.

Zheng, M., Yang, S.-L. and Zou, G. (1988) Reserpine increases proenkephalin mRNA content in rat corpus striatum. *Acta Pharmacol. Sinica,* 9: 97 – 100.

Zhou, Q., Grandy, D.K., Thambi, L., Kushner, J.A., Van Tol, H.H.M., Cone, R., Pribnow, D., Salon, J., Bunzow, J.R. and Civelli, O. (1990) Cloning and expression of human and rat D-1 dopamine receptors. *Nature,* 347: 76 – 80.

G.W. Arbuthnott and P.C. Emson (Eds.)
Progress in Brain Research, Vol. 99
© 1993 Elsevier Science Publishers B.V. All rights reserved.

CHAPTER 13

Neurochemically specialized projection neurons of the striatum respond differentially to psychomotor stimulants

S. Berretta[1], H.A. Robertson[2] and A.M. Graybiel[1]

[1]*Massachusetts Institute of Technology, Department of Brain and Cognitive Sciences, Cambridge, MA 02139, U.S.A. and
[2]Dalhousie University, Department of Pharmacology, Halifax, Nova Scotia, Canada*

The projection neurons of the striatum are uniformly GABAergic, and are of the densely spiny category. Despite their morphological similarities and the commonality of principal neurotransmitter expressed by these neurons, different subtypes of striatal projection neurons have been identified in a wide variety of species through examination of neuropeptide cotransmitters/modulators expressed by these cells: enkephalin-like peptide, neurotensin, and substance P and dynorphin (see Graybiel, 1990; Reiner and Anderson, 1990, for reviews). Not only do different groups of striatal projection neurons express different neuropeptides, they also express, to different degrees, D_1-like and D_2-like dopamine receptor mRNAs. D_1 receptor mRNA expression is prominent in substance P/dynorphin-positive neurons, but D_2 receptor mRNAs are expressed in enkephalinergic projection neurons (Le Moine et al., 1990, 1991; Gerfen et al., 1990; Meador-Woodruff et al., 1991).

There is evidence for varying degrees of co-expression of neuropeptides, as well as of D_1 and D_2 dopamine receptor mRNAs in striatal projection neurons (Penny et al., 1986; Reiner and Anderson, 1990; Besson et al., 1990; Gerfen et al., 1990, 1991; Meador-Woodruff et al., 1991). Nevertheless, projection neurons of the substance P/dynorphin-positive subclass and of the enkephalin-positive subclass are considered fundamentally differentiable in terms of their efferent connections. Substance P/dynorphin-positive neurons project strongly to the internal pallidum and to the substantia nigra pars reticulata, regions that give rise to direct basal ganglia outputs ("direct pathways") to the thalamus and midbrain. Enkephalin-positive striatal neurons project strongly to the external pallidum, and thus provide input to the subthalamic loops ("indirect pathways") that modulate activity in the output pathways of the basal ganglia.

In the course of studying the effects of psychomotor stimulants on immediate-early gene expression in the rat striatum (Graybiel et al., 1990; Moratalla et al., 1992a,b), we noted that even the highest doses of drugs used did not induce Fos-like immunoreactivity in every striatal neuron (Berretta et al., 1991a,b). This observation led to the question whether psychostimulants affect only a particular and identifiable subtype of striatal neurons. We have tested for such selectivity by analyzing the expression of Fos-like protein in different kinds of striatal interneurons and projection neurons identified with immunostains and histochemical stains (Berretta et al., 1992).

We identified subclasses of projection neurons by immunostaining for enkephalin-like immunoreactivity and for DARPP-32-like immunoreactivity. DARPP-32 is a phosphatase inhibitor associated with neurons bearing D_1-like receptors (Ouimet et al., 1984; Walaas and Greengard, 1984; Hemmings and Greengard, 1986; Schalling et al., 1990), almost certainly including substance P/dynorphin-positive neurons. For the interneurons, we identified presumptive cholinergic neurons by size following Nissl staining, parvalbumin-containing interneurons with a polyclonal antiserum, and somatostatin/NADPH diaphorase/nitrous oxide-containing interneurons by staining for the diaphorase with the Simms method (Vincent et al., 1983; Vincent and Johansson, 1983; Dawson et al., 1991a,b). In both sets of experiments, we carried out double immunostaining and histological staining to identify which striatal neurons expressed Fos-like protein as detected with polyclonal antisera to a peptide fragment of Fos protein.

Our evidence on the immediate-early gene response patterns generated by these neurons leads to three general conclusions:

First, for the Fos-like protein assayed, it is mainly the projection neurons of the striatum that are responsive to acute in vivo doses of cocaine and amphetamine. We found very few interneurons responding to these stimuli by expressing Fos-like protein.

Second, among the projection neurons of the striatum, it is DARPP-32-positive neurons that respond to psychomotor drugs administered in vivo by activating Fos-like protein. At all doses tried, for both cocaine and amphetamine, double-immunostaining showed the presence of Fos-like protein in the nucleus of many DARPP-32-positive neurons and a lack of Fos-like protein in DARPP-32-negative neurons. In untreated animals, there were almost no Fos-positive neurons. We have since demonstrated that the neurons responsive to amphetamine are, in fact, dynorphin-immunoreactive (Hiroi, Berretta and Grabiel, unpublished observations).

Third, almost no enkephalin-positive striatal neurons generate Fos-like protein in response to in vivo administration of cocaine or amphetamine. Typical values for the numbers of enkephalin-positive neurons responding were 2:2500. This negative result obtained despite the fact that we demonstrated coexpression of DARPP-32 in large numbers of enkephalin-positive neurons, perhaps as many as one-half.

Cocaine and amphetamine are both indirect catecholamine agonists that, through different mechanisms, result in increases in extracellular catecholamines. Cocaine binds to the dopamine

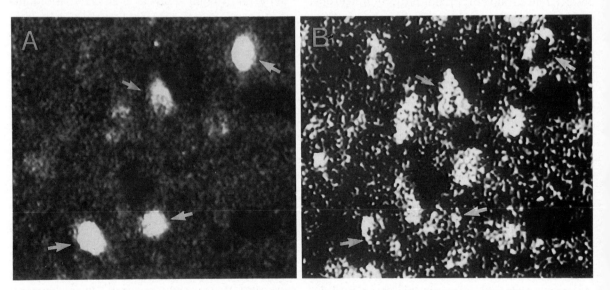

Fig. 1. Confocal images showing a field of striatal neurons with Fos-positive nuclei (A) and expressing DARPP-32-like immunoreactivity (B). Arrows point to doubly labeled neurons. From material reported in Berretta et al. (1992).

transporter (Ritz et al., 1987; Kilty et al., 1991; Shimada et al.,1991), blocking uptake of dopamine. Amphetamine is a powerful releaser of dopamine and other catecholamines. We and others have shown that the relatively selective D_1-like dopamine receptor antagonist, SCH 23390, blocks induction of Fos-like protein by cocaine and amphetamine (Graybiel et al., 1990; Young et al., 1991; Hope and Nestler, 1991; Hope et al., 1992). Serotonergic effects on immediate-early gene expression in the striatum have also been found with psychomotor stimulant exposure (Bhat and Baraban, 1992; Bhat et al., 1992), but a major action of the drugs through stimulation of D_1-like dopamine receptors is strongly suggested. Our results also support such receptor selectivity, as the induction of Fos-like protein was blocked by preadministration of SCH 23390 at doses as low as 0.1 mg/kg (Berretta et al., 1992), and as Fos-like immunostaining occurred exclusively in neurons expressing DARPP-32, a D_1-associated molecule.

These patterns suggest that stimulation of dopamine receptors by indirect agonists initiates an intracellular cascade driven by D_1-like dopamine receptors and leading to the induction of Fos-like protein. This effect is, however, restricted to a subpopulation of striatal neurons that (a) excludes the interneurons and (b) excludes the enkephalinergic projection neurons. The presence of DARPP-32 immunostaining was only partly correlated with the pattern of Fos-like protein induction: many enkephalinergic neurons expressed DARPP-32, but almost none were induced to express Fos-like protein. Enkephalinergic striatal neurons express dopamine D_2 receptor mRNA (Le Moine et al., 1990) and thus probably express D_2 receptors as well. Even if the DARPP-32-positive enkephalinergic neurons also express D_1 dopamine receptors capable of initiating a Fos response, such neurons might be prevented from activating the D_1 cascade by virtue of the D_2-like dopamine receptors they coexpress (De Camilli et al., 1979; Stoof and Kebabian, 1981; Vallar and Meldolesi, 1989). This suggestion would be in good accord with the findings of Surmeier et al. (1991) and Meador-Woodruff et al.

(1991), who report considerable coexpression of D_1 and D_2 mRNAs by striatal projection neurons.

At the systems level of analysis, our findings suggest striking selectivity in the capacity for psychomotor stimulants to activate Fos-like protein in the major classes of striatal projection neurons. The main population of projection neurons activated to express the transcription factor we monitored are the cells of origin of the direct output pathways of the striatum, which have the final effect of activation of premotor cortex and related cortical areas. The enkephalinergic cells of origin of the indirect pathways, which have the effect of inhibition of this motor circuit, are not activated. This result suggests that – as reflected by the Fos-like immediate-early gene expression we monitored – indirect dopamine agonists such as cocaine and amphetamine could create an imbalance between the direct and indirect pathways of the basal ganglia: there is an interesting parallel between this pattern and the behavioral hyperactivity generated by the psychomotor stimulants.

The induction of Fos-like protein is only one of several transcriptional events occurring in striatal neurons in response to psychomotor stimulants. We have shown that acute administration of cocaine and amphetamine rapidly induced expression of junB and NGFI-A as well as c-fos mRNAs (Moratalla et al., 1990, 1991, 1992a, 1993), and Young et al. (1991) have shown that other Fos-like proteins may be activated. We do not know the striatal cell types expressing these other transcription factors, and we have no information for any of the genes about the class of projection neurons expressing neurotensin. More generally, we do not know the relation between activation of any of these transcription factors and the ultimate physiological status of the responsive neurons. It is clear from our findings, however, that some transcriptional effects of psychomotor stimulants on the basal ganglia may be more directly targeted to the direct paths of the basal ganglia than to the indirect paths. This imbalance may provide clues to understanding the profound behavioral effects of these drugs, including their actions as stimulants of movement.

Finally, our findings support the existence of a high degree of functional specialization of the projection neurons of the striatum. Even when only one transcriptional response to one set of agonist drugs is considered, the in vivo response of the striatal projection neurons is highly fractionated. This complexity probably only hints at the interacting cascades triggered in striatal neurons by their membrane receptors.

Acknowledgements

This work was supported by National Institutes of Health Javits Award RO1 25529, the Human Frontier Science Program, and the National Parkinson Disease Foundation, Inc.

References

Berretta, S., Christie, R., Robertson, H.A. and Graybiel, A.M. (1991a) Molecular characteristics of striatal neurons that express Fos on stimulation by direct dopamine agonists. *Soc. Neurosci. Abstr.,* 17: 853.

Berretta, S., Robertson, H.A. and Graybiel, A.M. (1991b) Immediate-early gene expression induced by the psychostimulant cocaine is specific to subpopulations of striatal projection neurons. *Eur. J. Neurosci. (Suppl.),* 4: 166.

Berretta, S., Robertson, H.A. and Graybiel, A.M. (1992) Dopamine and glutamate agonists stimulate neuron-specific transcriptional activation of c-*fos* in the striatum. *J. Neurophysiol.,* 68: 767 – 777.

Besson, M.-J., Graybiel, A.M. and Quinn, B. (1990) Coexpression of neuropeptides in the cat's striatum: an immunohistochemical study of substance P, dynorphin B and enkephalin. *Neuroscience,* 39: 33 – 58.

Bhat, R.V. and Baraban, J.M. (1992) Activation of transcription factor genes in striatum by cocaine is mediated by blockade of both 5-TH and DA uptake. *Soc. Neurosci. Abstr.,* 18: 1432.

Bhat, R.V., Cole, A.J. and Baraban, J.M. (1992) Role of monoamine systems in activation of *zif*268 by cocaine. *J. Psychiatr. Neurosci.,* 17: 94 – 102.

Dawson, T.M., Bredt, D.S., Fotuhi, M., Hwang, P.M. and Snyder, S.H. (1991a) Nitric oxide synthase and neuronal NADPH diaphorase are identical in brain and peripheral tissues. *Proc. Natl. Acad. Sci. U.S.A.,* 88: 7797 – 7801.

Dawson, V.L., Dawson, T.M., London, E.D., Bredt, D.S. and Snyder, S.H. (1991b) Nitric oxide mediates glutamate neurotoxicity in primary cortical cultures. *Proc. Natl. Acad. Sci. U.S.A.,* 88: 6368 – 6371.

De Camilli, P., Macconi, D. and Spada, A. (1979) Dopamine inhibits adenylate cyclase in human prolactin-secreting pituitary adenomas. *Nature,* 278: 252 – 254.

Gerfen, C.R., Engber, T.M., Mahan, L.C., Susel, Z., Chase, T.N., Monsma Jr., F.J. and Sibley, D.R. (1990) D1 and D2 dopamine receptor-regulated gene expression of striatonigral and striatopallidal neurons. *Science,* 250: 1429 – 1432.

Gerfen, C.R., McGinty, J.F. and Young III, W.S. (1991) Dopamine differentially regulates dynorphin, substance P, and enkephalin expression in striatal neurons: in situ hybridization histochemical analysis. *J. Neurosci.,* 11: 1016 – 1031.

Graybiel, A.M. (1990) Neurotransmitters and neuromodulators in the basal ganglia. *Trends Neurosci.,* 13: 244 – 254.

Graybiel, A.M., Moratalla, R. and Robertson, H.A. (1990) Amphetamine and cocaine induce drug-specific activation of the c-*fos* gene in striosome-matrix and limbic subdivisions of the striatum. *Proc. Natl. Acad. Sci. U.S.A.,* 87: 6912 – 6916.

Hemmings Jr., H.C. and Greengard, P. (1986) DARPP-32, a dopamine- and cyclic AMP-regulated phosphoprotein: regional, tissue and phylogenetic distribution. *J. Neurosci.,* 6: 1469 – 1481.

Hope, B.T. and Nestler, E.J. (1991) Effects of chronic cocaine on c-*fos* and other immediate early genes and on AP1 binding in rat nucleus accumbens. *Soc. Neurosci. Abstr.,* 17: 150.3.

Hope, B.T., Kosofsky, B., Hyman, S.E. and Nestler, E.J. (1992) Regulation of immediate early gene expression and AP-1 binding in the rat nucleus accumbens by chronic cocaine. *Proc. Natl. Acad. Sci. U.S.A.,* 88: 5764 – 5768.

Kilty, J.E., Lorang, D. and Amara, S.G. (1991) Cloning and expression of a cocaine-sensitive rat dopamine transporter. *Science,* 254: 578 – 579.

Le Moine, C., Normand, E., Guitteny, A.F., Fouque, B., Teoule, R. and Bloch, B. (1990) Dopamine receptor gene expression by enkephalin neurons in rat forebrain. *Proc. Natl. Acad. Sci. U.S.A.,* 87: 230 – 234.

Le Moine, C., Normand, E. and Bloch, B. (1991) Phenotypical characterization of the rat striatal neurons expressing the D_1 dopamine receptor gene. *Proc. Natl. Acad. Sci. U.S.A.,* 88: 4205 – 4209.

Meador-Woodruff, J.H., Mansour, A., Healy, D.J., Kuehn, R., Zhou, Q.-Y., Bunzow, J.R., Akil, H., Civelli, O. and Watson Jr., S.J. (1991) Comparison of the distributions of D_1 and D_2 dopamine receptor mRNA in rat brain. *Neuropsychopharmacology,* 5: 231 – 242.

Moratalla, R., Robertson, H.A., DiZio, P.A. and Graybiel, A.M. (1990) Parallel induction of *jun* B and c-*fos* evoked in the striatum by the psychomotor stimulant drugs cocaine and amphetamine. *Soc. Neurosci. Abstr.,* 16: 953.

Moratalla, R., Robertson, H.A. and Graybiel, A.M. (1991) The immediate-early gene *NGFI*-A (*zif*268, *egr*1) is selectively induced in the striosomal system following acute amphetamine treatment. *Eur. J. Neurosci. (Suppl.),* 4: 274.

Moratalla, R., Robertson, H.A. and Graybiel, A.M. (1992a) Dynamic regulation of *NGFI*-A (*zif*268, *egr*1) gene expression in the striatum. *J. Neurosci.,* 12: 2609 – 2622.

Moratalla, R., Vickers, E.A., Robertson, H.A., Cochran, B.H. and Graybiel, A.M. (1993) Coordinate expression of c-*fos* and *jun* B is induced in the rat striatum by cocaine. *J. Neurosci.,* 13: 423 – 433.

Ouimet, C.C., Miller, P.E., Hemmings Jr., H.C., Walaas, S.I. and Greengard, P. (1984) DARPP-32, a dopamine- and adenosine 3′:5′-monophosphate-regulated phosphoprotein enriched in dopamine-innervated brain regions. III. Immunocytochemical localization. *J. Neurosci.,* 4: 111 – 124.

Penny, G.R., Afsharpour, S. and Kitai, S.T. (1986) The glutamate decarboxylase-, leucine enkephalin-, methionine enkephalin- and substance P-immunoreactive neurons in the neostriatum of the rat and cat: evidence for partial population overlap. *Neuroscience,* 17: 1011 – 1045.

Reiner, A. and Anderson, K.D. (1990) The patterns of neurotransmitter and neuropeptide co-occurrence among striatonigral projection neurons: conclusions based on recent findings. *Brain Res. Rev.,* 15: 251 – 265.

Ritz, M.C., Lamb, R.J., Goldberg, S.R. and Kuhar, M.J. (1987) Cocaine receptors on dopamine transporters are related to self-administration of cocaine. *Science,* 237: 1219 – 1223.

Schalling, M., Djurfeldt, M., Hökfelt, T., Ehrlich, M., Kurihara, T. and Greengard, P. (1990) Distribution and cellular localization of DARPP-32 mRNA in rat brain. *Mol. Brain Res.,* 7: 139 – 149.

Shimada, S., Kitayama, S., Lin, C.-L., Patel, A., Nanthakumar, E., Gregor, P., Kuhar, M. and Uhl, G. (1991) Cloning and expression of a cocaine-sensitive dopamine transporter complementary DNA. *Science,* 254: 576 – 578.

Stoof, J.C. and Kebabian, J.W. (1981) Opposing roles for D-1 and D-2 dopamine receptors in efflux of cyclic AMP from rat neostriatum. *Nature,* 294: 366 – 368.

Surmeier, D.J., Wilson, C.J., Stefani, A. and Kitai, S.T. (1991) Dopaminergic modulation of sodium currents in retrogradely-identified rat striatonigral neurons. *Soc. Neurosci. Abstr.,* 17: 851.

Vallar, L. and Meldolesi, J. (1989) Mechanisms of signal transduction at the dopamine D₂ receptor. *Trends Pharmacol. Sci.,* 10: 74 – 77.

Vincent, S.R. and Johansson, O. (1983) Striatal neurons containing both somatostatin and avian pancreatic polypeptide (APP)-like immunoreactivities and NADPH diaphorase activity: a light and electron microscopic study. *J. Comp. Neurol.,* 217: 264 – 270.

Vincent, S.R., Johansson, O., Hökfelt, T., Skirboll, L., Elde, R.P., Terenius, L., Kimmel, J. and Goldstein, M. (1983) NADPH-diaphorase: a selective histochemical marker for striatal neurons containing both somatostatin and avian pancreatic polypeptide (APP)-like immunoreactivities. *J. Comp. Neurol.,* 217: 252 – 263.

Walaas, S.I. and Greengard, P. (1984) DARPP-32, a dopamine- and adenosine 3′:5′-monophosphate-regulated phosphoprotein enriched in dopamine-innervated brain regions I. Regional and cellular distribution in the rat brain. *J. Neurosci.,* 4: 84 – 98.

Young, S.T., Porrino, L.J. and Iadarola, M.J. (1991) Cocaine induces striatal c-*fos*-immunoreactive proteins via dopaminergic D1 receptors. *Proc. Natl. Acad. Sci. U.S.A.,* 88: 1291 – 1295.

SECTION III

Responses to Signals

G.W. Arbuthnott and P.C. Emson (Eds.)
Progress in Brain Research, Vol. 99
© 1993 Elsevier Science Publishers B.V. All rights reserved.

CHAPTER 14

Functionally selective neurochemical afferents and efferents of the mesocorticolimbic and nigrostriatal dopamine system

Marianne Amalric[1] and George F. Koob[2]

[1] *Laboratoire de Neurobiologie Cellulaire et Fonctionnelle, Marseille, France and* [2] *Department of Neuropharmacology, The Scripps Research Institute, La Jolla, CA, U.S.A.*

Introduction

The limbic structures (nucleus accumbens, amygdala) as well as the striatum receive afferents from the two main dopaminergic systems of the CNS (the mesocorticolimbic and the nigrostriatal pathways, respectively) and form an interface between cortical inputs and thalamic, limbic and hypothalamic outputs. These structures are the locus of neuronal activities integrating sensory information in order to perform motor acts involving both unconditioned or conditioned behaviors. A considerable body of evidence now exists showing that the forebrain dopamine pathways play a crucial role in the expression of conditioned as well as unconditioned responding. It was thus of interest to try to compare the different functional involvement of these pathways in behavioral control. In fact, both the nucleus accumbens (N. Acc.) and the striatum (dorsal part) receive dopaminergic inputs from the mesencephalon and glutamate afferents from a large number of cortical areas. Furthermore, efferent outputs containing mainly GABAergic neurons are known to project respectively to the ventral and dorsal parts of the globus pallidus.

The role of the mesocorticolimbic dopamine system in locomotor activation produced by psychomotor stimulants

The neural substrates for the behavioral expression of mesocorticolimbic dopamine (DA) activity have been the focus of intense investigation. It has been suggested that psychostimulant-induced locomotion may result from a facilitation of the dopaminergic transmission in the nucleus accumbens and more generally within the ventral striatum. This hypothesis is based on experimental results involving intra-accumbens injection of DA agonists, and local intracerebral injection of dopamine receptor antagonists.

Indirect sympathomimetics such as amphetamine and cocaine are known to act primarily by enhancing the amount of neurotransmitter released within central catecholamine synapses (Iversen and Fray, 1982), while direct sympathomimetics, like apomorphine bind directly to dopamine (DA) receptors (Corrodi et al., 1973). When injected in rats, these stimulants produce a profound increase in locomotor activity as measured by photocell activity in a familiar cage environment (Joyce and Koob, 1981;

Swerdlow et al., 1986). Dopaminergic transmission is differentially affected when different doses of the indirect agonist (amphetamine) are injected. Low doses of amphetamine increase the total amount of locomotor activity and initiate a varied behavioral pattern, whereas high doses induce repetition of invariant sequences of behavior, described as "stereotyped behavior". These doses act at different neural sites, and their behavioral actions are differently modulated by an alteration of dopaminergic transmission at these sites.

Effects of dopaminergic lesions on psychostimulant locomotor activation

Dopaminergic terminal lesions following the injection of neurotoxin 6-hydroxydopamine (6-OHDA) into the N. Acc. region block amphetamine-stimulated locomotion in rats tested in photocell activity cages (Kelly et al., 1976; Costall et al., 1977; Joyce and Koob, 1981) or in an open-field (Hong and Levine, 1976; Taghzouti et al., 1985). However, the same local destruction of DA terminals in the N. Acc. induces a "supersensitive" locomotor response to the direct agonist apomorphine injection. This supersensitive response reaches its maximal intensity within 10–15 days after the lesion as a consequence to a post-synaptic DA receptor supersensitivity, reflected by biochemical data as an increase in DA receptor B_{max} in the denervated region (Staunton et al., 1982). Locomotor activity elicited by various doses of apomorphine is greatly potentiated in 6-OHDA lesions of the N. Acc. (Swerdlow et al., 1986; Koob and Swerdlow, 1988). These results suggest that post-synaptic DA receptors within the N. Acc. are a substrate of stimulant-enhanced locomotion. Furthermore, direct administration of amphetamine to the region of the N. Acc. produces increases in locomotor activity, while the same administration in a more dorsal region of the striatum does not produce locomotor effects but rather produces stereotyped behaviors (Costall et al., 1973; Statton and Solomon, 1984), as will be discussed later in this chapter.

Effects of dopamine receptor blockade on psychostimulant locomotor activation

The locomotor activation produced by psychostimulants is antagonized by DA receptor blockade in rats pretreated either with systemic injections of DA receptor antagonists (neuroleptics) (for review, see Lyon and Robbins, 1975) or with local injections into the N. Acc. (Pijnenburg et al., 1975). The central DA receptor antagonist α-flupenthixol, acting at the two major DA receptor subtypes D_1 and D_2, injected systemically has been shown to antagonize the locomotor hyperactivity produced by cocaine or D-amphetamine in rats (Vaccarino et al., 1986). The same effect has been seen after the local injection of another mixed D_1/D_2 DA receptor antagonist, haloperidol, directly into the N. Acc. (Pijnenburg et al., 1975), which further reveals a role of central DA transmission in the ventral striatum in the locomotor-activating properties of psychostimulants.

Role of the D_1/D_2 DA receptor subtypes

In order to examine the differential involvement of the two DA receptor subtypes on the locomotor activation induced by stimulants, the locomotor activation produced by amphetamine in animals pretreated with either the selective DA D_1 receptor antagonist, SCH 23390, or the selective D_2 receptor antagonist, raclopride, was studied. Low doses (10–20 μg/kg, s.c.) of SCH 23390 potently reversed the amphetamine-induced hyperlocomotion while raclopride (50–200 μg/kg, s.c.) only reduced amphetamine action during the first 30 min at low doses, and over 60 min at a dose of 200 μg/kg, a dose known to induce catalepsy (Fig. 1). Consistent with these results, cocaine-induced hyperactivity also has been shown to be inhibited by low doses of SCH 23390, while the selective D_2 antagonist metoclopramide or the classic neuroleptic haloperidol only reverse the cocaine activating effect at hypokinetic doses (Cabib et al., 1991).

However, the supersensitive response to apomor-

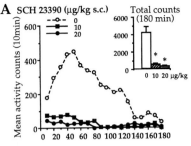

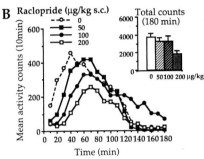

Fig. 1. Effects of different doses of the D_1 antagonist SCH 23390 and the D_2 antagonist raclopride on locomotor activity induced by subcutaneous (s.c.) 1.0 mg/kg of D-amphetamine. SCH 23390 completely blocked the locomotor stimulant effects of amphetamine, whereas raclopride only altered the locomotor effects during the first 60 min. $n = 8$ for each drug group. SCH 23390 and raclopride were injected s.c. 30 min prior to the amphetamine. (Taken with permission from Ouagazzal et al., 1993.)

phine in rats following 6-OHDA lesions of the N. Acc. is blocked by low doses of either SCH 23390 or spiperone (a D_2 DA receptor antagonist) injected alone (Amalric et al., 1986), and others have reported an inability of SCH 23390 or spiperone alone to significantly block apomorphine-stimulated locomotion in bilateral medial forebrain bundle 6-OHDA-lesioned rats (Arnt, 1985). While these discrepant results might reflect different lesion parameters, they suggest that denervation of the N. Acc. causes a loss of specificity among N. Acc. DA receptor subtypes. In intact animals, however, D_1 and D_2 receptors may play opposing roles in the regulation of psychostimulant-induced locomotor activation, which is known to be mediated by an increased DA transmission in the ventral striatum.

The role of mesocorticolimbic dopamine in environmentally induced activation

Non-drug-induced locomotor activation is also attenuated by destruction of the dopamine projection to the region of the nucleus accumbens. 6-Hydroxydopamine lesions of the nucleus accumbens produce decreases in locomotor activity associated with feeding in food-deprived rats (Koob et al., 1978). Similar 6-hydroxydopamine lesions to the region of the nucleus accumbens produce decreases in locomotor activity in an open field test (Joyce et al., 1983; Taghzouti et al., 1985) and decrease acquisition of schedule-induced polydipsia (Robbins and Koob, 1980) (for review, see Le Moal and Simon, 1991).

Similar lesions have also been shown to produce a syndrome of perseveration with reduced distraction caused by irrelevant information and a decrease in behavioral switching and flexibility (Robbins and Everitt, 1982; Le Moal and Simon, 1991). In learning tasks, animals with similar lesions show impairment in spontaneous alternation, disturbances in acquisition of spatial habits, and difficulty in reversing previously learned habits (Robbins and Everitt, 1982; Le Moal and Simon, 1991). These deficits suggest a role for the mesolimbic system in attentional function (Robbins and Everitt, 1982; Le Moal and Simon, 1991; see also Robbins and Everitt, 1992).

The role of mesocorticolimbic dopamine in psychostimulant reward

The mesocorticolimbic dopamine system has not only been implicated in the activating properties of psychostimulants but also appears to play a critical role in the reinforcing properties of these drugs (for reviews, see Le Moal and Simon, 1991; Koob, 1992; Robbins and Everitt, 1992). Mesocorticolimbic dopamine has been implicated in brain stimulation reward and the facilitation of brain stimulation reward produced by psychostimulants (Stellar and Rice, 1989). Dopamine receptor antagonists raise thresholds for brain stimulation reward (Bird and Kornetsky, 1990) and psychomotor stimulants decrease thresholds for brain stimulation reward (Kornetsky and Bain, 1982; for review, see Stellar and Rice, 1989). Local intracerebral microinjections into the nucleus accumbens of a mixed D_1/D_2 dopamine antagonist also decreases brain stimulation reward (Williams et al., 1987).

Even more compelling is the evidence supporting a role for the mesocorticolimbic dopamine in the direct reinforcing actions of psychomotor stimulants as measured by intravenous drug self-administration (for review, see Koob, 1992). Dopamine receptor antagonists when injected systemically decrease the interinjection interval or increase the number of drug infusions, a response similar to lowering the dose of cocaine (Yokel and Wise, 1975; Ettenberg et al., 1982). Experiments investigating the effects on cocaine self-administration of antagonists selective for D_1 (Koob et al., 1987) and D_2 (Woolverton and Virus, 1989; Bergman et al., 1990) receptors suggest that both can decrease the reinforcing properties of cocaine. However, D_2 antagonists, in contrast to selective D_1 antagonists, decrease responding maintained by food as well as responding maintained by cocaine (B. Caine and G. Koob, unpublished results), and recent studies suggest that a D_2 antagonist at low doses, but not the D_1 antagonist, can selectively impair the ability to respond (Amalric et al., 1993). These results suggest that D_1 receptors in the nucleus accumbens may be particularly important for the reinforcing properties of cocaine.

A specific role for the mesocorticolimbic dopamine system in the reinforcing actions of cocaine was the observation that 6-hydroxydopamine lesions of the region of the nucleus accumbens produced extinction-like responding and a significant and long-lasting decrease in intravenous self-administration of cocaine and amphetamine (Lyness et al., 1979; Roberts et al., 1980). 6-Hydroxydopamine lesions in the region of the nucleus accumbens also produced significant decreases in the highest ratio for which the rats would respond for cocaine in a progressive ratio schedule of reinforcement, suggesting that the reinforcing value of co-

caine is decreased following disruption of nucleus accumbens DA activity (Koob et al., 1987).

The role of efferent projections from the region of the nucleus accumbens in the activation and reinforcement produced by the mesocorticolimbic dopamine system

A series of studies have characterized the functional efferent output of the nucleus accumbens using locomotor activity as the dependent variable (Jones and Mogenson, 1980; Mogenson et al., 1980; Mogenson and Nielson, 1983). Dopamine injected into the nucleus accumbens produces locomotor hyperactivity and this locomotor response was reversed by injecting γ-aminobutyric acid (GABA) into the region of the ventral pallidum (Jones and Mogenson, 1980). Activation of the ventral tegmental area with injection of the GABA antagonist picrotoxin also increases locomotor activity and this hyperactivity was also attenuated by injections of GABA into the pallidum (Mogenson et al., 1980). Blockade of dopamine stimulation of the nucleus accumbens also was observed with ventral pallidal injection of the GABA transaminase inhibitor, ethanolamine O-sulfate (Pycock and Horton, 1976).

Similar results were obtained using a different model of dopamine receptor activation, i.e., the augmented locomotor response to systemic injections of dopamine agonists in animals with 6-OHDA-induced lesions of the dopamine input to the nucleus accumbens. This model has the advantage of an exaggerated locomotor response produced by activation of a select group of dopamine receptors, presumably only those having been denervated.

Animals receiving 6-OHDA lesions of the nucleus accumbens showed a significantly potentiated locomotor response to apomorphine. Electrolytic lesions and ibotenic acid lesions of the substantia innominata/ventral pallidum (SI/VP) significantly depressed the locomotor response to apomorphine in dopamine-denervated rats (Larrson, 1980;

Swerdlow et al., 1984). Similar results were obtained with microinjection of low doses of the GABA agonist muscimol into the SI/VP (Swerdlow et al., 1987). The locomotor response to amphetamine and heroin is also significantly decreased by muscimol injections into the SI/VP, however, the locomotor activation produced by caffeine and corticotropin releasing factor is not blocked by SI/VP injections of muscimol (Swerdlow and Koob, 1985).

The question of the circuitry involved in further processing of the locomotor stimulation associated with activation of DA receptors in the nucleus accumbens remains an area of current research. Efferent projections from the ventral pallidum include a major cholinergic projection which traverses through the medial prefrontal cortex (MPC) and then spreads caudally to innervate most of the neocortex (Divac et al., 1978), a projection to the pedunculopontine nucleus (PPN) (Swanson et al., 1984) which is considered a homolog in the rat to the mesencephalic locomotor region (Grillner and Shik, 1973; Skinner and Garcia-Rill, 1984), and a projection to the dorsomedial thalamus (DMT) (Young et al., 1984).

Both the PPN and the DMT have been implicated in mediating the locomotor activity produced by activation of dopaminergic function in the region of the nucleus accumbens. Substantia innominata-induced activation is attenuated by lesions of the PPN (Swanson et al., 1984) and electrolytic lesions of the DMT attenuated the supersensitive locomotor response to systemic apomorphine in rats with 6-OHDA lesions of the nucleus accumbens (Swerdlov et al., 1986).

Relatively little information has been obtained regarding the efferent anatomical substrates through which the nucleus accumbens may process drug reinforcement. Since previous work has established the substantia innominata-ventral pallidum as an important connection in the expression of behavioral stimulation produced by activation of the nucleus accumbens, a logical hypothesis was that the region of the ventral pallidum may also be involved in the processing of the reinforcing properties of cocaine and heroin.

Rats receiving bilateral ibotenic acid lesions of the region of the substantia innominata-ventral pallidum showed significantly decreased baseline cocaine and heroin self-administration, and when the rats were subjected to a progressive ratio procedure, lesions of the substantia innominata-ventral pallidum produced a significant decrease in the highest ratio obtained for both cocaine and heroin (Hubner and Koob, 1990). These results suggest that the substantia innominata-ventral pallidum may be an important site in the processing of the reinforcing effects of drugs and that the nucleus accumbens-ventral pallidum connection may be a common pathway for both stimulant and opiate reinforcement.

The specific anatomical nomenclature for the functional output of the nucleus accumbens has varied somewhat. Recent anatomical data suggest that a major output from the nucleus accumbens projects to the anterior lateral ventral pallidum (Alheid and Heimer, 1988). However, lesions and injections in the above mentioned studies fall more in the sublenticular part of the substantia innominata which is caudal and just ventral to the globus pallidus. This region is continuous with the bed nucleus of the stria terminalis and the centromedial part of the amygdala and thus forms part of the "extended amygdala" (Alheid and Heimer, 1988). Future studies will be necessary to delineate exactly what part of the basal forebrain forms the output of the nucleus accumbens. Indeed, some of the components of the medial nucleus accumbens may also represent a rostral part of the extended amygdala (Alheid and Heimer, 1988).

The role of the nigrostriatal dopamine system in response initiation and motor behavior

The nigrostriatal dopamine system has long been associated with motor function and response initiation. Destruction of this system results in the severe motor disturbances of Parkinson's disease which include tremor, dystonic-like involuntary movements, akinesia and other motor disturbances such as mask-like face and akathisia (De Long, 1990).

This is a progressive degenerative syndrome that can be successfully treated, at least in its earlier stages, with the dopamine precursor L-Dopa (Marsden, 1992).

Large bilateral 6-OHDA lesions of nigrostriatal dopamine system can reproduce some of these deficits. Rats become akinetic to the point of aphagia and adipsia and will die unless intubated (Ungerstedt, 1971). These animals also have severe deficits in learning a conditioned avoidance task and these deficits can also be reversed with L-Dopa treatment (Zis et al., 1974).

The role of the nigrostriatal dopamine system in psychomotor stimulant-induced stereotyped behavior

Smaller lesions restricted to the striatum itself do not reproduce this global syndrome (Koob et al., 1984) but do block the stereotyped behavior associated with administration of high doses of D-amphetamine (Creese and Iversen, 1974; Kelly et al., 1976; Iversen, 1977; Koob et al., 1984). Rats injected systemically (subcutaneously) with D-amphetamine in doses of 3 mg/kg and above show intense repetitive movements such as sniffing in one place, licking, biting and gnawing. This intense restricted repetitive behavior is blocked by 6-OHDA-induced lesions of the corpus striatum and results in intense locomotor activity (Koob et al., 1984). Both the stereotyped behavior and locomotor activity is blocked by bilateral lesions to both the corpus striatum and nucleus accumbens (Koob et al., 1984).

More recently subregions of the corpus striatum have been implicated in this stereotyped behavior by studies with local intracerebral injections of D-amphetamine (Kelley et al., 1989). D-amphetamine injected into the ventrolateral striatum produced pure oral stereotypy of licking, biting and self-gnawing (Kelley et al., 1989). This intense oral stereotypy was not reproduced by injections more dorsal and lateral.

The role of the nigrostriatal system in non-drug-induced motor performance-conditioned reaction time

Dopamine in the neostriatum is involved in critical aspects of sensorimotor processes. The neostriatum, the "input stage" of the basal ganglia, receives all the major inputs to the basal ganglia, which includes the dopaminergic projection from the substantia nigra and a large number of projections from neocortical areas. New functional models of basal ganglia circuitry have recently been proposed to account for the vast spectrum of motor disorders, such as Parkinson's and Huntington's diseases, associated with basal ganglia dysfunction. Current evidence suggests that the basal ganglia are organized into basic parallel arrangements of basal ganglia-thalamo-cortical circuits, which receive information from specific cortical areas and project back to certain of those areas after intermediate processing within the basal ganglia and the thalamus (Alexander et al., 1986; De Long, 1990). According to this more recent view, the functions of the neostriatum involve not only sensorimotor aspects of movement programming, but conditional aspects of planning movement, emotional (limbic) and cognitive processes. Furthermore, the widespread dopaminergic innervation of the striatum converging to striatal neurons innervated by specific and discrete cortical areas has suggested a novel way in which dopamine can process sensory and cognitive functions to influence motor control (Divac, 1972; Groves, 1983; Lidsky et al., 1985).

The dopamine systems are known to play an important role in the initiation and sequencing of conditioned or learned motor acts (Iversen, 1977). Increases in dopamine release in the ventral and dorsal striatum are associated with the presentation of motivationally relevant stimuli (Salamone et al., 1989). The measure of the catecholamine synthesis rates in different brain regions, estimated by the in vivo conversion of the endogenous catecholamine precursor tyrosine to dopamine and norepinephrine in the brains of rats performing an operant task, has revealed that increases in the rate of dopamine synthesis were only observed in neurons which terminate in the dorsal striatum but not in the mesolimbic or hypothalamic dopamine neurons (Heffner and Seiden, 1980). Furthermore, dopamine release modulates aspects of motor function, including local rates of responding and the duration of responding. The responses that are more sensitive to disruption after interference with striatal dopamine are complex learned instrumental responses elicited by conditioned stimuli (for review, see Salamone, 1991). The involvement of striatal dopamine in the coordination of learned motor acts in a temporal sequence has been suggested by behavioral experiments using reaction time paradigms for analyzing motor programming (Robbins and Brown, 1990). Early studies of reaction time performance in patients with Parkinson's disease showed significant lengthening in reaction time (Evarts et al., 1981; Marsden, 1982; Pullman et al., 1988). Others have suggested that these patients have impairments in the automatic execution of a learned motor plan (Marsden, 1982).

Effects of dopaminergic lesion on conditioned reaction time performance

The motor deficits in patients with Parkinson's disease have been suggested to be the consequence of an extensive loss of dopamine in the striatum, although other neurochemical deficits in noradrenergic, serotoninergic and cholinergic innervations of the neocortex could also be detected in parkinsonian patients (Scatton et al., 1982; Agid et al., 1987). Experimental studies in animals with midbrain neurotoxin lesions have shown dramatic behavioral deficits such as akinesia, catalepsy (maintenance of an abnormal posture) and impairments in operant measures of motor performance which closely resemble the deficits seen in humans with Parkinson's disease.

In order to specify further the role of the different dopamine pathways in the brain on the execution of a learned motor plan, the performance of rats

trained in an operant reaction time task was examined after specific destruction of dopamine neurons by 6-OHDA perfusion into the nucleus accumbens or the dorsal part of the neostriatum (caudate-putamen nucleus of primates and humans). The rats were trained to hold a lever down and release it with a fast movement, with a circumscribed reaction time, after the presentation of a visual cue (conditioned stimulus, CS). The experimental paradigm shown in Fig. 2 has been described in detail (Amalric and Koob, 1987). Briefly, each trial was initiated by the rat by pressing down the lever and waiting during a variable and random period of time (0.25 – 1.0 sec) for the presentation of the light stimulus. If the rats failed and released the lever before the light (anticipatory response), no reward was given and a new trial was initiated. If the rats met this first criterion, they then had to release the lever within a restriction

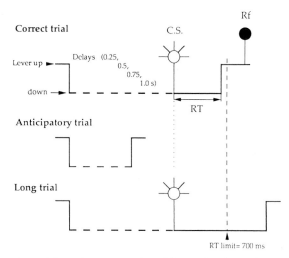

Fig. 2. Schematic representation of the reaction time task procedure. Rats are trained to press a lever down and wait for a visual cue (a light located above the lever). This conditioned stimulus (CS) occurs at random after four different delays (0.25 – 1.0 sec). The animals had then to release the lever in a fast movement controlled in a reaction time (RT). RTs were measured as the time period from the CS to the lever release. If the rat failed and released the lever before the CS (anticipatory error), no reward was given and a new trial had to be initiated. If the rat waited for the cue, then released the lever after the RT limit restriction (500 – 1000 msec), the trial was also not rewarded. Each correct trial was reinforced with a 45 mg Noyes food pellet and the daily session ended after 100 trials.

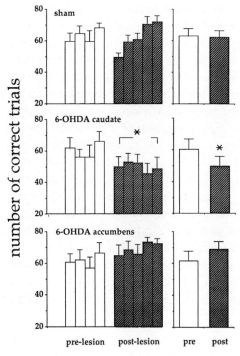

Fig. 3. Performance of the rats on reaction time task after 6-OHDA lesions either in the caudate nucleus (dorsal striatum, $n = 8$) or the nucleus accumbens ($n = 8$). Sham animals were infused with vehicle (a solution of ascorbate, 0.1 mg/ml) either in the nucleus accumbens ($n = 6$) or the caudate nucleus ($n = 5$). Data are presented together for the three groups as the mean number of the successful trials + S.E.M. during the four sessions preceding surgery and the five sessions following surgery (from day 9 to day 13 post-lesion). * Significant differences between post-lesion performance and baseline performance ($P < 0.05$, Newman-Keuls test). (Taken with permission from Amalric and Koob, 1987.)

time limit of 700 msec after the CS onset to be reinforced by a food pellet.

The results were expressed either as a number of correct responses (lever releases within 700 msec) by session or as the percentage success of the reaction time (i.e., number of correct responses divided by the number of CS). The number of incorrect responses, either anticipatory responses or long responses (release of the lever after 700 msec) were counted separately. The reaction time was the time period measured from the CS onset to the lever release. The rats were tested daily during 100 trials per session. Preoperative baseline values were ob-

tained after 25 – 30 sessions. Rats received bilateral injection of 6-OHDA or vehicle solution (sham) either into the N. Acc. or into the caudate nucleus and were tested again for four sessions 9 – 13 days postoperatively.

The results were consistent with the hypothesis that striatal dopamine depletion produces deficits in the ability to initiate motor responses after a stimulus. As seen in Figs. 3 and 4, lesions of the dopaminergic terminals of the nigrostriatal pathway in the dorsal striatum (59% decrease in posterior striatal DA) significantly lengthened reaction times. This deficit in performance in the lesioned rats was not accompanied by a general disruption in the ability to perform the task as seen with a bilateral destruction of the ascending dopaminergic pathway. Spirduso et al. (1985) have also found that rats with unilateral lesion of the striatum showed movement initiation deficits, as shown by a slowing in reaction times in the paw contralateral to the lesion, in a reactive capacity task. In a similar model of unilateral striatal DA depletion, animals trained to quickly orient their head either towards or away from an unpredictable, brief visual stimulus presented to either side of their head, were significantly slower to initiate responses contralateral to the dopamine-lesioned side (Carli et al., 1989). However, they were unimpaired in the detection of ipsilateral or contralateral stimuli (to the dopamine-lesioned side) which further suggests that there were no primary contralateral sensory deficits but a more specific motor impairment to initiate the response (Carli et al., 1989).

The deficits observed in our RT task were specific to a dopamine depletion of the dorsal striatum (caudate nucleus) as the lesion of the N. Acc. (75% DA depletion) failed to alter reaction time performance at any time post-lesion (Amalric and Koob, 1987). Carli et al. (1989) have also found that unilateral DA depletion from the ventral striatum failed to affect reaction time in their visual orientation task. The reaction time task thus appears to be a sensitive test to reveal deficits with less than a complete depletion of the dorsal striatum. Whether this performance deficit reflects a partial depletion of a large part of

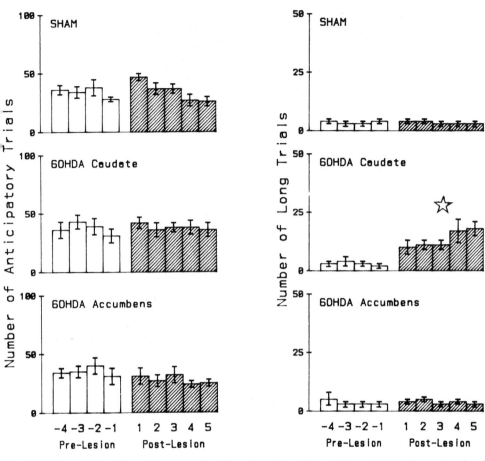

Fig. 4. Further analysis of the performance of rats from Fig. 3 (Amalric and Koob, 1987) in the reaction time (RT) task after 6-OHDA lesions of the caudate nucleus (dorsal striatum) and nucleus accumbens. Left: number of anticipatory trials (release of the lever before the visual conditioned stimulus). Right: number of long trials (release of the lever after the time limit restriction of 1 sec following the conditioned stimulus). Star represents a significant difference from pre-lesion performance. (Redrawn with permission from Amalric and Koob, 1987.)

the striatum or a large depletion of one specific subregion remains to be investigated. Brown and Robbins (1989) have examined the effects of discrete unilateral lesions of the medial and lateral parts of the striatum with localized excitotoxic lesions using ibotenic acid in a similar reaction time paradigm to that used by Carli and colleagues. Lesions of either the medial or lateral striatum produced an ipsilateral bias in the response orientation. Lateral striatal lesions produced no change in the latency for the initiation of responses to the visual cues, while in contrast, the medial striatal lesions resulted in a significant lengthening of contralateral reaction time (Brown and Robbins, 1989). This dissociation of behavioral results supports the existence of distinct processes of response selection mediated by the striatum and supports not only the concept of functional heterogeneity within the striatum but demonstrate the functional effects of hypothetical segregated parallel corticostriatal loops (Robbins and Brown, 1990).

Effects of DA receptor blockade on reaction time performance

The behavioral functions of neostriatal DA in sensorimotor function and motivation have been the focus of intense research using drugs acting directly or indirectly to facilitate or alter DA transmission. Dopamine receptor antagonists disrupt motor control in rats (Falk, 1969; Fowler et al., 1984). For example, low doses of neuroleptic drugs can impair preparatory behaviors in instrumental lever pressing responses without affecting food consummatory behaviors (Fadda et al., 1983; Blackburn et al., 1987). Comparatively little work has been directed to the exploration of the specific role of DA receptors on performance in an operant reaction time task. In the conditioned motor task previously described, Amalric and Koob (1987) have shown that the treatment of rats with the mixed D_1/D_2 DA receptor antagonist, α-flupenthixol, injected intraperitoneally significantly impaired reaction time

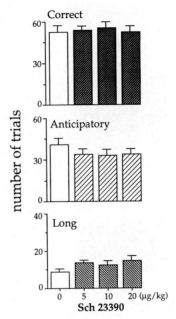

Fig. 6. Performance of rats in the reaction time task, after pretreatment with SCH 23390, injected subcutaneously (s.c.) 30 min before the test. A correct trial is a lever release before the reaction time limit restriction (700 msec after the CS). An anticipatory error is a release of the lever before the visual conditioned stimulus. A long error is a release of the lever after the time limit restriction. (Taken with permission from Amalric et al., 1993.)

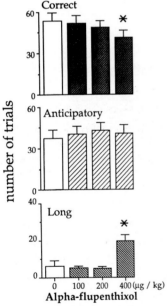

Fig. 5. Performance of rats in the reaction time task after intraperitoneal pretreatment with the dopamine mixed D_1/D_2 antagonist α-flupenthixol ($n = 7$ except for 400 μg/kg dose where $n = 6$). Asterisks indicate a significant difference from 0 (saline) dose. A correct trial is a lever release before the reaction time restriction (1 sec after the conditioned stimulus). An anticipatory error is a release of the lever before the visual conditioned stimulus. A long error is a release of the lever after the time limit restriction. (Redrawn with permission from Amalric and Koob, 1987.)

performance in rats. As shown in Fig. 5, the 200 and 400 μg/kg doses of α-flupenthixol reduced the percentage of correct responses as compared to baseline performance. Reaction times were also significantly lengthened following the injection of the higher dose. The drug also decreased the number of trials attempted by the rats during the session. This effect reflected an overall deficit in performance, as manifested by a complete cessation of responding after 37 trials at the 400 μg/kg dose. However, the animals appeared to be still motivated by the food reinforcement as they were able to eat food pellets freely given by the experimenter.

Previous work using a discriminative motor control task has shown similar deficits in rats (Falk, 1969; Fowler et al., 1984, 1986). In these studies, chlorpromazine, haloperidol and clozapine produced dose-related decreases in time spent on the task. This was estimated by the amount of time the animal was in contact with a force transducer that had to be pressed for 2 sec to obtain a reinforcer. Haloperidol was found to decrease the response rate, increase the mean emitted peak force necessary to press down the lever, and increase the response duration overall (Faustman and Fowler, 1981; Fowler et al., 1986). These results suggest that the dopamine receptor antagonists impaired performance by affecting the tendency to initiate responding instead of affecting the capacity to maintain steady forelimb force once a response was started (Fowler et al., 1984).

Role of the D_1/D_2 receptor subtypes

Most of the dopamine receptor antagonist drugs are antagonists at both receptor subtypes. However, it has now become clear that there is more than one DA receptor subtype and the main subdivisions of DA receptors into D_1 and D_2 receptor sites (Kebabian and Calne, 1979; Leff and Creese, 1983) has opened the question of their functional differences in behavioral experiments. Several studies investigating the effects of DA receptor selective antagonists on lever pressing for food or water, which again is a measure of a learned response with reinforcement, have shown that both D_1 and D_2 antagonists in addition to performance effects appear to lead to a decrease in effectiveness of reward in operant tasks (Clark and White, 1987, followed by Miller et al., 1990).

A potential differential role of the two dopaminergic receptors D_1 or D_2 in the execution of the reaction time motor task is shown in Figs. 6 and 7. The pretreatment with the D_1 DA receptor antagonist (SCH 23390; 5 – 10 μg/kg, s.c.) did not modify the performance at any dose tested. The animals performed the reaction time task with the same rate of correct trials as during control sessions following vehicle injection or during pre-testing sessions. In contrast, the pretreatment with the D_2 DA receptor antagonist (raclopride; 50 – 200 μg/kg, s.c.) dose-dependently decreased the number of correct trials which were wholly attributable to increases in the time to release the lever after the visual cue (Amalric et al., 1993).

The slowing in reaction time induced by raclopride resembles closely the deficits with α-flupenthixol (Amalric and Koob, 1987) and with systemic haloperidol (unpublished data). More importantly, this same profile of increases in reaction time was observed after intracaudate injection of haloperidol and after dopamine depletions of the dorsal striatum (Amalric and Koob, 1987). Clearly, the impairment of the reaction time task, controlled by dopaminergic activity in the dorsal striatum, following D_2 receptor blockade would be dependent on the doses of the drugs employed. Higher doses of SCH 23390 pronounced motor disturbances and catalepsy (Ioro et al., 1983; Creese and Chen, 1985; Hojrth and Carlsson, 1988) and animals will completely stop responding in any operant situation. In contrast, lower doses of SCH 23390 within the same

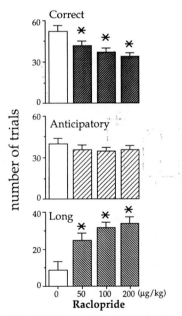

Fig. 7. Performance of rats in the reaction time task after pretreatment with raclopride injected s.c. 30 min before the test (legends: same as in Fig. 6). Asterisks indicate significant difference from control values ($P < 0.05$, paired t-test) following significant analysis of variance. (Taken with permission from Amalric et al., 1993.)

dose range as tested in the present study have been found to selectively reverse dopamine-mediated behaviors known to involve an activation of the mesolimbic DA system. As previously shown (Fig. 1), SCH 23390 significantly reduced the stimulant effect of D-amphetamine or cocaine (Cabib et al., 1991) on locomotion and the hyperlocomotor activity following apomorphine injection in rats with 6-OHDA lesions of the mesolimbic DA nerve terminals in the N. Acc. (Mailman et al., 1984; Amalric and Koob, 1987). Furthermore, low doses of SCH 23390 selectively decreased cocaine self-administration without disrupting responding for

food on a multiple schedule of reinforcement (Caine et al., 1990). Together these results suggest that low doses of the D_1 antagonist, SCH 23390, may selectively inhibit mesocorticolimbic DA hyperactivity.

In contrast, a preferential involvement of D_2 receptors in the expression of nigrostriatal dopaminergic functions has been suggested according to the results of Breese et al. (1987) and Delfs and Kelley (1990). Furthermore, low doses of D_2 antagonists produce response decrements in operant tasks (Amalric and Koob, 1989; Liao and Fowler, 1990; Phillips et al., 1991a) when injected systematically or directly into the dorsal striatum (Phillips et

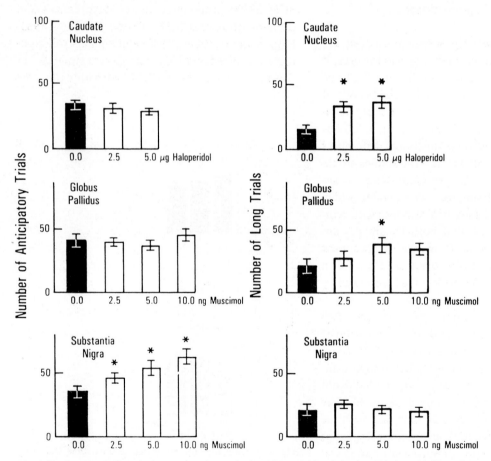

Fig. 8. Performance of rats in the reaction time task after bilateral microinjection of haloperidol into the caudate nucleus (dorsal striatum, $n = 10$) or muscimol into the globus pallidus ($n = 9$) or the substantia nigra ($n = 9$). Left: number of anticipatory trials (release of the lever before the visual conditioned stimulus). Right: number of long trials (release of the lever after the time limit restriction of 500 msec following the conditioned stimulus). Asterisks indicate significant difference from control values ($P < 0.05$), Newman-Keuls test) following significant analysis of variance. (Taken with permission from Amalric and Koob, 1989.)

al., 1991b; Pretsell and Robbins, 1992). The dopaminergic nigrostriatal system has been shown to be a sensitive site for sensorimotor integration involved in the execution of the reaction time motor task. The D_2 dopaminergic receptors thus appeared to be more specifically involved than the D_1 receptors in the reaction time performance.

Role of efferent projections from the neostriatum in motor behavior

Anatomical studies have described efferent connections from the dorsal striatum to the dorsal globus pallidus (GP), entopeduncular nucleus (EP) and substantia nigra reticulata (SNr). The SNr and the EP are anatomically and functionally similar respective to their input and output projections, and have been found to mediate behaviors such as postural asymmetry and catalepsy induced by a DA receptor activation within the striatum (Scheel-Kruger et al., 1981; Pycock and Phillipson, 1984). The cortical inputs in the striatum remain segregated through the output structures of the striatum (EP/SNr) and the thalamus to project back to these same cortical areas (Alexander et al., 1986), and this reciprocal relationship has important functional implications. The striatal output nuclei exert a tonic, GABA-mediated, inhibitory effect on their target nuclei in the thalamus (for review, see Pycock and Phillipson, 1984). Within the different cortico-striato-thalamo-cortical loops, the inhibitory outflow appears to be differentially modulated by two opposing but parallel pathways that pass from the striatum to the output nuclei. The "direct" pathway arises from striatal neurons containing both GABA and substance P and project directly to the EP and SNr. The "indirect" pathway, on the other hand, arises from striatal neurons containing both GABA and enkephalin, which influence EP and SNr activity through a sequence of connections involving the dorsal pallidum and the subthalamic nucleus (De Long, 1990).

To determine the respective contributions of the efferent projections from the dorsal striatum in the mediation of the conditioned reaction time motor performance, the effects of a GABA receptor agonist (muscimol) injected into the SNr and the GP were tested on rats previously trained in the reaction time task. These effects were then compared with those obtained after pharmacological blockade of dopaminergic receptors with intrastriatal injections of haloperidol. The increase in reaction time produced by DA receptor blockade of the dorsal striatum was mimicked by injection of muscimol in nanogram quantities in the region of the dorsal pallidum, but not in the SNr (Amalric and Koob, 1989). Fig. 8 shows that haloperidol injection into the striatum significantly increased the number of long trials. A similar effect was observed after activation of GABA receptors in the globus pallidus. In contrast, a significant dose-dependent increase in the number of anticipatory trials was observed after muscimol injection in the SNr, producing a facilitatory motor effect evidenced by shortened reaction times.

GABA activation in the striato-nigral pathway has been found to mediate striatal-DA behaviors. Local injection of muscimol in the SNr induces stereotyped behavior (Kilpatrick et al., 1980) and reverses striatal haloperidol-induced muscular rigidity (Ellenbroek et al., 1985). The facilitatory effects on the reaction time performance after increased GABAergic activity in the "direct" striatal output (SNr/EP) is consistent with the hypothesis that hyperkinetic motor disorders of hemiballismus and dyskinesias might be the result of a reduction in the SNr and entopeduncular inhibitory projection to the thalamus. The overall effect would be to disinhibit thalamo-cortical neurons and facilitate the responsiveness of cortical neurons involved in motor control (De Long, 1990). Altogether, our results suggest that GABA in the SNr modulates some striatal dopaminergic function via the "direct" striato-nigral pathway by inhibition of the efferent SNr neurons.

More importantly, our results show that stimulation of GABA receptors in the GP more closely reflects the effects of a dopaminergic receptor blockade in the striatum. Other behavioral studies have found that postural asymmetries of the head and the trunk and circling behavior in rats could be elicited by local injection of GABA agonists in the GP (Scheel-Kruger, 1986). The catalepsy induced by DA receptor antagonism could be reversed by microinjection of the GABA antagonist picrotoxin into the GP (Scheel-Kruger, 1986). Costa et al. (1978) have shown that systemic injection of DA antagonists increased GABA turnover in the GP and the nucleus accumbens. More recently, in "parkinsonian" animals (monkeys treated with MPTP) 2-deoxyglucose radioautography revealed a prominent increase in 2-deoxyglucose uptake in the lateral segment of the globus pallidus (homologous to the rat GP) with no change in the SNr (Mitchell et al., 1989). These results were interpreted as an increased synaptic activity in the putaminopallidal ("indirect" pathway) but not the caudatonigral ("direct" pathway) pathway which suggests a relatively greater involvement of the putaminopallidal pathway in relation to motor manifestation of parkinsonism (Mitchell et al., 1986). The present results further suggest that a dysfunction of the striatal dopaminergic system appears to be expressed via the pallidal GABAergic efferents. They are consistent with the hypothesis that an increase in the transmission through the "indirect" (striatopallidal) pathway disinhibiting the excitatory projection to the SNr/EP through the subthalamic nucleus is leading to excessive inhibition of thalamocortical neurons. The overall result would be a hypokinetic motor disorder of which Parkinson's disease is the best-known example (De Long, 1990). These results emphasize an important functional role for the globus pallidus as an output of the striatum, which most probably is involved in the pathophysiology of motor disorders of the basal ganglia.

Summary and conclusions

In summary, evidence is presented that the mesocorticolimbic and nigrostriatal dopamine systems form functionally selective afferents to different parts of the basal ganglia and these inputs are paralleled by functionally selective outputs. The ventral striatal region of the nucleus accumbens and olfactory tubercle has a dopamine input that is critical for locomotor activation produced by psychomotor stimulant drugs and some non-drug states. These regions also appear critical for the reinforcing actions of psychomotor stimulants such as cocaine and amphetamine, and these regions may also be involved in the activation associated with non-drug rewards. Both psychomotor stimulant-induced locomotor activation and reinforcement may selectively involve dopamine D_1 receptors. The functional efferents of this system appear to involve the region of the ventral pallidum and more specifically GABAergic mechanisms of the posterior medial (sublenticular) ventral pallidum. The relationship of this circuitry with the revised concept of the "extended amygdala" is an area of current work.

The nigrostriatal dopamine system forms a functionally selective afferent system to the dorsal striatum and appears to be critical for the focused stereotyped behavior associated with high doses of psychomotor stimulants. This dopamine input also appears to be involved in non-drug-induced conditioned reaction time performance and may selectively involve dopamine D_2 receptors. The functional efferents of this system appear to involve both direct and indirect GABAergic connections to the substantia nigra reticulata and dorsal pallidum, respectively. Activation of the GABAergic connection to the dorsal pallidum (indirect connection) appears to mimic the action of dopamine in the dorsal striatum, whereas activation of the GABAergic connection to the substantia nigra reticulata (direct connection) appears to modulate striatal dopamine function. These results show an important functional role for the globus pallidus in the output of the dorsal striatum and emphasize the parallel functional processing of both dorsal and ventral striatum.

Acknowledgements

Preparation of this manuscript was supported in part by the National Institute on Drug Abuse Grant number 04398. We thank the Molecular and Experimental Medicine Word Processing Department for manuscript preparation.

References

Agid, Y., Ruberg, M., Dubois, B. and Pillon, B. (1987) Anatomical and biochemical concepts of subcortical dementia. In: S.M. Stahl, S.D. Iversen and E.C. Goodman (Eds.), *Cognitive Neurochemistry*, Oxford University Press, Oxford, pp. 248 – 271.

Alexander, G.E., De Long, M.R. and Strick, P.L. (1986) Parallel organization of functionally segregated circuits linking basal ganglia and cortex. *Annu. Rev. Neurosci.*, 9: 357 – 381.

Alheid, G.F. and Heimer, L. (1988) New perspectives in basal forebrain organization of special relevance for neuropsychiatric disorders: the striatopallidal, amygdaloid, and corticopetal components of substantia inominata. *Neuroscience*, 27: 1 – 39.

Amalric, M. and Koob, G.F. (1987) Depletion of dopamine in the caudate nucleus but not nucleus accumbens impairs reaction time performance in rats. *J. Neurosci.*, 7: 2129 – 2134.

Amalric, M. and Koob, G.F. (1989) Dorsal pallidum as a functional motor output of the corpus striatum. *Brain Res.*, 483: 389 – 394.

Amalric, M., Koob, G.F., Creese, I. and Swerdlow, N.R. (1986) ''Selective'' D-1 and D-2 receptor antagonists fail to differentially alter supersensitive locomotor behavior in the rat. *Life Sci.*, 39: 1985 – 1993.

Amalric, M., Berhow, M., Polis, I. and Koob, G.F. (1993) Selective effects of low dose D2 dopaminergic receptor antagonism in a reaction time task in rats. *Neuropsychopharmacology*, 8: 195 – 200.

Arnt, J. (1985) Hyperactivity induced by stimulation of separate D1 and D2 receptors in rats with bilateral 6-OHDA lesions. *Life Sci.*, 37: 717 – 723.

Bergman, J., Kamien, J.B. and Spealman, R.D. (1990) Antagonism of cocaine self-administration by selective dopamine D1 and D2 antagonist. *Behav. Pharmacol.*, 1: 355 – 363.

Bird, M. and Kornetsky, C. (1990) Dissociation of the attentional and motivational effects of pimozide on the threshold for rewarding brain stimulation. *Neuropsychopharmacology*, 3: 33 – 40.

Blackburn, J.R., Phillips, A.G. and Fibiger, H.C. (1987) Dopamine and preparatory behavior: I. Effects of pimozide. *Behav. Neurosci.*, 101: 352 – 360.

Breese, G.R., Duncan, G.E., Napier, T.G., Bondy, S.C., Ioro, L.C. and Mueller, R.A. (1987) 6-Hydroxydopamine treatments enhance behavioral responses to intracerebral microinjections of D1 and D2 dopamine agonists into the nucleus accumbens and striatum without changing dopamine antagonist binding. *J. Pharmacol. Exp. Ther.*, 240: 167 – 176.

Brown, V.J. and Robbins, T.W. (1989) Elementary processes of responses selection mediated by distant regions of the striatum. *J. Neurosci.*, 9: 3761 – 3765. (Abstract.)

Cabib, S., Castellano, C., Cestari, V., Filibeck, V. and Puglisi-Allegra, S. (1991) D1 and D2 receptor antagonists differently affect cocaine-induced locomotor hyperactivity in the mouse. *Psychopharmacology*, 105: 335 – 339.

Caine, S.B., Berhow, M., Amalric, M. and Koob, G.F. (1990) The D1 antagonist SCH 23390 and the D2 antagonist raclopride selectively decrease behavior maintained by cocaine or food in the rat. *Soc. Neurosci. Abstr.*, 16: 25a.

Carli, M., Jones, G.H. and Robbins, T.W. (1989) Effects of dorsal and ventral striatal dopamine depletion on visual neglect in the rat: a neural and behavioural analysis. *Neuroscience*, 29: 309 – 327.

Clark, D. and White, F.J. (1987) Review: D1 dopamine receptor: the search for a function? A critical evaluation of the D1/D2 dopamine receptor classification and its functional implication. *Synapse*, 1: 347 – 388.

Corrodi, H., Fuxe, K. and Hökfelt, T. (1973) Effect of ergot drugs on central catecholamine neurons: evidence for a stimulation of central dopamine neurons. *J. Pharm. Pharmacol.*, 25: 409 – 412.

Costa, E., Cheney, D.L., Mao, C.C. and Moroni, F. (1978) Action of antischizophrenic drugs on the metabolism of gamma-aminobutyric acid and acetylcholine in globus pallidus, striatum and n. accumbens. *Fed. Proc.*, 37: 2408 – 2414.

Costall, B., Naylor, R.W. and Olley, J. (1973) Stereotypy and anti-cataleptic action of amphetamine after intracerebral injection. *Eur. J. Pharmacol.*, 18: 83 – 94.

Costall, B., Marsden, C.D., Naylor, R.J. and Pycock, C.J. (1977) Stereotyped behavior patterns and hyperactivity induced by amphetamine and apomorphine after discrete 6-hydroxy-dopamine lesions of extrapyramidal and mesolimbic nuclei. *Brain Res.*, 123: 89 – 111.

Creese, I. and Chen, A. (1985) Selective D1 dopamine receptor increase following chronic treatment with SCH 23390. *Eur. J. Pharmacol.*, 109: 127 – 128.

Creese, I. and Iversen, S.D. (1974) A role of forebrain dopamine systems in amphetamine-induced stereotyped behavior in the rat. *Psychopharmacology*, 39: 345 – 347.

Delfs, J.M. and Kelley, A.E. (1990) The role of D1 and D2 dopamine receptors in oral stereotypy induced by dopaminergic stimulation of the ventrolateral striatum. *Neuroscience*, 39(1): 59 – 67.

De Long, M. (1990) Primate models of movement disorders of basal ganglia origin. *Trends Neurosci.*, 13: 281 – 285.

Divac, I. (1972) Neostriatum and functions of prefrontal cortex. *Acta Neurobiol.*, 32: 461 – 477.

Divac, I., Kosmal, A., Björklund, A. and Lindvall, D. (1978) Subcortical projections to the prefrontal cortex in the rat as revealed by the horseradish peroxidase technique. *Neuroscience*, 3: 785 – 796.

Ellenbroek, B., Schwarz, M., Sontag, K.H. and Cools, A. (1985) The importance of the striato-nigro-collicular pathway in the expansion of haloperidol-induced tonic electromyographic activity. *Neurosci. Lett.*, 56: 189 – 194.

Ettenberg, A., Pettit, H.O., Bloom, F.E. and Koob, G.F. (1982) Heroin and cocaine intravenous self-administration in rats:

mediation by separate neural systems. *Psychopharmacology,* 78: 204–209.

Evarts, E., Teravainen, H. and Calne, D.B. (1981) Reaction time in Parkinson's disease. *Brain,* 104: 167–186.

Fadda, F., Argiolas, A., Melis, M.R., DeMontis, G. and Gessa, G.L. (1983) Suppression of voluntary ethanol consumption in rats by gammabutyrolactone. *Life Sci.,* 32: 1471–1477.

Falk, J.L. (1969) Drug effects on discriminative motor control. *Physiol. Behav.,* 4: 421–427.

Faustman, W.O. and Fowler, S.C. (1981) Use of operant response duration to distinguish the effects of haloperidol from non-reward. *Pharmacol. Biochem. Behav.,* 15: 327–329.

Fowler, S.C., Ford, K.E., Gramling, S.E. and Nail, G.L. (1984) Acute and subchronic effects of neuroleptics on quantitative measures of discriminative motor control in rats. *Psychopharmacology,* 84: 368–373.

Fowler, S.C., La Cerra, M.M. and Ettenberg, A. (1986) Effects of haloperidol on the biophysical characteristics of operant responding: implications for motor and reinforcement processes. *Pharmacol. Biochem. Behav.,* 25: 791–796.

Grillner, S. and Shik, M.I. (1973) On the descending control of the lumbrosacral spinal cord from the mesencephalic locomotor region. *Acta Physiol. Scand.,* 87: 320–333.

Groves, P.M. (1983) A theory of the functional organization of the neostriatum and the neostriatal control of voluntary movement. *Brain Res. Rev.,* 5: 109–132.

Heffner, T.G. and Seiden, L.S. (1980) Synthesis of catecholamines from [^{3}H] tyrosine in brain during the performance of operant behavior. *Brain Res.,* 183: 403–419.

Hojrth, S. and Carlsson, A. (1988) In vivo receptor binding neurochemical and function studies with the dopamine D1 receptor antagonist SCH 23390. *J. Neural Transm.,* 72: 83–97.

Hong, S.C. and Levine, L. (1976) Stimulation of prostaglandin synthesis by bradykinin and thrombin and their mechanisms of action on MC5-5 fibroblasts. *J. Biol. Chem.,* 251: 5814–5816.

Hubner, C.B. and Koob, G.F. (1990) The ventral pallidum plays a role in mediating cocaine and heroin self-administration in the rat. *Brain Res.,* 508: 20–29.

Ioro, L.C., Barnett, A., Leitz, F.H., Hauser, V.P. and Korduba, C.A. (1983) SCH 23390 a potential benzazepine antipsychotic with unique interaction on dopaminergic systems. *J. Pharmacol. Exp. Ther.,* 226: 462–468.

Iversen, S.D. (1977) Brain dopamine system and behavior. In: L.L. Iversen, S.D. Iversen and S.H. Snyder (Eds.), *Handbook of Psychopharmacology, Vol. 8,* Plenum, New York, pp. 334–384.

Iversen, S.D. and Fray, P.J. (1982) Brain catecholamines in relation to affect. In: *Neural Basis of Behavior,* Spectrum, New York, pp. 229–269.

Jones, D.L. and Mogenson, G.J. (1980) Nucleus accumbens to globus pallidus GABA projection subserving ambulatory activity. *Am. J. Physiol.,* 238: R63–R69.

Joyce, E.M. and Koob, G.F. (1981) Amphetamine-, scopolamine-, and caffeine-induced locomotor activity following 6-hydroxydopamine lesions of the mesolimbic dopamine system. *Psychopharmacology,* 73: 311–313.

Joyce, E.M., Stinus, L. and Iversen, S.D. (1983) Effect of injections of 6-OHDA into either nucleus accumbens septi or frontal cortex on spontaneous and drug-induced activity. *Neuropharmacology,* 22: 1141–1145.

Kebabian, J.W. and Calne, D.B. (1979) Multiple receptors for dopamine. *Nature,* 277: 93–96.

Kelley, A.E., Gauthier, A.M. and Lang, C.G. (1989) Amphetamine microinjections into distinct striatal subregions cause dissociable effects on motor and ingestive behavior. *Behav. Brain Res.,* 35: 27–39.

Kelly, P., Seviour, P. and Iversen, S. (1976) Selective 6-OHDA induced destruction of mesolimbic dopamine neurons: abolition of psychostimulant induced locomotor activity in rats. *Eur. J. Pharmacol.,* 40: 45–56.

Kilpatrick, I.C., Starr, M.S., Fletcher, A., James, T.A. and MacLeod, N.K. (1980) Evidence for a GABAergic nigrothalamic pathway in the rat I. Behavioural and biochemical studies. *Exp. Brain Res.,* 40: 45–54.

Koob, G.F. (1992) Drugs of abuse: anatomy, pharmacology, and function of reward pathways. *Trends Pharmacol. Sci.,* 13: 177–184.

Koob, G.F. and Swerdlow, N.R. (1988) Functional output of the mesolimbic dopamine system. *Ann. N.Y. Acad. Sci.,* 537: 216–227.

Koob, G.F., Riley, S.J., Smith, S.C. and Robbins, T.W. (1978) Effects of 6-hydroxydopamine lesions of the nucleus accumbens septi and olfactory tubercle on feeding, locomotor activity, and amphetamine anorexia in the rat. *J. Comp. Physiol. Psychol.,* 92: 917–927.

Koob, G.F., Simon, H., Herman, J.P. and Le Moal, M. (1984) Neuroleptic-like disruption of the conditioned avoidance response requires destruction of both the mesolimbic and nigrostriatal dopamine systems. *Brain Res.,* 303: 319–329.

Koob, G.F., Le, H.T. and Creese, I. (1987) D-1 receptor antagonist SCH 23390 increases cocaine self-administration in the rat. *Neurosci. Lett.,* 79: 315–321.

Koob, G.F., Vaccarino, F.J., Amalric, M. and Bloom, F.E. (1987) Positive reinforcement properties of drugs: search for neural substrates. In: J. Engel and L. Oreland (Eds.), *Brain Reward Systems and Abuse,* Raven Press, New York, pp. 35–50.

Kornetsky, C. and Bain, G. (1982) Biobehavioral bases of the reinforcing properties of opiate drugs. *Ann. N.Y. Acad. Sci.,* 398: 240–259.

Larrson, E.L. (1980) Cyclosporin-A and dexamethasone suppress all responses by selectively acting at distinct sites of the triggering processes. *J. Immunol.,* 124: 2828.

Leff, S.E. and Creese, I. (1983) Dopamine receptors re-explained. *Trends Pharmacol. Sci.,* 4: 463–467.

Le Moal, M. and Simon, H. (1991) Mesocorticolimbic

dopaminergic network: functional and regulatory roles. *Physiol. Rev.*, 71: 155 – 234.

Liao, R.M. and Fowler, S.C. (1990) Haloperidol produces within session increments in operant response duration in rats. *Pharmacol. Biochem. Behav.*, 36: 199 – 201.

Lidsky, T.I., Buchwald, N.A., Manetto, C. and Schneider, J.S. (1985) A consideration of sensory factors involved in the motor functions of the basal ganglia. *Brain Rev. Res.*, 9: 133 – 146.

Lyness, W.H., Friedle, N.M. and Moore, K.E. (1979) Destruction of dopaminergic nerve terminals in nucleus accumbens: effect of D-amphetamine self-administration. *Pharmacol. Biochem. Behav.*, 11: 663 – 666.

Lyon, M. and Robbins, T.W. (1975) The action of central nervous system stimulant drugs: a general theory concerning amphetamine effects. In: W. Essman and L. Valzelli (Eds.), *Current Developments in Psychopharmacology, Vol. 2,* Spectrum Publications, New York, pp. 79 – 163.

Mailman, R.D., Schulz, D.W., Lewis, M.H., Staples, L., Rollema, H. and Dehaven, D.L. (1984) SCH 23390, a selective D1 dopamine antagonist with potent D2 behavioral actions. *Eur. J. Pharmacol.*, 101: 159 – 160.

Marsden, C.D. (1982) The mysterious motor function of the basal ganglia. *Neurology,* 32: 514 – 539.

Marsden, C.D. (1992) Dopamine and basal ganglia disorders in humans. *Semin. Neurosci.,* 4: 171 – 178.

Miller, R., Wickens, J.R. and Beninger, R.J. (1990) Dopamine D1 and D2 receptors in relation to reward and performance. A case for the D1 receptor as a primary site for therapeutic action of neuroleptic drugs. *Prog. Neurobiol.*, 34: 143 – 183.

Mitchell, I.J., Cross, A.J., Sambrook, M.A. and Crossman, A.R. (1986) Neural mechanisms mediating 1-methyl-4-phenyl 1,2,3,6-tetrahydropyridine induced parkinsonism in the monkey: relative contributions of the striato-pallidal and striato-nigral pathways as suggested by 2-deoxyglucose uptake. *Neurosci. Lett.*, 63: 61 – 65.

Mitchell, I.J., Clarke, C.E., Boyce, S., Robertson, R.G., Peggs, D., Sambrook, A. and Crossman, A.R. (1989) Neural mechanisms underlying parkinsonian symptoms based upon regional uptake of 2-deoxyglucose in monkeys exposed to 1-methyl, 4-phenyl, 1,2,3,6-tetrahydropyridine. *Neuroscience,* 32: 213 – 226.

Mogenson, G.J. and Nielson, M.A. (1983) Evidence that an accumbens to subpallidal GABAergic projection contributes to locomotor activity. *Brain Res. Bull.*, 11: 309 – 314.

Mogenson, G.J., Wu, M. and Jones, D.L. (1980) Locomotor activity elicited by injections of picrotoxin into the ventral tegmental area is attenuated by injections of GABA into the globus pallidus. *Brain Res.*, 191: 569 – 571.

Ouagazzal, A., Nieoullon, A. and Amalric, M. (1993) Effects of dopamine D1 and D2 receptor blockade on MK-801-induced hyperlocomotion in rats. *Psychopharmacology,* 107: in press.

Phillips, G., Willner, P. and Muscat, R. (1991a) Suppression of facilitation of operant behavior by raclopride is dependent on concentration of sucrose reward. *Psychopharmacology,* 105: 239 – 246.

Phillips, G., Willner, P. and Muscat, R. (1991b) Anatomical substrates for neuroleptic-induced reward attenuation and neuroleptic-induced response decrement. *Behav. Pharmacol.*, 2: 129 – 141.

Pijnenburg, A.J.J., Woodruff, G.N. and Van Rossum, J.M. (1975) Antagonism of apomorphine and D-amphetamine-induced stereotyped behavior by injection of low doses of haloperidol into the caudate nucleus and the nucleus accumbens. *Psychopharmacologia,* 45: 61 – 65.

Pretsell, D.O. and Robbins, T.W. (1992) D1 and D2 receptor subtypes in the rat striatum: modulation of reaction time performance. British Association for Psychopharmacology-European Behavioural Pharmacology Society, Cambridge, Aug. 12. *J. Psychopharmacol.,* 172 (abstract.)

Pullman, S.L., Watts, R.L., Juncos, J.L., Chase, T.N. and Sanes, J.N. (1988) Dopaminergic effects on simple and choice reaction time performance in Parkinson's disease. *Neurology,* 38: 249 – 254.

Pycock, C.J. and Horton, R. (1976) Evidence for an accumbens-pallidal pathway in the rat and its possible gabaminergic control. *Brain Res.*, 110: 629 – 634.

Pycock, C.J. and Phillipson, O.T. (1984) A neuroanatomical and neuropharmacological analysis of basal ganglia output. In: L.L. Iversen, S.D. Iversen and S.H. Snyder (Eds.), *Handbook of Psychopharmacology, Vol. 18, Drugs, Neurotransmitters and Behavior,* Plenum, New York, pp. 191 – 278.

Robbins, T.W. and Brown, V.J. (1990) The role of the striatum in the mental chronometry of action: a theoretical review. In: J.P. Huston and E.G. Jones (Eds.), *Reviews in the Neurosciences, Vol. 2,* Freund Publishing House, pp. 181 – 213.

Robbins, T.W. and Everitt, B.J. (1982) Functional studies of the central catecholamines. *Int. Rev. Neurobiol.*, 23: 303 – 365.

Robbins, T.W. and Everitt, B.J. (1992) Functions of dopamine in the dorsal and ventral striatum. *Semin. Neurosci.,* 4: 119 – 127.

Robbins, T.W. and Koob, G.F. (1980) Selective disruption of displacement behaviour by lesions of the mesolimbic dopamine system. *Nature,* 285: 409 – 412.

Roberts, D.C.S., Koob, G.F., Klonoff, P. and Fibiger, H.C. (1980) Extinction and recovery of cocaine self-administration following 6-hydroxydopamine lesions of the nucleus accumbens. *Pharmacol. Biochem. Behav.*, 12: 781 – 787.

Salamone, J.D. (1991) Behavioral pharmacology of dopamine systems: a new synthesis. In: P. Willner and J. Scheel-Krüger (Eds.), *The Mesolimbic Dopamine System: from Motivation to Action, Vol. 23,* Wiley, New York, pp. 599 – 613.

Salamone, J.D., Keller, R.W., Zigmond, M.J. and Stricker, E.M. (1989) Behavioral activation in rats increases striatal dopamine metabolism measured by dialysis perfusion. *Brain Res.*, 487: 215 – 224.

Scatton, B., Rouquier, L., Javoy-Agid, F. and Agid, Y. (1982) Dopamine deficiency in the cerebral cortex in Parkinson's dis-

226

ease. *Neurology,* 32: 1039 – 1040.

Scheel-Kruger, J. (1986) Dopamine GABA interactions: evidence that GABA transmits, modulates and mediates dopaminergic functions in the basal ganglia and the limbic system. *Acta Neurol. Scand.,* 73: 9 – 54.

Scheel-Kruger, J., Magelund, G. and Olianas, M.C. (1981) Role of GABA in the striatal output systems: globus pallidus, nucleus entopeduncularis, substantia nigra and nucleus subthalamicus. In: G. Di Chiara and G.L. Gessa (Eds.), *GABA and the Basal Ganglia,* Raven Press, New York, pp. 165 – 186.

Skinner, R.D. and Garcia-Rill, E. (1984) The mesencephalic locomotor region (MLR) in the rat. *Brain Res.,* 323: 385 – 389.

Spirduso, W.W., Gilliam, P.E., Schallert, T., Upchart, M., Vaugn, D.M. and Wilcox, R.E. (1985) Reactive capacity: a sensitive behavioral marker of movement initiation and nigrostriatal dopamine function. *Brain Res.,* 335: 45 – 54.

Statton, L.M. and Solomon, P.R. (1984) Microanalysis of D-amphetamine into the nucleus accumbens and caudate putamen. *Physiol. Psychol.,* 12: 159 – 162.

Staunton, D., Magistretti, P., Koob, G.F., Shoemaker, W. and Bloom, F.E. (1982) Dopaminergic supersensitivity induced by denervation and chronic receptor blockade is additive. *Nature,* 229: 72 – 74.

Stellar, J.R. and Rice, M.B. (1989) Pharmacological basis of intracranial self-stimulation reward. In: J.M. Liebman and S.J. Cooper (Eds.), *The Neuropharmacological Basis of Reward,* Clarendon Press, Oxford, pp. 14 – 65.

Swanson, L.W., Mogenson, G.J., Gerfen, C.R. and Robinson, P. (1984) Evidence for a projection from the lateral preoptic area and substantia innominata to the "mesencephalic locomotor region" in the rat. *Brain Res.,* 295: 161 – 178.

Swerdlow, N.R. and Koob, G.F. (1985) Separate neural substrates of the locomotor-activating properties of amphetamine, caffeine and corticotropin releasing factor (CRF) in the rat. *Pharmacol. Biochem. Behav.,* 23: 303 – 307.

Swerdlow, N.R., Swanson, L.W. and Koob, G.F. (1984) Electrolytic lesions of the substantia innominata and lateral preoptic area attenuate the "supersensitive" locomotor response to apomorphine resulting from denervation of the nucleus accumbens. *Brain Res.,* 306: 141 – 148.

Swerdlow, N.R., Vaccarino, F.J., Amalric, M. and Koob, G.F. (1986) The neural substrates for the motor-activating properties of psychostimulants. A review of recent findings. *Pharmacol. Biochem. Behav.,* 25: 232 – 248.

Swerdlow, N.R., Amalric, M. and Koob, G.F. (1987) Nucleus accumbens opiate-dopamine interactions and locomotor activation in the rat: evidence for a pre-synaptic locus. *Pharmacol. Biochem. Behav.,* 26: 765 – 769.

Taghzouti, K., Simon, H., Louilot, A., Herman, J.P. and Le Moal, M. (1985) Behavioral study after local injection of 6-hydroxydopamine into the nucleus accumbens in the rat. *Brain Res.,* 344: 9 – 20.

Ungerstedt, U. (1971) Adipsia and aphagia after 6-hydroxydopamine-induced degeneration of the nigrostriatal dopamine system. *Acta Physiol. Scand.* (Suppl.), 367: 96 – 122.

Vaccarino, F.J., Amalric, M., Swerdlow, N.R. and Koob, G.F. (1986) Blockade of amphetamine- but not opiate-induced locomotion following antagonism of dopamine function in the rat. *Pharmacol. Biochem. Behav.,* 24: 61 – 65.

Williams, J.T., Christie, M.J., North, R.A. and Roques, B.P. (1987) Potentiation of enkephalin action by peptidase inhibitors in rat locus coeruleus in vitro. *J. Pharmacol. Exp. Ther.,* 243: 397 – 401.

Woolverton, W.L. and Virus, R.M. (1989) The effects of a D1 and a D2 dopamine antagonist on behavior maintained by cocaine or food. *Pharmacol. Biochem. Behav.,* 32(3): 691 – 697.

Yokel, R.A. and Wise, R.A. (1975) Increased lever pressing for amphetamine after pimozide in rats: implications for a dopamine theory of reward. *Science,* 187: 547 – 549.

Young, W.S., Alheid, G.F. and Heimer, L. (1984) The ventral pallidal projection to the mediodorsal thalamus: a study with fluorescent retrograde tracers and immunohistofluorescence. *J. Neurosci.,* 4: 1626 – 1638.

Zis, A.P. Fibiger, H.C. and Phillips, A.G. (1974) Reversal by L-Dopa of impaired learning due to destruction of the dopaminergic nigroneostriatal projection. *Science,* 185: 960 – 962.

G.W. Arbuthnott and P.C. Emson (Eds.)
Progress in Brain Research, Vol. 99

CHAPTER 15

Reward-related activity in the monkey striatum and substantia nigra

Wolfram Schultz, Paul Apicella, Tomas Ljungberg, Ranulfo Romo and Eugenio Scarnati

Institut de Physiologie, Université de Fribourg, CH-1700 Fribourg, Switzerland

Introduction

The basal ganglia are often considered as parts of the motor system. This concept is derived from the movement disorders arising in parkinsonism, chorea and hemiballism, from the projections of the primary motor and somatosensory cortex to the putamen and subthalamic nucleus, and from movement-related neuronal activity in several basal ganglia nuclei. The motor role of the basal ganglia can be extended to include preparatory activity preceding the execution of limb and eye movements which reflects neuronal access to stored information about forthcoming events and thus constitutes a higher function than primary movement processes. However, there are a number of indications suggesting a larger involvement of the basal ganglia in behavioral processes. In particular, the basal ganglia, notably the striatum, receive input from several limbic structures, such as the amygdala and the orbitofrontal and cingulate cortex. In addition, results from lesioning and psychopharmacological experiments indicate that the functions of the nigrostriatal, mesolimbic and mesocortical dopamine systems encompass a larger spectrum of behavioral processes than a primary motor role suggested by the movement disorders. In particular, they appear to participate in motivational processes determining behavioral activity.

In order to assess the involvement of the basal ganglia in motivational processes, we studied the activity of neurons in the dorsal and ventral striatum and of dopamine neurons in the substantia nigra in relation to the delivery of primary rewards. Examples of primary rewards are food objects or fluids that are approached by subjects through innate or instinctive behavior, or are learned very early during ontogenesis. Primary rewards may serve to establish and sustain learned appetitive behavior, in which case they are called positive reinforcers. Thus, primary rewards are key components in the motivational control of behavior.

Methods

The studies were performed on *Macaca fascicularis* monkeys that performed various behavioral tasks under computer control for obtaining food or liquid reward. The activity of single neurons was recorded during task performance with moveable microelectrodes while monitoring arm and mouth muscle activity and eye movements through chronically implanted electrodes, lick detectors and closed-circuit video systems.

Behavioral procedures

The behavioral apparatus was positioned at reaching distance in the right half of the frontal wall of a completely enclosed primate chair. It contained an immovable, touch-sensitive key upon which the animal rested one hand prior to trial start. In tasks using liquid reward, the apparatus contained a yellow, rectangular light-emitting diode mounted at 27° lateral to the midsagittal plane at eye level of the animal. A small lever was positioned 40 mm below this light. A round light-emitting diode of 3 mm diameter was located 10 mm above the lever. A drop of apple juice delivered by an electronically controlled solenoid valve served as reward. In tasks using food rewards, the behavioral apparatus instead contained a food box mounted at the same position as the lights and the lever. The box had a frontal opening of 40 × 40 mm, and a cover in front of it prevented vision into its interior while permitting access of the animal's hand. Monkeys were deprived of fluid or food during weekdays. They were released into their home cages after each daily experiment of 3 – 4 h.

Striatal neurons. Animals performed in a delayed go-no-go task for liquid reward. A trial was initiated when the round light diode was illuminated for 1 sec with green or red color which served as instruction signal indicating a ''go'' or ''no-go'' situation, respectively. After a randomly varying interval of 3 ± 0.5 sec, the yellow, rectangular light was illuminated for 400 msec. In the go situation, the light served as a trigger stimulus in reaction to which the animal released the key, touched the lever and received a drop of apple juice. In the no-go situation, the animal had to remain on the resting key for a fixed duration of 2 or 3 sec after trigger light onset in order to receive the same reward. Go and no-go trials alternated randomly. Thus, reward was delivered in two behavioral situations which differed according to an arm movement being executed or withheld.

Dopamine neurons. Animals performed in a simple reaction time task in which the yellow trigger light served to elicit an arm movement from the resting key towards the lever in order to obtain liquid reward. Dopamine neurons were also investigated in two different food box tasks. In a simple reaction time task, the animal released the resting key when the food box opened and moved its hand into the box in order to collect a small morsel of apple or cookie. In the second task, employed with the same neurons, animals performed self-initiated arm movements in the absence of any external phasic stimulus to obtain a morsel of apple or cookie from the box. Since animals could not see the food inside the box, the touch of the food was the first external phasic stimulus to the animal in each trial, and there were no phasic reward-predicting stimuli preceding the contact with reward. The box did not contain food when animals moved too frequently (more than once every 5 sec), a measure that made the contact with reward an incompletely expected stimulus.

The different lights and the solenoid for delivering liquid reward were driven by output pulses from a laboratory computer which also controlled the behavioral performance. Key release was detected by a frequency-sensing circuit which reacted to a change in electrical capacity induced by the touch of the animal's hand. Entering the food box was monitored by interruption of an infrared light beam across the entrance of the food box. Manual contact with the food was detected by an electrical artifact produced when the wire holding the food was moved.

Data acquisition and evaluation

Following behavioral conditioning, animals were implanted under anesthesia and aseptic conditions with two cylinders for head fixation, a stainless steel chamber for holding the microelectrode, thin wire electrodes in arm and mouth muscles for recording electromyograms (EMGs) and periorbital electrodes for measuring eye movements. The activity of single neurons was recorded extracellulary with moveable tungsten miroelectrodes. Neuronal discharges were converted into standard digital pulses by means of an adjustable Schmitt-trigger, the output of which was continuously monitored on a digital oscilloscope together with the original wave form. EMGs and eye movements were collected during all neuronal recordings and converted to 12-bit digital signals. Filtered and rectified EMGs were also displayed on oscilloscopes and converted into digital pulses by an adjustable Schmitt-trigger. Licking movements were recorded by a touch-sensitive device connected to the spout. Digital signals derived from neuronal discharges, behavioral events, EMGs, licking movements and eye movements were sampled and displayed during the experiment by the computer. Only neurons tested with at least 15 trials in a given situation are reported. Recording positions in the striatum and substantia nigra were marked toward the end of the experiment by small electrolytic lesions and reconstructed on cresyl violet-stained coronal sections of the perfused brains.

Results

Responses of striatal neurons to the delivery of reward

The caudate nucleus, the putamen and the ventral striatum including the nucleus accumbens were predominantly investigated rostral to the anterior commissure and up to about 3 mm behind it. We defined the ventral striatum by the common, heavy innervation from the amygdala (Russchen et al., 1985) and the orbitofrontal and cingulate cortex (Selemon and Goldman-Rakic, 1985). The dorsal limit of this region extends from the ventral tip of the lateral ventricle to the internal capsule and descends farther laterally towards the inferior border of the putamen. Nucleus accumbens forms the medial portion of this area.

In the delayed go-no-go task, a drop of liquid was given each time the animal correctly executed or withheld an arm movement in reaction to the visual stimulus. Of 1593 neurons in caudate, putamen and ventral striatum, 115 showed increased activity in response to the delivery of liquid reward in both go and no-go trials (Apicella et al., 1991) (Fig. 1). Responding neurons were predominantly located in dorsal and ventromedial parts of anterior putamen, in dorsal and ventral caudate, and in nucleus accumbens. They were proportionally twice as frequent in ventral as compared to dorsal striatal areas. Responses occurred at a median latency of 337 msec and lasted for 525 msec, with insignificant differences between dorsal and ventral striatum. Reward responses could be differentiated from movement-related activity in the face area of posterior putamen

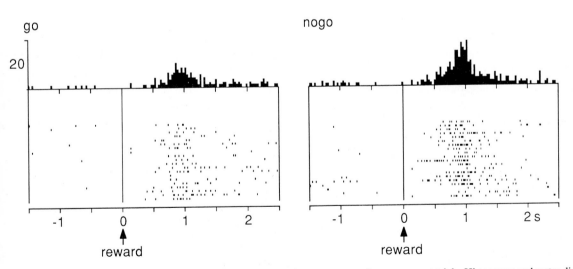

Fig. 1. Response to receipt of reward in dorsal putamen neuron in movement and no-movement trials. Histograms and raster displays of neuronal impulses are aligned on the electronic pulse driving the solenoid valve for reward delivery. Each dot denotes the time of an impulse, the distance to reward corresponding to their real-time interval. Each line of dots represents activity during performance in one trial. Go and no-go trials alternated randomly during the experiment. They were separated off-line and are shown in original sequence from above downward. Vertical calibration is 20 impulses/bin for both histograms.

where activity varied synchronously with individual mouth movements. Responses were directly related to the delivery of primary liquid reward and not to auditory stimuli associated with it, as shown by the absence of responses when liquid delivery was interrupted while maintaining the associated solenoid noise. In most reward-responsive neurons, responses also occurred when reward was delivered outside of the task, suggesting that they were not specific for the reinforcement of this particular task. Thus, neurons of dorsal and particularly ventral striatum are involved in processing information concerning the receipt of primary reward.

Activity of striatal neurons related to the expectation of reward

In the delayed go-no-go task, animals were instructed by a green light to perform a reaching movement when a trigger stimulus came on about 3 sec later (go situation). Movement was withheld after the same trigger light when the instruction cue had been red (no-go situation). Liquid reward was delivered upon correct performance in both situations. The individual task components became predictable to the animal after sufficient behavioral experience. Thus, the task included successive, separate time periods during which signals of behavioral significance were expected, the execution or inhibition of a reaching movement was prepared, and the delivery of reward was expected. The activity of 87 of 1173 neurons in caudate and putamen and 43 of 420 neurons in the ventral striatum showed sustained increases of activity which specifically *preceded* the delivery of reward, rather than occurring *after* the delivery of reward as in the reward responses mentioned above (Apicella et al., 1992) (Fig. 2). Reward expectation-related increases continued until the reward and were independent of the arm movement being executed or withheld. Thus, these activations occurred when the animal expected the predictable reward which was the common external event in both situations. In a series of additional tests, these activities were found to be prolonged when reward was delayed, disappeared within a few trials when reward was omitted and

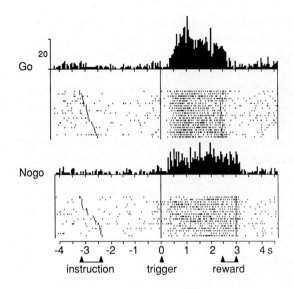

Fig. 2. Activation of a putamen neuron preceding delivery of reward in both go and no-go trials. The activation began after trigger onset and terminated upon reward delivery. In go trials, the early part of the activation coincided with the reaching movement. In no-go trials, the activation lasted during the total duration of movement inhibition. Note the absence of activation during the expectation of the trigger stimulus following instruction onset (left parts of upper and lower panels). Thus, this neuron was specifically activated during a time period during which reward was expected. Go and no-go trials alternated randomly during the experiment and were separated for analysis.

were temporally unrelated to mouth or eye movements. Changes in the appetitive value of the reward liquid modified the magnitude of activations, suggesting a possible relationship to the hedonic properties of the expected event. Activations also occurred when reward was delivered in a predictable manner outside of any behavioral task. These neurons are distinguished from other striatal neurons showing sustained activations during other periods of the task, such as during the expectation of the instruction or trigger stimuli independent of movement or no-movement reactions, and during the preparation of execution or inhibition of movements. Interestingly, most expectation- and preparation-related ventral striatal neurons were activated in relation to the expectation of reward (43 of 54 neurons = 80%), whereas a much lower proportion of this type of neurons in the dorsal cau-

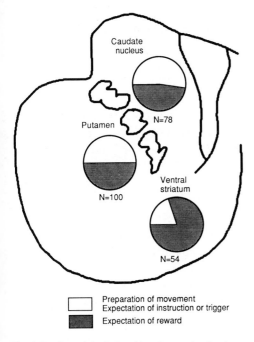

Preparation of movement
Expectation of instruction or trigger

Expectation of reward

Fig. 3. Preferential relationship of ventral striatal neurons to the expectation of reward. N, numbers of neurons in dorsal caudate, dorsal putamen and ventral striatum, respectively, that were activated during the expectation of instructions or trigger stimuli, during the preparation of behavioral reactions or during the expectations of reward. Shaded sectors indicate fractions of neurons activated during expectation of reward (36 of 78 neurons, 46% in dorsal caudate; 51 of 100, 51% in dorsal putamen; 43 of 54, 80% in ventral striatum).

date and putamen showed this preferential relationship (87 of 178 neurons = 49%) (Fig. 3).

These data show that striatal neurons are activated in relation to the expectation and preparation of individual environmental and behavioral events that occur predictably during task performance and are known to the animal through prior experience. These activations may reflect neuronal processes in which information acquired through past experience may be used for guiding the behavior of the subject. The presence of activations related to the expectation of reward suggests that these neurons have access to central representations of reward and thereby participate in the processing of information underlying the motivational control of goal-directed behavior.

Responses of dopamine neurons to food and fluid rewards

Dopamine neurons of substantia nigra (A9) and adjoining groups A8 and A10 discharged initially negative or positive impulses at low frequencies (0.5 – 7.0 imp./sec) and with polyphasic wave forms of relatively long durations (1.8 – 5.0 msec), in agreement with our previous experience (Schultz, 1986; Schultz and Romo, 1987; Romo and Schultz, 1990). In these characteristics, dopamine neurons contrasted with reticulata neurons of substantia nigra discharging impulses of < 1.1 msec duration at median rates of 70 – 90 imp./sec, with a few neurons discharging short impulses (< 1.0 msec) at low rates, and with presumptive fibers discharging very

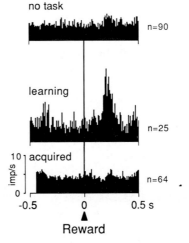

Fig. 4. Development of population response of dopamine neurons to the delivery of liquid reward during learning of a reaction time task. Population histograms were calculated from all neurons tested in two monkeys in each learning phase, independent of individual neuronal responses (n, numbers of neurons). Thus, there was a net response of the population of dopamine neurons to the delivery of liquid reward during learning, but not before when reward was regularly delivered (once every 2.5 – 3.5 sec) or after task acquisition when reward delivery was preceded by a known, predictive stimulus. For each population histogram, histograms from each neuron normalized for trial number were added and the resulting sum divided by the number of neurons. Vertical calibration indicates mean impulsive activity. (Reproduced from Ljungberg et al., 1992, with permission from The American Physiological Society.)

short impulses (0.1 – 0.3 msec). Neurons with these properties were antidromically activated from the striatum and were depressed in their activity by low doses of the dopamine receptor agonist apomorphine (Schultz, 1986; Schultz and Romo, 1987). These electrophysiological characterizations allow us to study the behavioral involvement of neurons containing the neurotransmitter dopamine in awake animals performing controlled behavioral tasks.

Dopamine neurons were recorded in monkeys that learned to perform a simple reaction time task in which they reached from the resting key towards the lever ahead of them when a small light came up. During the learning, which took 2 – 3 days, half of 25 dopamine neurons responded with a single impulse or a short burst of impulses when the drop of liquid reward arrived after correct task performance (Ljungberg et al., 1992) (Fig. 4). The same neurons did not respond when reward was delivered at regular intervals (2.5 – 3.5 sec) without performance of any task. However, neurons lost responses to primary reward after task performance was established and instead responded to the conditioned

light in more than half of 64 neurons. Thus, the response was transferred from primary reward during learning to the conditioned stimulus that predicted reward and had the capacity to elicit arm and eye movement reactions. These data show that a considerable portion of dopamine neurons respond to the most important appetitive stimuli in a given behavioral situation, this being primary liquid reward during learning and a stimulus-predicting reward and eliciting behavioral reactions after learning.

These results reflect the activity of the population of dopamine neurons, since different neurons were recorded during the various stages of learning. However, a similar differential relationship to primary rewards and conditioned stimuli was found when the activity of single dopamine neurons was compared across different behavioral situations. With self-initiated arm movements, animals released the resting key at a self-chosen moment, entered the food box and touched a morsel of food behind the cover without seeing it. Here, the contact with reward was not preceded by a predictive stimu-

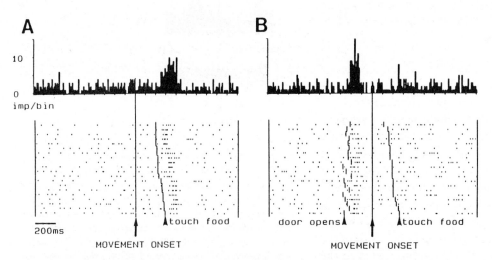

Fig. 5. Transfer of response from (A) primary food reward in the absence of predictive stimuli to (B) a conditioned stimulus predicting food reward in a single dopamine neuron. This neuron responded when the animal touched a morsel of apple during self-initiated movements not preceded by external phasic stimuli (A). With stimulus-triggered movements, the neuron responded instead to the conditioned stimulus of opening of the food-containing box predicting the reward and serving as trigger stimulus for the arm reaching movement (B). The sequence of trials is rearranged according to the time intervals between releasing the resting key ("movement onset") and touching the food inside the box. (Reproduced from Romo and Schultz, 1990, with permission from The American Physiological Society.)

lus and occurred in a partly unexpected manner. A non-habituating, phasic burst of impulses occurred in 130 of 154 dopamine neurons when the monkey's hand touched the food inside the box (Romo and Schultz, 1990) (Fig. 5A). The touch response was absent when the animal's hand touched the bare wire normally holding the food, when touching non-food objects, or during tactile exploration of the empty interior of the food box. Thus responses appeared to be related to the appetitive rather than the physical properties of the object being touched. Then some of the same neurons were tested in a simple reaction time task in which opening of the food box was the conditioned stimulus that predicted reward and elicited the arm movement. Of 72 dopamine neurons responding to the touch of food reward during self-initiated arm movements, 60 responded to box opening but entirely failed to respond to the touch of food in the box (Fig 5B). The response to door opening in this task was similar to the touch response during self-initiated movements in the same neurons in terms of latency, duration and magnitude. Apparently, the response was transferred in the same neuron from the primary food reward to the door opening when passing from self-initiated movements to those elicited by an external trigger stimulus.

Discussion

Primary rewards are key stimuli during learning and established behavior. They elicit approach behavior and, during learning, indicate to the subject that the task was correctly performed. Thus, they are key determinants for the frequency and intensity of behavioral reactions, the basic measure of motivation. When intrinsically neutral stimuli, such as a light or opening of a box, are repeatedly paired with primary rewards, they gain the capacity to elicit approach behavior. Recent animal learning theories propose that the effect of conditioned appetitive stimuli is related to a central representation of the primary reward that is evoked by a sufficiently well learned stimulus (Bolles, 1972; Bindra, 1974; Dickinson, 1980; Toates, 1986). Thus, the learned stimulus

predicting reward becomes an incentive stimulus by inducing an expectation of this prime motivational event and thereby directing the animal's behavior towards obtaining that goal.

This report presents evidence that dopamine neurons and neurons in the dorsal and ventral striatum show different relationships to the delivery of primary food and liquid rewards. Some striatal neurons respond unconditionally to the delivery of primary liquid rewards. These responses occurred in a well-established behavioral situation and may thus serve to indicate that reward has been received. This information can be used for reinforcing the stimulus-response relationship, a process that may occur outside of the striatum, since we have so far failed to find substantial numbers of striatal neurons with specific task reinforcement-related responses. Activating and depressing reward responses in other behavioral contexts have been observed in dorsal caudate during licking behavior (Rolls et al., 1983), after a pulse of rewarding milk or fruit juice (Soltysik et al., 1975; Schneider, 1987) and after a compound liquid reward-visual stimulus (Hikosaka et al., 1989).

Other neurons in the striatum are activated while the animal expects the predictable reward after occurrence of the conditioned incentive stimulus. Whereas the instruction may also be a conditioned stimulus, the trigger stimulus eliciting approach or withholding behavior is the main incentive stimulus because it is situated temporally closer to the reward. It can be inferred that the conditioned trigger stimulus evoked a representation of the reward and thus induces an expectation of this event. Interestingly, the neuronal activity lasts during the whole time after the trigger stimulus during which the reward is being expected, i.e., until the reward has been obtained. Thus, the activity of these striatal neurons is able to contribute important information for learned behavioral reactions that are executed on the basis of an expectation of predictable reward. In comparison with the dorsal striatum, it is particularly interesting that the ventral striatum with its prominent input from limbic cortical and subcortical structures contains a higher number of neurons

234

activated during the expectation of reward or responding to the delivery of reward.

Yet another relationship to reward is found with dopamine neurons. These neurons only respond to reward when it is not entirely predictable, such as during the trial-and-error learning of tasks with specific constraints and during self-initiated movements without preceding phasic reward-predicting stimuli. Because the responses are transferred after learning to the conditioned incentive stimulus eliciting the movement, it appears that dopamine neurons do not respond to primary reward unconditionally, like some striatal neurons, but that the response is due to the salient, alerting stimulus property of primary reward during learning. With progressive learning, stimulus salience is transferred to the conditioned incentive stimulus that predicts reward and has the capacity to elicit behavioral reactions, whereas the predictable reward is merely a confirmatory stimulus which, accordingly, fails to activate dopamine neurons. Thus, dopamine neurons appear to respond to the large class of salient, alerting stimuli, of which primary reward is an important, albeit not exclusive member. The response to primary reward then occurs under the condition that reward constitutes a salient stimulus. Reward responses during learning signal that the most important stimulus in this situation, primary reward, has occurred, but without encoding specific information about the behavioral reaction. Information about the presence of an alerting stimulus requesting a behavioral reaction would be conducted by the evoked impulses of dopamine neurons to the dopamine terminal areas, such as the dorsal and ventral striatum and the frontal cortex where impulse-dependent dopamine release (Gonon and Buda, 1985; Gonon, 1988) influences postsynaptic neurons involved in the specific details of the emergent behavioral reaction. Thus, the responses of dopamine neurons would be able to facilitate the learning of approach behavior by engaging arousing, motivational and activating processes that determine behavioral reactivity. A role of dopamine systems in incentive motivational processes and motivational arousal has been proposed on the basis of dopamine depletions and blockade of dopamine receptors (Wise, 1982; Beninger, 1983; Fibiger and Philips, 1986; Robbins et al., 1989).

Acknowledgements

The experiments were supported by the Swiss NSF (grants 3.533-0.83, 3.473-0.86, 31-28591.90), the United Parkinson Foundation (Chicago) and the Italian CNR. P. Apicella received postdoctoral fellowships from the Fondation pour la Recherche Médicale (Paris) and the Fyssen Foundation.

References

Apicella, P., Ljungberg, T., Scarnati, E. and Schultz, W. (1991) Responses to reward in monkey dorsal and ventral striatum. *Exp. Brain Res.,* 85: 491 – 500.

Apicella, P., Scarnati, E., Ljungberg, T. and Schultz, W. (1992) Neuronal activity in monkey striatum related to the expectation of predictable environmental events. *J. Neurophysiol.,* 68: 945 – 960.

Beninger, R.J. (1983) The role of dopamine in locomotor activity and learning. *Brain Res. Rev.,* 6: 173 – 196.

Bindra, D. (1974) A motivational view of learning, performance, and behavior modification. *Psychol. Rev.,* 81: 199 – 213.

Bolles, R.C. (1972) Reinforcement, expectancy and learning. *Psychol. Rev.,* 79: 394 – 409.

Dickinson, A. (1980) *Contemporary Animal Learning Theory,* Cambridge University Press, Cambridge.

Fibiger, H.C. and Phillips, A.G. (1986) Reward, motivation, cognition: psychobiology of mesotelencephalic dopamine systems. In: *Handbook of Physiology – The Nervous System, IV.* Am. Physiol. Soc., Bethesda, MD, pp. 647 – 675.

Gonon, F.G. (1988) Nonlinear relationship between impulse flow and dopamine released by rat midbrain dopaminergic neurons as studied by in vivo electrochemistry. *Neuroscience,* 24: 19 – 28.

Gonon, F.G. and Buda, M.J. (1985) Regulation of dopamine release by impulse flow and by autoreceptors as studied by in vivo voltammetry in the rat striatum. *Neuroscience,* 14: 765 – 774.

Hikosaka, O., Sakamoto, M. and Usui, S. (1989) Functional properties of monkey caudate neurons. III. Activities related to expectation of target and reward. *J. Neurophysiol.,* 61: 814 – 832.

Ljungberg, T., Apicella, P. and Schultz, W. (1992) Responses of monkey dopamine neurons during learning of behavioral reactions. *J. Neurophysiol.,* 67: 145 – 163.

Robbins, T.W., Cador, M., Taylor, J.R. and Everitt, B.J. (1989) Limbic-striatal interactions in reward-related processes. *Neu-*

rosci. Biobehav. Rev., 13: 155 – 162.

Rolls, E.T., Thorpe, S.J. and Maddison, S.P. (1983) Responses of striatal neurons in the behaving monkey. 1. Head of the caudate nucleus. *Behav. Brain Res.,* 7: 179 – 210.

Romo, R. and Schultz, W. (1990) Dopamine neurons of the monkey midbrain: contingencies of responses to active touch during self-initiated arm movements. *J. Neurophysiol.,* 63: 592 – 606.

Russchen, F.T., Bakst, I., Amaral, D.G. and Price, J.L. (1985) The amygdalostriatal projections in the monkey. An anterograde tracing study. *Brain Res.,* 329: 241 – 257.

Schneider, J.S. (1987) Ingestion-related activity of caudate and entopeduncular neurons in the cat. *Exp. Neurol.,* 95: 216 – 233.

Schultz, W. (1986) Responses of midbrain dopamine neurons to behavioral trigger stimuli in the monkey. *J. Neurophysiol.,* 56:

1439 – 1462.

Schultz, W. and Romo, R. (1987) Responses of nigrostriatal dopamine neurons to high intensity somatosensory stimulation in the anesthetized monkey. *J. Neurophysiol.,* 57: 201 – 217.

Selemon, L.D. and Goldman-Rakic, P.S. (1985) Longitudinal topography and interdigitation of corticostriatal projections in the rhesus monkey. *J. Neurosci.,* 5: 776 – 794.

Soltysik, S., Hull, C.D., Buchwald, N.A. and Fekete, T. (1975) Single unit activity in basal ganglia of monkeys during performance of a delayed response task. *Electroenceph. Clin. Neurophysiol.,* 39: 65 – 78.

Toates, F. (1986) *Motivational Systems,* Cambridge University Press, Cambridge.

Wise, R.A. (1982) Neuroleptics and operant behavior: the anhedonia hypothesis. *Behav. Brain Sci.,* 5: 39 – 87.

G.W. Arbuthnott and P.C. Emson (Eds.)
Progress in Brain Research, Vol. 99
© 1993 Elsevier Science Publishers B.V. All rights reserved.

CHAPTER 16

The organization of somatosensory activity in dorsolateral striatum of the rat

Lucy L. Brown[1] and Samuel M. Feldman[2]

[1] *Departments of Neurology and Neuroscience, Albert Einstein College of Medicine, Bronx, NY 10461 and* [2] *Center for Neural Science, New York University, New York, NY 10003, U.S.A.*

Introduction

The function of the striatum and its intrinsic mechanisms are of particular interest to neuroscience because this nuclear complex is removed from the primary input and output pathways and may mediate "higher order" functions. The existence of neurochemical compartmentalization (e.g., Graybiel, 1990; Gerfen, 1992) and a pattern of input and output projections (e.g., Goldman and Nauta, 1977; Graybiel and Ragsdale, 1978; Graybiel et al., 1979; Goldman-Rakic and Selemon, 1990) indicate an underlying organization that might provide the substrate for segregation or integration of sensorimotor and/or cognitive information. However, the characterization of striatal neurochemical compartmentalization goes well beyond our current understanding of striatal functional organization. Although a general topographical arrangement of corticostriate input has been described, which is essential for functional studies, the details of localization remain elusive, as does the function for striatal neurons. For example, nothing approaching the organization of sensory thalamus (e.g., Jones, 1985) has been observed in striatum. Striatal neurons have functional properties that are related to the cortical origin of their input: primate putamen receives input from sensory and motor cortex and neural discharge is related to skeletal movement (Liles and Updyke, 1985); caudate receives input from frontal and prefrontal cortex (including frontal eye fields),

and neural discharge accompanies visual memory-guided saccades (Hikosaka, 1991). But a fuller understanding of the functional properties of the neurons may benefit from a more complete understanding of the anatomical organization.

We have been concerned with the organization of somatosensory input to rat striatum: it is first-order functional information that can be easily defined and experimentally controlled. Anatomical studies in primate and cat have shown that the terminals from primary somatosensory cortex (SI) form a complex somatotopic map that is extensive anteroposteriorly. In primate putamen, a general dorsal-to-ventral organization of leg/arm/face has been described (Kunzle, 1975, 1977; Flaherty and Graybiel, 1991), which is similar to the organization seen in cat (Malach and Graybiel, 1986). But the somatotopy is not always distinct (Kunzle, 1977); and the organization appears to shift from one coronal section to the next (e.g., Malach and Graybiel, 1986; Flaherty and Graybiel, 1991). Electrophysiological studies, which have generally confirmed the organization described by the anatomical work (e.g., Crutcher and DeLong, 1984; Alexander and DeLong, 1985), also indicate that the localization is confounded by some "intermingling of arm neurons with leg and orofacial neurons" (Crutcher and DeLong, 1984). In the rat, a dorsolateral "sensorimotor zone", equivalent to primate putamen (West et al., 1990), extends anteroposteriorly through most of the striatum (McGeorge and Faull,

1989). However, although neurons in this dorsolateral zone respond to movement (e.g., West et al., 1990; Carelli and West, 1991), even the limited somatotopy described in primate putamen has not been seen. This poses a difficult problem, because the organization of sensorimotor cortex input to striatum, which seems to be elusive, especially in the rat, must be determined if we are to understand the nature of its function.

We have developed a functional probe to study rat striatum using [^{14}C] deoxyglucose (DG) autoradiography (Sokoloff et al., 1977), a metabolic mapping technique that offers some unique advantages in approaching the problem. Rather than looking at a limited number of cells, one is afforded the opportunity to examine simultaneously the effects of a stimulus on the entire nervous system, within the limitations of the technique. (For example, increased glucose utilization reflects activity primarily in axon terminals, rather than in cell bodies or axons.) Although the technique does not permit exploration of the effects of many stimuli on a single cell, the effects of a limited number of stimuli can be examined extensively throughout the nervous system. First-order information, somatotopic representation of cutaneous stimulation, was used to map corticostriatal input to dorsolateral striatum, because understanding of the "higher order" functions of striatum will depend upon our first understanding the organization of the simplest kinds of signals. Unanesthetized rats were restrained while a motor-driven nylon bristle applied controlled strokes to different body regions in different animals. Our autoradiographic analysis included an image analysis procedure for feature detection that made possible objective identification of regions of maximal glucose utilization during presentation of the localized somatosensory stimulus. The image analysis program also permitted that the localization of regions maximally affected be translated into a system of Cartesian coordinates. Rather than making tracings from histological material, the procedure made possible a quantitative analysis of location and size of striatal regions of maximal glucose utilization, and to use inferential statistics to test the reliability of any observed localization of function. Our deoxyglucose mapping studies have revealed an unexpected, bilateral organization of functional activity in striatum that may best be described as a combinational map (see also Brown, 1992.)

The use of feature detection to localize maximal striatal activity

Glucose utilization is heterogeneous and patchy in striatum, even under control conditions (Brown et al., 1987), and it is difficult for the eye to detect differences from control. Accordingly, a detection technique was necessary to achieve reliable and objective identification of features as the loci of changes related to somatosensory input. Analysis of digitized autoradiograms was done on an image analysis system (Quantimet 970) that was programmed to detect regions of contiguous pixels ("features") at preset levels of sensitivity ("grey levels"). Fig. 1 illustrates the basic feature detection procedure used. The threshold grey level was the sensitivity at which the most optically dense pixels (minimum = 5; maximum = 10) were detected (Fig. 1A). When the detect level was set at 8 – 12 grey levels above threshold (Fig. 1B), a large region of maximal glucose utilization was apparent in dorsolateral striatum that was different from medial and ventral regions. A feature was defined as an area of 30 or more contiguous pixels (10000 μm^2) detected at 8 – 12 grey levels above threshold. As many as 25 features (typically 10) were detected in a single coronal section at the grey levels used for detection (Fig. 1C). In a previous study we found that this procedure preserves the heterogeneity of striatal glucose utilization and identifies independent zones of maximal striatal activity (Brown et al., 1987).

Area (μm^2) and position were calculated for each feature. A grid overlay was included in the image analysis program to enable translation of the autoradiograms into a system of Cartesian coordinates (Fig. 1C). The brain was oriented in the field to allow definition of the midline as X_0 and the dorsal edge of striatum as Y_0. Feature position was de-

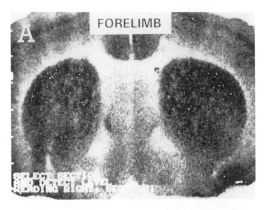

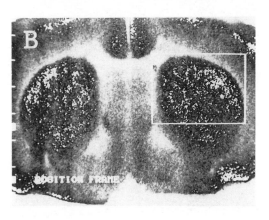

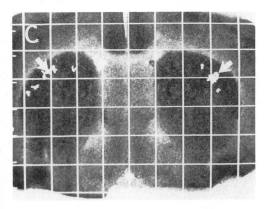

Fig. 1. Detection procedure for striatal features. Digitized autoradiogram of a coronal section from a rat that received stimulation of forelimb. Detected pixels are masked in white. *A*. Detection at two grey levels above theshold; at this grey level, only slightly more pixels are detected than at threshold. *B*. Detection at eight grey levels above threshold, the same level used for feature detection. *C*. Features in dorsal striatum. Detection is restricted to features that include clusters of at least 30 contiguous

fined as the location of its center of mass (centroid) relative to the established coordinate system. In addition, the anteroposterior (AP) level of each feature was established by localization of the section within the same stereotaxic coordinate system used to position the brain for sectioning. AP levels are referred to bregma (AP_0 mm), and were guided by the atlas of Paxinos and Watson (1986). The error in coordinate assignment caused by brain shape differences and angle of cut were rarely greater than 0.2 mm. Thus the centroid of each feature could be localized in three-dimensional space relative to bregma (AP_0), midline (X_0), and dorsal edge of striatum in a given section (Y_0).

The largest feature was initially detected at five grey levels above threshold. At this detect level, it was either the only feature detected, or was one of a group of two or three. Its size, at this level, was typically the minimum for feature definition. As the detect level was increased, the size of the largest feature continued to increase, and additional features were detected. Eventually, the detection level was sufficiently high that features began to merge, and the coordinates of the centroid of the newly detected largest feature changed. Accordingly, feature measurements were taken at the grey levels just below this, to preserve the identity of the largest feature, and to learn the extent of its size prior to losing identity. This feature is referred to as the *primary* feature. (Note that the largest feature on the right side of Fig. 1*C* (arrow) defines the region of highest glu-

pixels (10000 μm^2). The grid overlay makes possible alignment of the autoradiogram for location of feature centroids in a Cartesian coordinate system. The area of the largest feature on the right side (arrow) is 39000 μm^2 (two secondary features make the whole highlighted region 89000 μm^2). It defines the largest region of high glucose utilization contralateral to forelimb stimulation in this animal. The feature appears consistently across animals in response to the salient stimulus. Ipsilaterally, the largest feature is slightly offset from the contralateral location. Secondary features are also seen, both ipsi- and contralaterally, some of which are related to the salient stimulus; other reflect the fact that the animals are awake and alert, with the result that inputs other than the salient cutaneous stimulus had effects on regional glucose utilization.

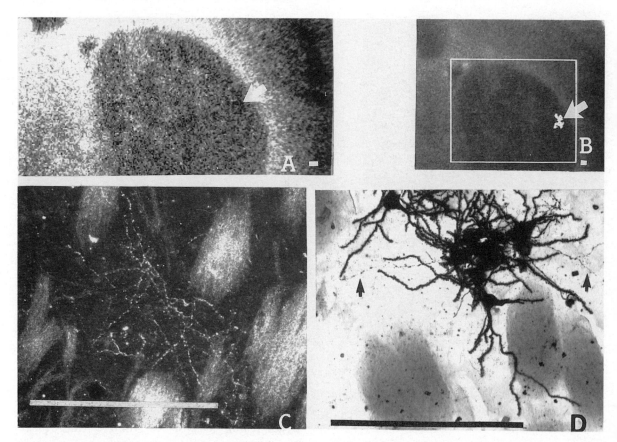

Fig. 2. Largest detected feature compared to corticostriate terminal endings and medium spiny neurons in rat striatum. *A*. Digitizer autoradiogram in a rat that received forelimb stimulation. The autoradiogram is digitized for glucose utilization, without detection masking. Note the regions of maximal glucose utilization in the dorsolateral quadrant of striatum. One is darker and larger than the rest (arrow). *B*. The same autoradiogram shown in *A*, at lower magnification. In this figure, the autoradiogram has been processed for feature detection at 10 grey levels above theshold. Only the largest feature, with an area of 49000 μm^2 is detected (arrow). *C*. Axon terminal cluster of a corticostriatal projection in dorsolateral striatum after iontophoretic application of PHA-L in forelimb SI cortex of a rat (40 μm section; Brown and Walkley, unpublished data). The long axis of the cluster is parallel to the external capsule and measures approximately 200 μm. *D*. Medium spiny cells in dorsolateral striatum of rat. Golgi preparation in a 40 μm section. The extent of axon collaterals (arrows) and dendritic arborization of a group of medium spiny cells in dorsolateral striatum is comparable to the cortical terminal field revealed by PHA-L (*C*) and to the size of the largest feature seen in contralateral striatum (*B*). Bars, 200 μm.

cose utilization contralateral to forelimb stimulation in this animal.) Smaller features are referred to as *secondary* features, a cluster of which was consistently related to the stimulation. Primary and secondary feature area and position were analyzed at 0.2 mm intervals, from the anterior pole of striatum (+ 2.2 mm) to 1.5 mm caudal to bregma (Paxinos and Watson, 1986). Because the animals are awake during the 45 min experimental session, many of the small features, seen both contra- and ipsilaterally,

were from inputs other than the salient stimulus; hence their localization varied widely from animal to animal.

The cellular substrate of striatal features

The source of increased glucose utilization appears to be metabolic activity in presynaptic axon terminals (e.g., Mata et al., 1980); hence the primary features identified in the striatum probably reflect the

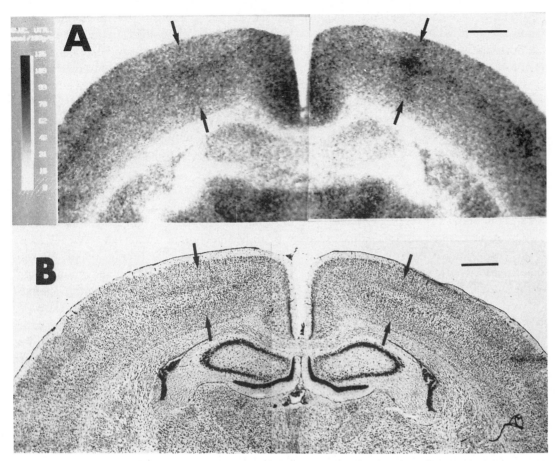

Fig. 3. Cortical activation during somatosensory stimulation. *A*. Digitized deoxyglucose autoradiogram of a coronal section through the cortex in an animal stimulated on the hindlimb. The image is coded for glucose utilization rate; the scale appears at the left. Arrows on the right indicate the region of increased glucose utilization contralateral to the somatosensory stimulation. Arrows on the left indicate a region of increase, ipsilateral to the stimulation, that may reflect cortico-cortical connections. *B*. Toluidine blue-stained alternate (20 μm) section to *A*. Arrows indicate the same regions as do the arrows in panel *A*. (Note that the sections are at slightly different magnifications.) The glucose utilization increase spans layers II – V, and is in the sensorimotor region for hindlimb defined by electrophysiological investigation (e.g., Hall and Lindholm, 1974; Chapin and Lin, 1984). The greatest increase is seen in layers IV and superficial V. Bars, 1.0 mm.

areas of largest clusters of axon terminals from cortex, with some contribution from axon collaterals of medium spiny neurons. Perhaps 95% of striatal neurons are medium spiny cells (Wilson, 1990), to which the terminal fields activated by the cutaneous stimulus are likely to project. Fig. 2*A* shows an autoradiogram digitized for glucose utilization, prior to initiation of detection procedures. In Fig. 2*B*, the same autoradiogram is seen at lower magnification, after image analysis processing, with the primary

feature masked at a 10 grey detect levels above pixel detect theshold. (As in Fig. 1, the stroke stimulus was applied to contralateral forelimb.) The size of the feature at this grey level was 49000 μm². (The primary contralateral feature in Fig. 1*C* was 39000 μm².) Note that primary features, which are derived from 20 μm sections, are comparable to the size of the terminal fields subtended by corticostriate axons that project to dorsolateral striatum, as seen in a 40 μm thick section stained for *Phaseolis vulgaris* leucoagglutinin (PHA-L) in Fig. 2*C*, and to the dendritic and axon collateral arborization of medium spiny cells in dorsolateral striatum seen in a Golgi preparation of a 40 μm thick section (Fig. 2*D*). This further suggests that the features may reflect activity in corticostriate terminals and axon collaterals of cell clusters to which they project.

Cortical effects of the somatosensory stimuli

Somatic stimulation of hindlimb, trunk, and forelimb affected the cortex in a predictable manner. The stimuli were continuous strokes of a nylon bristle (2.5 g; 3 – 4/sec) that covered a 2.0 cm path from anterior to posterior along a limb or the trunk. Primary somatosensory cortex was activated contralateral to the stimuli in a pattern consistent with activation of vertically arranged functional units. Layers II, III, IV and V showed increased glucose utilization in the granular region (Fig. 3). The pattern was evident even upon inspection of unprocessed autoradiograms. Some hindlimb and trunk animals also showed ipsilateral cortical effects (Fig. 3), which were not seen in forelimb animals. This is consistent with the known distribution of cortico-cortical connections in primate (Jones et al., 1979). The region of activation was typically 0.3 mm wide in coronal sections and extended continuously for 0.4 to 1.0 mm in the AP plane. The nature of the stimulus was such that a large part of the receptive field for the stimulated limb or trunk would be activated. The AP and mediolateral localization of hindlimb, trunk and forelimb activation in cortex was consistent with electrophysiological mapping studies (Hall and Lindholm, 1974; Chapin and Lin, 1984). Hindlimb was the most medial (centered 2.5 mm from the midline) and forelimb the most lateral (3.5 – 4.0 mm from the midline); the trunk area was situated between the two limbs mediolaterally (3.0 mm), but was more caudally located. This pattern and location of cortical activation confirms that the peripheral receptors activated functionally specific units of cortex, and identifies the primary source of cortical input to striatum in the animals studied. This is in contrast to electrical stimulation, which

can activate neural elements that do not necessarily function together physiologically. The pattern of activation seen in Fig. 3 is also unlike patterns revealed by anatomical anterograde tracing studies, because the latter often cover too large a region to be as functionally specific. In these studies, we had the opportunity to study the localization and pattern of activation in striatum that parallels the cortical activation during physiological stimulation.

Striatal effects

Maximal striatal activity, represented by features, was studied in coronal sections at seven AP levels from AP + 2.0 to − 1.0 (Paxinos and Watson, 1986). Differences from controls and among stimulation groups indicated that the activation spanned an AP region from + 1.0 to − 0.5 mm relative to bregma. Features of stimulated animals were larger than in control animals that were not restrained or stimulated in any way, and their positions were different from controls and from each other. Importantly, localization of a given body region was reliable at any one AP level, but the juxtaposition of the several stimulated regions varied from one AP level to another (Brown, 1992). A trend analysis showed that the major source of variance across the seven AP levels examined was best described by a sixth-order function, indicating that the representation of a single body region in striatum takes a somewhat helical AP course through dorsolateral striatum. The striatal location of the forelimb and hindlimb stimuli was also similar to activated striatal regions seen by Sharp and his colleagues (Sharp, 1984; Sharp et al., 1988), who stimulated the motor cortex to produce movement of the forelimb or hindlimb (Sharp, personal communication, and Brown and Sharp, unpublished data, Fig. 4).

Contralateral striatum

The striatal regions of primary features in hindlimb-, trunk- and forelimb-stimulated animals were clearly different at AP + 0.2 (Fig. 5*B*). They also reflected the organization of the cortex mediolaterally: hindlimb was most medial, trunk just

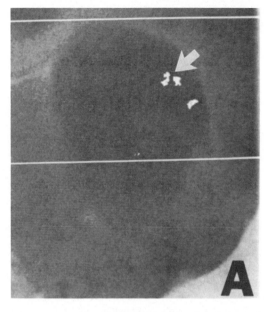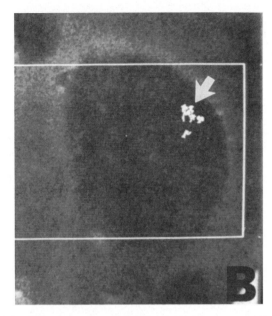

Fig. 4. *A*. Striatal localization of activation (arrows) associated with forelimb motor cortex stimulation, just below movement threshold (Brown and Sharp, unpublished data). *B*. Striatal localization of activation (arrow) associated with somatosensory stimulation of the forelimb. The two experimental conditions activate features in the same general region.

lateral to hindlimb, and forelimb most lateral. However, at other AP locations (e.g., AP $+1.0$, Fig. 5*D*), hindlimb animals were different from the other two, which were juxtaposed or intermingled. At bregma, features of all three groups were juxtaposed (Fig. 5*A*). A comparison of the arrangement at AP $+0.2$ with AP $+0.6$ shows that the relative positions of the groups were shifted between the two points: hindlimb was most dorsomedial at $+0.2$, but it shifted ventrally so that trunk became most dorsomedial at $+0.6$. Secondary features at this level reflected the relative positions of the primary features (Fig. 5*C*). However, secondary features at $+0.2$ intermingled with primary features from other body regions (Fig. 5*B*).

When all AP regions are considered together, the group mean mediolateral and dorsoventral positions of primary features show several important effects as a function of AP level. First, as seen in Fig. 6, each group does not show a simple linear repetition of its position from anterior to posterior, but shows deviations, either mediolaterally or dorsoventrally. Importantly, a trend analysis showed

that the most significant effect of AP with respect to dorsoventral location is best described by a sixth-order polynomial for each body region ($P < 0.02$, $P < 0.02$, $P < 0.004$). The individual deviations from one AP level to the next stay within 0.7 mm of each other, as all groups shift ventrolaterally from AP $+1.0$ to -0.5. Second, there is a significant group $\times$ AP interaction (dorsoventral position, $P < 0.01$) exemplified in Figs. 5 and 6. The interaction suggests that to predict the localization of activation in striatum associated with body region, one has to know not only the body region stimulated, but also the AP level examined. Fig. 6 also demonstrates how the juxtaposition of hindlimb and forelimb alternate from anterior to posterior. At AP $+0.6$ they are within 0.25 mm; at $+0.2$ they are over 1.0 mm apart; at 0.0 they are within 0.25 mm again. In the same regions the trunk alternates its relative position from being closest to hindlimb at AP $+0.6$, to being equidistant between hindlimb and forelimb ($+0.2$), to being closest to forelimb (0.0).

The localization of activation in striatum of

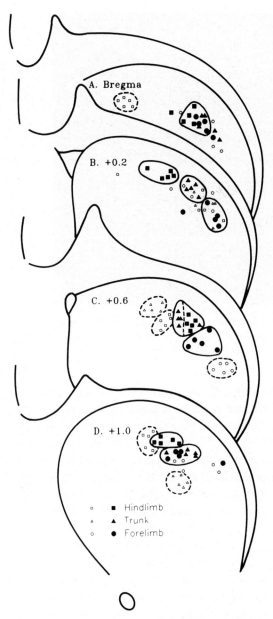

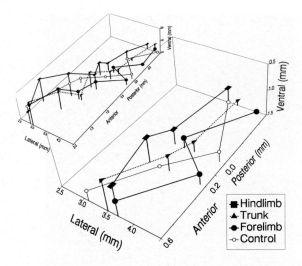

Fig. 6. Graphical representation of the mean positions of the hindlimb, trunk and forelimb areas of maximal activity in striatum. Upper graph: all AP levels sampled are shown. Hindlimb is the most dorsomedial point at all but one AP level. Forelimb is the most ventrolateral at four AP levels. Each group shows a different AP localization compared to control, and to each other. Lower graph: enlargement of four of the AP levels shown above. The relative positions of the different representations of body region are demonstrated. Relative to hindlimb and forelimb, trunk is dorsomedial to both at +0.6, between both at +0.2, and ventrolateral to both at 0.0.

animals stimulated on the hindlimb and forelimb simultaneously was similar to that seen in individually stimulated animals (Fig. 7). At bregma, where all body regions appeared to be intermingled in maps of individually stimulated animals, there were two features closely juxtaposed in the simultaneously stimulated animals (Fig. 8).

Fig. 5. Plots of centroids of primary (filled symbols) and secondary (open symbols) features from individual animals at four AP levels. *A*. At bregma (AP_0), forelimb and trunk features are intermingled over a wide area, and are close to hindlimb features. Secondary features from forelimb animals are spread out over the entire lateral field. (Secondary trunk features are not shown.) *B*. At this AP level the greatest separation of primary features for the three body regions is seen. Secondary hindlimb and trunk features are found ventrally, within either the forelimb or trunk primary feature field, while secondary forelimb features are found dorsally, within the trunk field. *C*. At 0.4 mm anterior to

the previous section, the hindlimb primary features are found ventrolateral to the more posterior position, and trunk features are dorsomedial. The forelimb primary features have also shifted dorsomedially, and are proximal to hindlimb features. Secondary features have similar relationships to each other as do their respective primary features. *D*. At AP +1.0, the hindlimb primary features are shifted dorsomedially to their previous position, the forelimb features are in similar positions, and trunk features are ventrolateral. This results in an intermingling of forelimb and trunk features, which are separated from hindlimb. The secondary features for hindlimb and trunk show separate clustering. (After Brown, 1992.)

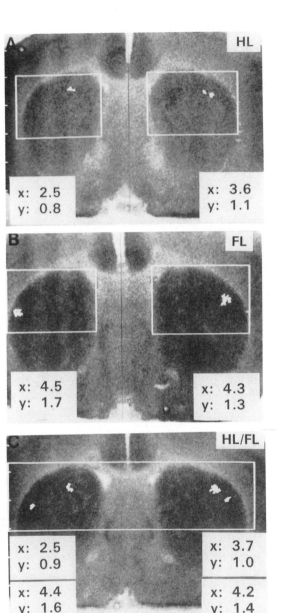

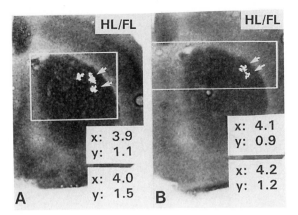

Fig. 8. *A.* and *B.* Digitized autoradiograms of animals stimulated on the hindlimb and forelimb simultaneously, as in Fig. 7. The AP level is at bregma, where plots of individually stimulated animals suggested juxtaposed or intermingling regions of activation for the three body regions stimulated. The features shown are typical of what was seen in all animals stimulated on the hindlimb and forelimb simultaneously. There was never a single large feature; rather, two or three were closely juxtaposed.

Fig. 7. Autoradiograms of coronal sections, digitized for grey level, with the areas of maximal striatal activity (features) masked in white. Right is contralateral to the somatosensory stimulation. The Cartesian coordinates are given for the centroid of the largest feature, or of the two largest features. The *X* position refers to mm lateral to the midline (X_0) in either direction; the *Y* position refers to mm ventral to the dorsal edge of the striatum (Y_0). *A.* Hindlimb stimulated animal: contralateral and ipsilateral features are in different locations. *B.* Forelimb stimulated animal: features are ventral and lateral to the hindlimb features shown in *A. C.* In an animal stimulated on hindlimb and forelimb simultaneously, the localization of features is similar to those seen in the two individually stimulated animals.

Ipsilateral striatum

Features were reliably localized in ipsilateral striatum as well. As in the representation of somatic input in contralateral striatum, the ipsilateral also varied from one AP level to another. The result was that bilateral representations of the same stimulus were in homotopic striatal regions at some AP levels, and heterotopic at others. But again, there was an orderly pattern to the localization, consistent across animals. At AP -0.5, all groups showed ipsilateral localization dorsal to contralateral, by 0.30 ± 0.07 mm ($P < 0.01$, matched *t*; Fig. 9). At AP $+0.2$, where the three body regions were most separate contralaterally, the ipsilateral features were in regions that might overlap with contralateral (Fig. 9). Thus, on each side, contralateral and ipsilateral body regions could be represented, and in similar or different regions, revealing another element in the shifting body map (Fig. 10).

A combinational map in striatum

Goldman-Rakic (1984) has suggested that in primates, "prefrontal fibers alternate in caudate nucleus with other sources of striatal afferents and

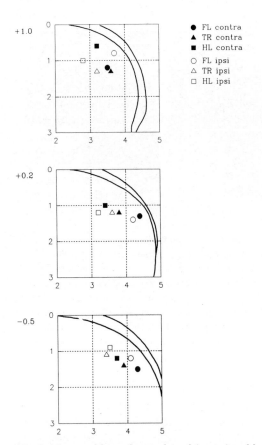

Fig. 9. Mean positions of contralateral (contra) and ipsilateral (ipsi) striatal activation sites demonstrate the magnitude and consistency of their separations and relative positions. At AP +1.0, contra and ipsi sites were separated by 0.4−0.5 mm. At AP +0.2, they were closely juxtaposed in each stimulation group, but ipsi sites were all medial to contra. At AP −0.5, contra and ipsi sites were different in all groups, and in each group a similar organization was seen with ipsi 0.3−0.5 mm dorsal to contra. HL, hindlimb; TR, trunk; FL, forelimb.

that interdigitation may thus represent a generalized anatomic mechanism for processing information from two or more cortical sources in the CNS''. Our data suggest that such an interactive scheme may apply to the organization of striatal afferents even within the sensorimotor domain alone. In the dorsolateral striatum of the rat, we have seen juxtapositions of functional activity that provide an anatomic substrate for integrating information from more than a single source within SI, such as hindlimb, trunk and forelimb regions. And that organization

is both specific and orderly. Thus the major source of inputs underlying the somatotopic map, the neocortex, appears to provide multiple combinations of input from different cortical sources, perhaps permitting all of the possible permutations and combinations of body region, including laterality, necessary to allow the organization of complex movement.

The neocortical projection pattern to striatum has several important characteristics. The axonal arborization appears to be cruciform axodendritic, with individual fibers coursing through tissue and making a number of contacts on dendrites en passant (see Wilson, 1990). Studies suggest that axons from any one cortical region project to a long AP field (Goldman and Nauta, 1977; McGeorge and Faull, 1989; Flaherty and Graybiel, 1991), covering most of the striatum. Within that cortical projection field the afferent terminals appear as clusters. In a model proposed by DeLong et al. (1983), the projection field has been described as a long striatal cylinder in which cortical input is integrated. In the metabolic mapping studies described here, the acti-

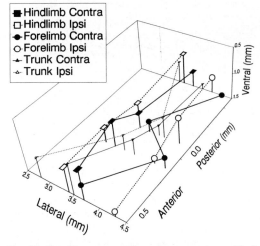

Fig. 10. Graphic representation of mean contra and ipsi sites at four AP levels. The figure demonstrates the varying combinational possibilities for laterality as well as for body region. At the most anterior position shown, contra trunk and ipsi hindlimb are juxtaposed, as are contra hindlimb and forelimb. At other AP levels, different juxtapositions exist.

vated regions had a clustered appearance, and also traversed an elongated AP region in striatum. However, the functional mapping revealed that the projection of afferents forms cylinders related to body region that may be somewhat helical through their AP course, with the juxtaposition of different cortical sources varying as a function of AP level. Wilson has suggested that there is a "combinational logic circuit in the neostriatum in which a single striatal neuron may be excited only when inputs from several cortical regions are activated" (Wilson, 1990). Our data demonstrate that functional elements might be combined in striatum to form a combinational map of input from SI, alone as well as with other cortical regions. The model is one of intersecting, possibly intertwining cylinders, rather than one of separate, parallel channels.

The model that projections from SI to striatum form a group of intertwining cylinders in their AP course is supported by data from other studies. In

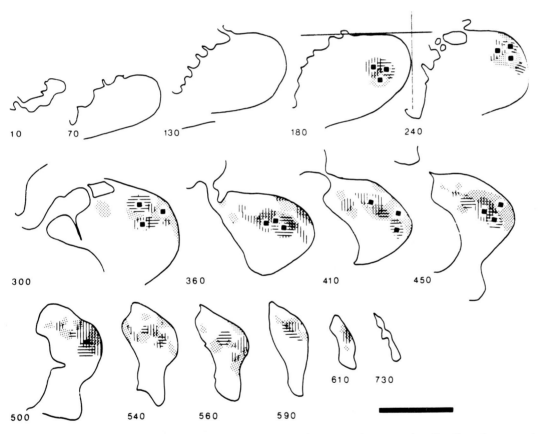

Fig. 11. "Projection drawings from frontal sections of the putamen in a cynomologous monkey. Data from three separate experiments show terminal labeling resulting from injections of [³H] amino acids in the hand representation of the ipsilateral cortical areas *3b* (vertical hatching), *1* (horizontal hatching) and *2* (stippled). Labeling in each case occupies the same part of putamen but many patches do not coincide" (Jones et al., 1977). Going from anterior to posterior, the hand representation taken as a whole shifts from medial (section 180) to dorsolateral (section 240). The major innervation then shifts medially (section 360), and then laterally (section 500). In sections 180–450, black squares have been added to the centers of the largest fields that represent *1, 2* and *3b* to demonstrate their shifting relationships. The relative position of the stippled to the two hatched patterns shifts from ventral (section 180) to lateral (section 300), then all overlap medially (section 360), then again laterally (section 450). The vertically hatched region shifts its relationship to the horizontal hatching from medial to ventral, then medial, then dorsal. The shifting positions of body region and modality may permit multiple combinations of inputs to striatum. Bar represents 5 mm. Section thickness was 50 μm. (Adapted from Jones et al., 1977.)

cat striatum, Malach and Graybiel (1986) found overlapping fields for proximal body regions such as the digits, or the upper forelimb and shoulder. However, they also described the striatal body map as anisotropic, apparently rotating from anterior to posterior. Jones et al. (1977) mapped the projection from the hand region of primate cortical areas *1, 2* and *3b* to the putamen. Fig. 11, reproduced from that report, shows how the hand area shifts from medial to lateral through its AP course, as the input from different subregions of SI alternate their positions relative to each other. Clearly the arrangement of somatotopic input to striatum does not follow the parallel arrangements seen in somatosensory thalamus or cortex.

In a study of awake rats, Carelli and West (1991) found that some cells in dorsolateral striatum responded to specific limb or head movements, but that 39% of the cells sampled fired in relation to "non-specific" body movements. However, such "non-specific" cells might be specific to some combination of inputs. For a combinational map to represent all of the necessary permutations and combinations of input elements would require that many of the intrinsic neurons respond preferentially to simultaneous or sequential inputs from specific groups of corticostriatal afferents that come from multiple cortical regions; others would preferentially respond to input from a single region.

In our functional mapping studies, six inputs to striatum were examined: ipsi- and contralateral forelimb, trunk and hindlimb. Looking only at combinational pairs, we estimate that primary features with centers separated by 300 μm or less might reasonably represent interactions of axon terminals on the dendritic field of a single cell, or on a cluster of related cells. Using group mean localization, such interaction is indicated for 11 of the 15 possible pairs of combinations of the six inputs, over the AP extent of dorsolateral striatum studied. (Of course, combinations of three or more inputs would offer even more combinatorial possibilities; and permutations of combined inputs might be differently encoded by the patterns of discharge of the corticostriate axons involved.)

The foregoing is based on consideration only of the largest regions of maximal glucose utilization seen in coronal sections, the primary features. But smaller, secondary features were also observed. We interpret these to be regions in which the activity of axon terminals is less than in regions characterized by the primary features, but which have the same cortical origin. Activity in regions characterized by both primary and secondary features might also account for some of the apparently non-specific somatotopic fields found in rats in electrophysiological studies (Carelli and West, 1991). It should be noted, however, that the DG data were extracted from a noisy system. The striatum of the awake rat is continually receiving afferent activity from many sources. (The striatum is a metabolically active region, while the globus pallidus is a metabolically inactive region; just the opposite of electrophysiological responses, which reflect cellular activity rather than the activity of axon terminals.) Some rats clearly had a primary feature in the dorsolateral striatum, with small features in all other striatal regions. Other rats showed features of nearly equal size in ventral or medial regions. Only a very limited region of the dorsolateral striatum was under experimental control in all animals − the region that received input from the salient experimental stimulus.

Conclusions

Unlike the parallel rods in VP thalamus (Rausell and Jones, 1991), the regions in dorsolateral striatum that are activated by somatosensory stimuli are better described as flexible cylinders that intertwine and braid throughout their AP striatal course. We also propose that the cylinders are porous, and that the points at which they intersect provide for the convergence and varied combinations of inputs. To generate further hypotheses for the model, it will be important to learn whether these flexible cylinders are continuous or discontinuous. What is the nature of the output of the cells within these flexible cylinders to neurons in pallidum and nigra? How does the input relate to striatal dopamine, opiates and substance P? It is likely that most of the activated points we have described will be found in the matrix, to which a large proportion of sensorimotor cortex projects (Gerfen, 1989). In developing this functional somatosensory probe, we anticipate as an important next step the investigation of the functional organization within chemically defined compartments of striatum.

References

Alexander, G.E. and DeLong, M.R. (1985) Microstimulation of the primate neostriatum. II. Somatotopic organization of striatal microexcitable zones and their relation to neuronal response properties. *J. Neurophysiol.*, 53: 1417 – 1443.

Brown, L.L. (1992) Somatotopic organization in rat striatum: evidence for a combinational map. *Proc. Natl. Acad. Sci. U.S.A.*, 89: 7403 – 7407.

Brown, L.L., Wolfson, L.I. and Feldman, S.M. (1987) Functional neuroanatomic mapping of the rat striatum: regional differences in glucose utilization in normal controls and after treatment with apomorphine. *Brain Res.*, 411: 65 – 71.

Carelli, R.M. and West, M.O. (1991) Representation of the body by single neurons in the dorsolateral striatum of the awake, unrestrained rat. *J. Comp. Neurol.*, 309: 231 – 249.

Chapin, J.K. and Lin, C.-S. (1984) Mapping the body representation in the SI cortex of anesthetized and awake rats. *J. Comp. Neurol.*, 229: 199 – 213.

Crutcher, M.D. and DeLong, M.R. (1984) Single cell studies of the primate putamen. I. Functional organization. *Exp. Brain Res.*, 53: 233 – 243.

DeLong, M.R., Georgopoulos, A.P. and Crutcher, M.D. (1983) Cortico-basal ganglia relations and coding of motor performance. *Exp. Brain Res.* (Suppl.), 7: 30 – 40.

Flaherty, A.W. and Graybiel, A.M. (1991) Corticostriatal transformations in the primate somatosensory system. Projections from physiologically mapped body-part representations. *J. Neurophysiol.*, 66(4): 1249 – 1263.

Gerfen, C.R. (1989) The neostriatal mosaic: striatal patch-matrix organization is related to cortical lamination. *Science*, 246: 385 – 388.

Gerfen, C.R. (1992) The neostriatal mosaic: multiple levels of compartmental organization. *Trends Neurosci.*, 15: 133 – 138.

Gerfen, C.R., Herkenham, M. and Thibault, J. (1987) The neostriatal mosaic: II. Patch- and matrix-directed mesostriatal dopaminergic and non-dopaminergic systems. *J. Neurosci.*, 7: 3915 – 3934.

Goldman, P.S. and Nauta, W.J.H. (1977) An intricately patterned prefronto-caudate projection in the rhesus monkey. *J. Comp. Neurol.*, 171: 369 – 386.

Goldman-Rakic, P.S. (1984) Modular organization of prefrontal cortex. *Trends Neurosci.*, 7: 419 – 424.

Goldman-Rakic, P.S. and Selemon, L.D. (1990) New frontiers in basal ganglia research. *Trends Neurosci.*, 13: 241 – 244.

Graybiel, A.M. (1990) Neurotransmitters and neuromodulators in the basal ganglia. *Trends Neurosci.*, 13: 244 – 254.

Graybiel, A.M. and Ragsdale Jr., C.W. (1978) Histochemically distinct compartments in the striatum of human, monkey and cat demonstrated by acetylcholinesterase staining. *Proc. Natl. Acad. Sci. U.S.A.*, 75: 5723 – 5726.

Graybiel, A.M., Ragsdale Jr., C.W. and Moon Edley, S. (1979) Compartments in the striatum of the cat observed by retrograde cell-labelling. *Exp. Brain Res.*, 34: 189 – 195.

Hall, R.D. and Lindholm, E.P. (1974) Organization of motor and somatosensory neocortex in the albino rat. *Brain Res.*, 66: 23 – 38.

Hikosaka, O. (1991) Role of the forebrain in oculomotor function. In: G. Holstege (Ed.), *Role of the Forebrain in Sensation and Behavior – Progress in Brain Research, Vol. 87,* Elsevier, Amsterdam, pp. 101 – 107.

Jones, E.G. (1985) *The Thalamus,* Plenum Press, New York, pp. 325 – 411.

Jones, E.G., Coulter, J.D., Burton, H. and Porter, R. (1977) Cells of origin and terminal distribution of corticostriatal fibers arising in the sensory-motor cortex of monkeys. *J. Comp. Neurol.*, 173: 53 – 80.

Jones, E.G., Coulter, J.D. and Wise, S.P. (1979) Commissural columns in the sensory-motor cortex of monkeys. *J. Comp. Neurol.*, 188: 113 – 136.

Kunzle, H. (1975) Bilateral projections from precentral motor cortex to the putamen and other parts of the basal ganglia. An autoradiographic study in *Macaca fascicularis. Brain Res.*, 88: 195 – 209.

Kunzle, H. (1977) Projections from the primary somatosensory cortex to basal ganglia and thalamus in the monkey. *Exp. Brain Res.*, 30: 481 – 492.

Liles, S.L. and Updyke, B.V. (1985) Projection of the digit and wrist area of precentral gyrus to the putamen: relation between topography and physiological properties of neurons in the putamen. *Brain Res.*, 339: 245 – 255.

Malach, R. and Graybiel, A.M. (1986) Mosaic architecture of the somatic sensory-recipient sector of the cat's striatum. *J. Neurosci.*, 6: 3436 – 3458.

Mata, M., Fink, D.J., Gainer, H., Smith, C.B., Davidsen, L., Savaki, H., Schwartz, W.J. and Sokoloff, L. (1980) Activity-dependent energy metabolism in rat posterior pituitary reflects sodium pump activity. *J. Neurochem.*, 34: 213 – 215.

McGeorge, A.J. and Faull, R.L.M. (1989) The organization of the projection from the cerebral cortex to the striatum in the rat. *Neuroscience*, 29: 503 – 537.

Paxinos, G. and Watson, C. (1986) *The Rat Brain in Stereotaxic Coordinates,* 2nd edn., Academic Press, San Diego, CA.

Rausell, E. and Jones, E.G. (1991) Histochemical and immunocytochemical compartments of the thalamic VPM nucleus in monkeys and their relationship to the representational map. *J. Neurosci.,* 11: 210 – 225.

Selemon, L.D. and Goldman-Rakic, P.S. (1985) Longitudinal topography and interdigitation of corticostriatal projections in the rhesus monkey. *J. Neurosci.,* 5: 776 – 794.

Sharp, F.R. (1984) Regional [^{14}C] 2-deoxyglucose uptake during forelimb movements evoked by rat motor cortex stimulation: cortex, diencephalon, midbrain. *J. Comp. Neurol.,* 224: 259 – 285.

Sharp, J.W., Gonzalez, M.F., Morton, M.T., Simon, F.R. and Sharp, F.R. (1988) Decreases of cortical and thalamic glucose metabolism produced by parietal cortex stimulation in the rat. *Brain Res.,* 438: 357 – 362.

Sokoloff, L., Reivich, M., Kennedy, C., DesRosiers, M.H., Pat-lak, C.S., Pettigrew, K.D., Sakurada, O. and Shinohara, M. (1977) The ^{14}C-deoxyglucose method for the measurement of local cerebral glucose utilization: theory, procedure, and normal values in the conscious and anesthetized albino rat. *J. Neurochem.,* 28: 897 – 916.

West, M.O., Carelli, R.M., Pomerantz, M., Cohen, S.M., Gardner, J.P., Chapin, J.K. and Woodward, D.O. (1990) A region in the dorsolateral striatum of the rat exhibiting single-unit correlations with specific locomotor limb movements. *J. Neurophysiol.,* 64: 1233 – 1246.

Wilson, C.J. (1990) Basal ganglia. In: G.M. Shepherd (Ed.), *The Synaptic Organization of the Brain,* 3rd edn., Oxford, New York, pp. 279 – 316.

G.W. Arbuthnott and P.C. Emson (Eds.)
Progress in Brain Research, Vol. 99
© 1993 Elsevier Science Publishers B.V. All rights reserved.

CHAPTER 17

Neurotransmitter receptors and ionic conductances regulating the activity of neurones in substantia nigra pars compacta and ventral tegmental area

M.G. Lacey

Department of Pharmacology, The Medical School, University of Birmingham, Birmingham B15 2TT, U.K.

Introduction

Midbrain dopamine neurones: location, projections and behavioural role

The dopamine-containing neurones of the midbrain are largely confined to the ventral tegmental area (VTA; A10), or, more laterally, within the substantia nigra pars compacta (SNc; A9) (Björklund and Lindvall, 1984, 1986). SNc neurones project predominantly to the dorsal striatum (caudate-putamen; Björklund and Lindvall, 1984, 1986), and dopamine released from their terminals appears critical for the control of voluntary movement – their degeneration results in the symptoms of Parkinson's disease (Hornykiewicz, 1966; Schultz, 1982). However, some of the more medial SNc neurones project to regions innervated by VTA neurones which comprise limbic (amygdala, septum, olfactory tubercule, nucleus accumbens) and cortical (medial prefrontal, anterior cingulate, entorhinal) areas (Swanson, 1982; Björklund and Lindvall, 1984, 1986). These have been implicated in behavioural reward and motivation, locomotor drive and cognition (Wise, 1983; Björklund and Lindvall, 1984, 1986; Fibiger and Phillips, 1986; Losonczy et al., 1987). The importance of dopamine in brain function suggests a critical modulatory role on integrative processes in the projection areas of dopamine neurones (Björklund and Lindvall, 1986).

Regulation of the activity of these neurones at the level of their cell bodies would influence these processes by altering impulse flow in ascending axons, thereby altering dopamine release from dopamine-containing nerve terminals.

The VTA and SNc do not contain exclusively dopamine cells, nor are they the only location of midbrain dopamine cells. Tyrosine hydroxylase-positive cells projecting to striatum (both dorsal and ventral portions) fall into two categories: (i) those projecting to the "matrix" (of which the ventral striatum, or nucleus accumbens is predominantly comprised) which are found in VTA, SNc (dorsal tier) and also the retrorubral field (A8), and which express calcium binding protein (Gerfen et al., 1987a,b); and (ii) those found in the ventral tier of the SNc, and also displaced into the pars reticulata in more caudal parts of the nucleus, and which project to "patch" regions of striatum (Gerfen et al., 1987b). Dopamine neurones have extensive, dopamine-containing (Björklund and Lindvall, 1975) dendritic trees which distribute within the area occupied by the dopamine cell bodies and also, in the case of the ventral tier SNc neurones, penetrating ventrally into the substantia nigra pars reticulata (SNr) (Fallon et al., 1978; Gerfen et al., 1987b).

Ventral midbrain neurones: functional studies

The first electrophysiological recordings of presumed dopamine-containing midbrain neurones were made extracellularly in vivo (Bunney et al., 1973), wherein it was shown that these cells were inhibited by the dopamine receptor agonist apomorphine, an effect that could be reversed by antipsychotic drugs (Bunney et al., 1973; Aghajanian and Bunney, 1977), which were subsequently shown to be dopamine D_2 receptor antagonists. The effect of apomorphine could be mimicked by the indirectly acting sympathomimetic amphetamine (Groves et al., 1975), indicating that dopamine neurones were able to "autoinhibit" themselves through dopamine released from their extensive dendritic trees (Björklund and Lindvall, 1975) acting on inhibitory "autoreceptors". Deployment of the push-pull cannula technique in vivo (Cheramy et al., 1981) and of measurement of release of preloaded [^{3}H]dopamine from midbrain slices (Geffen et al., 1976) confirmed that dopamine could indeed be released in the substantia nigra. However, changes in dopamine released from striatal terminals following introduction of agents via cannulae into the substantia nigra were generally inversely correlated with dopamine release in the nigra itself (Cheramy et al., 1981). This apparent independence of dendritic release of dopamine from electrical activity in the cell soma has provoked much discussion concerning its mechanism and function (Chesselet, 1984; Condé, 1992; see below). It may play a role in modulation of transmitter release (GABA) from descending striato-nigral fibres through actions on D_1 dopamine receptors on the terminals of these fibres (see Robertson, 1992), as well as to exert an (auto-) inhibitory influence on dopamine cell firing (see below).

In an extensive and influential series of papers, Grace and Bunney reported some properties of histochemically identified (Grace and Bunney, 1980, 1983a) dopamine-containing neurones recorded intracellularly in vivo. Many of the observations made with extracellular recordings were confirmed and embellished, including the ability of these cells to fire both regularly ("pacemaker-like") and in a bursting mode (Grace and Bunney, 1983a, 1984a,b), their inhibition by apomorphine (Grace

and Bunney, 1983a), and their projections to and receipt of inhibitory input from the striatum (Grace and Bunney, 1983a, 1985). In addition, the intracellular technique afforded detailed descriptions of the membrane potential changes occurring during spike generation, and the advancement of some hypotheses concerning the nature of the interplaying ionic mechanisms subserving firing activity (Grace, 1987), including suggestions of electrotonic coupling between dopamine cells (Grace and Bunney, 1983b). The problems posed by the in vivo preparation, mainly concerning the difficulty of obtaining and maintaining intracellular recordings, and limitations upon experimental manipulation of membrane potential and of the extracellular milieu, led others to explore the brain slice preparation for electrophysiological study of dopamine neurones. Early milestones include the report of firing patterns of presumed dopamine neurones recorded in brain slices using extracellular single unit recordings compared with those recorded in vivo (Sanghera et al., 1984), and of pharmacological characterisation of the action of dopamine in inhibiting the firing of extracellularly recorded SNc neurones (Pinnock, 1983, 1984a).

This article will attempt to summarise present knowledge on the cellular properties of midbrain dopamine neurones with the focus on the mechanisms underlying the modification of their behaviour by neurotransmitters. Most of the relevant studies in this regard have been performed in vitro, either in slices of adult rodent midbrain or in tissue culture. Where possible, these findings will be integrated with existing knowledge of basal ganglia circuitry and function with the object of achieving a synthesis of the mechanisms for regulating activity of dopamine neurones, either through physiological actions of endogenous neurotransmitters, or with drugs.

Electrophysiological properties of neurones in substantia nigra pars compacta and ventral tegmental area

Based on electrophysiological criteria, there are at least two types of cell in both the SNc and the VTA identifiable from in vitro experiments, and at least one of which is well characterised and dopamine-containing (Matsuda et al., 1987; Nakanishi et al., 1987; Lacey et al., 1989; Grace and Onn, 1989; Yung et al., 1991; Hainsworth et al., 1991; Johnson and North, 1992a,b; Nedergaard and Greenfield, 1992).

Dopamine cells

The predominant cell type (85 – 95% of the total, Lacey et al., 1989; Grace and Onn, 1989; Yung et al., 1991; Johnson and North, 1992b) usually exhibits spontaneous action potential firing at frequencies up to around 6 Hz (in brain slices), with an action potential duration of greater than 1 msec, and pronounced time-dependent inward rectification on hyperpolarisation (Fig. 1). Cells with some of these properties have also been seen in substantia nigra pars reticulata (SNr; Nakanishi et al., 1987).

Double-labelled cells of this type are tyrosine hydroxylase-positive (Grace and Onn, 1989; Yung et al., 1991), their electrophysiological properties resemble in many respects those identified as dopamine-containing projection neurones from foregoing in vivo studies (Grace and Bunney, 1980, 1983a; Tepper et al., 1987), and they are inhibited by dopamine or other D_2 receptor agonists (Lacey et al., 1987, 1988, 1989; Silva et al., 1990; Roeper et al., 1990; Hainsworth et al., 1991; Johnson and North, 1992a,b; see below). These may be considered dopamine cells. Dopamine cells often fire in bursts in vivo, as well as tonically (Bunney et al., 1973), but burst firing has not been observed in vitro in physiological media. However, manipulations that reduce potassium conductance, including extracellular barium (Grace and Bunney, 1984a; Harris et al., 1989), apamin (Shepard and German,

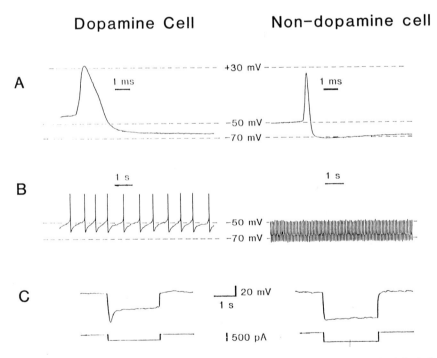

Dopamine Cell   Non-dopamine cell

Fig. 1. Dopamine cells (left) and non-dopamine cells (right) have different electrophysiological characteristics. Records of membrane potential from two representative cells of each type. *A.* Spontaneous action potentials in dopamine cells are greater than 1 msec in duration, whereas those of non-dopamine cells are less than 1 msec. *B.* Spontaneous firing in dopamine cells is generally regular and in the range of 1 – 8 Hz. Non-dopamine cells can fire up to 40 Hz or more. Action potential amplitude truncated. *C.* Hyperpolarising current pulses (lower records) produce time-dependent inward rectification of the membrane potential (upper records) in dopamine cells (left), but not in non-dopamine cells (right). (Adapted from Lacey et al., 1989, with permission.)

1988), tetraethylammonium, elevated extracellular potassium concentrations or intracellular caesium (Lacey, unpublished observations), can result in induction of burst firing (Fig. 2*B*). Furthermore, activation of NMDA-type glutamate receptors also appears to produce bursting (Charlety et al., 1991; Johnson et al., 1992b; see below). Thus it seems that dopamine cells are able to sustain a pacemaker-like firing that is intrinsically generated (for consideration of underlying ionic mechanisms, see Grace, 1987; Grace and Onn, 1989), possibly assisted by electrotonic coupling between cells (Grace and Bunney, 1983b, Fig. 2*A*). This may be converted to bursting behaviour by the action of neurotransmitters, with excitatory amino acids as prime candidates. Such interconversion may have considerable influence on the dynamics of dopamine release in the terminal fields of these cells (Gonon, 1988).

Non-dopamine cells

The second type of cell has a briefer action potential (< 1 msec), higher input resistance, higher frequencies of spontaneous action potential firing, which can sometimes be phasic or in bursts. If quiescent, they show a pronounced anode break (post-hyperpolarisation rebound) depolarisation leading to a "burst" of action potentials, and little or no time-dependent inward rectification on hyperpolarisation (Fig. 1). Such cells appear with an incidence of $5 - 15\%$, and are more common at the rostral ex-

tent of the SNc/VTA (Lacey et al., 1989; Grace and Onn, 1989; Yung et al., 1991; Johnson and North, 1992b). They are tyrosine hydroxylase-negative (Grace and Onn, 1989; Yung et al., 1991) and are probably GABA-containing (Yung et al., 1991). These cells are most likely to be interneurones (Lacey et al., 1989; Yung et al., 1991; Johnson and North, 1992b), although the possibility of them being projection neurones (either nigro-striatal, or analogous to SNr neurones, whose properties they resemble at least superficially; see Nakanishi et al., 1987) cannot be completely ruled out (Lacey et al., 1989; Grace and Onn, 1989; Yung et al., 1991). The non-dopamine "secondary" cells in the SNc (Lacey et al., 1989) and VTA (Johnson and North, 1992a,b) were neither inhibited nor hyperpolarised by dopamine, but, in contrast to the dopamine cells, were hyperpolarised by μ-opioid receptor agonists (see below). These pharmacological differences between the dopamine-containing cell type and the "secondary" cell constitute another important identifier of subtypes of cell in SNc and VTA.

Discrepancies

The above classification is not undisputed. Cells inhibited by neither opioids nor dopamine, with action potential durations similar to "secondary" cells, but with firing patterns more akin to the dopamine cells, comprised 7% of cells recorded in the VTA (Johnson and North, 1992b). Cells of similar,

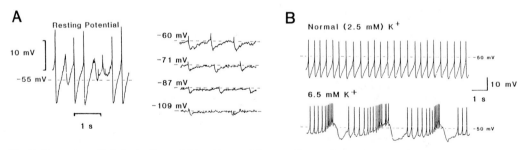

Fig. 2. Dopamine cells in brain slices exhibit evidence of electrotonic coupling and may be induced to burst firing. *A*. Records of membrane potential from the same cell at rest (left), and at four different, hyperpolarised potentials attained by current injection (right). Fast, low-amplitude spikes with an after-hyperpolarisation, visible at rest, are not abolished by hyperpolarisation like the full spikes, but rather are merely slowed down and attenuated. This indicates an electrotonically distant site of generation, possibly in adjacent dopamine neurones. *B*. Raising extracellular potassium concentration caused this cell to switch from a "pacemaker" to a "bursting" mode of firing. Action potential amplitude truncated.

but perhaps not identical properties to the minority class described above have been proposed to be of a second dopamine-containing class confined to the rostral portion of the guinea-pig substantia nigra, to the virtual exclusion of all other cell types (Nedergaard and Greenfield, 1992; Murphy and Greenfield, 1992). However, these cells have not been shown with double-labelling to contain dopamine, nor has their sensitivity to dopamine been convincingly demonstrated. Nonetheless, recordings from acutely dissociated cells identified by retrograde labelling as projecting to striatum showed them to be of two types resembling those described above, but both types displayed cathecholamine fluorescence (Hainsworth et al., 1991). Although the second class of cells was not described in another study with a similar approach to identifying nigrostriatal projection neurones in vitro (Silva et al., 1990), the possibility of subtypes of dopamine neurone, suggested by an in vivo electrophysiological study (Shepard and German, 1988), should be kept in mind. However, it is unlikely that the rostro-caudal contrast in dopamine cell properties proposed by Nedergaard and Greenfield (1992) could be accounted for by intrinsic differences between cells of the dorsal and ventral tiers of dopamine neurones (Fallon et al., 1978; Gerfen et al., 1987b). The pre-

sumed dopamine-containing neurones of the VTA (Calabresi et al., 1989; Lacey et al., 1990a; Johnson et al., 1992; Johnson and North, 1992a,b), which would be of the dorsal tier and which predominate rostrally (Gerfen et al., 1987b), appear to be of the same type as the confirmed dopamine-containing neurones of the substantia nigra (Grace and Onn, 1989; Yung et al., 1991), which may be recorded in caudal portions of the nucleus.

Actions of monoamines

Dopamine

Ever since the ground-breaking in vivo studies of the 1970s in which the "auto"-inhibitory action of dopamine receptor agonists on dopamine neurones was established (Bunney et al., 1973; Groves et al., 1975; Aghajanian and Bunney, 1977), the mechanism of this action of dopamine (and dopamine receptor agonists) has been pursued (Grace and Bunney, 1983a). It is now clear that dopamine (or D_2 receptor agonists) hyperpolarises neurones of the dopamine-containing type (above) in SNc and VTA, but not the "secondary", non-dopamine-containing cells, whether hyperpolarised by opioids or not (Lacey et al., 1989; Johnson and North, 1992a,b), thereby inhibiting action potential firing

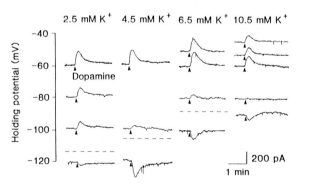
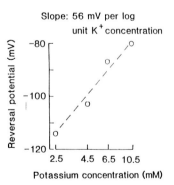

Fig. 3. Outward currents produced by dopamine in dopamine neurones are due to an increase in potassium conductance. *Left*: records of membrane currents in response to a brief application of dopamine (arrows) from a single cell recorded under voltage clamp at the potentials indicated. The reversal potential (where the outward currents became inward; dashed lines) was less negative in increasing extracellular potassium concentrations. *Right*: reversal potentials from the same experiment plotted against logarithm of potassium concentration. They fall on a line closely fitted by the Nernst equation, indicating potassium is the sole charge carrier of the dopamine current. (Adapted from Lacey et al., 1987, with permission.)

(Lacey et al., 1987, 1988, 1989; Mueller and Brodie, 1989; Silva et al., 1990; Roeper et al., 1990; Mereu et al., 1991; Hainsworth et al., 1991; Hicks and Henderson, 1992; Johnson and North, 1992b; see Fig. 4A). This effect appears a direct one upon dopamine neurones as it persisted in tetrodotoxin (TTX) and low calcium solutions, which block transmitter release from other neurones in the preparation (Lacey et al., 1987). The hyperpolarisation (or outward current under voltage clamp) is a consequence of an increase in membrane potassium conductance (Lacey et al., 1987, Fig. 3), utilising channels which appear to couple to the dopamine receptor through a pertussus toxin-sensitive GTP-binding protein (Innis and Aghajanian, 1987; Lacey et al., 1988; Fig. 4B). A comparable mechanism coupling to the D_2 receptor has been reported in pituitary melanotrophs (Israel et al., 1987), and comparisons may be drawn between this dopamine-mediated mechanism of inhibition and those mediated by other neurotransmitter receptors acting through increased potassium conductance (North, 1989). At least one other receptor (the $GABA_B$ receptor, see below) can operate these same channels in dopamine neurones (Lacey et al., 1988). The dopamine hyperpolarisation/outward current can be mimicked by apomorphine, 6,7 ADTN and quinpirole and antagonised by (−)-sulpiride (Lacey et al., 1987; Hainsworth et al., 1991) with an apparent affinity constant of 13 nM (Lacey et al., 1987), supporting results obtained with extracellular recording (Pinnock, 1983, 1984a) and consistent with involvement of a D_2 receptor. The D_1 receptor agonist SKF 38393 was ineffective, and the D_1 antagonist SCH 23390 did not affect the response to dopamine (Lacey et al., 1987). Indeed, following lesion-induced degeneration of striato-nigral fibres, only D_2 dopamine receptors remain in the substantia nigra, and these are considerably reduced in number following treatment with the selective dopamine

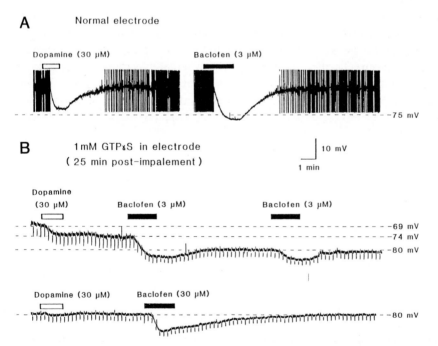

Fig. 4. Intracellular GTP-γ-S, the non-hydrolysable GTP analoque, renders irreversible the $GABA_B$ and D_2 receptor-mediated hyperpolarisation of dopamine cells. A. Dopamine and baclofen both reversibly inhibited and hyperpolarised cells recorded with 2 M KCl-filled electrode. B. In a different cell from A, GTP-γ-S in the electrode hyperpolarises the cell, and the effects of dopamine and baclofen were only partly reversible, implicating GTP in the coupling of the potassium channels to both $GABA_B$ and D_2 receptors. (From Lacey et al., 1988, with permission.)

neuronal toxin 6-hydroxydopamine (Quik et al., 1979; Filloux et al., 1987), further indicating that the dopamine receptors on dopamine neurones are of the D_2 type. However, the presence in the ventral midbrain of messenger RNA encoding for the cloned D2 and D3 receptors (Sokoloff et al., 1990), and the present unavailability of pharmacological agents to discriminate these receptors when expressed in cell lines, means that a definitive statement of the dopamine receptor subtype inhibiting dopamine neurones cannot yet be made.

In brain slice experiments the monoamine releaser amphetamine (Mercuri et al., 1989), the monoamine reuptake blocker cocaine (Lacey et al., 1990b; Brodie and Dunwiddie, 1990), and the monoamine synthesis precursor L-Dopa (Mercuri et al., 1990b) produce an inhibition of firing, accompanied by a small membrane hyperpolarisation or outward current, that is blocked by (−)-sulpiride. The effect of amphetamine was reduced by pretreatment of the preparation with the catecholamine synthesis inhibitor α-methyl-DL-tyrosine (Mercuri et al., 1989), indicating that its effects might be attributable to the action of endogenous dopamine. The action of L-Dopa was strongly attenuated by the dopa decarboxylase inhibitor carbidopa, consistent with it being converted to dopamine (Mercuri et al., 1990b). Cocaine, but not amphetamine, additionally potentiated the effect of exogenously applied dopamine (Mercuri et al., 1989; Lacey et al., 1990b; Brodie and Dunwiddie, 1990), presumably by blocking dopamine reuptake. The actions of all these agents was insensitive to TTX, as is the release of [^{3}H]dopamine from substantia nigra in vivo (Cheramy et al., 1981). The action of cocaine suggests that dopamine is being tonically released within the slice preparation (in a manner independent of sodium TTX-sensitive action potential firing), and that blocking its uptake permits it to open potassium channels by acting on the D_2 receptor. However, as sulpiride does not increase dopamine cell firing rate in brain slices when monoamine reuptake is not impaired (Lacey et al., 1990b), this tonic dopamine release is probably taken up too avidly to exert an "autoinhibitory" effect. Such release is likely to be from

dendrites, possibly regulated by dendritically located calcium conductances (see Nedergaard and Greenfield, 1992, for discussion). The effect of amphetamine was independent of extracellular calcium levels (Mercuri et al., 1989), suggesting that it may release dopamine in a manner independent of the physiological releasing mechanism, whereas that of L-Dopa was not, indicating it increases the concentration of intracellular dopamine which is then released in a calcium-dependent manner (Mercuri et al., 1990b). Dopamine-containing dendro-dendritic synapses have been reported in both substantia nigra (Groves and Linder, 1983) and VTA (Bayer and Pickel, 1990). These may be the sites of the autoinhibitory action of dopamine (Bunney et al., 1973; Groves et al., 1975; Aghajanian and Bunney, 1977), of indirectly acting dopamine agonists (above) and also of the slow, sulpiride-sensitive inhibitory synaptic potential evoked by focal electrical stimulation in VTA neurones (Johnson and North, 1992b).

Noradrenaline

There is evidence for a minor projection to the ventral midbrain from the noradrenergic nucleus locus coeruleus (Björklund and Lindvall, 1986) and also some β- (but not α-) adrenergic ligand binding sites in the substantia nigra (Palacios and Walmsley, 1984). However, the only reports of actions of noradrenaline on dopamine neurones in vitro describe an inhibition or hyperpolarisation antagonised by (−)-sulpiride, merely indicating that noradrenaline acts through the D_2 dopamine receptor, rather than an adrenoceptor, within an order of magnitude of the potency of dopamine itself (Pinnock, 1983; Lacey et al., 1987).

5-Hydroxytryptamine (serotonin)

There is a projection to the substantia nigra and VTA from the 5-hydroxytryptamine (5-HT)-containing neurones of the dorsal (and also medial) raphe nucleus (Dray et al., 1976a; Phillipson, 1979). 5-HT immunoreactivity is high in the ventral midbrain (Steinbusch, 1981) and is present in elements making synaptic contacts with dopamine-containing dendrites (Herve et al., 1987; Nedergaard et al., 1988). Stimulation of the dorsal raphe nucleus in vivo produces an inhibition, but also occasionally excitation, in substantia nigra neurones (Dray et al., 1976a). Similarly, variable and undramatic ("subtle") effects have been obtained with direct iontophoretic application of 5-HT or 5-HT receptor agonists onto dopamine neurones in vivo (Kelland et al., 1990). It has been shown that dorsal raphe stimulation, coincident with antidromic activation of nigro-striatal dopamine neurones, selectively blocks the presumed dendritic component of the extracellularly recorded antidromic spike waveform in these neurones, without affecting spontaneous firing rate per se. This effect was blocked by metergoline, an antagonist at $5-HT_1$ and $5-HT_2$ receptors, and also $(-)$-sulpiride, suggesting this refractoriness was due to the consequence of dopamine release from, and acting in an inhibitory manner upon, dopamine cell dendrites (Trent and Tepper, 1991). In support of this interpretation is the suggestion that 5-HT, acting through a cinanserin-sensitive receptor ($5-HT_2$ type?) enhances a dendritically located calcium conductance in substantia nigra neurones (Nedergaard et al., 1988), although no electrophysiological consequence (e.g., hyperpolarisation) of the resultant dopamine release predicted by the work of Trent and Tepper was reported (Nedergaard et al., 1988). Nonetheless, neurochemical evidence suggests that 5-HT may indeed promote dopamine release in the ventral midbrain (Williams and Davies, 1983). 5-HT has been reported to cause a small depolarisation in some dopamine neurones in brain slices (Nedergaard et al., 1991). This may be mediated by an enhancement of the hyperpolarisation-activated inward current I_h (Lacey and North, 1988), in a manner similar to that demonstrated in nucleus parabrachealis (Bobker and Williams, 1989) and thalamic (McCormick and Pape, 1990) neurones, through an action on receptors of neither the $5-HT_{1A}$ or $5-HT_2$ type (Nedergaard et al., 1991).

5-HT binding sites in substantia nigra are largely of the $5-HT_{1B}$ (in mouse and rat) or $5-HT_{1D}$ (in other mammals) type (Waeber et al., 1990), where they have been shown to negatively couple to adenyl cyclase (Bouhelal et al., 1988; Hoyer and Schoeffter, 1988). Their numbers are diminished following excitotoxic striatal lesions, but not after lesion of dopamine neurones with 6-hydroxydopamine (Waeber et al., 1990), indicating that they are on terminals of striatonigral projection neurones. Additionally, agonists at the homologous $5-HT_{1D}$ receptor elicit dopamine-mediated behaviours (Higgins et al., 1991). Synaptic potentials mediated by $GABA_B$ receptors in dopamine neurones of both the substantia nigra and VTA were reduced in amplitude by 5-HT (Sugita et al., 1992), presumably acting presynaptically on a receptor of the $5-HT_{1B}$ type (Johnson et al., 1992a; see below). Thus 5-HT can both have pre- and postsynaptic actions on dopamine neurones.

Systemic administration of several antagonists of $5-HT_3$ receptors have been shown to reduce the release of dopamine, measured by microdialysis in vivo, from projection areas of dopamine neurones (Di Chiara, 1990), and also to reduce the numbers of midbrain dopamine neurones exhibiting spontaneous firing in vivo (Minabe et al., 1991). There is as yet no direct evidence to support the suggestion that this is due to blockade of excitatory $5-HT_3$ receptor-mediated tone on dopamine neurones (Di Chiara, 1990); rather this effect is more likely due to actions on afferents to dopamine neurones, and not necessarily within the midbrain.

Actions of acetylcholine

There are choline acetyltransferase-immunoreactive terminals within SNc (Beninato and Spencer, 1988) which make contact with tyrosine hydroxylase-positive dendritic elements (Bolam et al., 1991). This innervation may arise from the cholinergic neurones of the pedunculopontine nucleus (PPN) (Woolfe and Butcher, 1986; Clarke et al., 1987). Dopamine neurones exhibit both [^{3}H]nicotine binding (Clarke and Pert, 1985) and express nicotinic receptor α subunit messenger RNA (Deutch et al., 1987), but evidence for muscarinic binding sites in SNc and VTA, particularly on dopamine neurones, is poor (Nonoka and Moroji, 1988).

Nicotinic effects

Excitation of dopaminergic neurones in both SNc and VTA in the rat in vivo has been reported following iontophoresis or systemic injection of nicotine (Lichtensteiger et al., 1982; Clarke et al., 1985; Grenhoff et al., 1986; Mereu et al., 1987). Furthermore, excitation of substantia nigra neurones following activation of pedunculopontine neurones was blocked by the nicotinic receptor antagonist mecamylamine, indicating a functional cholinergic input from this region (Clarke et al., 1987).

An excitation – caused by a depolarisation – in response to acetylcholine (in the presence of the acetylcholinesterase inhibitor neostigmine), nicotine or carbachol (using scopolamine to block the muscarinic action of acetylcholine and carbachol, see below) was reported in VTA neurones using intracellular recording in brain slices (Calabresi et al., 1989; Fig. 5). This nicotinic response showed many characteristics of those described in other preparations: it was due to an inward current with a reversal potential of around − 10 mV and appeared due to direct activation of receptors on dopamine neurones, as it was unaffected by TTX or calcium channel blockers (Calabresi et al., 1989; Fig. 5B). It showed cross desensitisation between agonists, was blocked by D-tubocurarine and the nicotinic channel blocker hexamethonium, the latter in a voltage-dependent manner (Calabresi et al., 1989; Fig. 5C). In slices pretreated with ϰ-bungarotoxin, nicotinic responses were reduced by over 50%, but were unchanged by α-bungarotoxin pretreatment (Calabresi et al., 1989), indicating that the nicotinic

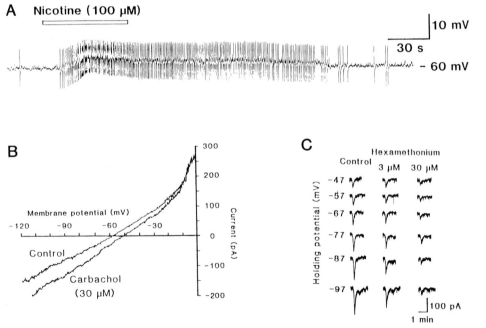

Fig. 5. Dopamine neurones have functional nicotinic cholinergic receptors. *A*. Nicotine caused a depolarisation and action potential firing (amplitude truncated). Note desensitisation to nicotine while still present (open bar). *B*. Steady-state current – voltage relationships of a voltage-clamped cell in control, and in carbachol (in presence of scopolamine 3 μM, TTX 1 μM, cobalt 2 mM, caesium 2 mM and TEA 30 nM to block muscarinic receptors and reduce membrane rectification). Carbachol inward current was reduced to zero at around − 10 mV. *C*. Inward currents in response to brief applications of acetylcholine at different holding potentials. The acetylcholine response was blocked by hexamethonium more effectively at more hyperpolarised potentials. (Adapted from Calabresi et al., 1989, with permission.)

receptor involved was of the "neuronal" or "ganglionic" type, rather than resembling those at the neuromuscular junction (Loring and Zigmond, 1988). This cellular response in VTA neurones may underly the behaviourally rewarding effects of nicotine ingestion through tobacco consumption (Henningfield et al., 1983; Grenhoff et al., 1986; Di Chiara and Imperato, 1988).

Muscarinic effects

Electrophysiological evidence for functional muscarinic receptors on dopamine neurones from in vivo experiments is limited to a report of a weak excitation of some neurones by iontophoretic application of acetylcholine which was blocked by atropine (Scarnati et al., 1986). However, muscarinic receptors in substantia nigra and/or VTA may play a role in enhancing dopamine-dependent behaviours (Niijima and Yoshida, 1988; Parker et al., 1991). Additionally, rewarding electrical stimulation of the lateral hypothalamus, which involves activation of dopamine neurones in the VTA, is impaired with atropine, implicating muscarinic cholinergic innervation of dopamine neurones in reward processes (Kofman et al., 1990).

In brain slices, acetylcholine and carbachol, in addition to causing a nicotinic excitation, also consistently depolarised and excited dopamine cells of both substantia nigra and VTA in a manner mimicked by muscarine (Calabresi et al., 1989; Lacey et al., 1990a). Under voltage clamp at around -60 mV, the inward current caused by muscarine was antagonised in an apparently competitive manner by pirenzepine, with an estimated equilibrium dissociation constant (K_D) of 14 nM (Lacey et al., 1990a), indicating the involvement of an M_1, rather than M_2 type of muscarinic receptor (Hammer et al., 1980). Potassium-evoked release of dopamine from "dendrosomes" of substantia nigra is enhanced by acetylcholine – the sensitivity of this response to pirenzepine suggests that it too is due to activation of an M_1-like receptor (Marchi et al., 1991). Of the m1 – 5 cloned muscarinic receptors, only the message for the m5 type was detectable in the substantia nigra and VTA, and mostly within neurones that also expressed dopamine D_2 messenger RNA (Weiner et al., 1990). The binding affinity of pirenzepine for the m5 receptor when expressed in Chinese hamster ovary cells was estimated at around 600 nM, whereas that for m1 receptors was around 15 nM (Buckley et al., 1989), indicating that the receptor mediating the functional response most closely resembled the cloned m1 type, rather than m5. Thus there appears to be a discrepancy between the pharmacology of pirenzepine in the expressed cloned m5 receptors and its likely homologue in mature mammalian brain.

The ionic mechanism of the muscarinic excitation of dopamine neurones has not been fully established. Despite several precedents from other neuronal subtypes (see Christie and North, 1988, for review), clear evidence for a reduction in membrane potassium conductance could not be obtained. Thus, although the muscarinic inward current reduced in amplitude with membrane hyperpolarisation from rest, accompanied by a conductance decrease in the range of -50 to -70 mV, it did not reverse polarity at around the predicted potassium equilibrium potential in solutions containing $2.5 - 20.5$ mM potassium ions (Fig. 6A), as would be expected if the M_1-like receptor closed "leak" potassium channels as, for example, in nucleus accumbens neurones (Uchimura and North, 1990). No change in action potential after-hyperpolarisation (Madison et al., 1987) was observed, nor was there any clear evidence either for the presence of the M-current (Adams et al., 1982), or any effect of muscarine on such a current (Lacey et al., 1990a). While the muscarinic depolarisation/inward current was insensitive to TTX, it was reversibly blocked with a low-calcium, high-magnesium solution, which would be expected to block calcium entry into cells. This might be taken to suggest that the response was due to release of other transmitters (albeit by a mechanism independent of sodium spikes), or, alternatively, that calcium entry into dopamine neurones was required to generate the muscarinic inward current. The action of muscarine is likely to be direct upon dopamine cells as they manufacture messenger RNA for muscarinic receptors (Weiner et

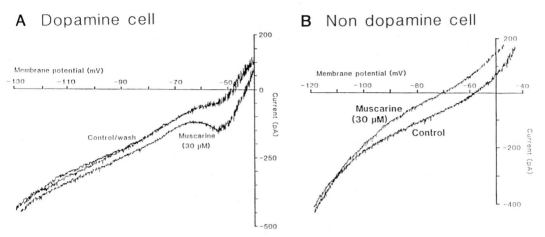

Fig. 6. Muscarine activates different ionic mechanisms in dopamine and non-dopamine cells. Steady-state current – voltage curves in presence and absence of muscarine in each of the two different cell types. *A*. Muscarine caused an inward current in a dopamine cell, which did not reverse in the range – 40 to – 130 mV and was accompanied by a clear conductance change only around resting potential (zero current). *B*. Muscarine caused an outward current in a non-dopamine cell, accompanied by a conductance increase, which reversed close to the predicted potassium equilibrium potential. (*A* from Lacey et al., 1990a, with permission.)

al., 1990), and the muscarinic receptor-mediated release of dopamine from dendrosomes is almost certainly a direct action (Marchi et al., 1991). M_1 receptors (Gil and Wolfe, 1985), and also cloned m1 and m5 receptors, readily couple to phosphatidylinositol (PI) turnover (Hulme et al., 1990), a process which requires extracellular calcium for its maintenance (Berridge and Irvine, 1989). It is therefore at least plausible that M_1-like receptors on dopamine neurones operate through PI turnover to increase a (calcium-dependent?) voltage-dependent, non-specific cation conductance such as demonstrated in intestinal smooth muscle (Benham and Bolton, 1985). A similar response to muscarine has been observed in the SH-SY5Y human neuroblastoma cell line, where two possible mechanisms have been suggested: the inward current is either a calcium current generated by calcium release from intracellular stores, or due to an electrogenic pump (Forsythe et al., 1992). All these hypotheses will require further testing.

In contrast to the muscarinic excitation of dopamine cells, the few "secondary" cells of the SNc tested were hyperpolarised by muscarine (Lacey, unpublished observations). This action was due to an outward current which reverses at potentials near

the predicted equilibrium potential for potassium ions (Fig. 6*B*), suggesting it was due to a potassium conductance increase. Such an action of muscarine has been reported in several types of excitable cells where receptors of the M_2 type couple via a GTP-binding protein to an inwardly rectifying potassium channel (Christie and North, 1988; North, 1989).

Inhibitory amino acids

Gamma-aminobutyric acid (GABA)

Fast inhibitory transmission in the brain mediated by the action of GABA on neuronal $GABA_A$ ionotropic receptors appears to be a widespread, if not ubiquitous phenomenon. Midbrain dopamine neurones have been shown to receive a GABA-mediated synaptic input from striatum in vivo (Precht and Yoshida, 1971; Grace and Bunney, 1985). $GABA_A$ receptor-mediated synaptic potentials, both evoked and spontaneously occurring, have been demonstrated in vitro in dopamine neurones of both substantia nigra (Mereu et al., 1991; Fig. 7) and VTA (Johnson and North, 1992a,b; Sugita et al., 1992), and also the "secondary" neurones of the VTA (Johnson and North, 1992b). This action of GABA appears conventional, in that it is probably mediated by a chloride conductance increase (Nakanishi et al., 1987; Lacey et al., 1988; Johnson and North, 1992b), and is sensitive to bicuculline (Lacey et al., 1988) and picrotoxin (Mereu et al., 1991; Johnson and North, 1992b). A proportion of such synaptic potentials have been shown to be sensitive to μ-opioid receptor agonists (Johnson and North, 1992a; Fig. 7), and these probably arise from local circuit interneurones (Johnson and North, 1992a; see below). In contrast to conclusions drawn from in vivo studies (Precht and Yoshida, 1971; Grace and Bunney, 1985), it has been proposed that of the other possible sources of GABA$_A$-mediated synaptic events in dopamine neurones, those arising from striatal inputs may be discounted (Johnson et al., 1992). This is because they are insensitive to inhibition by 5-HT (Sugita et al., 1992; Johnson et al., 1992a), and presynaptic 5-HT$_{1B}$ receptors are known to be present on striatonigral terminals and to mediate inhibition by 5-HT of GABA$_B$ receptor-mediated input in brain slices (Sugita et al., 1992; Johnson et al., 1992a).

A slow hyperpolarising synaptic potential, blocked by the GABA$_B$ antagonist 2-hydroxysaclofen and with a reversal potential close to the predicted potassium equilibrium potential, can be evoked with short trains of stimuli applied close to dopamine neurones recorded in slices both in SNc (Häusser and Yung, 1991) and VTA (Johnson and North, 1992b; Johnson et al., 1992a). This GABA$_B$ receptor-mediated synaptic event can be largely abolished by 5-HT acting on presynaptic 5-HT$_{1B}$ receptors (see above and Johnson and North, 1992b; Johnson et al., 1992a). In common with many other neurones (North, 1989), SNc dopamine neurones are hyperpolarised by the GABA$_B$ receptor agonist baclofen (Pinnock, 1984b), an action which involves coupling of a GTP-binding protein to an increase in potassium conductance (Lacey et al., 1988). The potassium channels opened by GABA$_B$ receptors are also utilised by D$_2$ receptors (Lacey et al., 1988). The equilibrium dissociation constant at this receptor of the GABA$_B$ antagonist CGP 35348 has been estimated as 18 μM (Seabrook et al., 1990), comparable to that in other preparations (Seabrook et al., 1990; Olpe et al., 1990). The "secondary" cells of the SNc also possess functional GABA$_B$ receptors (Lacey et al., 1989).

GABA$_B$ and GABA$_A$ receptor-mediated synaptic events in dopamine neurones may be distinguished by their respective sensitivity or insensitivity to the presynaptic inhibitory action of 5-HT (Sugita et al., 1992; Johnson et al., 1992a; above). This intruiging finding provides good evidence for GABA-mediated input to dopamine neurones of different origin utilising different sets of postsynaptic receptors, and therefore presumably for these receptors having disparate locations on the neuraxis. Similar

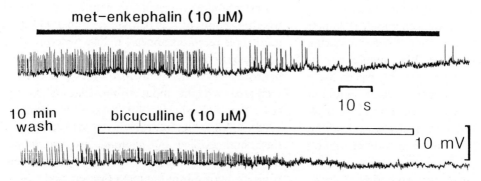

Fig. 7. Spontaneous GABA-mediated synaptic potentials in dopamine cells are inhibited by met-enkephalin. Two records of membrane potential from the same cell, separated by 10 min, which was exhibiting spontaneous, transient (synaptic) depolarisations. These were blocked reversibly by met-enkephalin (upper record) and then by the GABA$_A$ receptor antagonist bicuculline. Electrode contained 2 M KCl: Cl$^-$ loading of the cell renders GABA$_A$-mediated events depolarising. Lack of effect of met-enkephalin on membrane potential indicates a presynaptic action.

conclusions have been drawn in amygdala (Sugita et al., 1992) and hippocampus (Otis and Mody, 1992). While the majority of $GABA_B$ receptor-utilising input may arise from striatonigral fibres possessing presynaptic $5\text{-}HT_{1B}$ receptors, a proportion (around 20%) appeared insensitive to 5-HT (Sugita et al., 1992) and thus may originate elsewhere. A non-midbrain location would seem likely as, unlike $GABA_A$ synaptic potentials, $GABA_B$ events could not be elicited by elevated potassium concentration, probably eliminating GABA-containing intrinsic neurones as a source of this input (Sugita et al., 1992; Johnson et al., 1992a). It remains possible that GABA input to dopamine cells from other sources, such as the globus pallidus (Smith and Bolam, 1990), or collaterals of projection neurones or even interneurones (Grace and Bunney, 1985) within the substantia nigra pars reticulata, could utilise $GABA_B$ receptors and $GABA_A$ receptors as well.

Glycine and taurine

Glycine levels in substantia nigra and VTA are among the highest in the brain; calcium-dependent glycine release from ventral midbrain has been demonstrated in vitro, as have high- and low-affinity uptake systems, and its ability to release dopamine from substantia nigra, both in vivo (Cheramy et al., 1981) and in vitro (see Ottersen and Storm-Mathisen, 1984, for review). Additionally, and somewhat paradoxically, electrophysiological studies performed on dopamine neurones in vivo have demonstrated an inhibitory action of both glycine (Dray et al., 1976b) and taurine (Dray and Straughan, 1976) when applied by iontophoresis. All these actions of glycine (apart from at the uptake sites) can be blocked by strychnine. It has been suggested that there may be a class of glycine-containing interneurone-innervating dopamine cells (Dray et al., 1977; Ottersen and Storm-Mathisen, 1984). There is evidence for calcium-dependent taurine release from the striatonigral pathway, as well as a high-affinity taurine uptake site in substantia nigra (Della Corte et al., 1990), but otherwise evidence for a functional role of taurine in ventral midbrain is a little less compelling than that for glycine.

Glycine inhibits substantia nigra dopamine neurones in vitro in a strychnine-sensitive manner through an increase in conductance to chloride ions (Mercuri et al., 1988). This action was unaffected by blockers of $GABA_A$ receptor-mediated responses or by blockade of synaptic transmission (Mercuri et al., 1990a). It was proposed that glycine additionally increased potassium conductance, as the reversal potential showed some dependence on extracellular potassium concentration (Mercuri et al., 1988, 1990a), but an alternative explanation has since been proffered (Häusser et al., 1992). Taurine also increases chloride conductance in dopamine neurones by a direct action and, as this effect is also blocked by strychnine and a maximal effect of one amino acid occludes the effect of the other, it may be that both amino acids act on the same set of ionotropic receptors (Häusser et al., 1992), as has been proposed for other neuronal types (Krishtal et al., 1988; Tokutomi et al., 1989). However, it remains an open question as to whether either amino acid has a neurotransmitter role in afferents to dopamine cells and, if a strychnine-sensitive synaptic event is identified, which of these two amino acids will be the mediator.

Excitatory amino acids

Reports of neurones in mammalian brain that are not excited by glutamate or aspartate, the principal fast excitatory transmitter candidates, are hard to find. Examples of those that are are plentiful, and demonstrations of neurones receiving synaptic input mediated by glutamate receptors (named after their preferred selective agonists) of the kainate, quisqualate/AMPA and NMDA types are becoming increasingly common (Collingridge and Lester, 1989; Nicoll et al., 1990). It would not be surprising if intensive study would show this to be the case for dopamine neurones as well. Iontophoretic application of glutamate was shown to excite dopamine neurones in vivo (Grace and Bunney, 1984b), as was electrical stimulation of the pedunculo-pontine nucleus, an action blocked by iontophoresis of (non-selective) glutamate receptor antagonists (Scarnati et al., 1986). A pedunculopontine-nigral pathway has been demonstrated anatomically, but as it is not considered cholinergic (Lee et al., 1988), this does not support the report of a functional (nicotinic) response in SNc following pedunculopontine nucleus stimulation (Clarke et al., 1987; above). The subthalamic nucleus is another likely source of input onto dopamine neurones from glutamate-containing fibres (Graybiel, 1990). Stimulation of the subthalamic nucleus resulted in fast excitatory synaptic potentials in neurones in substantia nigra pars reticulata neurones in brain slices, some of which (type II) were probably dopamine cells (Nakanishi et al., 1987). A third source of excitatory amino acid input to the ventral midbrain is an aspartate-containing projection from the medial prefrontal cortex (Christie et al., 1985; see below).

Fast excitatory picrotoxin-resistant postsynaptic currents in dopamine cells of the SNc resulting from focal stimulation of brain slices have been demonstrated using whole-cell patch clamp recording (Mereu et al., 1991). They were generally comprised of two components, a fast non-NMDA receptor-mediated component blocked by 6-cyano-7-dinitroquinoxaline-2,3-dione (CNQX), and a slow NMDA receptor-mediated component which was blocked by DL-2-amino-phosphonovalerate (APV), enhanced by removal of extracellular magnesium or addition of glycine, but blocked by the NMDA receptor "glycine site" antagonist 7-chlorokynurenic acid. Spontaneous "miniature" synaptic currents were also observed, but acting through only the non-NMDA receptor type (Mereu et al., 1991). These observations have essentially been confirmed in recordings from both dopamine cells and secondary cells/interneurones in VTA, with the exception of the spontaneous synaptic events in dopamine cells, which were mediated by GABA rather than glutamate (Johnson and North, 1992a,b; above). A 34% percent reduction of the excitatory amino acid-mediated synaptic potential could be obtained with met-enkephalin (Johnson and North, 1992a), indicating that a proportion of the excitatory amino acid-containing afferents possess presynaptic opioid receptors.

Iontophoresis of the broad spectrum excitatory amino acid antagonist kynurenic acid (Collingridge and Lester, 1989) onto dopamine neurones in vivo produced an increased regularisation of their firing pattern at the expense of bursting (Charlety et al., 1991). This effect could be mimicked by cold block of the prefrontal cortex (Svensson and Tung, 1989), a possible source of excitatory amino acid projections to dopamine neurones (Christie et al., 1985). The conclusion from these findings, that the burst firing seen in vivo, but generally not in vitro (above), is a result of excitatory amino acid input has been reinforced by a recent description of the induction of burst firing in dopamine neurones by NMDA in brain slices (Johnson et al., 1992b). In what may prove to be a novel mechanism associated with both NMDA receptor activation and control of the dopamine neurone firing pattern, the refractory interburst interval appears due to a hyperpolarisation produced by an ouabain-sensitive outward sodium pump current, reinforced by the consequent voltage-dependent block by magnesium of the NMDA depolarisation. Interestingly this effect could also be induced by aspartate, but not glutamate, kainate or quisqualate (Johnson et al., 1992b). The NMDA receptor involved might be a subtype (Kutsuwada et al., 1992) with a particular preference for aspartate, the proposed transmitter in the prefrontal cortical-ventral midbrain pathway (Christie et al., 1985).

Peptides

Opioids

The distribution of immunohistochemical markers for opioid peptides and their precursors suggests that both the prodynorphin products dynorphin and leucine-enkephalin are found colocalised with GABA in terminals of striato-nigral projection neurones (Zamir et al., 1984; Petrusz et al., 1985; Graybiel, 1990), and predominantly in substantia nigra pars reticulata. Additionally, the proenkephalin product methionine-enkephalin (and perhaps leucine-enkephalin as well) is likely to be in both terminals and cell bodies within SNc and VTA (Petrusz et al., 1985). Numbers of μ-opioid receptor (which preferentially bind met-enkephalin) in ventral midbrain are unaffected by 6-hydroxydopamine lesion of dopamine cells, but are reduced by 50% in VTA by excitotoxic lesions of intrinsic neurones. Thus they are present on both non-dopamine cells and also on extrinsically derived terminals (Dilts and Kalivas, 1989), at least some of which are striato-nigral projections (Abou Khalil et al., 1984). Electrophysiological studies in vivo have shown dopamine neurones to be excited by morphine, particularly when given intravenously as opposed to iontophoretically (Gysling and Wang, 1983; Matthews and German, 1984), and correspondingly terminal dopamine release, particularly in nucleus accumbens, is enhanced (Di Chiara and Imperato, 1988). This excitation of dopamine neurones by morphine could represent the cellular mechanism of the rewarding effects of opioids.

Studies in brain slices have shown that dopamine neurones are not directly affected by agonists at μ- and δ-opioid receptors (Lacey et al., 1989; Johnson and North, 1992a,b), whereas non-dopamine "secondary" cells are generally hyperpolarised by μ-, but not δ- or $\varkappa$-opioid receptor activation (Lacey et al., 1989; Johnson and North, 1992a; Fig. 8A), through a conductance increase, probably to potassium ions, as has been shown in other cell types (North and Williams, 1985; North, 1989). However, spontaneous GABA-mediated synaptic potentials in dopamine cells are potently inhibited by μ-opioid receptor-selective agonists (Johnson and North, 1992a; Fig. 7) and the most parsimonious explanation for this disinhibitory effect is that opioids act on the intrinsic, presumed interneuronal non-dopamine cells to stop them firing and releasing GABA onto dopamine cells (Johnson and North, 1992a). Evoked synaptic potentials activating excitatory amino acid, $GABA_A$ and $GABA_B$ receptors were also reduced in amplitude by 25 – 35% by met-enkephalin (Johnson and North, 1992a), this action probably being through presynaptic receptors on terminals of fibres of extrinsic origin. These data provide persuasive evidence for actions of exogenously administered opioids within substantia nigra, with possibly profound behavioural consequences in providing a stimulus to dopamine neurones that appears important in the rewarding effects of opioids (Wise, 1983; Wise and Bozarth, 1987; Di Chiara and Imperato, 1988; Johnson and North, 1992a). Nonetheless, a physiological role of endogenous opioids in synaptic transmission in this part of the basal ganglia, or for that matter in any part of the central nervous system, remains to be demonstrated.

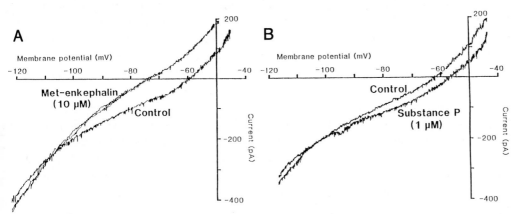

Fig. 8. Voltage dependence of the action of two neuropeptides, met-enkephalin and substance P, on a non-dopamine cell. Steady-state current – voltage relationships from the same cell, both in control and in the presence of peptide. A. Met-enkephalin caused an outward current becoming inward at around the predicted potassium equilibrium potential, accompanied by conductance increase, suggestive of it opening potassium channels. B. Substance P caused an inward current, also reversing at around the same potential as in A, accompanied by conductance decrease, indicating that it may close potassium channels.

Neurokinins

There is a great deal of neuroanatomical evidence for a tachykinin (substance P and neurokinin A/substance K)-containing pathway from striatum to substantia nigra, with at least some of the tachykinins being colocalised with GABA in nerve terminals (see Bolam and Smith, 1990, and Mendez et al., 1992, for both recent contributions and literature reviews). Substance P-like immunoreactivity is found in terminals contacting both dopamine-containing cell bodies and dendrites (Bolam and Smith, 1990; Mendez et al., 1992), and also GABA-containing neurones in SNc (Mendez et al., 1992). Substance P, neurokinin A (substance K), and to a lesser extent both neuropeptide K and neurokinin B, can be released from substantia nigra both in vivo and in brain slices (Jessell, 1978; Diez Guerra et al., 1988). Injection of a stable substance P analogue into the VTA produces increased locomotion, which may be blocked by the dopamine receptor antagonist haloperidol, and is accompanied by increased dopamine metabolism in limbic and cortical regions (Elliott et al., 1986). Based on in vivo experiments using the push-pull cannula technique, it has been proposed that in the substantia nigra, substance P acts indirectly to cause dopamine release, via a pars reticulata-thalamo-cortico-striatal loop, whereas neurokinin A directly activates dopamine neurones to cause both dendritic and terminal release of dopamine (Baruch et al., 1988).

Iontophoretic application of both substance P (Pinnock and Dray, 1982) and substance K (neurokinin A; Innis et al., 1985) excites a small proportion (no more than 50%) of both SNc (dopamine) and pars reticulata (non-dopamine) cells. In brain slices, around 50% of both dopamine and non-dopamine cells in both substantia nigra and VTA were depolarised and excited by substance P (0.1 – 1 μM; Lacey, unpublished observations). The ionic mechanism for this effect on non-dopamine cells may be a potassium conductance decrease (Fig. 8B), but has yet to be ascertained in dopamine neurones. Recently developed pharmacological tools permit characterisation of three tachykinin receptor types (Elliott et al., 1991; Watling, 1992). The be-

havioural consequences of infusion of neurokinin receptor subtype-selective agonists into the ventral midbrain suggest that dopamine neurones of the VTA are activated by NK_1 and NK_3 receptors, whereas those of the substantia nigra are sensitive to NK_2 receptor agonists (Elliott et al., 1991). However, in brain slices around 75% of substantia nigra dopamine cells were depolarised through NK_3 (neurokinin A-preferring) receptors, with selective agonists at NK_1 and NK_2 (more substance P-preferring) receptors ineffective (Keegan et al., 1992). This discrepancy between the pharmacology of single cells (Keegan et al., 1993) and behavioural and neurochemical data from the whole animal (Elliott et al., 1991) requires further investigation. Whether the neurokinin receptor subtypes on either the interneurones or the pars reticulata cells are different from those on the dopamine cells, or whether these receptors play a role in synaptic transmission in the striato-nigral pathway, also remains to be seen.

Cholecystokinin

Cholecystokinin (CCK) is found colocalised with dopamine in a large proportion of dopamine neurones, particularly in the VTA (Hökfelt et al., 1980). Some of these cells also contain neurotensin (Seroogy et al., 1987; see below). Extensive colocalisation of messenger RNA for tyrosine hydroxylase and CCK has also been demonstrated in midbrain neurones (Savasta et al., 1989). Of the two CCK receptor subtypes presently recognised, binding sites of the CCK-A (formerly "peripheral" type) subtype are present in high concentrations in the dopamine-rich areas of ventral midbrain (Hill et al., 1990). The dopamine-CCK colocalisation and potential for functional interaction, combined with the development of potent and selective CCK-A and B receptor antagonists, has stimulated hopes of novel approaches to antipsychotic therapy in this field (see Crawley, 1991). CCK-sulphated octapeptide has been shown to both excite dopamine neurones and potentiate the inhibitory effect of the dopamine receptor agonist apomorphine in vivo (Hommer et al., 1986). However, although CCK can modulate dopamine release from nucleus accumbens, when injected into the VTA very little change in dopamine release in nucleus accumbens was detected, casting doubt on the importance of CCK effects on dopamine neurones at the level of the cell body (see Crawley, 1991, for review).

CCK (at low nanomolar concentrations) has been reported to both excite extracellularly recorded VTA neurones in vitro and to potentiate the inhibitory effects of dopamine in brain slices (Brodie and Dunwiddie, 1987; Stittsworth and Mueller, 1990), similar to findings in vivo (above). However, apart from these two reports, this author is unaware of publication of any investigation into the mechanism and pharmacology of either the CCK excitation or its potentially fascinating interaction with dopamine. At considerably higher concentrations than those found effective by Brodie and Dunwiddie (1987) or Stittsworth and Mueller (1989), CCK was seen to depolarise and excite a small proportion of dopamine cells, both in VTA and substantia nigra (Fig. 9), but a potentiation of the dopamine hyperpolarisation was not observed (Lacey, unpublished observations). Thus cellular electrophysiology has yet to make a major contribution to a further understanding of the function or mechanism of action of CCK in substantia nigra or VTA.

Neurotensin

Neurotensin-like immunoreactivity is found in a subset of midbrain dopamine-containing neurones, and these are predominantly in the VTA (Hökfelt et al., 1984). Around 90% of these cells also contain CCK (Seroogy et al., 1987). Neurotensin-containing terminals of striatonigral fibres have also been demonstrated, but they terminate in substantia nigra pars reticulata and pars lateralis rather than pars compacta or the VTA (Sugimoto and Mizuno, 1987). Neurotensin binding sites are present on midbrain dopamine neurones (Palacios and Kuhar, 1981; Dilts and Kalivas, 1989) and neurotensin applied in the ventral midbrain can cause dopamine release from both ventral midbrain (presumably from dopamine cell dendrites) and caudate nucleus (Faggin et al., 1990). In brain slices, most dopamine neurones of both substantia nigra (Pinnock, 1985; Keegan et al., 1990; Shi and Bunney, 1991) and VTA (Seutin et al., 1989) are excited by neurotensin in the low nanomolar range, as a result of a long-lasting membrane depolarisation (Pinnock, 1985). This ef-

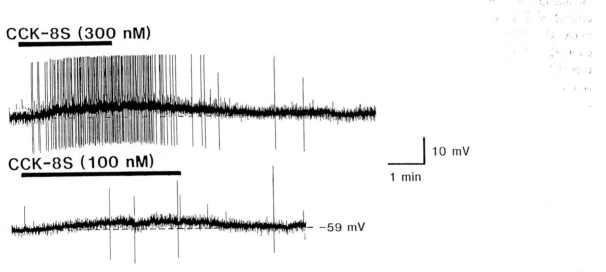

Fig. 9. Cholecystokinin-sulphated octapeptide (CCK-8S) can depolarise and excite dopamine neurones in a concentration-dependent manner. Records of membrane potential from a dopamine cell hyperpolarised to prevent spontaneous action potential firing. CCK-8S (100, 300 nM) caused a small depolarisation. CCK-8S (30 nM) was without effect on this cell.

fect appears independent of transmitter release (Pinnock, 1985; Keegan et al., 1990) and may prove to be due to a decrease in membrane potassium conductance (Keegan et al., 1993). This effect could be mimicked by several fragments of neurotensin including NT 8 – 13 (but not NT 1 – 8; Pinnock, 1985; Seutin et al., 1989; Keegan et al., 1990), and also neuromedin N, a product of the same messenger RNA as neurotensin (Keegan et al., 1990; Shi and Bunney, 1991). At concentrations below around 10 nM, neurotensin has been reported to attenuate the inhibitory effect of dopamine on dopamine cell firing, whereas at concentrations above 100 nM it causes a biphasic response (Shi and Bunney, 1991). These paradoxical effects remain unexplained. It may be that inroads into the question of how neurotensin might regulate dopamine cell activity under physiological conditions must await the availability of stable and selective non-peptide agonists and antagonists, such as those for the other neuropeptide classes discussed above.

Other regulators of dopamine cell activity

ATP-gated potassium channels

Potassium channels gated (closed) by intracellular adenosine triphosphate (ATP-K channels) are critical to the control by glucose of insulin secretion in pancreatic B cells. A chemically diverse group of compounds often called potassium channel activators (KCAs) open these channels, and antidiabetic sulphonylurea drugs close them, and not just in B cells, but in a range of tissues, including central neurones (Ashcroft and Ashcroft, 1990). The region of brain with perhaps the highest density of binding sites for the sulphonylurea glibenclamide is the substantia nigra, albeit predominantly the pars reticulata (Mourre et al., 1990). The release of GABA from slices of ventral midbrain is analogous to that of insulin from pancreatic B cells in that it is stimulated by glucose and sulphonylureas, and reduced by KCAs and anoxia (which probably lowers intracellular ATP; Amoroso et al., 1990; Schmid Antomarchi et al., 1990). The release of GABA was inversely related to efflux of $^{86}Rb^+$,

suggesting that there are functional ATP-K channels on GABA-containing terminals in ventral midbrain (Schmid Antomarchi et al., 1990; Amoroso et al., 1990).

Using whole-cell patch clamp recording from acutely dissociated substantia nigra dopamine cells, GABA-mediated synaptic potentials (considered to arise from isolated terminals attached to the recorded cells) were abolished by the KCA cromakalim, presumably acting presynaptically (Häusser et al., 1991). Furthermore, cromakalim, or low intracellular ATP concentrations, caused hyperpolarisation of the dopamine cells which was reversed with glibenclamide, suggesting that dopamine cells themselves also had ATP-K channels (Häusser et al., 1991). Previously it had been reported that dopamine cells had potassium channels that could be closed by the sulphonylurea tolbutamide, and that they were the same ones that could be opened by D_2 or $GABA_B$ receptor activation (Roeper et al., 1990). However, this finding has since been disputed by others who have been unable to reproduce it using whole cell recording from brain slices. (Hicks and Henderson, 1992). Additionally, in brain slices the membrane potential of the type of cells generally considered to contain dopamine was rather insensitive to both anoxia and the KCA diazoxide (Murphy and Greenfield, 1992). However, these same authors provided evidence for functional ATP-K channels on another type of cell in the rostral part of the substantia nigra whose electrophysiological properties differ from those most others consider dopamine-containing (Murphy and Greenfield, 1992; see above). Taken together, the data on the direct regulation of dopamine cells by ATP-K channels is presently contradictory, even controversial, and it seems somewhat premature to suggest that "the K_{ATP} channel plays a vital part in the aetiology of Parkinson's disease" (Murphy and Greenfield, 1992).

Ethanol

VTA dopamine neurones are exited by ethanol applied in millimolar concentrations in brain slices, apparently by a direct action (Brodie et al., 1990).

The mechanism of this effect is not established, although a decrease in action potential after-hyperpolarisation may be involved, nor is it clear if ethanol can act by interfering with GABA-mediated transmission onto dopamine neurones (Harris et al., 1992). This action may be important for the rewarding effects of ethanol (Harris et al., 1992).

Conclusions

The use of in vitro electrophysiological techniques has permitted new vistas to be opened onto the ionic and receptor mechanisms subserving synaptic transmission in dopamine neurones, as in other areas of mammalian brain. Functional correlates of receptors described previously by neurochemical techniques have been demonstrated; also functional receptors have been demonstrated whose existence was little suspected (muscarinic and glycine/taurine). While several of the mechanisms of neurotransmitter action are not unique to dopamine neurones, and have been previously demonstrated in other brain regions (Nicoll et al., 1990), work on dopamine neurones has produced some original findings with implications for mechanisms of chemical transmission in other neurones. These include the demonstration that D_2 receptors can couple to an increase in potassium conductance (Lacey et al., 1987), that muscarinic M_1-like receptors may increase neuronal excitability through means other than a potassium conductance decrease (Lacey et al., 1990a), that projection cells may be disinhibited by actions of opioids in interneurones (Lacey et al., 1989; Johnson and North, 1992a) and the discrimination of GABA-mediated input between post-synaptic GABA receptor subtypes (Sugita et al., 1992). Other interesting, but perhaps less well established phenomena include the synergy between CCK and dopamine (Brodie and Dunwiddie, 1987), the idea that ligand-gated potassium channels may also be sulphonylurea-sensitive and ATP-gated (Roeper et al., 1990) and that NMDA receptor activation may cause an outward current due to an ion exchange pump (Johnson et al., 1992b).

Although not all studies have attempted to discriminate between substantia nigra and VTA, where comparisons are possible there is as yet very little reason to suppose that mesolimbo-cortical dopamine neurones, originating in the VTA, possess either different membrane properties or neurotransmitter receptors from nigrostriatal neurones. Their basic electrophysiological characteristics appear the same, both for dopamine and non-dopamine interneurones (Lacey et al., 1989; Grace and Onn, 1989; Yung et al., 1991; Johnson and North, 1992b); dopamine cells from both areas are hyperpolarised by D_2 receptor activation, but not affected by opioids, whereas the reverse is true for non-dopamine cells (Lacey et al., 1989; Johnson and North, 1992b); dopamine cells from both regions are depolarised by acetylcholine acting on both nicotinic and muscarinic receptors (Lacey et al., 1991); and they all receive synaptic input mediated by GABA, acting on $GABA_A$ and $GABA_B$ receptors (Mereu et al., 1991; Johnson and North, 1992b; Johnson et al., 1992a), and glutamate (or aspartate), acting on NMDA and non-NMDA type receptors (Mereu et al., 1991; Johnson and North, 1992b). Any emerging differences would be potentially exploitable in the context of selective therapeutic manipulation of the different ascending dopamine systems. One possibility would be for discovery of novel antipsychotic drugs which, in sparing the nigrostriatal dopamine system, would be expected to produce fewer extrapyramidal side effects. Extrapolating from cellular studies of dopamine neurones in vitro, it seems likely that apparent differences in drug actions observed in vivo upon midbrain dopamine neurones projecting to different forebrain targets may reflect their different afferent and efferent connections, and participation in different neuronal circuitry in which other elements might be differentially drug-sensitive, rather than intrinsic differences between the cells themselves. This may account for the apparent mesolimbic selectivity of "atypical" antipsychotic drugs (Reynolds, 1992). The application of cellular electrophysiological techniques, in combination with pharmacological dissection of synaptic events, to areas efferent and afferent to midbrain dopamine neurones promises to build up a more complete picture of their function and regulation, and of the interaction of the component neurones and nuclei of the basal ganglia.

References

Abou Khalil, B., Young, A.B. and Penney, J.B. (1984) Evidence for the presynaptic localization of opiate binding sites on striatal efferent fibers. *Brain Res.,* 323: 21 – 29.

Adams, P.R., Brown, D.A. and Constanti, A. (1982) M-currents and other potassium currents in bullfrog sympathetic neurones. *J. Physiol., (Lond.),* 330: 537 – 572.

Aghajanian, G.K. and Bunney, B.S. (1977) Dopamine "autoreceptors": pharmacological characterisation by microiontophoretic single cell recording studies. *Naunyn Schmiedebergs Arch. Pharmacol.,* 297: 1 – 7.

Amoroso, S., Schmid Antomarchi, H., Fosset, M. and Lazdunski, M. (1990) Glucose, sulfonylureas, and neurotransmitter release: role of ATP-sensitive K^+ channels. *Science,* 247: 852 – 854.

Ashcroft, S.J. and Ashcroft, F.M. (1990) Properties and functions of ATP-sensitive K-channels. *Cell Signal,* 2: 197 – 214.

Baruch, P., Artaud, F., Godeheu, G., Barbeito, L., Glowinski, J. and Cheramy, A. (1988) Substance P and neurokinin A regulate by different mechanisms dopamine release from dendrites and nerve terminals of the nigrostriatal dopaminergic neurons. *Neuroscience,* 25: 889 – 898.

Bayer, V.E. and Pickel, V.M. (1990) Ultrastructural localisation of tyrosine hydroxylase in the rat ventral tegmental area: relationship between immunolabelling density and neuronal associations. *J. Neurosci.,* 10: 2996 – 3010.

Benham, C.D. and Bolton, T.B. (1985) Acetylcholine activates an inward current in single mammalian smooth muscle cells. *Nature,* 316: 345 – 347.

Beninato, M. and Spencer, R.F. (1988) The cholinergic innervation of the rat substantia nigra: a light and electron microscopic immunohistochemical study. *Exp. Brain Res.,* 72: 178 – 184.

Berridge, M.J. and Irvine, R.F. (1989) Inositol phosphates and cell signalling. *Nature,* 341: 197 – 205.

Björklund, A. and Lindvall, O. (1975) Dopamine in dendrites of substantia nigra neurons: suggestions for a role in dendritic terminals. *Brain Res..,* 83: 531 – 537.

Björklund, A. and Lindvall, O. (1984) Dopamine-containing systems in the CNS. In: A. Björklund and T. Hökfelt (Eds.), *Handbook of Chemical Neuroanatomy, Vol. 2: Classical Transmitters in the CNS, Part I,* Elsevier, Amsterdam, pp. 55 – 122.

Björklund, A. and Lindvall, O. (1986) Catecholaminergic brain stem regulatory systems. In: V.B. Mountcastle and F.E. Bloom (Eds.), *Handbook of Physiology, Section 1: The Nervous System. Vol. IV: Intrinsic Regulatory Systems of the Brain,* American Physiological Society, Bethesda, MD, pp. 155 – 236.

Bobker, D.H. and Williams, J.T. (1989) Serotonin augments the cationic current Ih in central neurons. *Neuron,* 2: 1535 – 1540.

Bolam, J.P. and Smith, Y. (1990) The GABA and substance P input to dopaminergic neurones in the substantia nigra of the rat. *Brain Res.,* 529: 57 – 78.

Bolam, J.P., Francis, C.M. and Henderson, Z. (1991) Cholinergic input to dopaminergic neurons in the substantia nigra: a double immunocytochemical study. *Neuroscience,* 41: 483 – 494.

Bouhelal, R., Smounya, L. and Bockaert, J. (1988) 5-HT1B receptors are negatively coupled with adenylate cyclase in rat substantia nigra. *Eur. J. Pharmacol.,* 151: 189 – 196.

Brodie, M.S. and Dunwiddie, T.V. (1987) Cholecystokinin potentiates dopamine inhibition of mesencephalic dopamine neurons in vitro. *Brain Res.,* 425: 106 – 113.

Brodie, M.S. and Dunwiddie, T.V. (1990) Cocaine effects in the ventral tegmental area: evidence for an indirect dopaminergic mechanism of action. *Naunyn Schmiedebergs Arch. Pharmacol.,* 342: 660 – 665.

Brodie, M.S., Shefner, S.A. and Dunwiddie, T.V. (1990) Ethanol increases the firing rate of dopamine neurons of the rat ventral tegmental area in vitro. *Brain Res.,* 508: 65 – 69.

Buckley, N.J., Bonner, T.I., Buckley, C.M. and Brann, M.R. (1989) Antagonist binding properties of five cloned muscarinic receptors expressed in CHO-K1 cells. *Mol. Pharmacol.,* 35: 469 – 476.

Bunney, B.S., Walters, J.R., Roth, R.H. and Aghajanian, G.K. (1973) Dopaminergic neurones: effect of antipsychotic drugs and amphetamine on single cell activity. *J. Pharmacol. Exp. Ther.,* 185: 560 – 571.

Calabresi, P., Lacey, M.G. and North, R.A. (1989) Nicotinic excitation of rat ventral tegmental neurones in vitro studied by intracellular recording. *Br. J. Pharmacol.,* 98: 135 – 139.

Charlety, P.J., Grenhoff, J., Chergui, K., De La Chappelle, B., Buda, M., Svensson, T.H. and Chouvet, G. (1991) Burst firing of mesencephalic dopamine neurons is inhibited by somatodendritic application of kynurenate. *Acta Physiol. Scand.,* 142: 105 – 112.

Cheramy, A., Leviel, V. and Glowinski, J. (1981) Dendritic release of dopamine in the substantia nigra. *Nature,* 289: 537 – 542.

Chesselet, M.F. (1984) Presynaptic regulation of neurotransmitter release in the brain: facts and hypothesis. *Neuroscience,* 12: 347 – 375.

Christie, M.J. and North, R.A. (1988) Control of ionic conductances by muscarinic receptors. *Trends Pharmacol. Sci. (Suppl.): Subtypes of Muscarinic Receptors, III,* pp. 30 – 34.

Christie, M.J., Bridge, S., James, I.B. and Beart, P.M. (1985) Excitotoxic lesions suggest an aspartatergic from rat medial prefrontal cortex to ventral tegmental area. *Brain Res.,* 333: 169 – 172.

Clarke, P.B. and Pert, A. (1985) Autoradiographic evidence for nicotine receptors on nigrostriatal and mesolimbic dopaminergic neurons. *Brain Res.,* 348: 355–358.

Clarke, P.B., Hommer, D.W., Pert, A. and Skirboll, L.R. (1985) Electrophysiological actions of nicotine on substantia nigra single units. *Br. J. Pharmacol.,* 85: 827–835.

Clarke, P.B., Hommer, D.W., Pert, A. and Skirboll, L.R. (1987) Innervation of substantia nigra neurons by cholinergic afferents from pedunculopontine nucleus in the rat: neuroanatomical and electrophysiological evidence. *Neuroscience,* 23: 1011–1019.

Collingridge, G.L. and Lester, R.A.J. (1989) Excitatory amino acid receptors in the vertebrate central nervous system. *Pharmacol. Res.,* 41: 143–210.

Condé, H. (1992) Organization and physiology of the substantia nigra. *Exp. Brain Res.,* 88: 233–248.

Crawley, J.N. (1991) Cholecystokinin-dopamine interactions. *Trends Pharmacol. Sci.,* 12: 232–236.

Della Corte, L., Bolam, J.P., Clarke, D.J., Parry, D.M. and Smith, A.D. (1990) Sites of [^{3}H] taurine uptake in the rat substantia nigra in relation to the release of taurine from the striatonigral pathway. *Eur. J. Neurosci.,* 2: 50–61.

Deutch, A.Y., Holliday, J., Roth, R.H., Chun, L.L. and Hawrot, E. (1987) Immunohistochemical localization of a neuronal nicotinic acetylcholine receptor in mammalian brain. *Proc. Natl. Acad. Sci. U.S.A.,* 84: 8697–8701.

Di Chiara, G. (1990) In-vivo brain dialysis of neurotransmitters. *Trends Pharmacol. Sci.,* 11: 116–121.

Di Chiara, G. and Imperato, A. (1988) Drugs abused by humans preferentially increase synaptic dopamine concentrations in the mesolimbic system of freely moving rats. *Proc. Natl. Acad. Sci. U.S.A.,* 85: 5274–5278.

Diez Guerra, F.J., Sirinathsinghji, D.J. and Emson, P.C. (1988) In vitro and in vivo release of neurokinin A-like immunoreactivity from rat substantia nigra. *Neuroscience,* 27: 527–536.

Dilts, R.P. and Kalivas, P.W. (1989) Autoradiographic localization of mu-opioid and neurotensin receptors within the mesolimbic dopamine system. *Brain Res.,* 488: 311–327.

Dray, A. and Straughan, D.W. (1976) Synaptic mechanisms in the substantia nigra. *J. Pharm. Pharmacol.,* 28: 400–405.

Dray, A., Gonye, T.J., Oakley, N.R. and Tanner, T. (1976a) Evidence for the existence of a raphe projection to the substantia nigra in rat. *Brain Res.,* 113: 45–57.

Dray, A., Goyne, T.J. and Oakley, N.R. (1976b) Caudate stimulation and substantia nigra activity in the rat. *J. Physiol. (Lond.),* 259: 825–849.

Dray, A., Goyne, T.J. , Oakley, N.R., Simmonds, M.A. and Tanner, T. (1977) Regulation of nigro-striatal dopaminergic transmission in the rat. *Neuropharmacology,* 16: 511–518.

Elliott, P.J., Alpert, J.E., Bannon, M.J. and Iversen, S.D. (1986) Selective activation of mesolimbic and mesocortical dopamine metabolism in rat brain by infusion of a stable substance P analogue into the ventral tegmental area. *Brain Res.,* 363: 145–147.

Elliott, P.J., Mason, G.S., Stephens Smith, M. and Hagan, R.M. (1991) Behavioural and biochemical responses following activation of midbrain dopamine pathways by receptor selective neurokinin agonists. *Neuropeptides,* 19: 119–126.

Faggin, B.M., Zubieta, J.K., Rezvani, A.H. and Cubeddu, L.X. (1990) Neurotensin-induced dopamine release in vivo and in vitro from substantia nigra and nucleus caudate. *J. Pharmacol. Exp. Ther.,* 252: 817–825.

Fallon, J.H., Riley, J.N. and Moore, R.Y. (1978) Substantia nigra dopamine neurons: separate populations project to neostriatum and allocortex. *Neurosci. Lett.,* 7: 157–162.

Fibiger, H.C. and Phillips, A.G. (1986) Reward, motivation, cognition: psychobiology of mesentelencephalic dopamine systems. In: V.B. Mountcastle and F.E. Bloom (Eds.), *Handbook of Physiology, Section 1: The Nervous System, Vol. IV, Intrinsic Regulatory Systems of the Brain,* American Physiological Society, Bethesda, MD, pp. 647–675.

Filloux, F.M., Walmsley, J.K. and Dawson, T.M. (1987) Dopamine D_2 auto- and postsynaptic receptors in the nigrostriatal system of the rat brain: localization by quantitative autoradiography with sulpiride. *Eur. J. Pharmacol.,* 138: 61–68.

Forsythe, I.D., Lambert, D.G., Nahorski, S.R. and Lindsell, P. (1992) Elevation of cytosolic calcium by cholinoceptor agonists in SH-SY5Y human neuroblastoma cells: estimation of the contribution of voltage-dependent currents. *Br. J. Pharmacol.,* 107: 207–214.

Geffen, L.B., Jessell, T.M., Cuello, A.C. and Iversen, L.L. (1976) Release of dopamine from dendrites in rat substantia nigra. *Nature,* 260: 258–260.

Gerfen, C.R., Baimbridge, K.G. and Thibault, J. (1987a) The neostriatal mosaic: III. Biochemical and developmental dissociation of patch-matrix mesostriatal systems. *J. Neurosci.,* 7: 3935–3944.

Gerfen, C.R., Herkenham, M. and Thibault, J. (1987b) The neostriatal mosaic: II. Patch- and matrix-directed mesostriatal dopaminergic and non-dopaminergic systems. *J. Neurosci.,* 7: 3915–3934.

Gil, G.W. and Wolfe, B.B. (1985) Pirenzepine distinguishes between muscarinic receptor-mediated phosphoinositide breakdown and inhibition of adenylate cyclase. *J. Pharmacol. Exp. Ther.,* 232: 608–616.

Gonon, F.G. (1988) Nonlinear relationship between impulse flow and dopamine released by rat midbrain dopaminergic neurons as studied by in vivo electrochemistry. *Neuroscience,* 24: 19–28.

Grace, A.A. (1987) The regulation of dopamine neuron activity as determined by in vivo and in vitro intracellular recordings. In: L.A. Chiodo and A.S. Freeman (Eds.), *The Neurophysiology of Dopamine Systems,* Shore Publications, Detroit.

Grace, A.A. and Bunney, B.S. (1980) Nigral dopamine neurons: intracellular recording and identification with L-Dopa injection and histofluorescence. *Science,* 210: 654–656.

Grace, A.A. and Bunney, B.S. (1983a) Intracellular and extracellular electrophysiology of nigral dopaminergic neurons, 1. Identification and characterization. *Neuroscience,* 10:

301 – 315.

Grace, A.A. and Bunney, B.S. (1983b) Intracellular and extracellular electrophysiology of nigral dopaminergic neurons, 3. Evidence for electrotonic coupling. *Neuroscience*, 10: 333 – 348.

Grace, A.A. and Bunney, B.S. (1984a) The control of firing pattern in nigral dopamine neurons: burst firing. *J. Neurosci.*, 4: 2877 – 2890.

Grace, A.A. and Bunney, B.S. (1984b) The control of firing pattern in nigral dopamine neurons: single spike firing. *J. Neurosci.*, 4: 2866 – 2876.

Grace, A.A. and Bunney, B.S. (1985) Opposing effects of striatonigral feedback pathways on midbrain dopamine cell activity. *Brain Res.*, 333: 271 – 284.

Grace, A.A. and Onn, S.P. (1989) Morphology and electrophysiological properties of immunohistochemically identified rat dopamine neurons recorded in vitro. *J. Neurosci.*, 9: 3463 – 3481.

Graybiel, A.M. (1990) Neurotransmitters and neuromodulators in the basal ganglia. *Trends Neurosci.*, 13: 244 – 253.

Grenhoff, J., Aston Jones, G. and Svensson, T.H. (1986) Nicotinic effects on the firing pattern of midbrain dopamine neurons. *Acta Physiol. Scand.*, 128: 351 – 358.

Groves, P.M. and Linder, J.C. (1983) Dendro-dendritic synapses in substantia nigra: descriptions based on analysis of serial sections. *Exp. Brain Res.*, 49: 209 – 217.

Groves, P.M., Wilson, C.J., Young, S.J. and Rebec, G.V. (1975) Self-inhibition by dopaminergic neurons. *Science*, 190: 522 – 529.

Gysling, K. and Wang, R.Y. (1983) Morphine-induced activation of A10 dopamine neurons in the rat. *Brain Res.*, 277: 119 – 127.

Hainsworth, A.H., Roeper, J., Kapoor, R. and Ashcroft, F.M. (1991) Identification and electrophysiology of isolated pars compacta neurons from guinea pig substantia nigra. *Neuroscience*, 43: 81 – 93.

Hammer, R., Berrie, C.P., Birdsall, N.M.J., Burgen, A.S.V. and Hulme, E.C. (1980) Pirenzepine distinguishes between different subclasses of muscarinic receptor. *Nature*, 283: 90 – 92.

Harris, N.C., Webb, C. and Greenfield, S.A. (1989) A possible pacemaker mechanism in pars compacta neurons of the guinea-pig substantia nigra revealed by various ion channel blocking agents. *Neuroscience*, 31: 355 – 362.

Harris, R.A., Brodie, M.S. and Dunwiddie, T.V. (1992) Possible substrates of ethanol reinforcement: GABA and dopamine. *Ann. N.Y. Acad. Sci.*, 654: 61 – 70.

Häusser, M.A. and Yung, W.H. (1991) Functional role of pre- and post-synaptic GABA-B receptors of substantia nigra. *Third IBRO Congress Abstracts, Montreal*, p. 138.

Häusser, M.A., de Weille, J.R. and Lazdunski, M. (1991) Activation by cromakalim of pre- and post-synaptic ATP-sensitive K^+ channels in substantia nigra. *Biochem. Biophys. Res. Commun.*, 174: 909 – 914.

Häusser, M.A., Yung, W.H. and Lacey, M.G. (1992) Taurine and glycine activate the same Cl^- conductance in substantia nigra dopamine neurones. *Brain Res.*, 571: 103 – 108.

Henningfield, J.E., Miyasato, K. and Jasinski, D.R. (1983) Cigarette smokers self-administer intravenous nicotine. *Pharmacol. Biochem. Behav.*, 19: 887 – 890.

Herve, D., Pickel, V.M., Joh, T.H. and Beaudet, A. (1987) Serotonin axon terminals in the ventral tegmental area of the rat: fine structure and synaptic input to dopaminergic neurons. *Brain Res.*, 435: 71 – 83.

Hicks, G.A. and Henderson, G. (1992) The effects of dopamine on rat substantia nigra zona compacta neurones studied using the whole cell recording technique. *Br. J. Pharmacol.*, 105 (Suppl.): 6P.

Higgins, G.A., Jordan, C.C. and Skingle, M. (1991) Evidence that the unilateral activation of 5-HT1D receptors in the substantia nigra of the guinea pig elicit contralateral rotation. *Br. J. Pharmacol.*, 102: 305 – 310.

Hill, D.R., Shaw, T.M., Graham, W. and Woodruff, G.N. (1990) Autoradiographical detection of cholecystokinin-A receptors in primate brain using ^{125}I-Bolton-Hunter CCK-8 and 3H-MK-329. *Neuroscience*, 10: 1070 – 1081.

Hökfelt, T., Skirboll, L.R., Rehfeld, J., Goldstein, M., Markey, K. and Dann, O. (1980) A subpopulation of mesencephalic dopamine neurones projecting to limbic areas contain a cholecystokinin-like peptide: evidence from immunohistochemistry combined with retrograde tracing. *Neuroscience*, 5: 2093 – 2124.

Hökfelt, T., Everitt, B.J., Theodorsson-Norheim, E. and Goldstein, M. (1984) Occurrence of neurotensin-like immunoreactivity in subpopulations of hypothalamic, mesencephalic, and medullary catecholamine neurons. *J. Comp. Neurol.*, 222: 543 – 559.

Hommer, D.W., Stoner, G., Crawley, J.N., Paul, S.M. and Skirboll, L.R. (1986) Cholecystokinin-dopamine coexistence: electrophysiological actions corresponding to cholecystokinin receptor subtype. *J. Neurosci.*, 6: 3039 – 3043.

Hornykiewicz, O. (1966) Dopamine and brain function. *Pharmacol. Rev.*, 18: 925 – 964.

Hoyer, D. and Schoeffter, P. (1988) 5-HT1D receptor-mediated inhibition of forskolin-stimulated adenylate cyclase activity in calf substantia nigra. *Eur. J. Pharmacol.*, 147: 145 – 147.

Hulme, E.C., Birdsall, N.J. and Buckley, N.J. (1990) Muscarinic receptor subtypes. *Annu. Rev. Pharmacol. Toxicol.*, 30: 633 – 673.

Innis, R.B. and Aghajanian, G.K. (1987) Pertussis toxin blocks autoreceptor-mediated inhibition of dopaminergic neurons in rat substantia nigra. *Brain Res.*, 411: 139 – 143.

Innis, R.B., Andrade, R. and Aghajanian, G.K. (1985) Substance K excites dopaminergic and non-dopaminergic neurons in rat substantia nigra. *Brain Res.*, 335: 381 – 383.

Israel, J.M., Kirk, C. and Vincent, J.D. (1987) Electrophysiological responses to dopamine of rat hypophysial cells in lactotroph-enriched primary cultures. *J. Physiol. (Lond.)*,

390: 1–22.

Jessell, T.M. (1978) Substance P release from the rat substantia nigra. *Brain Res.*, 151: 469–478.

Johnson, S.W. and North, R.A. (1992a) Opioids excite dopamine neurons by hyperpolarization of local interneurons. *J. Neurosci.*, 12: 483–488.

Johnson, S.W. and North, R.A. (1992b) Two types of neurone in the rat ventral tegmental area and their synaptic inputs. *J. Physiol. (Lond.)*, 450: 455–468.

Johnson, S.W., Mercuri, N.B. and North, R.A. (1992a) 5-Hydroxytryptamine$_{1B}$ receptors block the GABA$_B$ synaptic potential in rat dopamine neurons. *J. Neurosci.*, 12: 2000–2006.

Johnson, S.W., Seutin, V. and North, R.A. (1992b) Burst firing in dopamine neurons induced by *N*-methyl-D-aspartate: role of electrogenic sodium pump. *Science,* 258: 665–667.

Keegan, K.D., Woodruff, G.N. and Pinnock, R.D. (1990) The pharmacology of neurotensin and neurotensin analogues on dopamine neurones in the rat substantia nigra pars compacta. *Br. J. Pharmacol.*, 101 (Suppl.): 579P.

Keegan, K.D., Woodruff, G.N. and Pinncok, R.D. (1992) The selective NK$_3$ receptor agonist senktide excites a subpopulation of dopamine-sensitive neurones in the rat substantia nigra pars compacta in vitro. *Br. J. Pharmacol.*, 105: 3–5.

Keegan, K.D., Woodruff, G.N. and Pinnock, R.D. (1993) Sensitivity of the neurotensin response of rat substantia nigra neurones in vitro to toxins and ion channel blockers. *J. Physiol. (Lond.)*, 459: 53P.

Kelland, M.D., Freeman, A.S. and Chiodo, L.A. (1990) Serotonergic afferent regulation of the basic physiology and pharmacological responsiveness of nigrostriatal dopamine neurons. *J. Pharmacol. Exp. Ther.*, 253: 803–811.

Kofman, O., McGlynn, S.M., Olmstead, M.C. and Yeomans, J.S. (1990) Differential effects of atropine, procaine and dopamine in the rat ventral tegmentum on lateral hypothalamic rewarding brain stimulation. *Behav. Brain Res.*, 38: 55–68.

Krishtal, O.A., Osipchuk, Y.V. and Vrublensky, S.V. (1988) Properties of glycine-activated conductances in rat brain neurones. *Neurosci. Lett.*, 84: 271–276.

Kutsuwada, T., Kashiwabuchi, N., Mori, H., Sakimura, K., Kushiya, E., Araki, K., Meguro, H., Masaki, H., Kumanishi, T., Arakawa, M. and Mishina, M. (1992) Molecular diversity of the NMDA receptor channel. *Nature*, 358: 36–41.

Lacey, M.G. and North, R.A. (1988) An inward current activated by hyperpolarization (Ih) in rat substantia nigra zona compacta neurones in vitro. *J. Physiol. (Lond.)*, 406: 18P.

Lacey, M.G., Mercuri, N.B. and North, R.A. (1987) Dopamine acts on D$_2$ receptors to increase potassium conductance in neurones of the rat substantia nigra zona compacta. *J. Physiol. (Lond.)*, 392: 397–416.

Lacey, M.G., Mercuri, N.B. and North, R.A. (1988) On the potassium conductance increase activated by GABA$_B$ and dopamine D$_2$ receptors in rat substantia nigra neurones. *J.*

Physiol. (Lond.), 401: 437–453.

Lacey, M.G., Mercuri, N.B. and North, R.A. (1989) Two cell types in rat substantia nigra zona compacta distinguished by membrane properties and the actions of dopamine and opioids. *J. Neurosci.*, 9: 1233–1241.

Lacey, M.G., Calabresi, P. and North, R.A (1990a) Muscarine depolarizes rat substantia nigra and ventral tegmental area neurones in vitro through M$_1$-like receptors. *J. Pharmacol. Exp. Ther.*, 253: 395–400.

Lacey, M.G., Mercuri, N.B. and North, R.A. (1990b) Actions of cocaine on rat dopaminergic neurones in vitro. *Br. J. Pharmacol.*, 99: 731–735.

Lacey, M.G., Calabresi, P. and North, R.A. (1991) Cholinergic excitation of A9 and A10 dopaminergic neurones in vitro through both muscarinic and nicotinic receptors. In: G. Bernardi, M.B. Carpenter, G. Di Chiara, M. Morelli and P. Stanzione (Eds.), *The Basal Ganglia, III*, Plenum, New York, pp. 275–284.

Lee, H.J., Rye, D.B., Hallanger, A.E., Levey, A.I. and Wainer, B.H. (1988) Cholinergic vs. noncholinergic efferents from the mesopontine tegmentum to the extrapyramidal motor system nuclei. *J. Comp. Neurol.*, 275: 469–492.

Lichtensteiger, W., Hefti, F., Felix, D., Huwyler, T., Melamed, E. and Schlumpf, M. (1982) Stimulation of nigrostriatal dopamine neurones by nicotine. *Neuropharmacology*, 21: 963–968.

Loring, R.H. and Zigmond, R.E. (1988) Characterization of neuronal nicotinic receptors by snake venom neurotoxins. *Trends. Neurosci.*, 11: 73–78.

Losonczy, M.F., Davidson, M. and Davis, K.L. (1987) The dopamine hypothesis of schizophrenia. In: H.Y. Meltzer (Ed.), *Psychopharmacology: the Third Generation of Progress*, Raven Press, New York, pp. 715–726.

Madison, D.V., Lancaster, B. and Nicoll, R.A. (1987) Voltage clamp analysis of cholinergic actions in the hippocampus. *J. Neurosci.*, 7: 733–741.

Marchi, M., Augliera, A., Codignola, A., Lunardi, G., Fedele, E., Fontana, G. and Raiteri, M. (1991) Cholinergic modulation of [^{3}H]dopamine release from dendrosomes of rat substantia nigra. *Naunyn Schmiedebergs Arch. Pharmacol.*, 344: 275–280.

Matsuda, Y., Fujimura, K. and Yoshida, S. (1987) Two types of neurons in the substantia nigra pars compacta studied in a slice preparation. *Neurosci. Res.*, 5: 172–179.

Matthews, R.T. and German, D.C. (1984) Electrophysiological evidence for excitation of rat ventral tegmental area dopamine neurons by morphine. *Neuroscience*, 11: 617–625.

McCormick, D.A. and Pape, H.-C. (1990) Noradrenergic and seronergic modulation of a hyperpolarization-activated cation current in thalamic relay neurones. *J. Physiol. (Lond.)*, 431: 319–342.

Mendez, I., Elisevich, K. and Flumerfelt, B. (1992) Substance P synaptic interactions with GABAergic and dopaminergic neurons in rat substantia nigra: an ultrastructural double-labeling immunocytochemical study. *Brain Res. Bull.*, 28: 557 – 563.

Mercuri, N.B., Calabresi, P. and Bernardi, G. (1988) Potassium ions play a role in the glycine-induced inhibition of rat substantia nigra zona compacta neurones. *Brain Res.*, 462: 199 – 203.

Mercuri, N.B., Calabresi, P. and Bernardi, G. (1989) The mechanism of amphetamine-induced inhibition of rat substantia nigra compacta neurones investigated with intracellular recording in vitro. *Br. J. Pharmacol.*, 98: 127 – 134.

Mercuri, N.B., Calabresi, P. and Bernardi, G. (1990a) Effects of glycine on neurons in the rat substantia nigra zona compacta: in vitro electrophysiological study. *Synapse*, 5: 190 – 200.

Mercuri, N.B., Calabresi, P. and Bernardi, G. (1990b) Responses of rat substantia nigra compacta neurones to L-Dopa. *Br. J. Pharmacol.*, 100: 257 – 260.

Mereu, G., Yoon, K.W., Boi, V., Gessa, G.L., Naes, L. and Westfall, T.C. (1987) Preferential stimulation of ventral tegmental area dopaminergic neurons by nicotine. *Eur. J. Pharmacol.*, 141: 395 – 399.

Mereu, G., Costa, E., Armstrong, D.M. and Vicini, S. (1991) Glutamate receptor subtypes mediate excitatory synaptic currents of dopamine neurons in midbrain slices. *J. Neurosci.*, 11: 1359 – 1366.

Minabe, Y., Ashby Jr., C.R. and Wang, R.Y. (1991) The effect of acute and chronic LY 277359, a selective 5-HT_3 receptor antagonist, on the number of spontaneously active midbrain dopamine neurons. *Eur. J. Pharmacol.*, 209: 151 – 156.

Mourre, C., Widmann, C. and Lazdunski, M. (1990) Sulfonylurea binding sites associated with ATP-regulated K^+ channels in the central nervous system: autoradiographic analysis of their distribution and ontogenesis, and of their localization in mutant mice cerebellum. *Brain Res.*, 519: 29 – 43.

Mueller, A.L. and Brodie, M.S. (1989) Intracellular recording from putative dopamine-containing neurons in the ventral tegmental area of Tsai in a brain slice preparation. *J. Neurosci. Methods*, 28: 15 – 22.

Murphy, K.P.S.J. and Greenfield, S.A. (1992) Neuronal selectivity of ATP-sensitive potassium channels in guinea-pig substantia nigra revealed by responses to anoxia. *J. Physiol. (Lond.)*, 453: 167 – 183.

Nakanishi, H., Kita, H. and Kitai, S.T. (1987) Intracellular study of rat substantia nigra pars reticulata neurons in an in vitro slice preparation: electrical membrane properties and response characteristics to subthalamic stimulation. *Brain Res.*, 437: 45 – 55.

Nedergaard, S. and Greenfield, S.A. (1992) Sub-populations of pars compacta neurons in the substantia nigra: the significance of qualitatively and quantitatively distinct conductances. *Neuroscience*, 48: 423 – 437.

Nedergaard, S., Bolam, J.P. and Greenfield, S.A. (1988) Facilitation of a dendritic calcium conductance by 5-hydroxytryptamine in the substantia nigra. *Nature*, 333: 174 – 177.

Nedergaard, S., Flatman, J.A. and Engberg, I. (1991) Excitation of substantia nigra pars compacta neurones by 5-hydroxytryptamine in-vitro. *Neuroreport*, 2: 329 – 332.

Nicoll, R.A., Malenka, R.C. and Kauer, J.A. (1990) Functional comparison of neurotransmitter receptor subtypes in mammalian central nervous system. *Physiol. Rev.*, 70: 513 – 565.

Niijima, K. and Yoshida, M. (1988) Activation of mesencephalic dopamine neurons by chemical stimulation of the nucleus tegmenti pedunculopontinus pars compacta. *Brain Res.*, 451: 163 – 171.

Nonoka, R. and Moroji, T. (1988) Quantitative autoradiography of muscarinic cholinergic receptors in the rat brain. *Brain Res.*, 451: 163 – 171.

North, R.A. (1989) Drug receptors and the inhibition of nerve cells. *Br. J. Pharmacol.*, 98: 13 – 28.

North, R.A. and Williams, J.T. (1985) On the potassium conductance increased by opioids in rat locus coeruleus neurones. *J. Physiol. (Lond.)*, 364: 265 – 280.

Olpe, H.R., Karlsson, G., Pozza, M.F., Brugger, F., Steinmann, M., Van Riezen, H., Fagg, G., Hall, R.G., Froestl, W. and Bittinger, H. (1990) CGP 35348: a centrally active blocker of $GABA_B$ receptors. *Eur. J. Pharmacol.*, 187: 27 – 38.

Otis, T.S. and Mody, I. (1992) Differential activation of $GABA_A$ and $GABA_B$ receptors by spontaneously released transmitter. *J. Neurophysiol.*, 67: 227 – 234.

Ottersen, O.P. and Storm-Mathisen, J. (1984) Neurons containing or accumulating transmitter amino acids. In: A. Björklund, T. Hökfelt and M.J. Kuhar (Eds.), *Handbook of Chemical Neuroanatomy, Vol. 3: Classical Transmitters and Transmitter Receptors in the CNS, part II*, Elsevier, Amsterdam, pp. 141 – 246.

Palacios, J.M. and Kuhar, M.J. (1981) Neurotensin receptors are located on dopamine containing neurones in rat midbrain. *Nature*, 294: 587 – 588.

Palacios, J.M. and Walmsley, J.K. (1984) Catecholamine receptors. In: A. Björklund, T. Hökfelt and M.J. Kuhar (Eds.), *Handbook of Chemical Neuroanatomy, Vol. 3: Classical Transmitters and Transmitter Receptors in the CNS, part II*, Elsevier, Amsterdam, pp. 325 – 351.

Parker, G.C., Rugg, E.L. and Winn, P. (1991) Cholinergic stimulation of substantia nigra: abolition of carbachol-induced eating by unilateral 6-hydroxydopamine lesion of nigrostriatal dopamine neurones. *Exp. Brain Res.*, 87: 597 – 603.

Petrusz, P., Merchenthaler, I. and Maderdrut, J.L. (1985) Distribution of enkephalin-containing neurons in the central nervous system. In: A. Björklund and T. Hökfelt (Eds.), *Handbook of Chemical Neuroanatomy, Vol. 4: GABA and Neuropeptides in the CNS, part I*, Elsevier, Amsterdam, pp. 273 – 334.

Phillipson, O.T. (1979) Afferent projections to the ventral tegmental area of Tsai and interfascicular nucleus: a horseradish peroxidase study in the rat. *J. Comp. Neurol.*, 187: 117 – 144.

Pinnock, R.D. (1983) Sensitivity of compacta neurones in the rat substantia nigra slice to dopamine agonists. *Eur. J. Pharmacol.*, 96: 269 – 276.

Pinnock, R.D. (1984a) The actions of antipsychotic drugs on

dopamine receptors in the rat substantia nigra. *Br. J. Pharmacol.*, 81: 631 – 635.

Pinnock, R.D. (1984b) Hyperpolarizing action of baclofen on neurons in the rat substantia nigra slice. *Brain Res.*, 322: 337 – 340.

Pinnock, R.D. (1985) Neurotensin depolarizes substantia nigra dopamine neurones. *Brain Res.*, 338: 151 – 154.

Pinnock, R.D. and Dray, A. (1982) Differential sensitivity of presumed dopaminergic and non-dopaminergic neurones in rat substantia nigra to electrophoretically applied substance P. *Neurosci. Lett.*, 29: 153 – 158.

Precht, W. and Yoshida, M. (1971) Blockage of caudate-evoked inhibition of neurons in the substantia nigra by picrotoxin. *Brain Res.*, 32: 229 – 233.

Quik, M., Emson, P.C. and Joyce, E. (1979) Dissociation between the presynaptic dopamine-sensitive adenylate cyclase and [^{3}H]spiperone binding sites in rat substantia nigra. *Brain Res.*, 167: 355 – 365.

Reynolds, G.P. (1992) Developments in the drug treatment of schizophrenia. *Trends Pharmacol. Sci.*, 13: 116 – 121.

Robertson, H.A. (1992) Dopamine receptor interactions: some implications for the treatment of Parkinson's disease. *Trends Neurosci.*, 15: 201 – 206.

Roeper, J., Hainsworth, A.H. and Ashcroft, F.M. (1990) Tolbutamide reverses membrane hyperpolarisation induced by activation of D_2 receptors and $GABA_B$ receptors in isolated substantia nigra neurones. *Pflügers Arch.*, 416: 473 – 475.

Sanghera, M.K., Trulson, M.E. and German, D.C. (1984) Electrophysiological properties of mouse dopamine neurons: in vivo and in vitro studies. *Neuroscience*, 12: 793 – 801.

Savasta, M., Ruberte, E., Palacios, J.M. and Mengod, G. (1989) The colocalization of cholecystokinin and tyrosine hydroxylase mRNAs in mesencephalic dopaminergic neurons in the rat brain examined by in situ hybridization. *Neuroscience*, 29: 363 – 369.

Scarnati, E., Proia, A., Campana, E. and Pacitti, C. (1986) A microiontophoretic study on the nature of the putative synaptic neurotransmitter involved in the pedunculopontine-substantia nigra pars compacta excitatory pathway of the rat. *Exp. Brain Res.*, 62: 470 – 478.

Schmid Antomarchi, H., Amoroso, S., Fosset, M. and Lazdunski, M. (1990) K^+ channel openers activate brain sulfonylurea-sensitive K^+ channels and block neurosecretion. *Proc. Natl. Acad. Sci. U.S.A.*, 87: 3489 – 3492.

Schultz, W. (1982) Depletion of dopamine in the striatum as an experimental model of Parkinsonism: direct effects and adaptive mechanisms. *Prog. Neurobiol.*, 18: 121 – 166.

Seabrook, G.R., Howson, W. and Lacey, M.G. (1990) Electrophysiological characterization of potent agonists and antogonists at pre- and postsynaptic $GABA_B$ receptors in rat brain slices. *Br. J. Pharmacol.*, 101: 949 – 957.

Seroogy, K.B., Mehta, A. and Fallon, J.H. (1987) Neurotensin and cholecystokinin coexistence within neurons of the ventral mesencephalon: projections to forebrain. *Exp. Brain Res.*, 68:

277 – 289.

Seutin, V., Massotte, L. and Dresse, A. (1989) Electrophysiological effects of neurotensin on dopaminergic neurones of the ventral tegmental area of the rat in vitro. *Neuropharmacology*, 28: 949 – 954.

Shepard, P.D. and German, D.C. (1988) Electrophysiological and pharmacological evidence for the existence of distinct subpopulations of nigrostriatal dopaminergic neurons in the rat. *Neuroscience*, 27: 537 – 546.

Shi, W.X. and Bunney, B.S. (1991) Effects of neurotensin on midbrain dopamine neurons: are they mediated by formation of a neurotensin – dopamine complex? *Synapse*, 9: 157 – 164.

Silva, N.L., Pechura, C.M. and Barker, J.L. (1990) Postnatal rat nigrostriatal dopaminergic neurons exhibit five types of potassium conductances. *J. Neurophysiol.*, 64: 262 – 272.

Smith, Y. and Bolam, J.P. (1990) The output neurones and the dopaminergic neurones of the substantia nigra receive a GABA-containing input from the globus pallidus in the rat. *J. Comp. Neurol.*, 296: 47 – 64.

Sokoloff, P., Giros, B., Martres, M.P., Bouthenet, M.L. and Schwartz, J.C. (1990) Molecular cloning and characterization of a novel dopamine receptor (D_3) as a target for neuroleptics. *Nature*, 347: 146 – 151.

Steinbusch, H.W.M. (1981) Distribution of serotonin-immunoreactivity in the central nervous system of the rat – cell bodies and terminals. *Neuroscience*, 6: 557 – 618.

Stittsworth, J.D.J. and Mueller, A.L. (1990) Cholecystokinin octapeptide potentiates the inhibitory response mediated by D_2 dopamine receptors in slices of the ventral tegmental area of the brain in the rat. *Neuropharmacology*, 29: 119 – 127.

Sugimoto, T. and Mizuno, N. (1987) Neurotensin in projection neurons of the striatum and nucleus accumbens, with reference to coexistence with enkephalin and GABA: an immunohistochemical study in the cat. *J. Comp. Neurol.*, 257: 383 – 395.

Sugita, S., Johnson, S.W. and North, R.A. (1992) Synaptic inputs to $GABA_A$ and $GABA_B$ receptors originate from discrete afferent neurons. *Neurosci. Lett.*, 134: 207 – 211.

Svensson, T.H. and Tung, C.S. (1989) Local cooling of prefrontal cortex induces pacemaker-like firing of dopamine neurons in rat ventral tegmental area in vivo. *Acta Physiol. Scand.*, 136: 135 – 136.

Swanson, L.W. (1982) The projections of the ventral tegmental area and adjacent regions: combined fluorescent retrograde tracer and immunofluorescence study in the rat. *Brain Res. Bull.*, 9: 321 – 353.

Tepper, J.M., Sawyer, S.F. and Groves, P.M. (1987) Electrophysiologically identified nigral dopaminergic neurons intracellularly labeled with HRP: light-microscopic analysis. *J. Neurosci.*, 7: 2794 – 2806.

Tokutomi, N., Kaneda, M. and Akaike, N. (1989) What confers specificity on glycine for its receptor site? *Br. J. Pharmacol.*, 97: 353 – 360.

Trent, F. and Tepper, J.M. (1991) Dorsal raphe stimulation

modifies striatal-evoked antidromic invasion of nigral dopaminergic neurons in vivo. *Exp. Brain Res.*, 84: 620 – 630.

Uchimura, N. and North, R.A. (1990) Muscarine reduces inwardly rectifying potassium conductance in rat nucleus accumbens neurones. *J. Physiol. (Lond.)*, 422: 369 – 380.

Waeber, C., Schoeffter, P., Hoyer, D. and Palacios, J.M. (1990) The serotonin 5-HT1D receptor: a progress review. *Neurochem. Res.*, 15: 567 – 582.

Watling, K.J. (1992) Nonpeptide antagonists herald a new era in tachykinin research. *Trends Pharmacol. Sci.*, 13: 266 – 269.

Weiner, D.M., Levey, A.I. and Brann, M.R. (1990) Expression of muscarinic acetylcholine and dopamine receptor mRNAs in rat basal ganglia. *Proc. Natl. Acad. Sci. U.S.A.*, 87: 7050 – 7054.

Williams, J.T. and Davies, J.A. (1983) The involvement of 5-hydroxytryptamine in the release of dendritic dopamine from slices of rat substantia nigra. *J. Pharm. Pharmacol.*, 35: 734 – 737.

Wise, R.A. (1983) Brain neuronal systems mediating reward processes. In: J.E. Smith and J.D. Lane (Eds.), *The Neurobiology of Opiate Reward Processes*, Elsevier, Amsterdam, pp. 405 – 437.

Wise, R.A. and Bozarth, M.A. (1987) A psychomotor stimulant theory of addiction. *Psychol. Rev.*, 94: 469 – 492.

Woolfe, N.J. and Butcher, L.L. (1986) Cholinergic systems in the rat brain. III. Projections from the pontomesencephalic tegmentum to the thalamus, tegmentum, basal ganglia and basal forebrain. *Brain Res. Bull.*, 16: 603 – 637.

Yung, W.H., Häusser, M.A. and Jack, J.J.B. (1991) Electrophysiology of dopaminergic and non-dopaminergic neurones of the guinea-pig substantia nigra pars compacta in vitro. *J. Physiol. (Lond.)*, 436: 643 – 668.

Zamir, N., Palkovits, M., Weber, E., Mezey, E. and Brownstein, M.J. (1984) A dynorphinergic pathway of Leu-enkephalin production in rat substantia nigra. *Nature*, 307: 643 – 645.

G.W. Arbuthnott and P.C. Emson (Eds.)
Progress in Brain Research, Vol. 99
© 1993 Elsevier Science Publishers B.V. All rights reserved.

CHAPTER 18

The generation of natural firing patterns in neostriatal neurons

Charles J. Wilson

Department of Anatomy and Neurobiology, University of Tennesse, Memphis, TN 38163, U.S.A.

Introduction

In one of the first single unit recording studies of the mammalian neostriatum, Albe-Fessard and co-workers (1960) observed that spontaneously active neostriatal neurons in unanesthetized (decerebrate) animals fired at low rates in an irregular, somewhat bursty pattern. They further observed that upon onset of chloralose anesthesia, the bursts of activity were more pronounced and began to occur rhythmically at 3 – 10 Hz. A later study by Sedgwick and Williams (1967) showed that this rhythmic bursting was also characteristic of light barbiturate anesthesia, and that deeper anesthesia could lead to slowing and complete cessation of firing. Using intracellular recordings, Sedgwick and Williams were able to demonstrate prolonged depolarizing potentials that underlay the bursts of firing in the lightly anesthetized animals, and they postulated that these arose from a rhythmic excitatory synaptic input to the neostriatum, acting in conjunction with inhibitory processes that terminated the bursts (Sedgwick and Williams, 1967). Numerous studies published over the past 25 years have repeated these observations, usually emphasizing the low firing rates of the neurons, the large number of neurons with practically no spontaneous firing (in both anesthetized and unanesthetized preparations), and the rhythmic bursting of neurons under light anesthesia (e.g., Bloom et al., 1965; Purpura and Malliani, 1967; Connor, 1970; Hull et al., 1970; Feltz and Albe-Fessard, 1972; Liles, 1974; Richardson et al., 1977; Katayama et al., 1980; Wilson and Groves, 1981; Aldridge and Gilman, 1990; Calabresi et al., 1990; Wilson, 1992).

Three different neostriatal firing patterns

Two issues arising from these observations: (1) the mechanisms responsible for the low spontaneous activity of striatal neurons; and (2) those responsible for the rhythmicity of activity in chloralose- or barbituate-anesthetized animals, have been addressed in a number of studies since 1960. Although considerable progress has been made, these studies have been hampered by the problem of cell identity, from which the other issues could not be disentangled. Despite its relative homogeneity (compared to, for example, the cerebral cortex or the retina), the existence of a number of morphologically distinct cell types has been known since the time of Cajal. Neurophysiologists confronted with the variations of spontaneous activity recorded from unidentified neurons in the neostriatum have necessarily considered the existence of different cell types as a possible explanation, and a number of strictly neurophysiological schemes for distinguishing cell types have been devised. The simplest and most easily justified of these on anatomical grounds are those that use antidromic activation to identify projection neurons, and thus distinguish projection cells from interneurons. Although occasionally antidromic activation has been successfully used in this way (e.g.,

Liles, 1974; Fuller et al., 1975; Kimura, 1990), most authors have reported that very few striatal neurons are antidromically activated by electrical stimulation along the known course of their axons, despite the fact that most striatal cells are projection neurons (Preston et al., 1980; Chang et al., 1981; Wilson, 1983a).

An alternative approach to cell classification, based on variations in the pattern of spontaneous firing seen among neurons recorded in awake or anesthetized animals, has been proposed several times in the last 25 years by a number of authors. One of the earliest of these was that by Connor (1970), suggesting that some neurons, showing relatively high rates of spontaneous activity, may represent a different cell type. In Connor's study, the separate identity of the cells was supported by the observation that more rapidly firing neurons were more likely to show inhibitory responses to iontophoretically applied dopamine. Subsequent studies showed that cells with relatively continuous (tonic) spontaneous activity were also more likely to be activated by excitatory amino acids (Feltz and Albe-Fessard, 1972), and were much less likely to be antidromically activated by stimulation of the substantia nigra or entopeduncular nucleus (Liles, 1974). More recently, these tonically active neurons have been shown to respond differently to sensory stimuli or during performance of a learned task. Anderson (1977) described slowly (1 – 12 Hz) firing tonically active neurons and irregularly phasic neurons in the striatum of awake monkeys, and noted that fewer tonically active neurons fired in relation to chair tilts requiring postural adjustments. Kimura et al. (1984) described similar firing patterns in the neostriatum of monkeys, and reported that while the more common phasically active neurons responded in a time-locked manner to performance of a learned movement, tonically active neostriatal cells were more likely to respond to external stimuli than are the signals eliciting movements. Tonically firing cells also have been shown to fire in relation to sensory stimuli associated with other phases of the task, such as reward presentation (Apicella et al., 1991). These responses are not purely sensory in

nature, but are always associated with sensory stimuli that carry information relevant to the task. As in anesthetized animals, the tonically active neurons are never antidromically activated by electrical stimulation along the output pathways of the striatum (Kimura, 1990), suggesting that they may be instances of a morphologically distinct type of neuron with an axon restricted to the neostriatum (Kimura et al., 1984, 1990).

A third firing pattern, consisting of short stereotyped bursts of action potentials at very high frequency, has also been described, although very rarely. One of the first descriptions of this pattern of firing is that of Richardson et al. (1977), who suggested that it may arise from an inhibitory interneuron. These cells have apparently been only rarely observed in studies of the neostriatum, and are even more rarely described in the published reports. The most complete study of this cell type is that of Kita (this volume).

Defining tonic and phasic

Despite the large number of published descriptions of the phasic and tonic firing patterns in the neostriatum, there have been few attempts to quantify the differences between them. This raises a technical ambiguity, because the cells are usually described as different on the basis of their firing *patterns*, but are often divided in practice into two groups on the basis of their firing *rates*. When patterns are used, the categorization is usually qualitative, and the criteria are not described. In fact, quantitative criteria for distinguishing between phasically firing and tonically firing neurons are rare in any part of the brain. A step in the right direction was made by Anderson (1977), who presented interval histograms of tonically and phasically firing striatal neurons and showed that the tonically firing neurons generally exhibit a later modal interval than phasic neurons (about 200 versus < 50 msec, see Figs. 2 and 3). Studies using awake behaving animals have employed an ensemble of criteria to distinguish the two cell types, including differences in extracellularly recorded action potential wave forms, mean firing rate, and a qualitative impression of the degree of burstiness of the firing pattern (e.g., Alexander and DeLong, 1985; Hikosaka et al., 1989; Kimura et al., 1990). These reports all illustrate the differences between the two cell types using examples, but so far they have not provided any single set of criteria that can be shown to unequivocally place each cell into one category or the other. This lack of an agreed-upon criterion for identification of tonic and phasic neurons may be responsible for the large discrepancy in the proportion of tonic and phasic neurons reported by various authors (about 40% tonic according to Kimura et al., 1990; about 8% according to Alexander and DeLong, 1985), although this may also be influenced by differences in location of recordings in the neostriatum or microelectrode sampling biases.

The clearest quantitative definition of bursting relies on the identification of two distinct modes in the interval histogram, one corresponding to intraburst intervals and one to the intervals between bursts (Cocatre-Zilgien and Delcomyn, 1992). Interval histograms of neostriatal neurons, including very obviously phasic neurons, generally do not clearly show two modes, although a suggestion of a contribution from late intervals is usually present (e.g., Aldridge et al., 1990). This is because interburst intervals are longer and more variable than interspike intervals within bursts, and so make a much smaller contribution to the interval histogram. Frankly bimodal interspike interval histograms have been described by Kimura et al. (1990), but for a subset of the tonically firing cell type (which by most definitions should have a unimodal interspike interval histogram). The causes and implications of this are not yet clear, but it illustrates the difficulty in designing a quantitative criterion with which to standardize the identification of cells. The quantitative studies of Aldridge et al. (1991) represent the best attempt so far to characterize the firing patterns of neostriatal neurons from extracellular recordings in awake animals. The tendency of neurons to burst was measured using the surprise index (Legéndy and Salcman, 1985). The population of cells was distributed continuously along most of the parameters measured, making it difficult to distinguish categor-

ical types of firing patterns. An exception was the plane defined by the coefficient of variation of intervals and the median interval, in which approximately 15% of cells formed a distinct cluster. These were characterized by the relative absence of bursts, low variability of intervals and median intervals between 120 and 300 msec. This approximates an approach used successfully by others (Poulain et al., 1988; Cocatre-Zilgien and Delcomyn, 1992) in which bursting and tonic firing patterns are found to be separable in the plane defined by the variance of intervals and the mean interval. Perhaps application of this approach could help to sort out the differences in categorization of neurons that currently haunts the extracellular recording technique.

Firing patterns of identified cells versus identification of cells by their firing pattern

Even if there were no problems in identification of phasic and tonic neurons in the neostriatum, the remaining heterogeneity among neostriatal neurons would still be a serious problem for neurophysiologists. While two or three firing patterns have been identified, there are at least 8 morphologically distinct cell types, some of which can be divided into subtypes (e.g., Chang et al., 1981; Kawaguchi et al., 1990). This suggests that there are either severe sampling biases that prevent detection of most cell types, or that there is one-to-many mapping of firing patterns to cell types. Some of the ambiguity may be removed by neurophysiological identification of neurons using criteria other than firing pattern (e.g., Nisenbaum et al., 1988).

A more direct alternative is the study of the natural firing patterns (recorded intracellularly) of neurons identified by intracellular staining in vivo, under circumstances that do not suppress spontaneous activity. This method not only avoids the ambiguities associated with the uncertain mapping between firing patterns and cell types, but also offers information concerning the mechanisms giving rise to the firing patterns. Moreover, it allows a connection to be made between the data obtained from extracellular recording studies of behaving animals, and the equally large body of data obtained from reduced preparations, such as striatal tissue slices and dissociated striatal neurons. While only a subset of striatal neuron types have so far been studied in this way, the information from these offers some insights into the generation of firing patterns commonly seen in behaving animals.

Spontaneous firing in anesthetized rats

The ideal preparation for the study of firing patterns would be an awake, unrestrained animal. As described above, anesthetics have long been known to profoundly alter the firing of neostriatal neurons. As a practical expedient, local anesthesia was employed in initial studies (Wilson and Groves, 1981). This preparation made intracellular recording possible without the most serious of the ill effects of anesthetics, but of course there was no way to as-

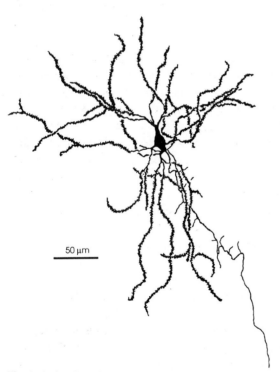

50 μm

Fig. 1. A drawing of a neostriatal spiny projection neuron injected intracellularly with HRP after recording its firing pattern extracellularly and intracellularly in an awake rat. The main axon, and the locations of collateral branches, are also shown (data from Wilson and Groves, 1981).

sociate firing patterns with behavioral state in this preparation. EEG recordings in these animals suggested that they were often asleep, and it was necessary to occasionally apply sensory stimulation to insure that data were collected from an awake animal. Thus some of the advantages of using unanesthetized preparations were already compromised for locally anesthetized animals. This, in addition to the need to apply electrical stimuli to the brain to test for antidromic activation, made it necessary to develop an acceptable anesthetized preparation. After trying a variety of anesthetics, it was found that the spontaneous activity in animals anesthetized with urethane most closely resembled that of awake animals, and subsequent intracellular recording studies of spontaneous and evoked activity performed in this laboratory have employed this preparation. Unless otherwise specified, the findings described here will be from rats anesthetized by a single dose of urethane (1.25 – 1.5 g/kg, i.p.) supplemented hourly with a mixture of ketamine and xylazine at about 1/3 the normal anesthetic dose (35 mg/ml each, i.m.).

Spiny projection neurons

Initial studies of the firing patterns of identified spiny neurons were reported by Wilson and Groves (1981). In these experiments, spontaneous activity was recorded extracellularly in locally anesthetized rats, after which an attempt was made to impale the neurons, record the same activity intracellularly and to stain the cells by intracellular injection of horseradish peroxidase. Of 128 neurons recorded extracellularly, 34 were successfully impaled and stained, and these all proved to be spiny neurons. A drawing of one of these neurons is shown in Fig. 1. Because all the cells were of the same type, comparisons between the firing patterns of spiny and aspiny neurons were not possible, but the variety of firing patterns observed among spiny cells could be described. The firing patterns were studied using interval histograms and autocorrelation histograms from the extracellularly recorded data, and when firing was not too seriously disturbed by damage

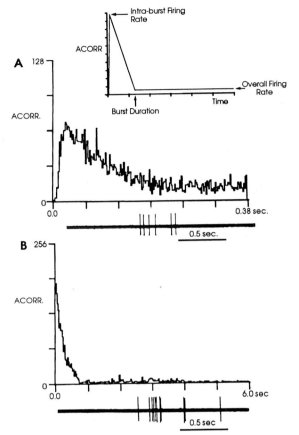

Fig. 2. Autocorrelation histograms and samples of the spontaneous firing patterns of two spiny projection neurons identified by intracellularly staining. *A*. The autocorrelation histogram of a phasically firing spiny neuron, computed using relatively short bin width to illustrate the internal structure of bursts. The absence of rhythmic firing is apparent in the absence of oscillations in firing probability over the duration of the episode of firing (the first 200 msec of the histogram). The cell's relative refractory period is seen as an initial trough of firing probability. Firing probability declines almost linearly from the peak at about 30 msec to a constant baseline level at about 200 msec. The inset shows the expected shape of the autocorrelation histogram for a cell firing in fixed duration bursts, with a random pattern within bursts, and a random pattern of burst occurrence. The similarity suggests that this is a good first approximation for the pattern of firing of neostriatal spiny neurons. *B*. The autocorrelation histogram for another spiny neuron showing even more strongly episodic firing, computed using a longer bin width, for visualizing temporal patterns in the occurrence of firing episodes. The burst duration for this cell was about 800 msec, and bursts had a weak tendency to recur at 2 – 4 sec intervals. Most spiny neurons showed either no detectable pattern in the occurrence of firing episodes, or a weak tendency for rhythmic recurrence of episodes, as shown here. (Data from Wilson and Groves, 1981.)

caused by the microelectrode, by analysis of spontaneous firing recorded intracellularly. Examples showing samples of spontaneous firing and autocorrelation histograms from identified spiny neurons are shown in Fig. 2*A, B*. It was clear from these recordings that the spiny neurons are among the phasically firing population of neostriatal cells. Many of the cells were silent, or nearly so, and cells for which spontaneous firing could be observed fired at very low rates. Many cells remained silent for seconds or minutes at a time, fired several action potentials over the course of 1 – 3 sec, and fell silent again.

The firing pattern within the episodes of firing is indicated by the form of autocorrelations composed using a short bin width, such as that shown in Fig. 2*A*. The early mode in the autocorrelation histogram corresponds to the modal interval seen in interval histograms from the same spike trains, and varied from 8 to 75 msec among neurons. Firing probability tapered off smoothly over the course of 0.1 – 3 sec to reach a relatively constant level indicative of the average firing rate for the cell. The existence of a prominent early peak in the autocorrelation histogram is indicative of the bursty firing pattern of the cells, that is, the existence of two distinctly different firing rates, one within bursts and one associated with the interburst interval. The autocorrelation histogram is much better than the interval histogram as a measure of bursty firing, as it represents the temporal relationship between all action potentials occurring in the same proximity in time, rather than merely the nearest neighbors. It can detect the existence of bursting even when bursts are few and irregular, as they are in the neurons shown in Fig. 2. The absence of any periodicity in the histogram over the time course of the burst indicates the absence of rhythmic firing during the burst. This was also characteristic of striatal spiny neurons, and distinguishes the bursts in these cells from more stereotyped bursty firing patterns, such as the complex spike bursts observed, for example, in cerebellar Purkinje cells or in hippocampal pyramidal cells. To emphasize this difference, it is probably preferable to refer to this firing pattern as

282

episodic, rather than bursty. It actually consists of distinct episodes of increased firing probability, but not stereotyped all-or-none patterns of action potential generation. Nonetheless, the terms episodic, bursty and phasic are all meant here to refer to the pattern of firing shown by the spiny neurons.

For purposes of interpretation of the autocorrelation histograms, it may be helpful to note that a fixed duration burst of random firing subject only to a relative refractory period, occurring at random inter-burst intervals, would produce a triangular autocorrelation histogram with its apex at the end of the refractory period, and its base superimposed on a constant firing probability, as shown in the inset to Fig. 2. The constant firing probability corresponds to the mean firing rate, averaged over the entire sample. In such a firing pattern, the duration of the burst could be read from the time at which firing probability intersected the baseline, and if the refractory period were short compared to the burst duration, the height of the apex of the triangle would provide an estimate of the firing rate within bursts. These conditions were not fully met by the firing patterns of neostriatal spiny neurons. Episodes of firing could be seen by inspection to be variable in duration, and the relative refractory period (as indicated by the initial trough in the autocorrelation histogram), while always smaller, was often within an order of magnitude of the duration of the firing episode. However, the qualitative resemblance of the autocorrelation histograms to that expected from simple fixed duration bursts suggested that a simple set of measurements based on this model might still be useful for comparing the firing patterns across the sample of neurons.

The timing of episodes of firing was studied using autocorrelation histograms calculated using long bin widths, allowing analysis of changes in firing probability over the course of 3 – 12 sec. An example of one of these, computed using a 6 sec period, is shown in Fig. 2B. The initial peak in the histogram represents a single burst of action potentials. This decays over a period of approximately 0.75 sec, corresponding to the average duration of the burst. The low level of firing probability at all times after that

is indicative of the low rate of bursting, and the absence of any strong periodicity in the occurrence. There is, in the cell shown in Fig. 2B, a slight tendency for bursts to recur at 2 – 4 sec intervals, as indicated by an increased firing probability over that interval. An estimate of burst strength was obtained by finding the difference between peak and basal firing probability, and dividing by the peak level. This yields a value ranging from 0 to 1, corresponding to no bursting and to firing restricted to bursts, respectively. For the example shown in Fig. 2B, the index was nearly 1, while the cell shown in Fig. 2A had a burst strength of about 0.8.

For the 21 spontaneously active neurons in the sample of spiny neurons studied by Wilson and Groves (1981), the durations of firing episodes

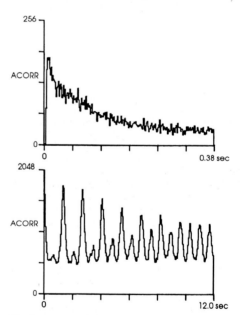

Fig. 3. Autocorrelation histograms for an identified spiny projection neuron firing in a rhythmic burst pattern. This was seen in a minority of spiny neurons. The upper histograms shows the within-burst firing pattern, which is not rhythmic but resembles that of other spiny neurons. The lower histogram is computed using a long bin width to show the rhythmic recurrence of episodes of firing with a 1.5 sec period. This spiny neuron had a tendency to fire more strongly on alternate 1.5 sec cycles, which is responsible for the appearance of a subharmonic in the histogram. This cell, and that in Fig. 2B, show the range of rhythmicity observed in 10 of the 21 spiny neurons recorded in awake rats. (Data from Wilson and Groves, 1981).

measured as described above varied from 0.1 to 3.0 sec (mean = 1.05, S.D. = 1.0), the burst strengths varied from 0.23 to 0.97 (mean = 0.64, S.D. = 0.25), while firing rates varied from 0.24 to 32.7/sec (mean = 5.54, S.D. = 7.38). While all identified spiny projection cells showed some indication of episodic firing, it was very weak in some cells. Three of the 21 cells had burst strengths less than 0.3, which would make them difficult to identify as episodically firing neurons if their identities were not known.

Although many spiny neurons in the sample of Wilson and Groves (1981) had irregularly occurring firing episodes, the autocorrelation histograms of some cells did show a tendency for rhythmic recurrence of firing episodes. Weak rhythmicity was detected in 10 of the 21 spontaneously active spiny cells, and two of the cells showed strong rhythmic firing. The frequency of these rhythms, and those in the larger sample of unidentified cells, was low, ranging from 0.5 to 3 Hz. Fig. 3 is an example showing autocorrelation histograms for a spiny neuron with strong rhythmic episodes of firing. This cell exhibited episodes of firing at approximately 1.5 Hz, and tended to fire more strongly on alternating cycles. Although this frequency is close to the respiratory rate of rats, firing of spiny neurons was unrelated to respiration, or to any other detectable movements of the animal or sensory stimuli in the room. It is similar to the rhythmic activity in the same frequency range seen in the thalamus of unanesthetized and urethane-anesthetized cats (Dossi et al., 1992).

Membrane potential shifts underlying the episodes of firing

Intracellular recording revealed that the episodes of firing in spiny projection neurons were the result of maintained plateau depolarizations that could last for several seconds (Wilson and Groves, 1981). Such depolarizing shifts had previously been reported in unidentified striatal neurons by Hull et al. (1970) in locally anesthetized cats, and rhythmic depolarizations had been seen to underly the rhythmic firing that is seen in animals lightly anesthetized

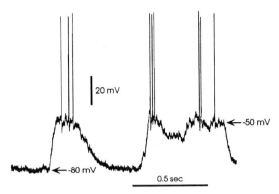

Fig. 4. Intracellular record of spontaneous membrane potential fluctuations and firing in an identified spiny projection neuron in an urethane-anesthetized rat. The episodes of firing can be seen to ride upon episodes of relatively constant subthreshold membrane depolarization. Individual action potentials arise from fluctuations in this noisy depolarized baseline. In the period between depolarizing episodes, the membrane potential is very polarized and fluctuations of membrane potential are diminished.

with barbituates (Sedgwick and Williams, 1967). In unanesthetized animals, and in animals anesthetized with urethane, spontaneous membrane potential shifts in neostriatal spiny cells are very dramatic, and their relationship to the firing pattern of the cells is readily apparent. An example showing a sample of the spontaneous membrane potential record from an identified spiny cell in an urethane-anesthetized rat is shown in Fig. 4. The membrane potential during the inter-episodic phase in these cells is very polarized, usually between − 80 and − 95 mV which, at least in slices, is near the potassium equilibrium potential. The threshold for action potentials, on the other hand, is between − 40 and − 50 mV, leaving a very large subthreshold range of membrane potentials that must be traversed for firing to occur. The membrane potential achieved during the depolarizing shifts does not cross the threshold for action potential generation, and that is why they do not give rise to rhythmic firing. Rather, the depolarizing shifts bring the membrane potential to within 5 − 10 mV of the firing threshold, enabling the smaller noisy depolarizing pertubations in membrane potential to fire the cell. The actual pattern of firing during the depolarizing epi-

284

sode appears random because the timing of action potentials is determined by these noisy depolarizations that are superimposed on the plateau depolarization. The duration of the episodes, and the timing of episodes of firing, are determined by the duration and timing of the depolarizing plateaux. Thus, an explanation of the firing patterns of neostriatal spiny neurons requires two different explanations, one for the generation of the enabling plateaux, and one for the superimposed noisy depolarizations.

The generation of the depolarizing plateau potentials

Based simply on the appearance of the membrane potential shifts seen in vivo, it might be expected that the spiny neuron is a bistable cell, with more than one equilibrium state. This would explain the bursting behavior, and could also help to explain the slow rhythmicity seen in these cells. However, it has not been possible to obtain any evidence for the existence of an equilibrium state associated with the depolarized state. For example, if a spiny neuron is depolarized by injection of current through the recording electrode, the cell will not show any tendency to maintain the depolarized state when the current is turned off. Likewise, hyperpolarizing current will not terminate a spontaneous depolarizing episode. This is in contrast to the behavior of other cells exhibiting bistable characteristics due to the existence of a second equilibrium potential (e.g., Hounsgaard et al., 1984). Because of this, it was not possible to reduce the study of the plateau potentials to an analysis of the properties of the spiny cell membrane. Spontaneous depolarizing potentials, on the other hand, being very unpredictable, were not ideal for analysis of the underlying mechanisms. Thus, most of what is known about the generation of the depolarizing episodes was not determined by studying spontaneous activity, but rather from experiments on the late components of the response to electrical stimulation of the cerebral cortex and the thalamus. Since the pioneering studies of Buchwald and his associates (Hull, 1970, 1973; Buchwald et al., 1973) it has been known that following the initial EPSP response to stimulation of cortical or tha-

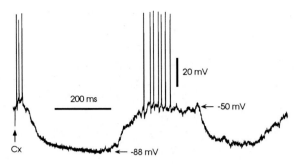

Fig. 5. The response of a spiny projection neuron to cerebral cortical stimulation in an urethane-anesthetized rat. The initial excitation is followed by a long-lasting hyperpolarization of the membrane, which is itself followed by a depolarizing episode which may elicit action potentials. This is followed by another hyperpolarizing phase. These late components of the response to cortical stimulation resemble the spontaneous shifts in membrane potential in the same neurons, and so may share a common mechanism. In this view, cortical stimulation may reset and transiently synchronize the mechanisms responsible for membrane potential state transitions in neostriatal cells.

lamic afferent pathways, neostriatal neurons often show a prolonged hyperpolarization, which is itself followed by a plateau-like depolarization. In some cases, this depolarization is followed by another hyperpolarizing period, which can be followed by another depolarization, which can under some circumstances continue for several cycles (Buchwald et al., 1973; Fig. 5). Katayama et al. (1980) showed that in lightly anesthetized animals these phases of the response to cortical stimulation (as seen by changes in firing rate) have the same time course as the spontaneous oscillations in firing rate, that cortical stimulation resets the spontaneous oscillations, and that spontaneous and evoked oscillations in firing rate are affected by anesthetics in the same way. At the time of Katayama's experiments, it was considered that the hyperpolarizing phase of the response of neostriatal neurons was caused by GABAergic mutual inhibition among the spiny cells. This opinion was formed both from consideration of the large local axonal arborization of the spiny neurons, and from the results of studies by Bernardi and his associates (Bernardi et al., 1975, 1976), who showed that systemic administration of

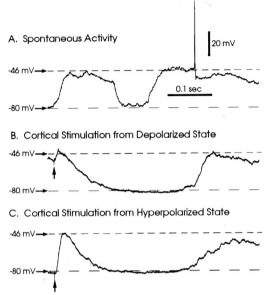

A. Spontaneous Activity

-46 mV →

20 mV

0.1 sec

-80 mV →

B. Cortical Stimulation from Depolarized State

-46 mV →

-80 mV →

C. Cortical Stimulation from Hyperpolarized State

-46 mV →

-80 mV →

Fig. 6. Spontaneous and evoked membrane potential shifts observe a common set of limiting membrane potentials. *A*. Spontaneous membrane potentials shifts in an identified spiny neuron. *B*. Stimulation of cortex during spontaneous depolarized state of the membrane. The stimulus intensity was adjusted so that the initial EPSP was just below the threshold for action potential generation. The hyperpolarizing phase attains approximately the same membrane potential as the spontaneous hyperpolarizations. The late depolarization does not summate with the spontaneous state of depolarization. *C*. The same stimulus, applied during a spontaneous hyperpolarized period. The hyperpolarizing phase does not summate with the spontaneous hyperpolarized state, and the late depolarization attains the same membrane potential as the spontaneous depolarized state. Note also the increased amplitude of the initial excitatory response, which at this membrane potential includes a large contribution from a reversed IPSP.

GABA antagonists could block the inhibitory phase of the response. It was therefore assumed that both the spontaneous quiet periods and the long-lasting evoked hyperpolarizing response were due to the action of feedback inhibition among striatal neurons.

The long-lasting hyperpolarization and the subsequent depolarizing plateau evoked by afferent stimulation was studied in identified neostriatal spiny projection neurons in urethane-anesthetized rats by Wilson et al. (1983b). An example showing the response to cortical stimulation is shown in Fig.

5. The initial EPSP response to stimulation of the cerebral cortex lasts approximately 50 msec and is followed by a long (150–400 msec) hyperpolarization, which is itself followed by a depolarization lasting approximately 100–200 msec. A comparison of the membrane potentials observed during the hyperpolarized and depolarized phases of the response and those observed during spontaneous membrane potential shifts, as shown in Fig. 6, illustrates their similarity. In Fig. 6*A*, spontaneous membrane potential shifts are shown, and the approximate limits of the shift in subthreshold membrane potential are indicated by the dotted lines. If the cortical stimulus is applied during the hyperpolarizing phase of the response (Fig. 6*C*) it is clear that the hyperpolarization evoked by afferent stimulation cannot hyperpolarize the neuron beyond the point achieved during the spontaneous membrane potential shifts. Likewise, the late depolarized phase does not summate with the spontaneous depolarizing episodes, even if the stimulus is presented during the depolarized phase of the spontaneous activity. These observations, like those of Katayama et al. (1980), support the view that the evoked membrane potential changes are an entrainment of the same mechanisms responsible for the spontaneous membrane potential shifts.

The mechanism responsible for the long-lasting hyperpolarization was investigated using acute lesions which interrupted the cortical and thalamic circuits responsible for the spontaneous input to the neostriatal spiny neurons, while leaving the axons of the cortical and thalamic neurons intact and available for stimulation (Wilson et al., 1983b). Large acute cortical aspirations were used to remove all ongoing corticostriatal spontaneous inputs, while allowing stimulation of intact corticostriatal axons by electrical pulses applied to the crus cerebri. Thalamic knife cuts rostral to the parafascicular nucleus were used to separate thalamostriatal neurons from their synaptic input and remove any ongoing thalamostriatal activity, while allowing electrical stimulation of the intact thalamostriatal axons rostral to the knife cut. If the hyperpolarizing phase of the response were due to the synchronous inhibition of corticostriatal or thalamostriatal inputs, and the resulting depolarization to a synchronous post-inhibitory re-excitation in these afferent neurons, these treatments would be expected to remove these phases completely. If, on the other hand, these were due to inhibitory and post-inhibitory rebound within the neostriatal circuitry (e.g., mutual inhibition and disinhibition of striatal spiny neurons), these lesions would have no such effect. The result, shown

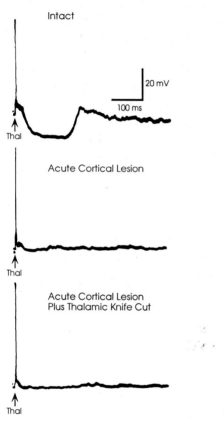

Fig. 7. Effects of acute lesions interrupting ongoing cortical and thalamic activity on the late components of the response to thalamic afferent fibers. The response to stimulation in intact animals included a late hyperpolarization and subsequent depolarization (top trace). Acute hemidecortication abolished the late components of the response (middle trace), as did a combination of acute hemidecortication and thalamic transection (bottom trace). Stimulation in all cases was applied to the thalamostriatal fibers rostral to the level of the transection. Acute decortication also abolished spontaneous membrane potential shifts, and the neurons were continuously in the hyperpolarized state. (Data from Wilson et al., 1983b.)

in Fig. 7, was that the late phases of the responses to all afferent input were abolished by acute decortication, with or without the thalamic knife cut. At the same time, the spontaneous depolarizing episodes and spontaneous firing of spiny neurons disappeared, and the cells became very stable, with membrane potentials comparable to the hyperpolarized state seen in intact animals.

The conclusion drawn from this experiment, that the depolarizing plateau potentials were driven by afferent input, rather than by the intrinsic properties of the membrane or by intrastriatal circuitry, was supported by a number of other observations. (1) The hyperpolarizing phase of the response to afferent stimulation showed a voltage sensitivity appropriate for a disfacilitation, rather than an inhibitory synaptic potential (Wilson et al., 1983a; Wilson, 1986). (2) The inhibitory phase of the response could be elicited alone, without excitation in the neostriatum, by antidromic stimulation of contralateral descending cortical outputs, which activate intracortical inhibitory circuits without directly exciting corticostriatal neurons (Wilson, 1986). (3) The spontaneous depolarizations and the late phases of the response to afferent stimulation both disappear in slices of the neostriatum, which is similar to the lesions described above in that corticostriatal and thalamostriatal axons have been separated from their somata and tonic input to the neostriatal neuron is absent (Lighthall and Kitai, 1983). (4) GABAergic inhibitory postsynaptic potentials that follow excitatory responses in the neostriatum are much shorter in duration than the hyperpolarizing phase of the late response to afferent stimulation, and are depolarizing at the resting membrane potential of neostriatal spiny cells (Misgeld et al., 1982; Lighthall and Kitai, 1983; Kita et al., 1985; see also Fig. 6). (5) While systemic administration of GABA antagonists does block the long lasting hyperpolarization, iontophoretic administration does not (Bernardi et al., 1976; Nisenbaum and Berger, 1992). (6) Corticostriatal neurons are inhibited during the long-lasting hyperpolarization, and fire during the late excitation, as would be required if the late components of the responses of neostriatal neurons were due to a decrease and subsequent increase in corticostriatal input.

The view of the spiny neuron which emerged from these studies was very different from the one depicted from early intracellular recording studies of the 1970s. In that previous view the neuron was pictured to be under the control of a tonic mutual inhibitory interaction with other spiny neurons. The very polarized membrane potential seen during the periods of silence and during the long-lasting inhibition that followed stimulation was explained as due to the action of this powerful inhibition. Instead, the polarized condition of the spiny neuron is now seen as its resting state in the absence of excitatory stimulation, and any deviation from that state is attributed to excitatory synaptic input. The rate of occurrence and the duration of depolarizing episodes (and episodes of firing) are, in this view, determined primarily by the pattern of excitatory synaptic input impinging on the spiny cell. The extremely polarized resting membrane potential, however, must be due to intrinsic properties of the cell.

What determines the resting membrane potential of spiny neurons?

In the membrane potential range normally observed in spiny neurons in slices of neostriatum (which is approximately the same as that observed in vivo during spontaneous silent periods), the membrane potential and the input resistance are dominated by a powerful voltage-dependent inwardly rectifying current. This current has been studied in voltage-clamp experiments: in unidentified cells of nucleus accumbens by Uchimura et al. (1989), and in identified neostriatal spiny neurons by Jiang and North (1991). The fast anomalous rectification in these neurons is carried by a barium-sensitive potassium conductance, which is responsible for at least half of the resting input conductance of the cells over the usual range of resting membrane potentials. The effect of this current on neurons as seen during current injections in slices is shown in the example in Fig. 8. As shown in that figure, an individual spiny projection neuron can exhibit a wide range of input resistances (typically about $10 - 80$ MΩ) over the range of subthreshold membrane potentials. Over the same range of membrane potentials, the apparent membrane time constant varies from about 3 to 20 msec.

Computer simulations of the spiny neuron including this fast inwardly rectifying potassium conductance (Wilson, 1992) reproduced most of the features of the spiny neuron shown in Fig. 8, especially if the inward rectifier conductance was placed on the dendrites, as well as on the soma. The results from a simulation passing current pulses into the soma of a morphologically accurate model of a spiny neuron

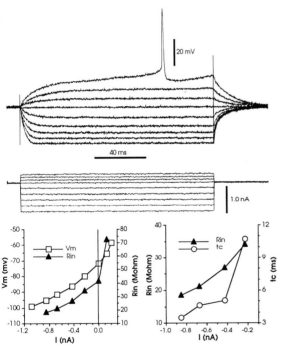

Fig. 8. The input resistance and time constant of identified spiny projection neurons in striatal tissue slices. Above are shown the responses of an identified cell to current pulses of various sizes, with the voltage records located above the current pulses. Note that closely spaced depolarizing current pulses produce larger incremental changes in membrane potential than the more widely spaced hyperpolarizing current pulses, and that the rate of charging of the membrane is different in the hyperpolarizing and depolarizing directions. These are illustrated in the graphs below, which show the steady-state membrane potential, input resistance and the time constant for the transients shown above. Time constants were calculated from the onset of the transient. (Data from Kawaguchi et al., 1989.)

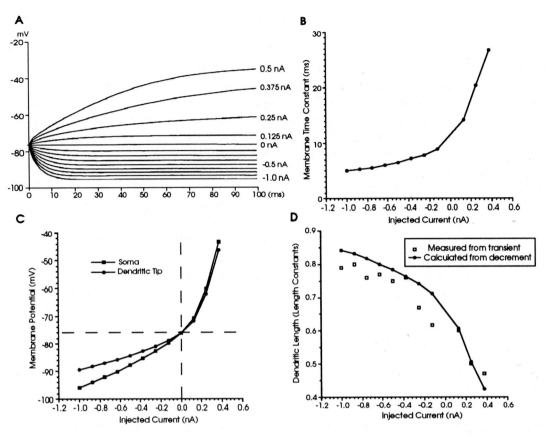

Fig. 9. Transient responses, steady-state I/V curves, time constants and dendritic lengths for a computer-simulated neostriatal spiny neuron including fast anomalous rectification. *A*. Simulated transient comparable to those in Fig. 8. The amplitudes of current pulses for some traces are shown at the right. *B*. Time constants measured from the late portion of the onset transients. The voltage dependence of time constants is similar to that seen in spiny neostriatal cells. *C*. Voltage/current plots for steady-state, calculated both for the soma (site of current injection) and the dendritic tips. Note that with depolarizing currents, there is little anomalous rectification and little attenuation of voltage along the dendrites, while the steady-state response to hyperpolarizing current pulses exhibits voltage attenuation that increases with hyperpolarization. *D*. Electrotonic length of the dendritic tree calculated from the attenuation shown in *C* and from fitting exponentials to the transients. (Data from Wilson, 1992.)

are shown in Fig. 9. The qualitative features of the response to current injection, including the slow ramp-like response to depolarizing currents, are present. This time-dependent ramp component of the response is generated because of an interaction between the membrane time constant and the inwardly rectifying potassium conductance. As the cell is depolarized, the membrane resistivity increases due to the deactivation of the inward rectifier. This increase in membrane resistivity causes the time constant to be increased, slowing the rate of depolarization. The increase in membrane resistivity also increases the overall input resistance of the cell, increasing the steady state level of depolarization toward which the constant current pulse is forcing the cell. Thus depolarization leads to more depolarization, but also to a slowing of the rate at which the new level of depolarization is achieved. The ramp would ultimately lead to a complete deactivation of the inward rectification and a steady-state membrane potential determined by the leak conductance. This would happen at a substantially depolarized level of membrane potential, at which other voltage-sensitive conductances would be expected to be activated, and so was considered outside the range of validity of the model, however. The effect of membrane potential on input resistance and time constant is shown for the model neuron in Fig. 9*B*, and matches that observed in identified spiny neurons (cf. Fig. 8).

An important result of the placement of the inwardly rectifying conductance on the dendritic membrane is its effect on the electrotonic length of the dendrites of the spiny neuron. This result is illustrated in Fig. 9*C, D,* which shows that the effective electrotonic length of the dendrites varied from a very compact 0.4 to a quite extended 0.8 length constant over the subthreshold range of membrane potentials (-100 to -45 mV). The assumptions of the method of measuring dendritic length by peeling exponentials is violated in the non-linear model of the spiny neuron presented here. The model violates several of the assumptions, including the assumption of electrotonic continuity at branch points (the famous 3/2 power rule) and the uniformity of membrane resistivity assumption (because membrane resistivity is dependent upon membrane potential, which varies over the surface of the neuron). Therefore, the effective electrotonic length was measured for the computer simulations using the steady-state attenuation from the soma to dendritic tips. When electrotonic length was measured from the simulated transients using the method of peeling exponentials and compared with that obtained from steady-state attenuation, the results were very similar, despite the violation of assumptions (Fig. 9*D*). Note that this effect of electrotonic length on membrane potential is only obtained from the model neuron when the inwardly rectifying conductance is placed on the dendrites, as well as the soma, of the cell. These results suggest that in real spiny neurons, as well as in those simulated on the computer, inward rectification is present on the dendrites.

The presence of the inward rectification on the dendrites can help to account for the low spontaneous activity of striatal cells by making the cells relatively insensitive to uncoordinated afferent activity. When excitatory input distributed over the surface of the neuron fires in an asynchronous fashion, individual excitatory events find the neuron in the hyperpolarized state, with its low input resistance, short time constant, and electrotonically extended dendritic tree. Excitation arriving in a coordinated fashion, and able to depolarize a region of the dendritic tree, can act cooperatively, increasing the input resistance and time constant and so increasing both the local amplitude of EPSPs, and also increasing the integration time of the dendrite. Most importantly, the local dendritic field becomes more compact, making all synapses in the vicinity (especially ones farther out on the same dendrite) more able to deliver charge to the soma. Individual synapses within a coordinated synaptic excitation, having overcome the barrier created by the inward rectification, are expected to be much more effective in depolarizing the soma. This positive feedback effect of the inward rectifier is probably responsible for the abrupt nature of the transitions between the depolarized and hyperpolarized state in both spontaneous and evoked activity.

While the properties of the hyperpolarized state of the spiny neuron are adequately explained by the absence of coordinated activity and the effect of inward rectification, the properties of the depolarized state are not. A characteristic feature of the depolarized state is the relatively constant subthreshold membrane potential maintained despite the presence of greatly increased synaptic noise (e.g., Fig. 4). In principle this could be explained if the synaptic input to neostriatal spiny neurons is tightly regulated and constant. A more likely possibility is that at membrane potentials corresponding to the depolarized state, another set of ionic channels is activated which decreases input resistance and maintains the preferred average membrane potential. This is probably not an equilibrium point, as already pointed out, but rather a ceiling placed on the membrane potential by an outwardly rectifying current. Outward rectification has been observed in striatal neurons at subthreshold membrane potentials, and has been offered as an explanation for the low spontaneous activity of the neurons (e.g., Calabresi et al., 1987). The most likely candidate for this current is the slowly inactivating potassium conductance that has been observed in voltage-clamp studies of dissociated striatal neurons (Surmeier et al., 1991, 1992). This conductance is activated in the appropriate voltage range for the depolarizing episodes, and inactivates over a time course measured in seconds. It can be detected both in dissociated striatal neurons and in tissue slices, and it has been studied in identified spiny neurons in slices, where it is seen to contribute to the ramp response to depolarizing current pulses (Bargas et al., 1989; Surmeier et al., 1992).

Action potential generation in the depolarized state

The depolarizing episode is an enabled state for action potential generation in the spiny neuron. It is necessary, but not sufficient to explain its pattern of firing, as can be seen by the fact that silent neurons have depolarizing episodes that do not attain threshold for firing (Wilson and Groves, 1981). Action potentials arising from the depolarized state of the cell are triggered by additional depolarizations which appear as noise superimposed on the enabling depolarization. Presumably, these depolarizations are fluctuations in the overall level of synaptic input responsible for the depolarized state, but it is also possible that they represent the action of some specialized input. What seems more certain is that they involve additional ionic conductances which are engaged in the membrane potential range between that of the depolarized state and the sodium spike threshold. These include both sodium and calcium conductances, acting in competition with the various potassium conductances that are engaged at these potentials (Kita et al., 1985a; Calabresi et al., 1987; Galarraga et al., 1989). These final steps in the generation of action potentials in spiny neurons are made all the more interesting by the discovery that the voltage sensitivity of both inward and outward currents active in this range of membrane potentials can be modulated by dopamine (Surmeier et al., 1992). This suggests the possibility that the firing of neostriatal neurons may be regulated at two relatively independent levels. The transitions in membrane potential between the disabled (hyperpolarized) and enabled (depolarized) states, as described above, are primarily controlled by synaptic input and by voltage-sensitive conductances that operate in the membrane potential range of -90 to -60 mV. While the determination of the preferred membrane potential in the enabled state may involve inward currents activated at more positive membrane potentials, the occurrence and duration of the state transitions probably do not involve them greatly. On the other hand, the rate and pattern of action potentials arising from the enabled state is likely to be greatly affected by a delicate interaction between several inward and outward currents. Because of the complex, extremely non-linear behavior of these currents, small changes in their kinetics and voltage sensitivity could create large changes in the intraepisodic firing rate of the cells. Thus firing rate during firing episodes and the rate and duration of occurrence of firing episodes could be controlled independently. This would help to explain why neostriatal spiny neurons continue to exhibit transitions between the disabled and enabled states even when they are no longer firing at all (Wilson and Groves, 1981). In this view, the occurrence of an episode of firing in a spiny cell would require not only convergent synaptic input to drive the membrane potential transition to the enabled state, but also the combination of ionic channel modulation by dopamine (and perhaps acetylcholine) to allow the expression of the state transition as action potentials in the efferent axon.

The functional importance of the timing of firing episodes, their duration, and the firing rate within an episode seem apparent, as these will determine the timing, duration, and strength of the pauses in the repetitive firing of pallidal and nigral neurons. It is less clear whether the fine structure of the intraepisodic firing pattern (that is, the precise timing of action potentials within the episode, whether short intervals follow long or the other way around) is important or not. Because spiny neurons usually do not fire rhythmically during episodes, it is possible in principle that the precise timing of action potentials contains information about the afferent signals and that this information is preserved in the firing pattern of target neurons in the globus pallidus and substantia nigra. Because of the large amount of convergence in the striato-pallidal and striato-nigral projections, preservation of the fine structure of firing of any one spiny cell's spike train in the target structures would probably require a high degree of fine-scale synchronization in the intra-episodic firing patterns across converging spiny neurons. Given the small size of the pertubations in membrane potential that lead to action potentials from the enabled membrane potential state, this seems unlikely. A more definitive statement should be possible from the results of studies of correlations in the firing of nearby neostriatal neurons, when such data become available.

Giant aspiny interneurons

Information on the firing patterns and physiological properties of the giant interneurons of Kölliker have become available with recent in vivo (Wilson et al., 1990) and in vitro (Jiang and North, 1991; Kawaguchi, 1992) studies. These neurons exhibit morphological features characteristic of neurons that stain using antibodies to choline acetyltransferase, and so are assumed to be cholinergic neurons. They have large somata and a very extended dendritic field, with the longest dendrites terminating nearly a millimeter from the soma. The axonal field

is even more extended, making these cells candidates for an associational interneuron in the striatum. These cells may connect the patch (striosome) and matrix compartments of the neostriatum, as their dendritic fields often extend into both compartments (Penney et al., 1988; Kawaguchi, 1992). A drawing of the dendritic tree of one of these neurons is shown in Fig. 10. The physiological characteristics of these cells in vivo are strongly in contrast to those of the spiny neurons, making identification of the cells easy in intracellular recordings. In their hyperpolarized state (and in slices) the membrane potential of spiny neurons is 30 – 40 mV from the threshold for action potentials. In giant aspiny neurons the baseline membrane potential is usually within 5 mV of threshold. The giant aspiny interneuron has a relatively slow (2 – 10 Hz) tonic but irregular pattern of firing in urethane-anesthetized animals, which is very unlike the firing pattern of the spiny neurons. Action potentials in the giant aspiny cell arise from brief spontaneous depolarizing potentials that occur in an all-or-none fashion. Generally, individually such spontaneous depolarizations are not large enough to trigger action potentials in the neuron, but two or more of these can summate to bring the giant neuron to threshold. An example showing a sample from the spontaneous firing of an identified giant cell is shown in Fig. 11A.

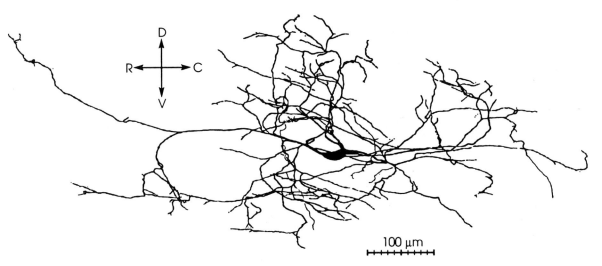

Fig. 10. A drawing of a giant aspiny neuron stained intracellularly with HRP. (Data from Wilson et al., 1990.)

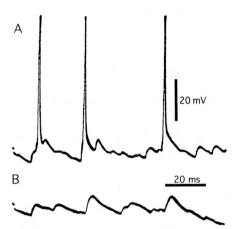

Fig. 11. Spontaneous fluctuations of membrane potential and firing of a giant aspiny neuron in an intact urethane-anesthetized rat recorded intracellularly in vivo. *A.* Spontaneous tonic activity arising from summation of small depolarizing potentials. *B.* The same activity but action potentials have been prevented by application of a small hyperpolarizing current. The underlying spontaneous depolarizing potentials remain. (From Wilson et al., 1992.)

The spontaneous depolarizations are best seen in Fig. 11*B*, which shows a recording from the same neuron taken while action potentials were prevented by passage of hyperpolarizing current. The spontaneous depolarizations have the voltage dependence and time course expected for unitary EPSPs located relatively close to the soma. Their identity as synaptic potentials is supported by the observation that their incidence is decreased under conditions known to decrease firing in corticostriatal and thalamostriatal neurons. Their incidence is reduced, for example, in hemidecorticate animals, and during the period of corticostriatal silence that follows cortical or thalamic stimulation (and is responsible for the late hyperpolarizing phase of the spiny neuron response). While these suggest that the depolarizations may be unitary synaptic potentials evoked by afferent fibers, they do not help to identify the source of the afferents. This is because both of these treatments reduce input in the thalamostriatal pathway, as well as in the corticostriatal pathway. An alternative approach to identification of the source of the excitatory input responsible for these depolari-

zations is a comparison of the spontaneous synaptic potentials with those evoked by stimulation of particular afferent pathways. A comparison of the EPSP evoked by thalamic stimulation with the spontaneous depolarizations is shown in Fig. 12*A* – *C*. The spontaneous activity of the neuron is shown in Fig. 12*A*, while the EPSP evoked with maximal stimulation is shown in Fig. 12*B*. The maximal amplitude of the evoked EPSP is much smaller than that observed in spiny neostriatal neurons, but is capable of firing an action potential in the aspiny interneuron. Examination of the maximal EPSP, shown at high gain in the lower trace of Fig. 12*B*, shows that the amplitude of the maximal EPSP is only slightly larger than the largest spontaneous depolarizations. With the stimulus intensity adjusted to be near threshold for a detectable synaptic response, the evoked EPSP can be seen to be intermittent (Fig. 12*C*). When present, the EPSP is variable from trial to trial and appears to consist of a

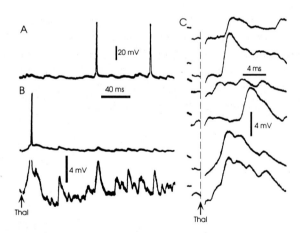

Fig. 12. A comparison of spontaneous depolarizing potentials in giant aspiny neurons with synaptic potentials evoked by stimulation of thalamostriatal fibers. *A.* Spontaneous depolarizing potentials and spontaneous firing of a giant neuron. *B.* Maximal EPSP evoked by thalamic stimulation, superimposed on a background of spontaneous depolarizing potentials. Low gain trace is shown above; high gain trace is below. *C.* A series of six EPSPs evoked in the same cell by thalamic stimulation at near-threshold levels. The amplitude and latency of the EPSP varies from trial to trial. The near-threshold EPSP consists of an increased probability of occurrence of all-or-none components resembling the spontaneous depolarizing potentials. (From Wilson et al., 1990.)

composite of smaller depolarizing potentials that resemble the spontaneous ones. This, combined with the reduced incidence of spontaneous depolarizing potentials after lesions to afferent pathways, strongly suggests that the smallest spontaneous depolarizations are unitary synaptic potentials evoked by afferent fibers from the thalamus, or the cerebral cortex, or both.

The contrast between the synaptic responses to afferents exhibited by the spiny neuron and the giant aspiny neuron is striking. Individual afferent synaptic inputs to the spiny neuron must be extremely weak. Reducing the intensity of cortical or thalamic inputs generally does not reveal a threshold in the spiny neuron, but rather the size of the evoked EPSP is gradually reduced until it disappears into the noise. This is interpreted to mean that spiny neurons receive very many weak afferent inputs, and individual afferent fibers do not pattern the firing of the spiny cell. The effects of individual afferents on the giant cell are much clearer, and the pattern of firing of the cell seems to be determined by the patterns of individual afferents, which appear to control it in groups of two or three. This accounts for the fact that the cells fire tonically, but not rhythmically. Rhythmic firing would be expected if the cells were tonically depolarized above their spike thresholds, in wich case the statistical features of the cells' firing patterns would be determined by their membrane properties, rather than by the fine structure of the pattern of afferent input. The firing of the giant cell, while not determined primarily by the properties of its membrane, is affected by its membrane properties. This is evident from a comparison of the pattern of spontaneous synaptic depolarizations and the pattern of cell firing. Although synaptic input is more or less continuous, the neurons show a prolonged relative refractory period that prevents firing at very high frequencies under resting conditions. This can be seen in the statistical pattern of cell firing, as shown in Fig. 13. This shows the interval histogram and autocorrelation histograms of a tonically firing neuron in the neostriatum of a rat. Although the cell's firing over a long time period (Fig. 13C) appears to be approximately random (as

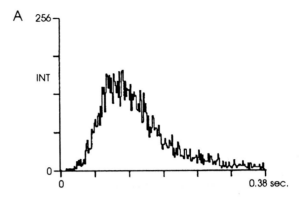

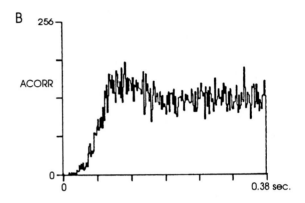

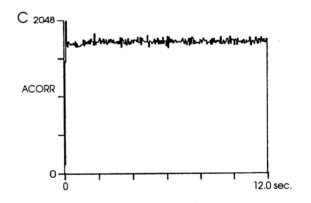

Fig. 13. Interval histogram and autocorrelation histogram of a tonically firing striatal neuron in the rat. *A*. Interval histogram showing a modal interval at about 100 msec. *B*. Autocorrelation histogram computed from the same spike train. Note the peak in firing probability at the time of the modal interval, indicating a tendency to fire after recovery from the relative refractory period, and the relatively constant firing probability thereafter. *C*. Autocorrelation histogram computed using a long bin width to show the absence of bursting or slow rhythms.

294

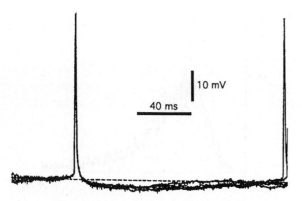

Fig. 14. Superimposed spontaneous action potentials from a giant aspiny neuron in an urethane-anesthetized, hemidecorticate rat, showing the spike afterhyperpolarization that follows individual spontaneous action potentials. This afterhyperpolarization corresponds in duration to the trough in the autocorrelation in Fig. 13. The tendency of the cell also shows an increased probability of firing for a period after termination of the afterhyperpolarization, which corresponds to the early peak in the autocorrelation histogram. These features of the firing pattern of aspiny neurons are apparently due to the cells' membrane properties, while the fine structure of the spike train is otherwise determined by the times of arrival of spontaneous depolarizing potentials. (From Wilson et al., 1990.)

indicated by the constant firing probability in the autocorrelation histogram), firing at intervals shorter than about 100 msec is relatively rare. This can be seen by examination of both the interval histogram and the autocorrelation histogram constructed using short bin widths (Fig. 13A,B). The autocorrelation histogram also reveals a heightened tendency of the cell to fire at the end of its refractory period. This firing pattern suggests that the giant cell may show a prolonged spike afterhyperpolarization which could be responsible for the relative refractory period. That this is the case is shown in the intracellular recordings in Fig. 14. In that figure, five spontaneous action potentials from an identified giant aspiny interneuron have been superimposed, and the afterhyperpolarization that follows a single spike is clearly visible. The increased tendency of the cell to fire at the end of the refractory period is indicated by the occurrence of spikes at this time in two of the five superimposed spontaneous cells. This tendency to fire at the end of the spike afterhyper-

polarization is probably due to the presence of inward currents activated by hyperpolarization in these neurons (Jiang and North, 1991; Kawaguchi, 1992). It should make the neuron resonate with afferents firing at around 8 – 10 Hz, and it is likely that there will be natural circumstances under which these neurons would fire rhythmically, although this has apparently not yet been observed.

Implications for striatal function

The striking differences in firing patterns, morphology, and synaptic connectivity of the spiny projection cell and the giant aspiny interneuron in the neostriatum offer some interesting contrasts in structure and function of central neurons. Despite the much larger dendritic tree of the aspiny neuron, it receives fewer afferent synaptic contacts than the spiny cell. Despite their much larger complement of excitatory synaptic inputs, the spiny projection neurons fire much less frequently than the giant interneurons. The spiny neuron utilizes a wide range of subthreshold membrane potentials for integration of synaptic inputs and for interaction of synaptic inputs with a layered set of voltage-dependent membrane non-linearities, each engaged over a different range of membrane potentials. The giant interneuron's membrane is restricted to a very narrow range of subthreshold potentials, and therefore a much more restricted set of membrane characteristics. The temporal pattern of action potentials in the spiny neurons probably does not reflect the precise temporal pattern of firing in any particular afferent fibers, but rather an envelope of afferent activity integrated over periods of tens or hundreds of milliseconds, and heavily filtered by the intrinsic properties of the cells. The giant aspiny interneurons, on the other hand, fire in an exact temporal relationship (although certainly not a one-to-one relationship) to the pattern of firing of individual afferent fibers with integration time measured in milliseconds. In addition to demonstrating the enormous variation in cellular properties that accompany the morphological differences between cell types in a single brain area, these differences suggest dramatically different computational functions for these two striatal neurons. The tight input-output linkage seen in the firing of the aspiny interneurons might seem to be for nothing, given the fact that the main synaptic target of these neurons is the spiny neuron, which apparently integrates its inputs over a much longer time epoch. However, the likely transmitter of the giant neuron is acetylcholine, which, like dopamine, can act to alter the membrane properties of the spiny neuron responsible for the transition between the enabled and disabled states, and so rapidly affect firing of the cell in the enabled state (see chapter by Surmeier and Kitai, this volume). Our need to identify the afferents that control the firing of aspiny neurons, and to discover the mechanism of action of acetylcholine on spiny neurons becomes even more urgent in light of these findings.

The replacement of inhibition as the primary influence governing the transition to firing in spiny neurons has implications that have not yet penetrated theoretical opinion on the basal ganglia. Most current models of the striatum depict this structure as a simple laterally inhibitory network, and most of the properties of these models arise from the action of the inhibition. The view of the neostriatum emerging from current neurophysiological work is one in which inhibition plays a small role in the transition of these neurons to the firing-enabled (depolarized) state, but may be important for interactions among nearby excited cells during the course of an episode of firing. Although the membrane properties responsible for the relative silence of neostriatal spiny neurons resemble inhibition superficially, they do not have the same temporal and spatial properties. Tonic inhibition should increase during the transition to firing as observed in any one neuron because the overall firing rate will increase in the cells responsible for inhibition. The membrane properties of spiny neurons lead to the opposite effect, with the excitability of cells growing rapidly as they are depolarized. Lateral inhibition also gives rise to spatial effects, such as relatively uninhibited zones near the edges of an excited group of cells and to inhibitory surround effects that will not occur in neurons whose firing is

limited by intrinsic membrane properties. A new generation of theoretical models of the neostriatum that incorporate current information on the mechanisms underlying the firing patterns of the spiny and aspiny neurons may yield valuable new insights into the functional properties of the basal ganglia.

Acknowledgements

Supported by NIH Grant NS20743 and Grant N00014-922-J-111-3 from the Office of Naval Research.

References

Albe-Fessard, D., Rocha-Miranda, C. and Oswaldo-Cruz, E. (1960) Activités évoquées dans le noyau caudé du chat en résponse à des types divers d'afférences. *Electroenceph. Clin. Neurophysiol.*, 12: 649 – 661.

Aldridge, J.W. and Gilman, S. (1990) Spontaneous neuronal unit activity in the primate basal ganglia and the effects of precentral cerebral cortical ablations. *Brain Res.*, 516: 46 – 56.

Aldridge, J.W. and Gilman, S. (1991) The temporal structure of spike trains in the primate basal ganglia: afferent regulation of bursting demonstrated with precentral cerebral cortical ablation. *Brain Res.*, 543: 123 – 138.

Anderson, J.E. (1977) Discharge patterns of basal ganglia neurons during active maintenance of postural stability and adjustment to chair tilt. *Brain Res.*, 143: 325 – 338.

Apicella, P., Scarnati, E. and Schultz, W (1991) Tonically discharging neurons of monkey striatum respond to preparatory and rewarding stimuli. *Exp. Brain Res.*, 84: 672 – 675.

Bargas, J., Galarraga, E. and Aceves, J. (1989) An early outward conductance modulates the firing latency and frequency of neostriatal neurons of the rat brain. *Exp. Brain Res.*, 75: 146 – 156.

Bernardi, G., Marciani, M.G., Morocutti, C. and Giacomini, P. (1975) The action of GABA on rat caudate neurones recorded intracellularly. *Brain Res.*, 92: 511 – 515.

Bernardi, G., Marciani, M.G., Morocutti, C. and Giacomini, P. (1976) The action of picrotoxin and bicuculline on rat caudate neurons inhibited by GABA. *Brain Res.*, 102: 379 – 384.

Bloom, F.E., Costa, E. and Salmoiraghi, G.C. (1965) Anesthesia and the responsiveness of individual neurons of the caudate nucleus of the cat to acetylcholine, norepinephrine and dopamine administered by microelectrophoresis. *J. Pharmacol. Exp. Ther.*, 150: 244 – 252.

Buchwald, N.A., Price, D.D., Vernon, L. and Hull, C.D. (1973) Caudate intracellular response to thalamic and cortical inputs. *Exp. Neurol.*, 38: 311 – 323.

Calabresi, P., Misgeld, U. and Dodt, H.U. (1987) Intrinsic membrane properties of neostriatal neurons can account for their low level of spontaneous activity. *Neuroscience,* 20: 293 – 303.

Calabresi, P., Mercuri, N.B., Stefani, A. and Bernardi, G. (1990) Synaptic and intrinsic control of membrane excitability of neostriatal neurons. I. An in vivo analysis. *J. Neurophysiol.,* 63: 651 – 662.

Chang, H.T., Wilson, C.J. and Kitai, S.T. (1981) Single neostriatal efferent axons in the globus pallidus: a light and electron microscopic study. *Science,* 213: 915 – 918.

Cocatre-Zilgien, J.H. and Delcomyn, F. (1992) Identification of bursts in spike trains. *J. Neurosci. Methods,* 41: 19 – 30.

Connor, J.D. (1970) Caudate nucleus neurones: correlation of the effects of substantia nigra stimulation with iontophoretic dopamine. *J. Physiol. (Lond.),* 208: 691 – 703.

Dossi, R.C., Nuñez, A. and Steriade, M. (1992) Electrophysiology of a slow (0.5 – 4 Hz) intrinsic oscillation of cat thalamocortical neurones in vivo. *J. Physiol. (Lond.),* 447: 215 – 234.

Feltz, P. and Albe-Fessard, D. (1972) A study of an ascending nigro-caudate pathway. *Electroenceph. Clin. Neurophysiol.,* 33: 179 – 193.

Fuller, D.R.G., Hull, C.D. and Buchwald, N.A. (1975) Intracellular responses of caudate output neurons to orthodromic stimulation. *Brain Res.,* 96: 337 – 341.

Galarraga, E., Bargas, J. and Aceves, J. (1989) The role of calcium in the repetitive firing of neostriatal neurons. *Exp. Brain Res.,* 75: 157 – 168.

Hikosaka, O., Sakamoto, M. and Usui, S. (1989) Functional properties of monkey caudate neurons I. Activities related to saccadic eye movements. *J. Neurophysiol.,* 61: 780 – 798.

Hounsgaard, J.H., Hultborn, B., Jespersen, B. and Kiehn, O. (1984) Intrinsic membrane properties causing a bistable behaviour of a-motoneurones. *Exp. Brain Res.,* 55: 391 – 394.

Hull, C.D., Bernardi, G. and Buchwald, N.A. (1970) Intracellular responses of caudate neurons to brain stem stimulation. *Brain Res.,* 22: 163 – 179.

Hull, C.D., Bernardi, G., Price, D.D. and Buchwald, N.A. (1973) Intracellular responses of caudate neurons to temporally and spatially combined stimuli. *Exp. Neurol.,* 38: 324 – 336.

Jiang, Z.-G. and North, R.A. (1991) Membrane properties and synaptic responses of rat striatal neurones in vitro. *J. Physiol. (Lond.),* 443: 533 – 553.

Katayama, Y., Tsubokawa, T. and Moriyasu, N. (1980) Slow rhythmic activity of caudate neurons in the cat: statistical analysis of caudate neuronal spike trains. *Exp. Neurol.,* 68: 310 – 321.

Kawaguchi, Y. (1992) Large aspiny cells in the matrix of the rat neostriatum in vitro − physiological identification, relation to the compartments and excitatory postsynaptic currents. *J. Neurophysiol.,* 67: 1659 – 1668.

Kawaguchi, Y., Wilson, C.J. and Emson, P.C. (1989) Intracellular recording of identified neostriatal patch and matrix spiny cells in a slice preparation preserving cortical inputs. *J. Neurophysiol.,* 62: 1052 – 1068.

Kawaguchi, Y., Wilson, C.J. and Emson, P.C. (1990) Projection subtypes of rat neostriatal matrix cells revealed by intracellular injection of biocytin. *J. Neurosci.,* 10: 3421 – 3438.

Kimura, M., Rajkowski, J. and Evarts, E.V. (1984) Tonically discharging putamen neurons exhibit set dependent responses. *Proc. Natl. Acad. Sci. U.S.A.,* 81: 4998 – 5001.

Kimura, M., Kato, M. and Shimazaki, H. (1990) Physiological properties of projection neurons in the monkey striatum to the globus pallidus. *Exp. Brain Res.,* 82: 672 – 676.

Kita, H., Kita, T. and Kitai, S.T. (1985a) Active membrane properties of rat neostriatal neurons in an in vitro slice preparation. *Exp. Brain Res.,* 60: 54 – 62.

Kita, T., Kita, H. and Kitai, S.T. (1985b) Local stimulation induced GABAergic response in rat striatal slice preparations: intracellular recording on QX-314 injected neurons. *Brain Res.,* 360: 304 – 310.

Lighthall, J.W. and Kitai, S.T. (1983) A short duration GABAergic inhibition in identified neostriatal medium spiny neurons. In vitro slices study. *Brain Res. Bull.,* 11: 103 – 110.

Liles, S.L. (1974) Single-unit responses of caudate neurons to stimulation of frontal cortex, substantia nigra and entopeduncular nucleus in cats. *J. Neurophysiol.,* 37: 254 – 265.

Misgeld, U., Wagner, A. and Ohno, T. (1982) Depolarizing IPSPs and depolarization by GABA of rat neostriatum cells in vitro. *Exp. Brain Res.,* 45: 108 – 124.

Nisenbaum, E.S. and Berger, T.W. (1992) Functionally distinct subpopulations of striatal neurons are differentially regulated by GABAergic and dopaminergic inputs. 1. In vivo analysis. *Neuroscience,* 48: 561 – 578.

Nisenbaum, E.S., Orr, W.B. and Berger, T.W. (1988) Evidence for two functionally distinct subpopulations of neurons within the rat striatum. *J. Neurosci.,* 8: 4138 – 4150.

Penny, G.R., Wilson, C.J. and Kitai, S.T. (1988) Relationship of the axonal and dendritic geometry of spiny projection neurons to the compartmental organization of the neostriatum. *J. Comp. Neurol.,* 269: 275 – 289.

Poulain, D.A., Brown, D. and Wakerley, J.B. (1988) Statistical analysis of patterns of electrical activity in vasopressin and oxytocin-secreting neurones. In: G. Leng (Ed.), *Pulsatility in Neuroendocrine Systems,* CRC Press, Boca Raton, FL, pp. 119 – 154.

Preston, R.J., Bishop, G.A. and Kitai, S.T. (1980) Medium spiny projection from the rat striatum: an intracellular horseradish peroxidase study. *Brain Res.,* 183: 253 – 262.

Purpura, D.P. and Malliani, A. (1967) Intracellular studies of the corpus striatum. I. Synaptic potentials and discharge characteristics of caudate neurons activated by thalamic stimulation. *Brain Res.,* 6: 325 – 340.

Richardson, T.L., Miller, J.J. and McLennan, H. (1977) Mechanisms of excitation and inhibition in the nigrostriatal system. *Brain Res.,* 127: 219 – 234.

Sedgwick, E.M. and Williams, T.D. (1967) The response of single units in the caudate nucleus to peripheral stimulation. *J. Physiol. (Lond.),* 189: 281 – 298.

Surmeier, D.J., Foehring, R., Stefani, A. and Kitai, S.T. (1991) Developmental expression of a slowly-inactivating voltage dependent potassium current in rat neostriatal neurons. *Neurosci. Lett.,* 122: 41 – 46.

Surmeier, D.J., Eberwine, J., Wilson, C.J., Cao, Y., Stefani, A. and Kitai, S.T. (1992) Cellular and molecular evidence for the co-localization of dopamine receptor subtypes in acutely isolated rat striatonigral neurons. *Proc. Natl. Acad. Sci. U.S.A.,* in press.

Surmeier, D.J., Xu, Z.C., Wilson, C.J., Stefani, A. and Kitai, S.T. (1992) Grafted neostriatal neurons express a late-developing transient potassium current. *Neuroscience,* 48: 849 – 856.

Uchimura, N., Cherubini, E. and North, R.A. (1989) Inward rectification in rat nucleus accumbens neurones. *J. Neurophysiol.,* 315: 498 – 500.

Wilson, C.J. (1986) Postsynaptic potentials evoked in spiny neostriatal projection neurons by stimulation of ipsilateral and contralateral neocortex. *Brain Res.,* 367: 201 – 213.

Wilson, C.J. (1992) Dendritic morphology, inward rectification, and the functional properties of neostriatal neurons. In: T. McKenna, J. Davis and S.F. Zornetzer (Eds.), *Single Neuron Computation,* Academic Press, San Diego, CA, pp. 141 – 171.

Wilson, C.J. and Groves, P.M. (1981) Spontaneous firing patterns of identified spiny neurons in the rat neostriatum. *Brain Res.,* 220: 67 – 80.

Wilson, C.J., Chang, H.T. and Kitai, S.T. (1982) Origins of postsynaptic potentials evoked in identified rat neostriatal neurons by stimulation in substantia nigra. *Exp. Brain Res.,* 45: 157 – 167.

Wilson, C.J., Chang, H.T. and Kitai, S.T. (1983a) Origins of post synaptic potentials evoked in spiny neostriatal projection neurons by thalamic stimulation in the rat. *Exp. Brain Res.,* 51: 217 – 226.

Wilson, C.J., Chang, H.T. and Kitai, S.T. (1983b) Disfacilitation and long-lasting inhibition of neostriatal neurons in the rat. *Exp. Brain Res.,* 51: 227 – 235.

Wilson, C.J., Chang, H.T. and Kitai, S.T. (1990) Firing patterns and synaptic potentials of identified giant aspiny interneurons in the rat neostriatum. *J. Neurosci.,* 10: 508 – 519.

G.W. Arbuthnott and P.C. Emson (Eds.)
Progress in Brain Research, Vol. 99
© 1993 Elsevier Science Publishers B.V. All rights reserved.

CHAPTER 19

Chemical modulation of synaptic transmission in the striatum

Paolo Calabresi[1], Nicola B. Mercuri[1] and Giorgio Bernardi[1,2]

[1]*Clinica Neurologica, Dipartimento Sanita, Universita di Roma "Tor Vergata", Rome, and* [2]*Istituto di Ricerca a Carottere Scientifico, Clinica S. Lucia, Rome, Italy*

Introduction

Intracellular recordings from in vivo (Buchwald et al., 1973; Kitai et al., 1976; Sugimori et al., 1978; Calabresi et al., 1990b) and in vitro preparations (Kita et al., 1984; Calabresi et al., 1987, 1990; Kawaguchi et al., 1989) have shown that medium spiny striatal neurons do not possess membrane mechanisms generating bursting activity and spontaneous firing discharge. For this reason the activation of firing activity in these GABAergic projecting neurons is mainly caused by synaptic inputs originating from cortical areas (Groves, 1983). Intracellular recordings in vivo from striatal neurons have shown that activation of cortex generates an EPSP (excitatory synaptic potential) followed by an IPSP (inhibitory synaptic potential) (Bernardi et al., 1976). The role of glutamate in the generation of cortically evoked EPSPs was suggested by electrophysiological studies (Herrling, 1985) and by biochemical evidence (Reubi and Cuenod, 1979). In contrast, the physiological mechanism generating the cortically evoked IPSPs was more debated. In fact, although it has been postulated that endogenous striatal GABA could be involved in the generation of these potentials (Bernardi et al., 1976; Herrling, 1984), other mechanisms (disfacilitation) were postulated to account for the generation of long-lasting inhibition of striatal neurons (Wilson et al., 1983).

However, the in vivo techniques did not allow a complete characterization of the possible pharmacological mechanisms involved in the modulation of striatal synaptic activity. For this reason we utilized a brain slice preparation in the study of the corticostriatal interaction and in the characterization of the receptors involved in the control of synaptic signals in the striatum.

Methodological aspects

Rats were used for the experiments. The preparation and the maintenance of the slices have been previously described (Calabresi et al., 1991a, 1992a). Coronal slices (200 – 300 μm) were prepared from tissue blocks of the brain with the use of a vibratome. These coronal slices included the neostriatum and the neocortex. A single slice was transferred to a recording chamber (vol. 0.5 ml) and submerged in a continuously flowing Krebs solution (36°C, 2 – 3 ml/min) gassed with a 95% O_2 and 5% CO_2 mixture. The composition of the solution was (in mM): 126 NaCl, 2,5 KCl, 1.2 NaH_2PO_4, 1.2 $MgCl_2$, 2.4 $CaCl_2$, 11 glucose and 24 $NaHCO_3$. Intracellular recording electrodes were filled with 2 M KCl (30 – 60 MΩ). For synaptic stimulation bipolar electrodes were used. To activate corticostriatal fibers the stimulating electrode was located either in the cortical areas close to the recording electrode or in the white matter between the cortex and the striatum. In some experiments we studied the effects of intrastriatal stimulation and in this case the stimulating electrode was positioned within the striatum close to the recording site.

Results

Pharmacological isolation of glutamate and GABA-mediated synaptic potentials

In order to quantify the glutamatergic component of the synaptic potentials evoked either by cortical or by intrastriatal stimulation, we applied in the external medium kynurenic acid (600 μM), a broad spectrum antagonist of excitatory amino acids. This glutamate receptor antagonist blocks both NMDA

and non-NMDA glutamate receptors. As shown in Fig. 1, kynurenic acid reversibly blocked the EPSP evoked by cortical stimulation, but it only partially reduced the potential evoked by intrastriatal stimulation suggesting that a component of the intrastriatally evoked potential is mediated by a transmitter other than glutamate. Bath application of bicuculline (100 μM), a GABA$_A$ receptor antagonist, did not greatly affect cortically evoked EPSPs, but it significantly reduced depolarizing potentials evoked by intrastriatal stimulation (Fig. 2). This finding shows that the synaptic potential evoked by intrastriatal stimulation is not only mediated by an

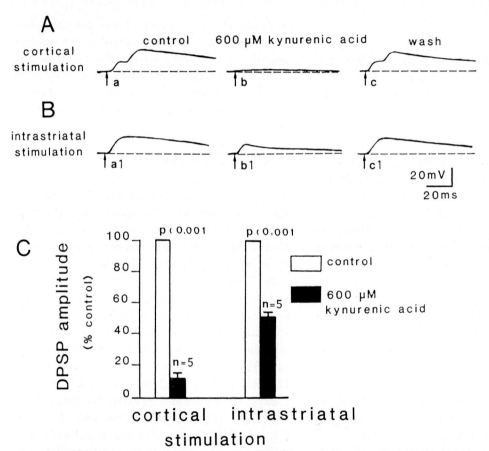

Fig. 1. Effect of kynurenic acid on cortically and intrastriatally evoked synaptic potentials. *A*. Under control condition, cortical stimulation evoked a depolarizing synaptic potential (a); this potential was almost completely abolished by 600 μM kynurenic acid (b); after the washout of this antagonist the potential recovered (c). *B*. Under control condition, intrastriatal stimulation produced a depolarizing potential (a); kynurenic acid produced only a partial reduction of this synaptic potential (b); the potential recovered after the wash-out of the drug (c). In the lower part of the figure *(C)* the graph represents data obtained from several neurons ($n = 5$). Note that synaptic potentials evoked by cortical stimulation were more sensitive to kynurenic acid (600 μM) than those produced by intrastriatal stimulation.

excitatory amino acid, but also by endogenous GABA released within the striatum. The depolarizing action of GABA, acting on $GABA_A$ receptors, was not only caused by the chloride-containing electrodes, but also by the high resting potential of neostriatal neurons (about -85 mV). In fact, at negative potentials, the activation of a chloride conductance causes a depolarizing driving force (Misgeld et al., 1982; Calabresi et al., 1991a; Mercuri et al., 1991).

In order to further characterize the role of glutamate in the corticostriatal transmission, we also studied the effect of CNQX (10 μM), a selective an-

tagonist of the non-NMDA glutamate receptors, on cortically evoked synaptic potentials. This antagonist, as well as kynurenic acid, produced a reversible inhibition of the EPSPs evoked by cortical stimulation. In contrast, APV (30 – 50 μM), an antagonist of the NMDA glutamate receptors, did not greatly affect the EPSP amplitude and duration (not shown). This experimental evidence indicates that, at least under control condition, the corticostriatal transmission is mainly mediated by glutamate receptors of the non-NMDA type. It is interesting to note that in the presence of either CNQX or kynurenic acid intrastriatal stimulation evoked

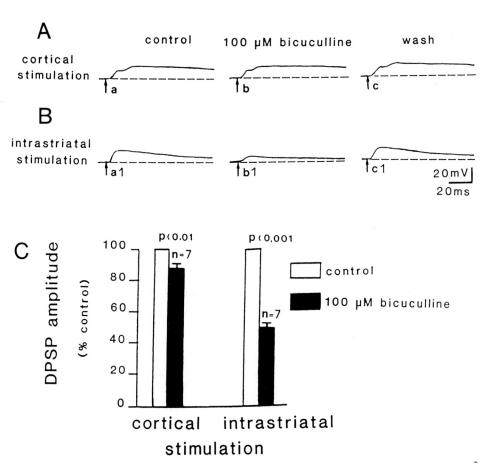

Fig. 2. Effect of bicuculline on cortically and intrastriatally evoked synaptic potentials. *A.* Under control condition, cortical stimulation produced a depolarizing synaptic potential (a); this potential was not greatly affected by 100 μM bicuculline (b); wash (c). *B.* The synaptic potential evoked by intrastriatal stimulation (a) was significantly reduced by bicuculline (b); wash (c). In the lower part of the figure *(C)* the graph shows data obtained from several neurons (n = 7). Note that synaptic potentials evoked by intrastriatal stimulation were more sensitive to bicuculline than those evoked by cortical stimulation.

depolarizing potentials which were fully blocked by bicuculline. This finding shows that, in the presence of glutamate receptor antagonists, it is possible to study in isolation GABA-mediated synaptic potentials.

Modulation of synaptic potentials by GABA$_B$ receptors

Since it has been shown that the activation of GABA$_B$ receptors causes a presynaptic reduction of the release of different transmitters in several brain structures (Bowery, 1989), we have characterized the effect of GABA$_B$ receptor stimulation in the striatum. As shown in Fig. 3, the application of GABA either by bath (1 mM) or by focal pressure ejection from a small pipette (10 – 100 mM) causes a membrane depolarization coupled with a reduction of both cortically and intrastriatally evoked synaptic potentials. The GABA-induced reduction

of synaptic potentials was caused neither by membrane depolarization nor by the fall in input resistance observed after the application of GABA. In fact, this effect on synaptic transmission persisted even in the presence of bicuculline, a condition in which the postsynaptic actions mediated by GABA$_A$ receptor activation are fully antagonized. This experimental evidence suggests that in the striatum, as in other brain structures, GABA activates not only GABA$_A$ receptors, but also bicuculline-insensitive GABA$_B$ receptors mediating presynaptic inhibition. In order to further test this hypothesis we studied the electrophysiological effects of baclofen (0.1 – 30 μM), a GABA$_B$ selective agonist, on striatal neurons. As shown in Fig. 4, this agonist reduced the EPSP evoked by cortical stimulation in the absence of changes of membrane potential and input resistance. The effects of baclofen were dose-dependent and were bicuculline-insensitive. Bac-

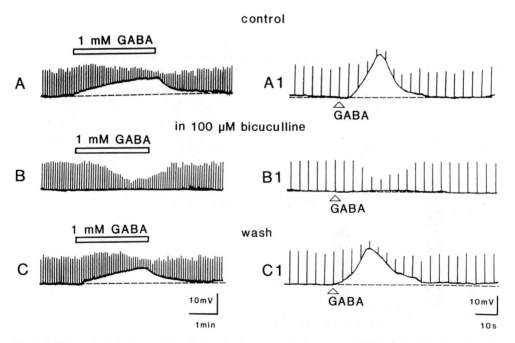

Fig. 3. GABA produces both pre- and postsynaptic effects on striatal neurons. *A.* Bath application of 1 mM GABA produced membrane depolarization in a striatal neuron (resting membrane potential was – 85 mV) and reduced cortically evoked synaptic potentials (upward deflections). *B.* Bath application of 100 μM bicuculline blocked the GABA-induced depolarization, but not the reduction of synaptic potentials. *C.* Recovery after the washout of bicuculline. *A1.* In another striatal neuron (resting membrane potential = – 87 mV) focal application of 10 mM GABA depolarized membrane potential and reduced synaptic potentials (upward deflections). *B1.* Also in this case bicuculline blocked the postsynaptic action of GABA, but not the GABA-induced presynaptic inhibition. *C1.* Recovery after the washout of bicuculline.

lofen reduced also the synaptic potentials evoked by intrastriatal stimulation in the presence of kynurenic acid suggesting that the activation of $GABA_B$ receptors reduces not only the synaptic release of glutamate, but also the release of GABA within the striatum (Calabresi et al., 1991a). Baclofen did not affect the postsynaptic responses of striatal neurons to exogenous glutamate and GABA and did not affect the postsynaptic membrane properties of striatal neurons (membrane potential and input resistance). These findings confirm that the baclofen-induced reduction of synaptic potentials is caused by presynaptic mechanisms. It is interesting to note that a pharmacological difference between $GABA_B$ receptors modulating the release of glutamate in comparison with those controlling the release of GABA was observed (Calabresi et al., 1991a). In fact, phaclofen (1 mM) and 2-OH-idroxysaclofen (100 – 300 μM), $GABA_B$ receptor antagonists, reduced the effect of baclofen on GABA-mediated potentials, but they did not antagonize the action of baclofen on glutamate-mediated EPSP. However, it has also been reported that in striatal slices the new $GABA_B$ receptor antagonists, CGP 35348 and 3-APHA, were more potent than phaclofen and were able to antagonize the reduction of glutamate-mediated synaptic potentials caused by SK&F 97541, a new $GABA_B$ agonist (Seabrook et al., 1990). Activation of $GABA_B$

receptors by endogenous GABA seems to be involved in the use-dependent modulation of both glutamate and GABA-mediated synaptic potentials in the striatum (Calabresi et al., 1991a). In fact, nipecotic acid, an inhibitor of the GABA uptake system, mimicked the presynaptic inhibitory effects of baclofen on both glutamate and GABA-mediated synaptic potentials (Calabresi et al., 1990a, 1991a). These findings suggest that endogenous striatal GABA by acting on $GABA_B$ receptors located on cortical glutamatergic terminals and on GABAergic terminals of striatal neurons exerts a feed-back control on glutamate and GABA release within the striatum.

Modulation of synaptic potentials by muscarinic receptors

An inhibitory effect of direct (muscarine and carbachol) and indirect (physostigmine) cholinergic agonists on intrastriatally evoked synaptic potentials was demonstrated in striatal slices (Dodt and Misgeld, 1986; Misgeld et al., 1986). The concentrations of cholinergic agonists necessary to produce this presynaptic inhibition were much lower than those required to induce postsynaptic effects on the recorded neurons (membrane depolarization and increase in input resistance). A prominent role of muscarinic receptors in the presynaptic regulation of synaptic potentials in striatal neurons recorded in

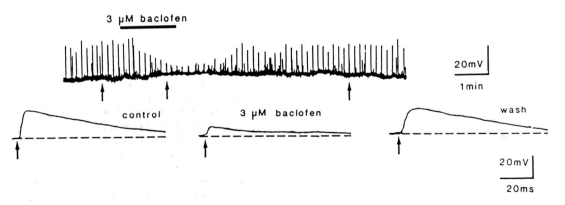

Fig. 4. Baclofen produces presynaptic inhibition in a striatal neuron, but it does not affect postsynaptic membrane properties. In the upper part of the figure is shown the chart record of the effect of 3 μM baclofen on synaptic potentials evoked by cortical stimulation (upward deflections). Note that baclofen did not affect resting membrane potential (-85 mV). In the lower part of the figure synaptic potentials are shown, recorded at higher speed before, during and after the application of baclofen.

in vitro brain slices was confirmed by Akaike et al. (1988). More recently Sugita et al. (1991) studied the effect of muscarinic agonists on pharmacologically isolated synaptic potentials mediated by GABA and by excitatory amino acids in neurons recorded from lateral amygdala, nucleus accumbens and striatum in vitro. They found that muscarine and acetylcholine reduced the amplitude of both GABA and glutamate-mediated synaptic potentials. Measurements of the equilibrium dissociation constants for the antagonists pirenzepine, AFDX-166, methoctramine and HHSD indicated that different muscarinic receptors are involved in the modulation of GABA and glutamate release (M_1 and probably M_3, respectively). We have recently studied the effects of muscarinic agonists on striatal neurons intracellularly recorded in vitro (Calabresi et al., 1991b). Low concentrations of muscarine (0.1 – 3 μM) produced a dose-dependent reduction of glutamate and GABA-mediated synaptic potentials in the striatum. These concentrations of muscarine did not affect intrinsic membrane properties and postsynaptic responses to exogenously applied glutamate and GABA. Neostigmine mimicked the muscarinic inhibition of synaptic potentials. High concentrations of muscarine (10 – 100 μM) produced membrane depolarizations (3 – 20 mV) in current-clamp recordings and inward currents (30 – 200 pA) in voltage-clamp mode. Voltage steps (1 – 3 sec) from the holding potential (– 75/ – 85 mV) showed inward membrane rectification. This rectification was reduced by low concentrations of barium (10 – 100 μM) and it was sensitive to different external potassium concentrations suggesting that potassium was its primary charge carrier. Muscarine decreased this inward rectification. Muscarinic currents were reversed at membrane potentials close to the potassium equilibrium potential, were blocked by barium and were not affected by TTX (1 – 3 μM). Scopolamine (1 – 10 μM) blocked both presynaptic inhibition (Fig. 5) and inward currents mediated by muscarine (not shown). These findings suggest that synaptic and intrinsic membrane properties of striatal neurons show differential sensitivity to muscarinic agonists.

Modulation of synaptic potentials by glutamate metabotropic receptors

Biochemical studies using cultured striatal neurons indicate that these neurons contain receptors of the metabotropic type (Sladeczek et al., 1985). This type of receptor seems to be linked to hydrolysis of inositol-containing phospholipids and it can be activated by t-ACPD at concentrations in the micromolar range. Although some excitatory effects following the activation of this type of receptor have been reported in the hippocampus (Charpak et al., 1990), the physiological effects of the activation of this

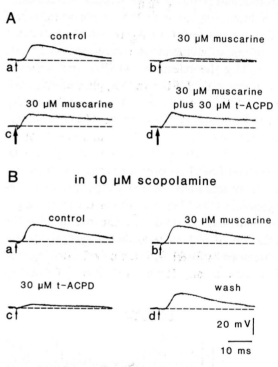

Fig. 5. Muscarine occludes the presynaptic action of t-ACPD. *A*. In a striatal cell, cortical stimulation evoked a synaptic potential (a); 30 μM muscarine greatly reduced the amplitude of this potential (b); under this condition, the increase of the intensity of stimulation partially restored the amplitude of the potential (c); under this condition 30 μM t-ACPD did not significantly alter the amplitude of the potential (d). *B*. The same neuron shown in *A* was recorded 10 min after the onset of the application of 10 μM scopolamine (a); under this condition 30 μM muscarine did not affect the amplitude of the synaptic potential (b) while 30 μM t-ACPD clearly reduced the synaptic potential (c); wash (d). 30 μM bicuculline was present throughout the experiment. The resting membrane potential of the cell was – 83 mV.

receptor in the striatum is still unknown. For this reason we have studied the effects of t-ACPD on synaptic transmission and membrane properties of striatal neurons (Calabresi et al., 1992b). As previously reported for muscarine, low concentrations (1 – 30 μM) of t-ACPD decreased glutamate-mediated synaptic potentials evoked in the striatum by the stimulation of corticostriatal fibers. This agonist decreased also GABA-mediated synaptic potentials evoked by intrastriatal stimulation and recorded in the presence of CNQX. This effect was less potent than the action of t-ACPD on glutamate-mediated synaptic potentials. While low concentrations of t-ACPD did not affect intrinsic membrane properties of striatal neurons and their postsynaptic responses to exogenous glutamate and GABA, higher concentrations (50 – 100 μM) of this agonist caused membrane depolarization and inward currents in several neurons. These data suggest that low concentrations of t-ACPD selectively reduce synaptic transmission while higher concentrations cause a direct excitatory action on striatal neurons. It is interesting to note that the presynaptic inhibitory action of t-ACPD is occluded by muscarine (Fig. 5) suggesting that muscarine and t-ACPD may activate a common mechanism in the modulation of striatal synaptic transmission. This mechanism, however, does not involve receptor specificity since scopolamine blocked the action of muscarine, but not the effect of t-ACPD (Fig. 5B). A presynaptic inhibitory action of t-ACPD on glutamate-mediated synaptic potentials has also been obtained by utilizing whole-cell recordings from striatal slices (Lovinger, 1991).

Modulation of glutamate-mediated synaptic potentials by D_2 dopamine receptors

Receptor binding studies have shown a decrease in striatal D_2 dopamine receptors after cortical ablation and subsequent degeneration of corticostriatal terminals (Garau et al., 1978; Schwarcz et al., 1978). Release-regulating D_2 dopamine receptors located on striatal glutamatergic nerve terminals have been demonstrated by in vitro release studies (Maura et al., 1988). Autoradiographic studies have

either reported the existence of presynaptic D_2 receptors (Filloux et al., 1988) or failed to observe the presence of striatal D_2 receptors on cortical afferents (Trugman et al., 1986; Joyce and Marshall, 1987). Although electrophysiological in vivo studies have also suggested a modulatory effect of dopamine on corticostriatal transmission (Brown and Arbuthnott, 1983; Mercuri et al., 1985), a pharmacological characterization of the mechanisms underlying this modulation was obtained by utilizing in vitro recordings. In previous studies, we have shown that in naive animals activation of D_1 dopamine receptors causes a reduction of membrane excitability by postsynaptic mechanisms, while activation of D_2 dopamine receptors does not induce significant electrophysiological effects. In contrast, in reserpinized animals activation of D_2 dopamine receptors by either bromocriptine or lisuride causes a dose-dependent reduction of synaptic potentials evoked by intrastriatal stimulation (Calabresi et al., 1988a,b). Recently, we have also studied the effects of activation of D_2 striatal dopamine receptors after chronic haloperidol treatment (Calabresi et al., 1992a). Haloperidol (2 mg/kg) was injected daily intraperitoneally for 30 days; after a 36 h treatment-free drug-washout period, the animals were sacrificed for the electrophysiological experiments. In slices obtained from haloperidol-treated rats, unlike naive animals, application of LY 151555 (0.1 – 10 μM) induced a potent inhibition of cortically evoked glutamatergic potentials. This effect was not coupled with changes of intrinsic membrane properties of the recorded cells and with alterations of the postsynaptic sensitivity to exogenously applied glutamate. For this reason we believe that the reduction of synaptic potentials was probably related to the activation of supersensitive D_2 dopamine receptors located on corticostriatal terminals and controlling the release of glutamate. In treated animals the glutamate-mediated synaptic potentials were not only reduced by LY 151777 (Fig. 6A), but also by dopamine (Fig. 6B) in the presence of SCH 23390, a D_1 receptor antagonist. Amphetamine, a dopamine releasing agent, was also able to decrease the EPSP amplitude in treated slices suggesting that

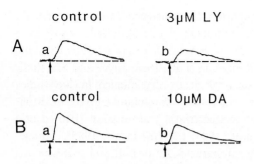

Fig. 6. Effect of LY 151777 and dopamine on glutamatergic potentials evoked by cortical stimulation after chronic neuroleptic treatment. *A*. A synaptic potential was recorded from a slice after chronic haloperidol treatment (see text) (a); 3 μM LY 151777 reduced the amplitude of this potential (b); *B*. A similar inhibitory action was caused by 10 μM dopamine.

supersensitive D_2 dopamine receptors located on cortical terminals can also be activated by endogenous dopamine. It is interesting to note that haloperidol treatment did not affect the reduction of synaptic potentials mediated by the activation of $GABA_B$ and muscarinic receptors. This finding suggests that this pharmacological treatment induces selective alterations of the dopaminergic receptors regulating the release of glutamate within the striatum. These alterations may modify the output signals from the striatum to the other structures of the basal ganglia and cause some of the motor dysfunctions observed in tardive dyskinesia (Casey, 1988).

Conclusions

Although medium spiny striatal neurons possess postsynaptic receptors for different transmitters, from electrophysiological experiments it is evident that most of these transmitters (acetylcholine, dopamine, GABA and glutamate itself) act to reduce the efficacy of corticostriatal glutamatergic transmission. This common modulatory action on the fast glutamatergic synaptic transmission seems to be justified by functional considerations. At rest, spiny neurons are silent and have very negative membrane potentials (Calabresi et al., 1987); in these cells glutamate is the main, if not the only, transmitter

that, at "physiological concentrations", is able to activate firing activity. The convergence of different transmitter systems on the mechanisms inhibiting the excitatory action of corticostriatal inputs is a reasonable manner to regulate the functional activity of the striatum. Furthermore, since an excess of excitatory amino acids in the striatum may cause neuronal death and produce neurochemical changes similar to those previously observed in some degenerative disorders (McGeer and McGeer, 1976), it is likely that the inhibitory action of different transmitters on the corticostriatal inputs may provide a crucial protection against the possible excitotoxicity caused by a massive glutamate release within the striatum.

Our data suggest that these different transmitters reduce glutamate-mediated synaptic potentials via a presynaptic mechanism, probably a decrease in neurotransmitter release. However, as we have previously suggested (Calabresi et al., 1992b), two alternative explanations must be considered: (1) glutamatergic synapses are electrotonically remote from the somatic recording site, consequently, changes in the postsynaptic neurons at the synaptic site occurred, but were not detected with intrasomatic recordings; and (2) activation of postsynaptic receptors may cause the production of metabolites which may leave the cell in which they are produced and act as messengers directed towards neighboring cells (Piomelli et al., 1987).

It has to be stressed that activation of several receptors subtypes ($GABA_B$, muscarinic and glutamate metabotropic receptors) reduces not only glutamate-mediated EPSPs, but also GABA-mediated synaptic potentials. The inhibitions of GABA release within the striatum seems to be in apparent contrast with the concomitant reduction of glutamatergic excitatory inputs. However, considering that in the striatum activation of $GABA_A$ receptors may induce a depolarizing driving force and even cause a short duration firing discharge, we believe that the concomitant inhibition of both glutamate and GABA-mediated synaptic potentials may strongly reduce the probability of striatal cells reaching the firing threshold.

Acknowledgements

This study was supported by CNR grants to P.C. (P.F. Fatma-Stress) and to G.B. (P.F. Chimice Fine).

References

Akaike, A., Sasa, M. and Takaori, S. (1988) Muscarinic inhibition as a dominant role in cholinergic regulation of transmission in the caudate nucleus. *J. Pharmacol. Exp. Ther.,* 246: 1129 – 1136.

Bernardi, G., Marciani, M.G., Morocutti, C. and Giacomini, P. (1976) The action of picrotoxin and bicuculline on rat caudate neurons inhibited by GABA. *Brain Res.,* 102: 379 – 384.

Bowery, N. (1989) GABA$_B$ receptors and their significance in mammalian pharmacology. *Trends Pharmacol. Sci.,* 10: 401 – 407.

Brown, J.R. and Arbuthnott, G.W. (1983) The electrophysiology of dopamine (D$_2$) receptors: a study of the action of dopamine on corticostriatal transmission. *Neuroscience,* 10: 349 – 355.

Buchwald, N.A., Price, D.D., Vernon, L. and Hull, C.D. (1973) Caudate intracellular response to thalamic and cortical inputs. *Exp. Neurol.,* 38: 311 – 323.

Calabresi, P., Misgeld, U. and Dodt, H.B. (1987) Intrinsic membrane properties of neostriatal neurons may account for their low level of spontaneous activity. *Neuroscience,* 20: 293 – 303.

Calabresi, P., Benedetti, M., Mercuri, N.B. and Bernardi, G. (1988a) Depletion of catecholamine reveals inhibitory effects of bromocriptine and lisuride on neostriatal neurons intracellularly recorded in vitro. *Neuropharmacology,* 27: 579 – 587.

Calabresi, P., Benedetti, M., Mercuri, N.B. and Bernardi, G. (1988b) Endogenous dopamine and dopaminergic agonists modulate synaptic excitation in neostriatum: intracellular studies from naive and catecholamine-depleted slices. *Neuroscience,* 27: 145 – 157.

Calabresi, P., Mercuri, N.B., De Murtas, M. and Bernardi, G. (1990a) Endogenous GABA mediates presynaptic inhibition of spontaneous and evoked excitatory synaptic potentials in the rat neostriatum. *Neurosci. Lett.,* 118: 99 – 102.

Calabresi, P., Mercuri, N.B., Stefani, A. and Bernardi, G. (1990b) Synaptic and intrinsic control of membrane excitability of neostriatal neurons. I. An in vivo analysis. *J. Neurophysiol.,* 63: 651 – 662.

Calabresi, P., Mercuri, N.B. and Bernardi, G. (1990c) Synaptic and intrinsic control of membrane excitability of neostriatal neurons. II. An in vitro analysis. *J. Neurophysiol.,* 63: 663 – 675.

Calabresi, P., De Murtas, M. and Bernardi, G. (1991a) Involvement of GABA systems in the feed-back regulation of glutamate and GABA-mediated synaptic potentials in rat neostriatum. *J. Physiol. (Lond.),* 440: 581 – 599.

Calabresi, P., Mercuri, N.B. and Bernardi, G. (1991b) Muscarinic modulation of synaptic and intrinsic membrane properties of striatal neurons. *Eur. J. Neurosci.,* S4: 116.

Calabresi, P., De Murtas, M., Mercuri, N.B. and Bernardi, G. (1992a) Chronic neuroleptic treatment: D$_2$ dopamine receptor supersensitivity and striatal glutamatergic transmission. *Ann. Neurol.,* 31: 366 – 373.

Calabresi, P., Mercuri, N.B. and Bernardi, G. (1992b) Activation of quisqualate metabotropic receptors reduces glutamate and GABA-mediated synaptic potentials in the rat striatum. *Neurosci. Lett.,* 139: 41 – 44.

Casey, D.E. (1988) Tardive dyskinesia. In: H.Y. Meltzer (Ed.), *Psychopharmacology, the Third Generation of Progress,* Raven Press, New York, pp. 1411 – 1419.

Charpak, S., Gahwiler, B.H., Do, K.O. and Knopfel, T. (1990) Potassium conductances in hippocampal neurones blocked by excitatory amino acids transmitters. *Nature,* 347: 765 – 767.

Dodt, H.U. and Misgeld, H.U. (1986) Muscarinic slow excitation and muscarinic inhibition of synaptic transmission in the rat neostriatum. *J. Physiol. (Lond.),* 380: 593 – 608.

Filloux, F., Liu, T.J., Hsu, C.Y., Hunt, M.A. and Wamsley, J.K. (1988) Selective cortical infarction reduces [³H] sulpiride binding in rat caudate-putamen: autoradiographic evidence for presynaptic D$_2$ receptors on corticostriate terminals. *Synapse,* 2: 521 – 531.

Garau, L., Govoni, S., Stefanini, E., Trabucchi, M. and Spano, P.F. (1978) Dopamine receptors: pharmacological and anatomical evidences indicated that two distinct populations are present in rat striatum. *Life Sci.,* 23: 1745 – 1750.

Groves, P.M. (1983) A theory of the functional organization of the neostriatum and the neostriatal control of voluntary movement. *Brain Res. Rev.,* 5: 109 – 132.

Herrling, P.L. (1984) Evidence for GABA as the transmitter for early cortically evoked inhibition of cat caudate neurons. *Exp. Brain Res.,* 55: 528 – 534.

Herrling, P.L. (1985) Pharmacology of the corticocaudate excitatory postsynaptic potential in the cat: evidence for its mediation by quisqualate or kainate receptors. *Neuroscience,* 14: 417 – 426.

Joyce, J.N. and Marshall, J.F. (1987) Quantitative autoradiography of dopamine D$_2$ sites in rat caudate-putamen: localization to intrinsic neurons and not to neocortical afferents. *Neuroscience,* 20: 773 – 795.

Kawaguchi, Y., Wilson, C.J. and Emson, P.C. (1989) Intracellular recording of identified neostriatal patch and matrix spiny cells in a slice preparation preserving cortical inputs. *J. Neurophysiol.,* 62: 1052 – 1068.

Kita, T., Kita, H. and Kitai, S.T. (1984) Passive electrical properties of rat neostriatal neurons in in vitro slice preparation. *Brain Res.,* 300: 129 – 139.

Kitai, S.T., Kocsis, J.D., Preston, R.J. and Sugimori, M. (1976) Monosynaptic inputs to caudate neurons identified by intracellular injection of horseradish peroxidase. *Brain Res.,* 109: 601 – 606.

Lovinger, D.M. (1991) Trans-1-aminocyclopentane-1,3-dicar-boxylix acid (t-ACPD) decreases synaptic excitation in rat stri-atal slices through a presynaptic action. *Neurosci. Lett.,* 129: 17–21.

Maura, G., Giardi, A. and Raiteri, M. (1988) Release-regulating D_2 dopamine receptors are located on striatal glutamatergic nerve terminals. *J. Pharmacol. Exp. Ther.,* 247: 680–684.

McGeer, E.G. and McGeer, P.L. (1976) Duplication of biochem-ical changes of Huntington's chorea by intrastriatal injections of glutamate and kainic acid. *Nature,* 263: 244–246.

Mercuri, N.B., Bernardi, G., Calabresi, P., Cotugno, A., Levi, G. and Stanzione, P. (1985) Dopamine decreases cell excitabil-ity in rat striatal neurons by pre- and postsynaptic mechan-isms. *Brain Res.,* 358: 110–121.

Mercuri, N.B., Calabresi, P., Stefani, A., Stratta, F. and Ber-nardi, G. (1991) GABA depolarizes neurons in the rat stria-tum. *Synapse,* 8: 38–40.

Misgeld, U., Wagner, A. and Ohno, T. (1982) Depolarizing IPSPs and depolarization by GABA of rat neostriatum cells in vitro. *Exp. Brain Res.,* 45: 108–114.

Misgeld, U., Calabresi, P. and Dodt, H.U. (1986) Muscarinic modulation in the striatum: possible involvement of calcium. *Exp. Brain Res.,* S14: 176–184.

Piomelli, D., Volterra, A., Dale, S., Siegelbaum, S.A., Kandel, E.R., Schwartz, J.H. and Belardetti, F. (1987) Lipoxygenase metabolites of arachidonic acid as second messengers for presynaptic inhibition of *Aplysia* sensory cells. *Nature,* 328: 38–43.

Reubi, J.C. and Cuenod, M. (1979) Glutamate release in vitro from corticostriatal terminals. *Brain Res.,* 176: 185–188.

Schwarcz, R., Creese, L., Coyle, J.T. and Snyder, S.H. (1978) Dopamine receptors localized on cerebral cortical afferents to rat corpus striatum. *Nature,* 271: 766–768.

Seabrook, G.R., Howson, W. and Lacey, M.G. (1990) Elec-trophysiological characterization of potent agonists and an-tagonists at pre- and post-synaptic $GABA_B$ receptors on neu-rones in rat brain slices. *Br. J. Pharmacol.,* 101: 949–957.

Sladeczek, F., Pin, J.P., Recasen, M., Bockaert, J. and Weiss, S. (1985) Glutamate stimulates inositol phosphate formation in striatal neurones. *Nature,* 317: 717–719.

Sugimori, M., Preston, R.I. and Kitai, S.T. (1978) Response properties and electrical constant of caudate neurons in the cat. *J. Neurophysiol.,* 41: 1662–1675.

Sugita, S., Uchimura, N., Jiang, Z.G. and North, R.A. (1991) Distinct muscarinic receptors inhibit release of GABA and ex-citatory amino acids in mammalian brain. *Proc. Natl. Acad. Sci. U.S.A.,* 88: 2608–2611.

Trugman, J.M., Geary, W.A. and Wooten, G.F. (1986) Locali-zation of D_2 dopamine receptors on intrinsic striatal neurons by quantitative autoradiography. *Nature,* 322: 267–269.

Wilson, C.J., Chang, H.T. and Kitai, S.T. (1983) Disfacilitation and long-lasting inhibition of neostriatal neurons in the rat. *Exp. Brain Res.,* 51: 227–235.

G.W. Arbuthnott and P.C. Emson (Eds.)
Progress in Brain Research, Vol. 99
© 1993 Elsevier Science Publishers B.V. All rights reserved.

CHAPTER 20

D₁ and D₂ dopamine receptor modulation of sodium and potassium currents in rat neostriatal neurons

D.J. Surmeier and S.T. Kitai

Department of Anatomy and Neurobiology, College of Medicine, University of Tennessee at Memphis, Memphis, TN 38163, U.S.A.

Introduction

The role of the dopaminergic nigrostriatal system in controlling the excitability of neostriatal neurons has been intensely studied since it became clear that the loss of this innervation was responsible for the psycho-motor symptoms of Parkinson's disease (Hornykiewcz, 1973). In years past, the actions of dopamine have been attributed to activation of two types of dopamine receptor. The application of molecular cloning techniques to characterizing these receptors has revealed that rather than two there are at least six dopamine receptors (D_1, D_{2s}, D_{2l}, D_3, D_4 and D_5) (Civelli et al., 1991). All share a similar structural motif that is characteristic of G protein-coupled catecholamine receptors. In situ hybridization and Northern blot analyses suggest that all six receptors are expressed in the neostriatum with the D_1 and D_2 subtypes being the predominant forms in the dorsal striatum (Bunzow et al., 1988; Meador-Woodruff et al., 1989,1991; Monsma et al., 1989, 1990; Dearry et al., 1990; Le Moine et al., 1990; Mansour et al., 1990; Sokoloff et al., 1990; Zhou et al., 1990; Sunahara et al., 1991; Tiberi et al., 1991; Weiner et al., 1991).

The existence of so many receptors has made understanding the actions of dopamine an even more daunting task than previously imagined, especially in light of our growing awareness of the biochemical heterogeneity of medium spiny neurons. Faced with this sort of complexity, simplifying hypotheses become particularly appealing. One such hypothesis that appears to make dopamine's actions in the striatum more tractable is that dopamine receptor subtypes are segregated in striatal projection neurons. There are two lines of study that support this hypothesis. First, Gerfen et al.'s (1990, 1992) work has shown that in 6-hydroxydopamine-lesioned or haloperidol-treated striatum, D_2-class agonists can selectively alter the levels of enkephalin mRNA in striatopallidal neurons whereas D_1-class agonists selectively alter the levels of substance P in striatonigral neurons. Second, both Gerfen and Le Moine et al., (1991) have reported that D_1 and D_2 receptor mRNAs are found only in striatonigral and striatopallidal neurons respectively (cf. Meador-Woodruff et al., 1991).

Although appealing, this model is difficult to reconcile with much of the biochemical, physiological and behavioral literature demonstrating interactions between D_1- and D_2-class receptors (i.e., receptors with a D_1 and D_2 pharmacological profile, respectively). For example, D_1- and D_2-class receptors are known to interact in the regulation of adenylate cyclase (Stoof and Kebabian, 1984), receptor affinity (Seeman et al., 1989) and Na/K ATPase (Bertorello et al., 1990). Both receptors also regulate proenkephalin mRNA abundance in striatopallidal neurons (Angulo, 1992) (in contrast to the situation in the 6-hydroxydopamine-lesioned striatum). Electrophysiological studies in vivo (Ohno et al., 1987; Hu and Wang, 1988) or in

310

slices (Akaike et al., 1987) have consistently found that both D_1 and D_2 agonists are capable of modulating the activity of individual neurons. At the behavioral level, D_1- and D_2-class receptors have long been known to synergistically control motor behavior (White et al., 1988; Robertson, 1992).

In spite of their combined weight, these studies do not provide unequivocal proof that dopamine receptors colocalize on striatal projection neurons. It is possible that the appearance of convergence is a consequence of the failure to separate direct post-synaptic effects from indirect effects mediated by adjacent neurons. A definitive separation of indirect and direct effects is virtually impossible in any preparation that preserves local tissue architecture or fails to isolate individual neurons. So, to directly attack the problem, we have studied acutely isolated striatal neurons in which there are no interactions with other neurons. In some of the work described below, we have retrogradely labeled striatonigral

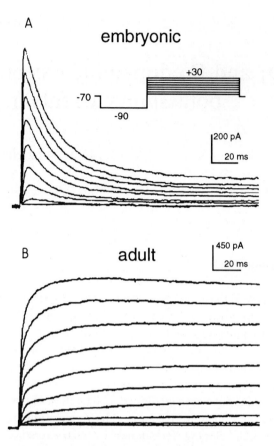

Fig. 2. Comparison of outward currents evoked by depolarizing voltage steps in cultured embryonic and acutely dissociated adult neostriatal neurons. *A*. Whole-cell currents evoked in an embryonic neuron following a conditioning step to -90 mV for 2 sec from the holding potential of -70 mV; the voltage protocol is shown in the inset. Note the rapid activation and inactivation time course. The cell was cultured from an E17 rat embryo and maintained in culture for 14 days. *B*. Whole-cell currents evoked in acutely dissociated adult neuron (P45) by the same voltage protocol used in *A*. Note that the currents peak much more slowly and exhibit little inactivation in the 200 msec pulse. Near threshold, the currents appear to have at least two kinetically distinct components.

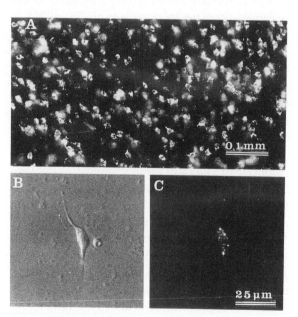

Fig. 1. *A*. Photomicrograph of a frontal section through the striatum of a retrogradely labeled rat viewed under epi-fluorescence. Note the numerous rhodamine labeled cell bodies. At the bottom: acutely isolated neurons from the striatum viewed under normal illumination (*B*) and under epi-fluorescence (*C*) showing a retrogradely labeled neuron.

neurons with rhodamine-impregnated microbeads to allow a single efferent population to be studied (Fig. 1). In these isolated neurons, we have used two approaches to determine the extent of receptor colocalization. First, whole-cell and cell-attached voltage-clamp were used to determine whether D_1 and D_2 agonists could modulate Na or K currents in individual neurons. Second, the RNA from individual neurons was amplified and used to probe Southern blots of dopamine receptor cDNA to provide a molecular characterization of the receptors mediating physiologically characterized responses.

D_1- and D_2-class dopamine receptors modulate potassium currents in isolated neostriatal neurons

In early postnatal (P1-7) and embryonic neostriatal neurons, the potassium currents activated by depolarizing commands are largely attributable to a rapidly inactivating A-current and a very slowly inactivating delayed rectifier (Fig. 2A). Dopamine (1 – 50 μM) does not appear to modulate these currents in spite of the fact that dopamine receptors are expressed in these neurons and they are coupled to second messenger systems (Weiss et al., 1985; Akins et al., 1990; Nishi et al., 1990). There are two possible explanations for this result: (1) either dopamine does not modulate potassium currents in neostriatal

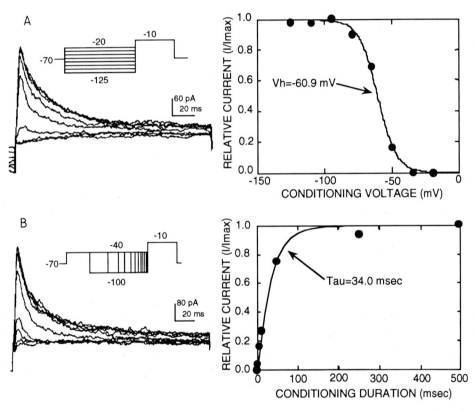

Fig. 3. The steady-state inactivation and inactivation recovery kinetics of potassium currents in embryonic neurons suggest that a single inactivating conductance is expressed. A. Steady-state inactivation was studied by holding the cell for 4 sec at potentials between − 125 and − 20 mV prior to delivery of a test pulse to − 10 mV. The currents evoked by this test pulse are shown at the left. At the right, the normalized (I'/I'_{max}) peak currents are plotted as a function of conditioning voltage, $I' = I - I\text{-}20$, where I-20 is the current measured at the time of the peak following a prepulse to − 20 mV. Although approximate, this procedure eliminated leak currents and most of the delayed rectifier currents from the measurements. The data were then fit with a Boltzmann function ($I'/I'_{max} = 1/(1 + \exp[(V - V_h)/V_c]$. In this case, $V_h = -60.9$ mV, $V_c = 6.9$ mV. B. The kinetics of recovery were studied by holding the cell at − 40 mV for 4 sec to inactivate all voltage-sensitive conductances and then stepping to − 100 mV for increasing periods of time to remove inactivation prior to the test pulse to − 10 mV. The currents evoked by the test pulse are shown at the left. At the right, the normalized peak currents (I'/I'_{max}) are plotted as a function of conditioning duration; $I' = I - I_o$, where I_o is the current evoked without a hyperpolarizing prepulse. The data points were fit with a recovery function ($I'/I'_{max} = 1 - \exp(-t/\tau)$), where t = conditioning duration and τ = 34.0 msec. The cell was cultured from a P1 rat and maintained in culture for 14 days.

neurons or (2) the current that is normally modulated is expressed later in development. The second explanation appears to be the correct one.

In neostriatal neurons acutely dissociated from older rats ($\geq$ 4 weeks postnatal), the whole-cell potassium currents activated by depolarizing steps are quite different from those seen in younger neurons (Surmeier et al., 1991). As shown in Fig. 2B, the outward currents evoked by a series of depolarizing commands from a holding potential of -90 mV appear to have multiple components and exhibit very little inactivation within the time frame of the 200 msec test pulse. Because these neurons had only short (10 – 50 μM) processes following acute isolation, these kinetic complexities were unlikely to have arisen from poor space-clamp. Experiments examining tail current reversals and the effects of C1 replacement (not shown) clearly suggested that these currents were carried primarily by potassium. With a few exceptions, recordings from neurons acutely dissociated from 1 – 2-week-old rats resembled those seen in cells cultured from embryos or early postnatal pups; recordings from 3 week-old rats were more heterogeneous. Because over 95% of the neurons in the neostriatum are medium spiny projection neurons, we assume that most of our acute recordings were from this class and that the changes in the whole-cell currents we observed reflect the maturation of this group.

Examination of the voltage dependence of steady-state inactivation and the kinetics of recovery from inactivation suggested that the difference between the immature and adult neurons was due to the presence in the adults of an additional conductance which exhibits steady-state inactivation at relatively hyperpolarized membrane potentials. In Fig. 3A (left), the currents evoked in an embryonic neuron by a test pulse to -10 mV following conditioning voltage steps are shown. In most juvenile neurons the only voltage-dependent potassium current exhibiting steady-state inactivation between -110 and -30 mV is the rapidly inactivating A-current. To the right of the current traces, the normalized peak currents are plotted as a function of conditioning voltage; these data were well-fit by a single Boltz-

mann function – suggesting that a single conductance was responsible for the transient current. The kinetics of recovery from inactivation also suggested that a single conductance was involved (Fig. 3B). In the recovery protocol, the cell was held at -40 mV for 4 sec and then subjected to hyperpolarizing conditioning pulses to -100 mV for increasing durations prior to the test pulse; the currents evoked by this test pulse are shown. A plot of the normalized peak current as a function of conditioning duration was well-fit with a single exponential having a time constant of 34 msec (Fig. 3B, right).

The inactivation properties of adult neurons suggested that another inactivating potassium conductance was expressed in addition to the A-current. In most adult neurons, the steady-state inactivation plots were significantly better fit with a sum of Boltzmann functions than with a single function. The whole-cell currents evoked in an exemplary cell by the test pulse in the steady-state inactivation protocol are shown in Fig. 4A. Note that as more depolarized conditioning pulses are given, the current becomes more rapidly inactivating, as if a more sustained component of the current was selectively inactivated. A plot of the normalized peak currents is shown to the right. The data fit well with a sum of Boltzmann's having half-inactivation voltages (V_h) of about -100 and -55 mV (each function is shown in the figure at the appropriate scale; the inset shows the two fitted functions on a normalized scale). The distribution of V_hs for the population of adult neurons was bimodal, with one mode near -95 mV, the other near -60 mV. The more depolarized mode very closely matches that of the embryonic A-current in similar recording conditions (Fig. 4A). The delayed rectifier currents in the adults do not appear to have contributed to the inactivation as they do not inactivate at potentials negative to their activation threshold and above this level they inactivate with a time constant of tens of seconds (not shown).

The kinetics of inactivation recovery also suggested that a third, slowly recovering current was expressed in adults. With short hyperpolarizing

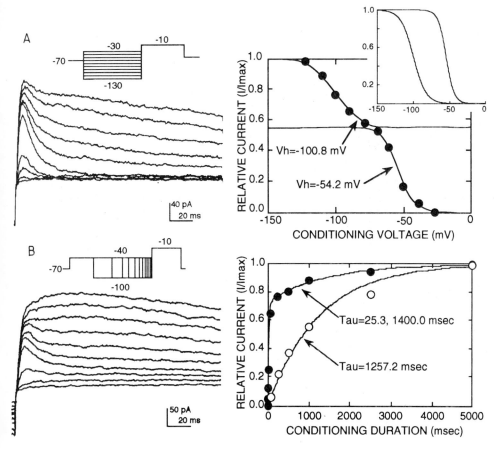

Fig. 4. The steady-state inactivation and inactivation recovery kinetics of potassium currents in adult neurons suggest that at least two inactivating conductances were expressed. *A*. Steady-state inactivation was studied as in Fig. 2; conditioning pulses were from -130 to -30 mV. The currents evoked by the test pulse (to -10 mV) are shown at the left. At the right, the normalized (I'/I'_{max}) peak currents are plotted as a function of conditioning voltage, $I' = I - I\text{-}30$; this gave a reasonable isolation of the inactivating currents. The data were well-fit only with a sum of Boltzmann functions (each function is plotted as a solid line) $(I'/I'_{max} = \beta(1/(1 + \exp((V - V_{h1})/V_{c1})) + (1 - \beta)(1/(1 + \exp((V - V_{h2})/V_{c2}));\beta = 0.452, V_{h1} = -100.8$ mV, $V_{c1} = 18.5$ mV, $V_{h2} = -54.2$ mV, $V_{c2} = 5.6$ mV. Inset shows the two Boltzmann functions on the same scale to allow easier comparison of their differences. *B*. The kinetics of recovery were studied as in Fig. 2. The currents evoked by the test pulse are shown at the left. At the right, the normalized peak currents (I'/I'_{max}) (closed circles) and currents at the end of the test pulse (open circles) are plotted as a function of conditioning duration. The peak data were well-fit only with a sum of recovery functions $(I'/I'_{max} = \beta(1 - \exp(-t/\tau_1) + (1 - \beta)(1 - \exp(-t/\tau_2)$, where t = conditioning duration, $\beta = 0.73$, $\tau_1 = 25.3$ msec, $\tau_2 = 1400.0$ msec; the sustained currents were fit with at single exponential with $\tau = 1257.2$ msec. The cell was dissociated from the neostriatum of a P28 rat.

prepulses, the current evoked by the test pulse was rapidly inactivating, resembling the A-current seen in younger neurons. With longer conditioning pulses, the evoked current becomes slowly inactivating. A plot of the normalized peak current as a function of conditioning duration is shown at the right (open circles). This recovery function was well-fit only with a sum of exponentials having time constants of about 25 and 1400 msec. The faster time constant was well within the range seen for embryonic A-current at this conditioning voltage. At the end of the test pulse where the A-current should have been nearly completely inactivated, the currents recovered mono-exponentially with a time

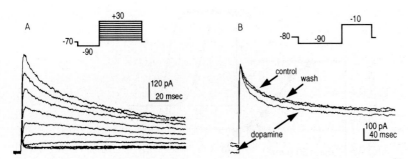

Fig. 5. Dopamine reduces a slowly inactivating component of whole-cell potassium current. *A*. Whole-cell potassium currents evoked in response to depolarizing voltage steps following a prepulse to − 100 mV. A schematic protocol is shown as an inset. *B*. The application of dopamine (25 µM) produced a reversible decrease in the slowly inactivating component of the current without affecting the peak current. Note also that the holding current at − 90 mV was altered by dopamine. This cell was dissociated from a P35 rat.

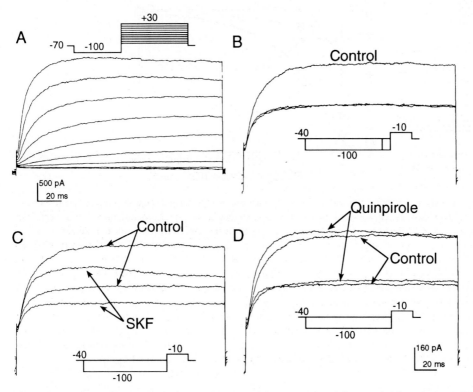

Fig. 6. D₁ agonists reduce a slowly inactivating potassium current in adult neostriatal neurons. *A*. Whole-cell potassium currents evoked in response to depolarizing voltage steps following a prepulse to − 100 mV. A schematic protocol is shown as an inset. *B*. Currents evoked in response to a standard inactivation recovery paradigm. Currents were evoked by a step to − 10 mV following a long prepulse (4 sec) to − 40 mV, a short prepulse to − 100 mV (50 msec) or a long prepulse to − 100 mV (2 sec). Note that there was no evidence for an A_f current in this cell, as it would have been apparent following the short hyperpolarizing step (cf. Fig. 4). *C*. SKF 38393 (5 µM) produced a profound reduction in the recovering current and that component of the current evoked following the prepulse to − 40 mV. Note the difference in kinetics of the currents evoked without a hyperpolarizing prepulse before and after SKF 38393. *D*. Quinpirole (5 µM) produced a moderate enhancement of the recovering current in this cell. This cell was dissociated from a P32 rat.

constant near that of the slower component of the peak currents. Although the kinetics of the slower current varied considerably, a similar slow component was found in nearly all adult neurons (32/35). If the bi-exponential recovery kinetics were due to two inactivated states of a single channel type, then the recovery time course should not have differed early and late in the test pulse – as observed. This suggests that two channel types contributed to the inactivating current in the adult currents.

In addition to voltage dependence and kinetics, the rapidly and slowly inactivating A-currents (A_f and A_s) seen in adults appear to differ in their sensitivity to 4-aminopyridine (4-AP) and dendrotoxin (DTX) (data not shown). Preliminary experiments suggest that the 4-AP K_i of A_s is at least an order of magnitude lower than that of A_f, being $150 - 250\ \mu M$ as opposed to $2 - 5$ mM (the K_i of the delayed rectifier is near 50 mM). Other experiments have shown that A_s is reduced by nanomolar concentrations of DTX, whereas A_f is unaffected by DTX in this concentration range. These results argue that A_f and A_s currents in the adult did not arise from a single population of channels with multiple gating modes.

In adult neurons possessing A_s, the application of dopamine reduces potassium currents activated by depolarization. In Fig. 5A, the whole-cell potassium currents activated by a series of depolarizing voltage steps are shown. Note that there are both

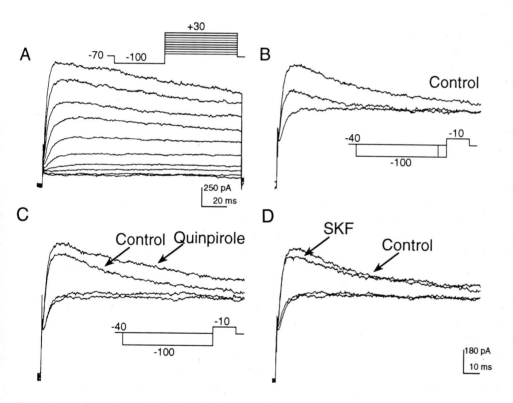

Fig. 7. D_2 agonists enhance a slowly inactivating potassium current in adult neostriatal neurons. A. Whole-cell potassium currents evoked in response to depolarizing voltage steps following a prepulse to -100 mV. A schematic protocol is shown as an inset. B. Currents evoked in response to a standard inactivation recovery paradigm. Currents were evoked by a step to -10 mV following a long prepulse (4 sec) to -40 mV, a short prepulse to -100 mV (50 msec) or a long prepulse to -100 mV (2 sec). Note that there was an A_f current in this cell. C. Quinpirole (5 μM) produced a clear enhancement of the recovering current in this cell. D. SKF 38393 (5 μM) produced a reduction in the recovering current without affecting that component of the current evoked following the prepulse to -40 mV. This cell was dissociated from a P28 rat.

rapidly and slowly inactivating components of the current, particularly at potentials above around -20 mV. In Fig. 5B, the effects of dopamine (25 μM) on the currents evoked by a step to -10 mV are shown. Dopamine reversibly decreased the more slowly inactivating part of the current but did not significantly affect the rapidly inactivating component, as the peak current was relatively unchanged by drug treatment.

The identification of the dopamine-modulated current was performed using an inactivation recovery protocol similar to those described above. In Fig. 6A, the whole-cell potassium currents evoked by depolarizing voltage steps are shown. There was little evidence of an A_f current in these traces. The currents evoked in an inactivation recovery protocol (shown in Fig. 6B) confirmed the absence of an A_f current and the presence of a prominent A_s current as only the long hyperpolarizing prepulse led to an augmentation in the current evoked by the step to -10 mV. The application of the specific D_1 agonist SKF 38393 (5 μM) reduced the recovering current and that residual portion of the A_s current not inactivated by the depolarizing test pulse. A similar pattern was seen in most of the cells examined (21/35).

In contrast, the application of the D_2 agonist quinpirole (5 μM) enhanced the slowly recovering A_s current. This is shown in Fig. 6D. The presence of complimentary D_1 and D_2 agonist responses in the same neuron suggests that receptors with a D_1 pharmacological profile and those with a D_2 profile colocalize. Similar responses to D_2 agonists were seen in about one third of the sampled population (11/35). In Fig. 7, the data from another cell exhibiting this same pattern of modulation is shown. The biophysical basis of the modulation of the D_2 agonists as well as the D_1 agonists remains to be fully worked out.

The role of the A_s current and dopaminergic modulation in regulating discharge behavior in medium spiny neurons is currently being explored. Tentatively, it appears that as in the case of acetylcholine (Akins et al., 1990b) the effects of the dopaminergic modulation should depend upon the membrane potential range in which the neuron is operating. If a medium spiny neuron is in the "down" state with a mean membrane potential near -80 mV, then a considerable fraction of the A_s current will be available. In this state, dopamine, acting through D_1 receptors, should decrease the strength of this current and facilitate the transition to the "up" state in response to depolarizing cortical inputs (see chapter by Wilson). In this way, dopamine, acting at D_1 receptors, can be viewed as destabilizing the down state making discharge more likely, in contrast to the apparent state stabilizing actions of acetylcholine (Akins et al., 1990b) and dopamine acting at the D_2 receptor.

D_1- and D_2-class receptors modulate sodium currents in striatonigral neurons

Sodium (Na) currents in neostriatal neurons play an important role in sub-threshold integration and spike generation (Kita et al., 1985; Calabresi et al., 1987). These currents are carried by a single class of channel with a high affinity for tetrodotoxin ($K_i = 8.5$ nM $\pm$ 4.2) and biophysical properties very similar to those described in other brain neurons (Gahwiler and Llano et al.,1988; Huguenard et al., 1988; Sah et al., 1988; Ogata and Tatebayashi, 1990). As described for monoamines in other tissues (Marchetti et al., 1986; Schubert et al., 1989), the application of dopamine ($10-50$ μM) produces a reversible decrease in the amplitude of Na currents evoked by depolarizing voltage steps. We examined this modulation in retrogradely labeled striatonigral neurons to determine the contribution of D_1- and D_2-class receptors to this modulation (Surmeier et al., 1992).

A large percentage (81%, 25/31) of the neurons tested responded to the specific D_1 agonist SKF 38393. In most of these cells (80%, 20/25), SKF 38393 ($1-5$ μM) reduced the amplitude of the evoked Na current (Fig. 8A). The modulation by SKF 38393 appeared to be mediated by D_1 receptors as it was blocked by the specific D_1 antagonist SCH 23390 (1 μM) (Fig. 7A; $n = 4$) and unaffected by the D_2 receptor antagonist $(-)$ sulpiride (5 μM) ($n = 6$). Bath application of 8-bromo-cAMP

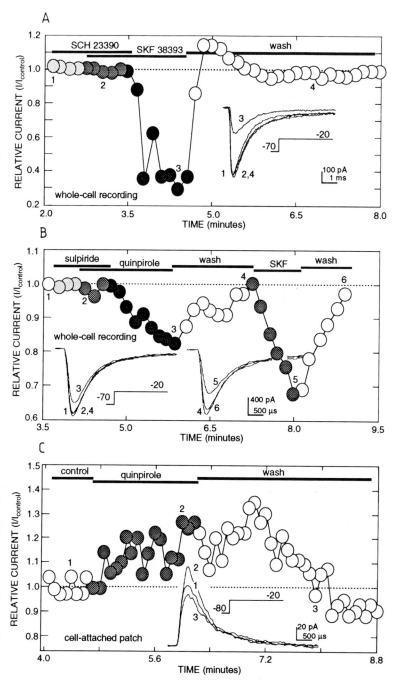

Fig. 8. Both the D_2 agonist quinpirole and the D_1 agonist SKF 38393 modulated the amplitude of evoked Na currents. *A.* The relative current amplitude evoked by a step to -20 mV from a holding potential of -70 mV is plotted as a function of time after initiating whole-cell recording. Inset shows the current traces from relevant points in the record, labeled $1-4$. The records show that the reduction in current produced by the specific D_1 agonist SKF 38393 (1 μM) is blocked by the D_1 receptor antagonist SCH 23390 (1 μM). *B.* Quinpirole (100 nM) produced a similar reduction that was antagonized by the D_2 receptor antagonist ($-$) sulpiride (1 μM). After recovery, the specific D_1 agonist SKF 38393 (1 μM) was applied. *C.* In cell-attached patch recordings, the D_2 agonist quinpirole (1 μM) enhanced Na currents evoked by a step to -20 mV from a holding potential of -80 mV.

318

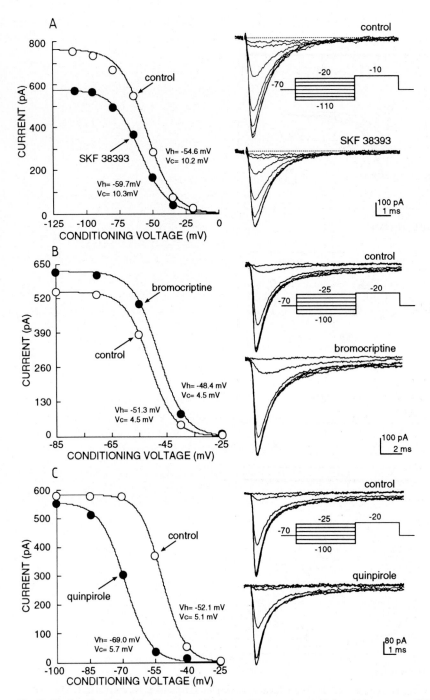

Fig. 9. The biophysical mechanisms by which D_1 and D_2 agonists modulated Na currents differed, suggesting at least three signaling pathways. *A*. SKF 38393 produced a reduction in peak current and a negative shift in the voltage dependence of steady-state inactivation. On the right, the currents evoked by a step to −10 mV in a standard inactivation protocol (shown in inset) are shown; at the top, the currents evoked under control conditions and, at the bottom, currents evoked in the presence of 1 μM SKF 38393. At the left, the peak currents are plotted as a function of prepulse potential; under both conditions, the data were well-fit with a Boltzmann function. Under control conditions (open circles): I_{max} = 764 pA, V_h = − 54.6 mV, V_c = 10.2 mV; in the presence of SKF 38393 (closed cir-

(1 mM) partially mimicked this effect ($n = 2$), suggesting that the modulation was mediated by D_1 receptors that were positively coupled to adenylate cyclase.

In 55% (23/42) of the neurons tested in whole-cell recordings, the application of D_2 agonists quinpirole ($n = 31$) or bromocriptine ($n = 11$) produced a time-locked decrease in evoked current amplitude (Fig. 8B). The decrease was not a consequence of the enhancement of an outward current as the application of the specific Na channel blocker tetrodotoxin eliminated the evoked current and the change produced by quinpirole ($n = 5$). As shown in Fig. 8B, the response to quinpirole (100 nM) was blocked by the D_2 receptor antagonist ($-$) sulpiride (1 μM, $n = 5$) suggesting that the modulation was mediated by D_2-like receptors.

In about 20% (8/42) of our whole-cell recordings, the application of D_2 agonists increased the amplitude of the current evoked from -70 mV. ($-$) Sulpiride antagonized this response, suggesting that it also was mediated by a D_2-like receptor ($n = 4$). Similar responses to D_2 agonists were observed in more than half (6/10) of cell-attached patch recordings with bath-applied agonists, as shown in Fig. 8C. D_2 agonists never decreased the evoked current in cell-attached patches. The D_1 agonist SKF 38393, on the other hand, decreased the evoked current in most patches (4/5), as in whole-cell recordings. In the cell-attached recording configuration, bath-applied agonists do not interact with the membrane containing the channels being modulated. As a consequence, the modulatory responses seen in this configuration must be dependent upon soluble second messengers produced by activation of receptors *outside* of the recorded patch. These experiments suggest that D_1 and D_2-like receptors can reciprocally

modulate Na currents through a soluble second messenger (presumably cAMP) in many striatonigral neurons. These results also suggest that the reduction in Na current produced by D_2 agonists is mediated by a membrane-delimited pathway, as it was not seen in cell-attached patches.

An examination of the biophysical mechanisms underlying the changes in evoked current revealed three patterns of modulation. The D_1 agonist SKF 38393 reduced the maximal Na current and shifted its steady-state inactivation voltage dependence toward more negative potentials, without changing the voltage dependence of activation. An example of these changes is shown in Fig. 9A; in ten cells, peak current was reduced an average of 22% and the half-inactivation voltage shifted an average of -5.6 mV. This modulation is similar to that produced by cAMP-dependent kinase phosphorylation of Na channels (Li et al., 1992). When D_2 agonists increased Na current, the biophysical changes were complementary to those of D_1 agonists. In the example of Fig. 9B, bromocriptine (500 nM) shifted inactivation voltage dependence toward more depolarized values and increased the maximal current. In four cells, the half-inactivation voltage shifted an average of 3.2 mV and the peak current increased an average of 19%. In contrast, the membrane-delimited modulation produced by D_2 agonists did not change peak current but did shift steady-state inactivation toward more negative potentials (Fig. 9C). In eight neurons where quinpirole (100–500 nM) reduced current amplitudes, the mean half-inactivation voltage shifted an average of -5.1 mV. The maximal current in these cells was not altered significantly nor was the voltage dependence of activation. The modulation produced by quinpirole was not seen in neurons cultured from

cles): $I_{max} = 576$ pA, $V_h = -59.7$ mV, $V_c = 10.3$ mV. The dotted line is the zero current level. *B*. Bromocriptine (500 nM) produced a positive shift in the voltage dependence of steady-state inactivation and increased the maximal current. Plots are as above. In control records: $I_{max} = 547.2$ pA, $V_h = -51.3$ mV, $V_c = 4.5$ mV; in bromocriptine records: $I_{max} = 612.4$ pA, $V_h = -48.4$ mV, $V_c = 4.5$ mV. *C*. Quinpirole (100 nM) produced a negative shift in steady-state inactivation voltage dependence without reducing peak current. Plots are as in *A*. Under control conditions (open circles): $I_{max} = 578$ pA, $V_h = -52.1$ mV, $V_c = 5.1$ mV; in the presence of quinpirole (closed circles): $I_{max} = 558$ pA, $V_h = -69.0$ mV, $V_c = 5.7$ mV. The voltage dependence of activation did not appear to be altered by SKF 38393, quinpirole or bromocriptine.

the embryonic striatum ($n = 8$; data not shown) suggesting that its mechanism of action differed from that reported for neuroleptics (Ogata and Tatebayashi, 1989).

These findings are not only contrary to a strict segregation of dopamine receptors but suggest that many striatonigral neurons co-express *two* D_2-like receptors, in addition to a D_1-like receptor. However, at present, the pharmacological tools necessary to differentiate D_2, D_3 and D_4 receptors are not available. As a consequence, we turned to a recently developed technique for amplifying the mRNA of single cells to characterize the receptors (Van Gelder et al., 1990; Eberwine et al., 1992). The top of Fig. 10A shows an ethidium bromide-stained gel containing cDNAs that were transferred to nitrocellulose for probing with radiolabeled antisense RNA (aRNA) from a single striatonigral neuron. The dopamine receptor cDNAs were constructed from the mRNA sequences coding for non-homologous regions of the third cytoplasmic domain of the receptors. At the bottom of Fig. 10A is shown the autoradiogram resulting from aRNA hybridization to the Southern blot. Positive hybridization to cDNAs for D_1, D_2 and D_3 dopamine receptors, the $GABA_A$ receptor and the sodium channel are apparent; longer development times also revealed hybridization to the neurofilament cDNA. All five of the striatonigral neurons subjected to aRNA amplification had detectable levels of D_1, D_2 and D_3 receptor mRNA. These receptor signals did not result from amplification of genomic DNA because aRNA populations did not hybridize to known middle repetitive sequences and hybridization intensity was not uniform. Other experiments ($n = 2$) have shown that retrogradely labeled cells possess mRNA for substance P but not enkephalin, in agreement with their identification as striatonigral neurons (Brownstein et al., 1977; Hong et al., 1977; Finley et al., 1981).

To further test the specificity of the dopamine receptor hybridization, regions of aRNA molecules coding for the third cytoplasmic domain of each receptor were amplified with the polymerase chain reaction (PCR) and subjected to size analysis. This

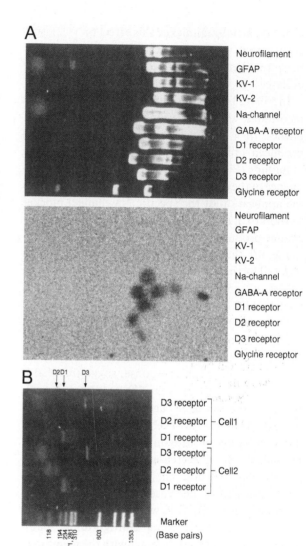

Fig. 10. Expression profiles and specific PCR of D_1, D_2 and D_3 dopamine receptors from single striatonigral neurons. *A*. The upper portion of this figure shows the ethidium bromide-stained agarose gel containing cDNAs for neurofilament, GFAP, potassium channels (KV-1, KV-2), sodium channel, $GABA_A$ receptor, D_1, D_2 and D_3 dopamine receptors and the glycine receptor. The lower portion of this figure shows the autoradiogram resulting from probing the Southern blot of the gel shown at the top with radiolabeled aRNA from a single neuron. *B*. An agarose gel containing the PCR amplified cDNAs for the D_1, D_2 and D_3 dopamine receptors from two neurons (Cell 1 and Cell 2). The marker lane contains ΦX174 DNA digested with *Hae III*, the size in base pairs of each band is as indicated. Arrows at the top of the gel show the approximate positions expected for the D_1, D_2 and D_3 receptor DNAs.

was accomplished by converting the aRNA into cDNA (using random primers to prime reverse transcription) (Eberwine et al., 1992) and then performing PCR using oligonucleotide primers that were specific for regions of the third cytoplasmic loop of the distinct receptor subtypes. For D_1 receptor aRNA, this should yield a cDNA of 203 base pairs; D_2 and D_3 receptor aRNAs should yield cDNAs of 170 and 400 base pairs respectively. In Fig. 10B, the ethidium bromide-stained gel of PCR-amplified cDNA made from the aRNA of two striatonigral neurons is shown. In cell 1, cDNA of the predicted sizes for D_1, D_2 and D_3 receptor mRNA was evident. In cell 2, cDNA of the predicted sizes was seen plainly for D_1 and D_3 receptors while that for the D_2 receptor was faint. As the D_2 PCR cDNA was from a region of the D_2 mRNA transcript that is normally spliced, the absence of an unspliced product in either cell provides further evidence that genomic DNA was not amplified. These experiments establish the specificity of the aRNA hybridization and the supposition that mRNA was amplified, not genomic DNA fragments.

Based upon our findings, it is difficult not to conclude that many striatonigral neurons express D_1, D_2 and D_3 dopamine receptors and that activation of these receptors produces functionally significant alterations in Na currents and excitability. An accurate estimate of the extent of receptor colocalization must await further work, but both physiological and molecular approaches indicate that well over half of the striatonigral population express all three receptors. It is plausible that in situ receptor hybridization experiments have failed to detect D_2 mRNA in striatonigral neurons (Gerfen et al., 1990; Le Moine et al., 1991) because it is present at levels below the technique's detection threshold; a similar situation may exist for the D_3 receptor (Sokoloff et al., 1991). Others, however, have reported considerable overlap suing these techniques (Meador-Woodruff et al., 1991). The functional significance of quantitative differences in receptor mRNA levels is difficult to know a priori because of the uncertain relationship between mRNA and receptor protein. This uncertainty can also be extended to the relationship between receptor protein and channel modulation because of the signal amplification afforded G protein-linked receptors, like the dopamine receptors (Gilman, 1987; Civelli et al., 1991).

The colocalization of both D_2 and D_3 receptors with D_1 receptors in a significant fraction of neostriatal neurons helps to explain the perplexing ability of D_1- and D_2-class agonists to act either synergistically or antagonistically. This duality has been seen in both biochemical and physiological studies. For example, it is well-established that D_2 agonists can reduce the elevation in cAMP levels produced by D_1 agonist activation of adenylate cyclase (Stoof and Kebabian, 1984). On the other hand, Greengard's group has shown that in isolated neostriatal neurons, D_1 and D_2 agonists can act synergistically to suppress Na/K ATPase activity (Bertorello et al., 1990).

Physiological studies using dopamine have revealed complex response patterns of excitation and inhibition of evoked activity (Bernardi et al., 1978; Herrling and Hull, 1980) that were attributed to indirect effects or co-activation of D_1 and D_2 receptors. However, the use of receptor-selective agonists has clarified the picture only for the D_1 receptor-mediated modulation where a reduction in evoked discharge has consistently been reported (Uchimura et al., 1986; Akaike et al., 1987; Calabresi et al., 1987; Hu and Wang, 1988). Calabresi et al. (1987) attributed this effect to a reduction of Na current, as we have confirmed. D_2 agonists, on the other hand, have been reported to either enhance evoked discharge (Akaike et al., 1987; Ohno et al., 1987) or to reduce activity (Hu et al., 1990). In part, the variation in responses to D_2 agonists may be attributable to differences in the nominal "holding potential". At hyperpolarized potentials (ca. -80 mV, as typically found in "good" slice recordings, the leftward shift in the steady-state inactivation of Na current will not be apparent; this modulation would only be evident if the cell was allowed to move to the "upstate" near -55 mV. Because D_1 agonists also reduce the peak conductance, the alteration in spike threshold produced by these agonists should not be dependent upon the recent potential history of the cell (Calabresi et al., 1987; Akaike et al., 1987). This could also explain why studies using extracellular recording techniques (e.g., Hu et al., 1990) in which the membrane potential is not controlled so readily find that D_2 agonists are inhibitory – the most common finding in the whole-cell recordings shown here.

Can any inferences be drawn about the D_2 receptor subtypes responsible for the membrane-delimited and soluble-signal modulations? First, while the D_2 receptor has been shown to inhibit cAMP accumulation (Civelli et al., 1991), the D_3 receptor appears not to couple to any known soluble second messenger system (D. Piomelli, personal communication). Also, the cooperative reduction in activity by D_1 and D_2 agonists is most commonly observed in the ventral striatum/nucleus accumbens (White and Wang, 1986), where the apparent density of D_3 receptors is highest (Sokoloff et al., 1990). This distribution can readily be reconciled with our results if one assumes that the membrane-delimited reduction in Na current produced by D_2 agonists was mediated by D_3 receptors and the non-membrane-delimited enhancement was mediated by D_2 receptors.

From a functional standpoint, being able to correlate these modulations with particular receptor subtypes buys us little. All of the receptors are activated by dopamine, albeit with somewhat different affinities. A key to understanding the interaction between these signaling pathways must lie in their spatial distribution. It makes little sense to have the receptors mediating opposing modulations within the same patch of membrane. What is more plausible is the existence of the receptor for the membrane-delimited D_2 pathway, which presumably would be relatively fast and spatially restricted in scope, and the D_1 receptor in the same patch of membrane. Both pathways would work together in suppressing Na current and reducing excitability. The fact that these were the most common modulations seen in neurons that were largely dendrite-less suggests that these two pathways (D_1 and D_3) may be preferentially located somatically and the D_2 receptor dendritically. This might also explain the difficulty in seeing D_2 mRNA with in situ techniques which are essentially limited to somatic mRNA. The use of receptor-selective fluorescent ligands (Ariano et al., 1989) to visualize receptors on intact neurons may allow this question to be settled.

Summary

The potassium and sodium currents in acutely isolated neostriatal neurons are modulated by activation of both D_1- and D_2-class receptors. The amplification of mRNA in individual neurons supports this conclusion and has shown that striatonigral neurons express not only D_1 and D_2 receptors, but D_3 receptors as well. The characteristics of the modulations produced by these receptors provide a foundation for both antagonistic and synergistic actions of D_1 and D_2 agonists in the neostriatum. Understanding precisely how these modulations interact in shaping excitability, however, will require a better characterization of spatial domains in which they operate.

Acknowledgements

This work was supported by N.I.H. grants NS 28889 to D.J.S., NS 20702 to S.T.K., N.I.A. grant AG 9900 to J.E. and O.N.R. grant N00014-92-J-1113 to C.J.W and D.J.S. We wish to thank Dr. Robert Foehring for comments on the manuscript; Angela Howe for her help in many of the experiments; and the following people for providing cDNA clones for use in this study: Drs. Ron Liem, William Catteral, Len Kaczmarek, Dolan Pritchett, Perry Molinoff and Neurogen Corp. We also thank Dr. Roman Artymyshan for providing the D_1 and D_2 receptor oligonucleotides used in the PCR.

References

Akaike, A., Ohno, Y., Sasa, M. and Takaori, S. (1987) Excitatory and inhibitory effects of dopamine on neuronal activity of the caudate neurons in vitro. *Brain Res.,* 418: 262 – 272.

Akins, P.T., Surmeier, D.J. and Kitai, S.T. (1990a) The M_1 muscarinic acetylcholine receptor in cultured rat neostriatum regulates phosphoinositide hydrolysis. *J. Neurochem.,* 54: 266 – 273.

Akins, P.T., Surmeier, D.J. and Kitai, S.T. (1990b) Muscarinic modulation of the transient potassium current in rat neostriatal neurons. *Nature,* 344: 240–242.

Angulo, J.A. (1992) Involvement of dopamine D_1 and D_2 receptors in the regulation of proenkephalin mRNA abundance in the striatum and accumbens of the rat brain. *J. Neurochem.,* 58: 1104–1109.

Ariano, M.A., Monsma, F.J., Barton, A.C., Kang, H.C., Haugland, R.P. and Sibley, D.R. (1989) Direct visualization and cellular localization of D_1 and D_2 dopamine receptors in rat forebrain by use of fluorescent ligands. *Proc. Natl. Acad. Sci. U.S.A.,* 86: 8570–8574.

Bernardi, G., Marciani, M.G., Morocutti, C., Pavone, F. and Stanzione, P. (1978) The action of dopamine on rat caudate neurones intracellularly recorded. *Neurosci. Lett.,* 8: 235–240.

Bertorello, A.M., Hopfield, J.F., Aperia, A. and Greengard, P. (1990) Inhibition by dopamine of (Na-K) ATPase activity in neostriatal neurons through D_1 and D_2 dopamine receptor synergism. *Nature,* 347: 386–388.

Brownstein, M.J., Mroz, M.J., Mroz, E.A., Tappaz, M.L. and Leeman, S.E. (1977) On the origin of substance P and glutamic decarboxylase (GAD) in the substantia nigra. *Brain Res.,* 135: 315–323.

Bunzow, J.R., Van Tol, H.H.M., Grandy, D.K., Albert, P., Salon, J., Christie, M., Machida, C.A., Neve, K.A. and Civelli, O. (1988) Cloning and expression of a rat D_2 dopamine receptor cDNA. *Nature,* 336: 783–787.

Calabresi, P., Mercuri, N., Stanzione, P., Stefani, A. and Bernardi, G. (1987a) Intracellular studies on the dopamine-induced firing inhibition of neostriatal neurons in vitro: evidence for D_1 receptor involvement. *Neuroscience,* 20: 757–771.

Calabresi, P., Misgeld, U. and Dodt, H.U. (1987b) Intrinsic membrane properties of neostriatal neurons can account for their low level of spontaneous activity. *Neuroscience,* 20: 293–303.

Civelli, O., Bunzow, J.R., Grandy, D.K., Zhou, Q.-Y. and Van Tol, H.H.M. (1991) Molecular biology of the dopamine receptor. *Eur. J. Pharmacol.,* 207: 277–286.

Dearry, A., Gingrich, J.A., Falardeau, P., Fremeau Jr., R.T., Bates, M.D. and Caron, M.G. (1990) Molecular cloning and expression of the gene for a human D_1 dopamine receptor. *Nature,* 347: 72–76.

Eberwine, J., Yeh, H., Miyashiro, K., Cao, Y., Nair, S., Finnell, R., Zettel, M. and Coleman, P. (1992) Analysis of gene expression in single live neurons. *Proc. Natl. Acad. Sci. U.S.A.,* 89: 3010–3014.

Finley, J.C.W., Maderdut, J.L. and Petrusz, P. (1981) The immunocytochemical localization of enkephalin in the central nervous system. *J. Comp. Neurol.,* 198: 541–565.

Gähwiler, B.H. and Llano, I. (1989) Sodium and potassium conductances in somatic membranes of rat Purkinje cells from organotypic cerebellar cultures. *J. Physiol. (Lond.),* 417:

105–122.

Gerfen, C.R. (1992) The neostriatal mosaic: multiple levels of compartmental organization. *Trends Neurosci.,* 15: 133–139.

Gerfen, C.R., Engber, T.M., Mahan, L.C., Susel, Z., Chase, T.N., Monsma, F.J. and Sibley, D.R. (1990) D_1 and D_2 dopamine receptor-regulated gene expression of striatonigral and striatopallidal neurons. *Science,* 250: 1429–1432.

Gerfen, C.R., McGinty, J.F. and Young, W.S. (1991) Dopamine differentially regulates dynorphin, substance P, and enkephalin expression in striatal neurons: in situ hybridization histochemical analysis. *J. Neurosci.,* 11: 1016–1031.

Gilman, A.G. (1987) G proteins: transducers of receptor-generated signals. *Annu. Rev. Biochem.,* 56: 615–649.

Herrling, P.L. and Hull, C.D. (1980) Iontophoretically applied dopamine depolarizes and hyperpolarizes the membrane of cat caudate neurons. *Brain Res.,* 192: 441–462.

Hong, J.S., Yang, H.Y., Racagni, G. and Costa, E. (1977) Projections of substance P containing neurons from neostriatum to substantia nigra. *Brain Res.,* 122: 541–544.

Hornykiewcz, O. (1973) Dopamine in the basal ganglia. Its role and therapeutic implications. *Br. Med. Bull.,* 29: 172–178.

Hu, X.-Y. and Wang, R.Y. (1988) Comparison of effects of D_1 and D_2 dopamine receptor agonists on neurons in the rat caudate putamen: an electrophysiological study. *J. Neurosci.,* 8: 4340–4348.

Huguenard, J.R., Hamill, O.P. and Prince, D.A. (1988) Developmental changes in Na conductance in rat neocortical neurons: appearance of a slowly inactivating component. *J. Neurophysiol.,* 59: 778–795.

Kita, H., Kita, T. and Kitai, S.T. (1985) Active membrane properties of rat neostriatal neurons in an in vitro slice preparation. *Exp. Brain Res.,* 60: 54–62.

Le Moine, C., Normand, E. and Bloch, B. (1991) Phenotypical characterization of the rat striatal neurons expressing the D_1 dopamine receptor gene. *Proc. Natl. Acad. Sci. U.S.A.,* 88: 4205–4209.

Li, M., West, J.W., Lai, Y., Scheur, T. and Catterall, W.A. (1992) Functional modulation of brain sodium channels by cAMP-dependent phosphorylation. *Neuron,* 8: 1151–1159.

Mansour, A., Meador-Woodruff, J.H., Bunzow, J., Van Tol, H., Civelli, O., Akil, H. and Watson, S.J. (1990) Localization of dopamine D_2 receptor mRNA and D_1 and D_2 receptor binding in the rat brain and pituitary: an in situ hybridization-receptor autoradiographic analysis. *J.Neurosci.,* 10: 2587–2600.

Marchetti, C., Carbone, E. and Lux, H.D. (1986) Effects of dopamine and noradrenaline on Ca channels of cultured sensory and sympathetic neurons of chick. *Pflügers Arch.,* 406: 104–111.

Meador-Woodruff, J.H., Mansour, A., Bunzow, J.R., Van Tol, H.H.M., Watson Jr., S.J. and Civelli, O. (1989) Distribution of D_2 dopamine receptor mRNA in rat brain. *Proc. Natl. Acad. Sci. U.S.A.,* 86: 7625–7628.

324

Meador-Woodruff, J.H., Mansour, A., Healy, D.J., Kuehn, R., Zhou, Q.-Y., Bunzow, J.R., Akil, H., Civelli, O. and Watson Jr., S.J. (1991) Comparison of the distributions of D_1 and D_2 dopamine receptor mRNAs in rat brain. *Neuropsychopharmacology,* 5: 231 – 242.

Monsma, F.J., McVittie, L.D., Gerfen, C.R., Mahan, L.C. and Sibley, D.R. (1989) Multiple D_2 dopamine receptors produced by alternative RNA splicing. *Nature,* 342: 926 – 929.

Monsma, F.J., McVittie, L.D., Gerfen, C.R., Mahan, L.C. and Sibley, D.R. (1990) Molecular cloning and expression of a D_1 dopamine receptor linked to adenylyl cyclase activation. *Proc. Natl. Acad. Sci. U.S.A.,* 87: 6723 – 6727.

Nishi, K., Akins, P.T., Surmeier, D.J. and Kitai, S.T. (1990) Muscarinic regulation of cyclic AMP metabolism in rat neostriatal cultures. *Brain Res.,* 534: 111 – 116.

Ogata, N. and Narahashi, T. (1989) Block of sodium channels by psychotropic drugs in single guinea-pig cardiac myoctes. *Br. J. Pharmacol.,* 97: 905 – 913.

Ogata, N. and Tatebayashi, H. (1990) Sodium current kinetics in freshly isolated neostriatal neurones of the adult guinea pig. *Pflügers Arch.,* 416: 594 – 603.

Ohno, Y., Sasa, M. and Takaori, S. (1987) Coexistence of inhibitory dopamine D_1 and excitatory D_2 receptors on the same caudate nucleus neurons. *Life Sci.,* 40: 1937 – 1945.

Robertson, H.A. (1992) Dopamine receptor interactions: some implications for the treatment of Parkinson's disease. *Trends Neurosci.,* 15: 201 – 206.

Sah, P., Gibb, A.J. and Gage, P.W. (1988) The sodium current underlying action potentials in guinea pig hippocampal CA1 neurons. *J. Gen. Physiol.,* 91: 373 – 398.

Schubert, B., Van Dongen, A.M.J., Kirsch, G.E. and Brown, A.M. (1990) Inhibition of cardiac Na^+ currents by isoproterenol. *Am. J. Physiol.,* 258: 977 – 982.

Seeman, P., Niznik, H.B., Guan, H.C., Booth, G. and Ulpian, C. (1989) Link between D_1 and D_2 dopamine receptors is reduced in schizrenia and Huntington diseased brain. *Proc. Natl. Acad. Sci. U.S.A.,* 86: 10156 – 10160.

Sokoloff, P., Giros, B., Martres, M.-P., Bouthenet, M.-L. and Schwartz, J.-C. (1990) Molecular cloning and characterization of a novel dopamine receptor (D_3) as a target for neuroleptics. *Nature,* 347: 146 – 151.

Stoof, J.C. and Kebabian, J.W. (1984) Two dopamine receptors: biochemistry, physiology and pharmacology. *Life Sci.,* 35: 2281 – 2296.

Sunahara, R.K., Guan, H.-C., O'Dowd, B.F., Seeman, P., Laurier, L.G., Ng, G., George, S.R., Torchia, J., Van Tol, H.H.M. and Niznik, H.B. (1991) Cloning of the gene for a human dopamine D_5 receptor with higher affinity for dopamine

than D_1. *Nature,* 350: 614 – 619.

Surmeier, D.J., Stefani, A., Foehring, R. and Kitai, S.T. (1991) Developmental expression of a slowly inactivating voltage-dependent potassium current in rat neostriatal neurons. *Neurosci. Lett.,* 122: 41 – 46.

Surmeier, D.J., Eberwine, J., Wilson, C.J., Stefani, A. and Kitai, S.T. (1992) Dopamine receptor subtypes co-localize in rat striatonigral neurons. *Proc. Natl. Acad. Sci. U.S.A.,* 89: 10178 – 10182.

Tiberi, M., Jarvie, K.R., Silvia, C., Falardeau, P., Gingrich, J.A., Godinot, U., Bertrand, L., Yang-Feng, T.L., Fremeau Jr., R.T. and Caron, M.G. (1991) Cloning, molecular characterization, and chromosomal assignment of a gene encoding a second D_1 dopamine receptor subtype: differential expression pattern in rat brain compared with the D_{1A} receptor. *Proc. Natl. Acad. Sci. U.S.A.,* 88: 7491 – 7495.

Uchimura, N., Higashi, H. and Nishi, S. (1986) Hyperpolarizing and depolarizing actions of dopamine via D-1 and D-2 receptors on nucleus accumbens neurons. *Brain Res.,* 375: 368 – 372.

Van Gelder, R.N., von Zastrow, M.E., Yool, A., Dement, W.C., Barchas, J.D. and Eberwine, J.H. (1990) Amplified RNA synthesized from limited quantities of heterogeneous cDNA. *Proc. Natl. Acad. Sci. U.S.A.,* 87: 1663 – 1667.

Weiner, D.M., Levey, A.I. and Brann, M.R. (1990) Expression of muscarinic acetylcholine and dopamine receptor mRNAs in rat basal ganglia. *Proc. Natl. Acad. Sci. U.S.A.,* 87: 7050 – 7054.

Weiner, D.M., Levey, A.I., Sunahara, R.K., Niznik, H.B., O'Dowd, B.F., Seeman, P. and Brann, M.R. (1991) D_1 and D_2 dopamine receptor mRNA in rat brain. *Proc. Natl. Acad. Sci. U.S.A.,* 88: 1859 – 1863.

Weiss, S., Sebben, M., Garcia-Sainz, J.A. and Bockaert, J. (1985) D_2-dopamine receptor mediated inhibition of cyclic AMP formation in striatal neurons in primary culture. *Mol. Pharmacol.,* 27: 595 – 599.

White, F.J. and Wang, R.Y. (1986) Electrophysiological evidence for the existence of both D_1 and D_2 dopamine receptors in the rat nucleus accumbens. *J. Neurosci.,* 6: 274 – 280.

White, F.J., Bednarz, L.M., Wachtel, S.R., Hjorth, S. and Brooderson, R.J. (1988) Is stimulation of both D_1 and D_2 receptors necessary for the expression of dopamine-mediated behaviors? *Pharmacol. Biochem. Behav.,* 30: 189 – 193.

Zhou, Q.-Y., Grandy, D.K., Thambi, L., Kushner, J.A., Van Tol, H.H., Cone, R., Pribnow, D., Salon, J., Bunzow, J.R. and Civelli, O. (1990) Cloning and expression of human and rat D_1 dopamine receptors. *Nature,* 347: 76 – 80.

G.W. Arbuthnott and P.C. Emson (Eds.)
Progress in Brain Research, Vol. 99
© 1993 Elsevier Science Publishers B.V. All rights reserved.

CHAPTER 21

The corticostriatal system on computer simulation: an intermediate mechanism for sequencing of actions

J.R. Wickens[1] and G.W. Arbuthnott[2]

[1]Department of Anatomy and Theoretical Neuroscience Research Group, Otago University Medical School, Dunedin, New Zealand and [2]MRC External Scientific Staff, Department of Preclinical Veterinary Sciences, University of Edinburgh, Summerhall, Edinburgh EH9 1QH, U.K.

Introduction

Several independent lines of evidence implicate the neostriatum in programming of sequences of actions: sequential movements are disturbed in parkinsonian patients, as evidenced by slowing of movements when they are performed as part of a sequence (Stelmach et al., 1987; Benecke et al., 1987). Cools et al. (1984) have shown that after bilateral injections of haloperidol into the caudate nucleus, cats walking on a treadmill show a deficit in the capacity to "program the serial ordering of non exteroceptively directed behavior". In primates, single unit recordings from the putamen have revealed the existence of neurones which are activated prior to the onset of actions when they are performed as part of a sequence, but not when the same actions are performed outside of the sequence (Kimura, 1990).

The probable involvement of the neostriatum in internally generating serially ordered sequences of actions (or thoughts), and the deficits in performing such sequences following dopamine depletion, suggest several questions: does the neostriatum contain a mechanism which can generate sequences of activity? How is the required sequence specified by the inputs into the striatum? What are the natural limits on the rate and length of the sequences that can be produced by this mechanism? What role does stria-

tal dopamine play in these limits, under normal conditions and in dopamine deficiency states?

Computer simulation can provide insight into the capabilities of neural mechanisms which exist in the neostriatum. It is increasingly being applied to research on the basal ganglia (Brotchie et al., 1991; Mitchell et al., 1991; Wickens et al., 1991). Simulations of neural circuits based on the neostriatum can lead to a better understanding of how membrane conductances at the level of single neurones can influence the macroscopic activity of populations of striatal neurones. In particular, they can show how changes in conductance parameters brought about by diffusely acting neurotransmitters such as dopamine can regulate the macroscopic behaviour of a network.

In the following sections a model is defined, based on a selection from present knowledge of the physiology of the component neurones of the striatum and the anatomy of their interconnections. The responses of the model neurones to direct current injections will be described. The neurones will then be connected into a simple network. It will be shown that the network is able to generate sequences of activity patterns in response to a sustained input. The temporal characteristics of the sequences the model is able to produce will then be discussed in relation to the temporal features of the sequential behaviours in which the neostriatum is implicated.

A

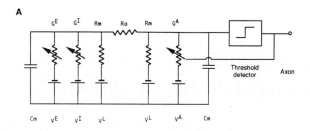

B

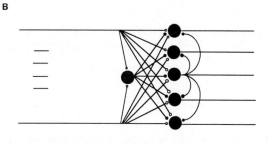

Corticostriatal afferents   Feedforward interneurone   Medium spiny output neurones

Fig. 1. The simplified model for the medium spiny neurones used in the simulation. The dendritic compartment is connected to the soma compartment by an axial resistance. The membrane potential at the soma is connected to a spike-generating region. When the membrane potential exceeds threshold, the spike-generating region initiates an action potential on the axon. Excitatory and inhibitory conductances on the dendrite are driven by corticostriatal afferents and the local collaterals of other medium spiny neurones (respectively). The after-hyperpolarization conductances are located on the soma, and activated by action potential firing of the neurone.

Methods

There were a number of stages in the modelling. The first stage involved developing a simplified model of a single neostriatal neurone. A two compartment model was used which incorporated excitatory and inhibitory synaptic conductances, and two forms of a potassium conductance activated by suprathreshold depolarization. With this model, the responses of a single cell to direct current injection and synaptic activation were examined. In the second stage, changes in the membrane potassium conductances were introduced into the model to simulate the effects of different levels of activity in dopaminergic afferents. The influence of different dopamine levels on the responses of the model neurone to

direct current injection was compared with experimental data obtained in vitro. In the third stage, the activity patterns produced in a network model consisting of a number of interconnected neurones were examined. The effects of different dopamine levels on these activity patterns were investigated. The way in which different sequences of activity could be produced by the network was analysed, and the role of a particular subset of feedforward inhibitory interneurones considered.

The model was implemented using the general simulation system (GENESIS, CalTech) script language interpreter (Wilson and Bower, 1989) and the computer simulations were run on a DEC 5000 workstation.

Modelling the medium spiny neurone

A simplified model of a medium spiny neurone was used in the computer simulation. It consisted of two compartments (dendrite and soma), a spike generat-

TABLE I

Parameter values used in striatal simulation

Label	Description	Units and values
G_{max}^{E}	Peak excitatory conductance	1.0 – 2.0 nS/synapse
G_{max}^{I}	Peak inhibitory conductance	80 nS/synapse
G_{max}^{A1}	Fast AHP conductance	25 nS
G_{max}^{A2}	Slow AHP conductance	0.25 – 1.5 nS
α^{E}	Time constant excitatory synapse	2.0 msec^{-1}
α^{I}	Time constant inhibitory synapse	10.0 msec^{-1}
α^{A1}	Fast AHP time constant	5.0 msec^{-1}
α^{A2}	Slow AHP time constant	250 – 500 msec^{-1}
V^{E}	Excitatory equilibrium potential	0 mV
V^{I}	Inhibitory equilibrium potential	– 75 mV
V^{A}	AHP equilibrium potential	– 90 mV
V^{L}	Leak equilibrium potential	– 80 mV
rm	Membrane resistivity	10.0 KΩ/cm^2
cm	Membrane capacitivity	1.0 μF/cm^2
ra	Axial resistance	300.0 Ω/cm
θ	Action potential threshold	– 45 mV

ing region, and a branching axon (see Fig. 1*A*). The physical dimensions of the dendrite and soma determined the passive electrical membrane properties of neostriatal neurons. The assumed values for the constants involved are given in Table I. The values used were approximations based on a review of available evidence. The following sections describe the arguments used in arriving at the final approximations.

Passive electrical properties

The dendritic tree of the medium spiny neurones was simplified to a single compartment and modelled as a cylinder of diameter 15 μm and length 400 μm. This gave a dendritic membrane area of 18850 μm^2. Assuming a membrane resistivity of 10000 Ω/cm^2 gives a membrane resistance for the dendritic compartment of 53 MΩ. If the membrane capacitivity is assumed to be 1 μF/cm^2, the membrane time constant is then approximately 10 msec.

From intracellular recordings from striatal cells, measurements using small currents reveal a membrane resistance of 17 – 39 MΩ and a membrane time constant of 4 – 15 msec (Sugimori et al., 1978; Kita et al., 1984; Bargas et al., 1988; Kawaguchi et al., 1989; Jiang and North, 1991). The membrane resistance calculated from the dimensions of the model neurone described above (53 MΩ) represents the "naive" value before the various membrane conductances which bring down the membrane resistance have been included.

Dendritic spines were not explicitly included in the model. However, the effect of spine neck resistance was taken into account in the choice of excitatory synaptic conductance, and their contribution to the membrane capacitance was included in the area of the dendritic compartment.

The dendritic compartment was connected to the soma compartment by an axial resistance, which was determined by the cord conductance of the dendritic cylinder. A cytoplasmic resistance of 300 Ω/cm was assumed, giving a total axial resistance of 68 MΩ from the soma to the dendrite.

Corticostriatal afferents

The corticostriatal pathway is one of the major efferent projections of the cerebral cortex. In almost every cortical area there exists a population of layer V pyramidal cells which project to the neostriatum. The axons of these cells converge to form an extensive and powerful source of excitatory drive to the neostriatal neurons.

In the model, 100 input lines were used to represent the corticostriatal afferent axons. Each afferent axon branched to every striatal neuron in the model, so each received 100 excitatory synapses. These were located on the distal end of the dendritic compartment. The conduction delay for each branch of the axon was constant, the value being randomly assigned according to a Gaussian distribution about a mean conduction time of 7.5 msec with a variance of 5.0 msec, truncated at zero.

The conductance increase brought about by the excitatory corticostriatal synapses was modelled as an alpha function:

$$G^E = G^E_{max} t \exp(1 - \alpha^E t)$$

This was assigned a peak value of approximately $G^E_{max} = 1.0$ nS at time $1/\alpha^E = 2.0$ msec. Since there are no direct measurements of conductance increases for unitary excitatory post-synaptic conductance increases in the striatum, indirect arguments had to be used to arrive at these values, as follows.

The time constant for excitatory synapses (α^E) was estimated from the time-to-peak of cortically evoked EPSPs. Park et al. (1980) recorded a time to peak of 1.64 msec. Akaike et al. (1988) measured a rise time in slices of 1.8 ± 0.2 msec. The time to peak for the conductance increase was therefore set to $1/\alpha^E = 2.0$ msec.

In order to estimate the peak excitatory synaptic conductance G^E_{max} the amplitude of the excitatory post-synaptic potentials (EPSPs) typically evoked by stimulation of corticostriatal afferents were considered. Striatal EPSPs evoked by cortical stimulation have a relatively large amplitude. Lighthall et al. (1981) reported values obtained in slices which varied between 2 and 18 mV (mean 6.3 mV). Also in slices, Akaike et al. (1988) reported mean peak amplitudes of 14.4 mV. In vivo, Bishop et al. (1982) recorded EPSPs from medium spiny neurones in response to cortical stimulation which varied from 2 to 14mV (see their fig. 3A).

In order to calculate the conductance increase at a single synapse from the size of the EPSP evoked by electrical stimulation, it is necessary to estimate the contribution of each synapse to the total EPSP amplitude. This will depend on the number of afferent fibers activated by the stimulus. This cannot be known with any certainty, but can be estimated by considering the distribution of corticostriatal cells in the cortex, on the one hand, and the likely spread of current from the stimulating electrode on the other.

Striatal neurones receive inputs from cells thinly spread over a wide area of cortex with each afferent neurone contributing only a few terminals to individual neostriatal cells. Jones et al. (1977) identified the cells of origin of the corticostriatal projection using retrograde horseradish peroxidase labelling and established that they were small- to medium-sized pyramidal cells which were evenly spread with gaps of up to several hundred microns between individual cells. The EPSP amplitudes produced by cortical stimulation are therefore unlikely to be the result of activating a very large number of corticostriatal afferents because the current spread using conventional stimulus intensities is limited (see Updyke and Liles, 1987). A reasonable estimate would be 10 synapses. Using the range of EPSP amplitudes reported above, this suggests that a single synapse could produce an EPSP between approximately 0.2 and 2.0 mV. An EPSP of this amplitude could be produced in the model by a single synapse with G_{max}^E between 0.2 and 2.0 nS.

Inhibitory synapses

Intracellular estimates of the duration of the local GABAergic inhibition seen in the striatum in vitro range from approximately 10 to 50 msec (Misgeld et al., 1982; Lighthall and Kitai, 1983). The inhibitory equilibrium potential reported by Misgeld et al. (1982) was between -57 and -62 mV. Jiang and

North (1991) report a similar reversal potential (-47 to -70 mV, mean -57 mV).

In the model, the time course of the inhibitory conductance increase was modelled as an alpha function with a time constant of $\alpha^I = 10.0$ msec. The peak conductance of inhibitory synapses was set to $G_{max}^I = 80.0$ nS. The equilibrium potential for inhibitory synapses was set to $V^I = -60$ mV.

Resting membrane potential

Misgeld et al. (1982) report resting membrane potentials around -67 mV. The true resting membrane potential is probably more negative than that. Akaike et al. (1988) report a resting membrane potential of -73.3 ± 4.2 mV (in slices). Also in slices, Jiang and North (1991) report resting membrane potentials of about -90 mV. An average value of -80.0 mV was used in the simulations. The value in vitro depends on the extracellular potassium concentration and is somewhat arbitrary.

Action potential threshold

Neostriatal neurones in vivo tend to fire in irregular phasic bursts of activity. Intracellular recordings from identified spiny neurones reveal noisy irregular periods of maintained $5-20$ mV membrane depolarizations (Wilson and Groves, 1980). These do not reliably produce firing of the neurones, though tend to be present when firing does occur. This seems to suggest a relatively high threshold, because tonic background excitatory input activity of significant amplitude only occasionally causes cell firing.

Misgeld et al. (1982) report firing levels ranging from -45 to -51 mV from resting membrane potentials around -67 mV. A value of -45 mV for the action potential threshold was used in the simulation.

The potassium conductances

Despite the high level of the excitatory inputs to the striatum, the striatal output neurones only rarely produce action potentials. Calabresi et al. (1990a,b) attributed this behaviour to persistent membrane potassium conductances, which reduce the excitability of the neostriatal neurones. A variety of different types of potassium conductance have been described in the literature. It is likely that several different types of potassium conductance are expressed in the neostriatal neuronal membranes. Only two will be considered in detail here: a transient potassium conductance similar to the A-current described in other neurons; and a calcium-activated potassium conductance.

A transient potassium current activated by depolarization above -50 mV has been analysed in neostriatal neurons by whole-cell voltage-clamp techniques (Surmeier et al., 1988). It is called "transient" because although it is activated by depolarization, maintained depolarization will lead to inactivation. It is blocked by 4-aminopyridine but not by inorganic calcium channel blockers, and has a reversal potential near the potassium equilibrium potential. These features are very similar to the features of the A-current described in other neurones.

The transient potassium current may show some deactivation at the resting membrane potential. A hyperpolarizing prepulse can reactivate the current, and this has the effect of prolonging the latency to the first action potential and decreasing the firing frequency during the pulse (Bargas et al., 1989). The transient potassium conductances described may also contribute to the fast component of the after-hyperpolarization potential (AHP) which has been observed in striatal neurons.

A slow AHP potential has been described in striatal neurons following the firing of a single action potential (Calabresi et al., 1987) or train of action potentials (Rutherford et al., 1988; Galarraga et al., 1989). Potassium channel blockers tetraethylammonium (TEA) or 4-aminopyridine (4-AP) block the AHP potentials triggered by direct current injection (Calabresi et al., 1987). The slow AHP is probably due to a calcium-activated potassium conductance and is blocked by cobalt (Galarraga et al., 1989).

The potassium conductances which give rise to AHPs are of particular significance for the generation of sequences. In order to make this clearly evident, without using a large number of parameters,

an extremely simple approximation of the AHP was used in the model. The AHP conductance was modelled as the sum of two alpha functions: a fast AHP conductance (to represent the effects of the transient potassium conductance) with a time to peak of $\alpha^{A1} = 5.0$ msec; and a slow AHP conductance (to represent the effects of the calcium-activated potassium conductance) of $\alpha^{A2} = 250.0$ msec. The alpha function for both conductances was activated after action potential firing of the neurone in question.

Dopamine has been shown to reduce the amplitude of the AHP in striatal neurones (Rutherford et al., 1988). The mechanism by which this is brought about is not yet known. However, two effects of dopamine are likely to be relevant: firstly, dopamine exerts an indirect effect on the rapidly inactivating potassium conductances via inhibition of the muscarinic effects of cholinergic interneurones (Akins et al., 1990). This involves a shift of the steady-state voltage dependence of the rapidly inactivating potassium current. Secondly, dopamine reduces a high-voltage-activated calcium current. This would be likely to reduce the calcium-activated potassium conductances which underlie the slow component of the AHP.

Although it is impossible at this stage to define the exact mechanism by which dopamine reduces the AHP, it is nonetheless useful to consider what effect reducing the AHP is likely to have on the responses of the medium spiny neurones in isolation, and the activity sequences generated by a network of such neurones. The effects of dopamine were thus incorporated into the model by varying the maximum conductance of the slow AHP channels.

Neostriatal network model

The neostriatum is a heterogeneous structure composed of a number of neurochemically distinct compartments (Gerfen, 1985). The present model is concerned with the largest, so-called "matrix" compartment.

Inhibitory domains

The vast majority of the neurones in the neostriatum are of one type, known as "medium spiny". According to Kemp and Powell (1971) these constitute 95% of the neurones in the neostriatum. There is a certain degree of uniformity in the shape of the dendritic and axonal arborizations of the medium spiny neurones. The medium spiny neurones have 4 – 7 main dendrites which radiate centripetally in all directions, branching repeatedly. The dendritic fields so formed appear as "randomly oriented spheres or flattened ovoids" (Fisher et al., 1986) up to 500 μm in diameter (Bishop et al., 1982). In addition to a long axon which extends into the globus pallidus or substantia nigra (Graveland and DiFiglia, 1985), each medium spiny neuron also produces a plexus of local axon collaterals which is mainly restricted to the space of the neurone's dendritic field.

The anatomical features just described suggest that the local axon collaterals of the medium spiny output neurones overlap extensively with the dendrites of neighbouring neurones. The axons branch repeatedly and form large symmetrical synapses on the proximal dendrites of nearby medium spiny neurones (Preston et al., 1980). These synapses are almost certainly inhibitory (Somogyi et al., 1981; Aronin et al., 1986; Kitai and Kitai, 1988; Pasik et al., 1988). This arrangement implies there is mutual inhibition between striatal neurones which lie within a distance of, at most, about 500 μm of each other (Wilson and Groves, 1980). However, the effective inhibitory synapses will probably be the ones located on the proximal dendrites, so the neurones making up the domain will be those that fall within a smaller sphere of 250 μm radius. This has been termed a "domain of inhibition" by Wickens et al. (1991). The existence of a mutually inhibitory relationship between striatal output neurones, though still somewhat speculative, is supported by electrophysiological evidence (Katayama et al., 1981).

The number of neostriatal neurones in a single domain can be estimated as follows. Schröder et al. (1975) estimate there are of the order of 100 million (10^8) small neurones in the human neostriatum. The density (ϱ) of small neurones counted in the human neostriatum was 11000/mm^3. Assuming, as above,

that the axons of a medium spiny neostriatal neurone can contact dendrites within a 250 μm radius (r). The number of neurones (n) in a domain will be given by:

$$n = \varrho\frac{4}{3}\pi r^3 = 720$$

In the network model, a single domain was simulated as a network of either 9 or 25 medium spiny neurones connected in a mutually inhibitory array. Each neurone inhibited all of the other neurones in the domain, but did not inhibit itself. This latter assumption may be partially justified by noting that inhibition of a striatal neurone by its own collaterals is not common (Hull et al., 1973).

Although for practical reasons it was necessary to limit the size of the network to 25 neurones for most simulations, it should be emphasized that each "neurone" in the model represents a selected single neurone, rather than any sort of average of many neurones. For the particular case of a network of mutually inhibitory neurones, in which very few are active at any one time, such a reduction in the size of the network has negligible effects on the behaviour of interest. Simulations with networks of 625 neurones have been conducted with essentially the same results, but for clarity in presentation, only the results from the 25 neurone network will be shown, and in some cases the results from a 9 neurone network will be used to illustrate particular points.

A total of 100 corticostriatal afferents were simulated for each neurone in the network. Each afferent fibre branched to supply every neurone in the domain, as described above. The excitatory conductance values were varied somewhat to observe the effects of different assumptions about the distribution of synaptic weights on the dynamic behaviour of the networks. The distribution used will be described in the appropriate section of the Results.

Feedforward inhibition

In addition to the feedback network formed by the domains of inhibition, a feedforward inhibitory interneurone (see Kita, this volume) was included in some models. This represented the subpopulation of

GABA (parvalbumin) interneurones, which in reality constitute about 3% of the total neuronal population of the striatum.

Preliminary anatomical descriptions suggest that the feedforward interneurones go specifically to make pericellular baskets around spiny neurones. The feedforward interneurones receive presumed excitatory (asymmetrical) synapses from the corticostriatal afferents, and probably receive more cortical input than the medium spiny neurones.

A single feedforward interneurone was included in some simulations (Fig. 1B). The feedforward interneurone received excitatory input from the branches of the same corticostriatal input lines that supplied the medium spiny neurones. The synapses with the feedforward interneurones were made twice the strength of the corticostriatal synapses upon medium spiny neurones.

The feedforward interneurones made inhibitory synapses with all neurones in the domain. Assuming the pericellular baskets to be a particularly potent source of inhibition, the conductance of the inhibitory synapses from the interneurones to the medium spiny neurones was made five times greater than the conductance of the inhibitory synapses from the medium spiny neurones to other medium spiny neurones.

Finally, the membrane resistance of the dendritic compartment of the feedforward interneurones was set to 100 MΩ and the capacitance was set to 100 pF. These assumptions were intended to reflect the reduced surface area of the aspiny dendrite of the feedforward interneurones as compared with medium spiny neurones.

Results

The parameter values used in all the simulations being described were those listed in Table I. Although simulations were performed on networks of different sizes the programme was organized so that the same file of constants was used by all models. Thus, no parameter value could be changed in one network, without the change affecting all networks.

This ensured consistency in assumptions across different levels of the model.

The response of a single model neurone to a direct current injection applied as a pulse of 100 msec duration is shown in Fig. 2. The current injected (0.7 nA) is just suprathreshold for action potential firing of the cell. The trajectory of the membrane potential follows the passive charging curve given by the time constants for the two compartments. An action potential is produced when the membrane potential exceeds threshold. The action potential is followed by a period of hyperpolarization. This has two components: a fast component with a time to peak of $\alpha^{A1} = 5.0$ msec and peak conductance $G_{max}^{A1} = 25.0$ nS, and a slow component with a time to peak of $\alpha^{A2} = 250.0$ msec and peak conductance of $G_{max}^{A2} = 0.25$ nS.

In order to display the exact time at which the action potential is generated, the state of the spike generating region has been weighted and added to the membrane potential of the soma compartment. This gives rise to the apparently instantaneous action potential shown in Fig. 2. It should be noted that the biophysical events which underlie action potential firing are not being simulated in the model. The membrane potential of the soma compartment during cell firing is not directly modified by the action potential because the generation of action potentials is not explicitly being modelled. The ac-

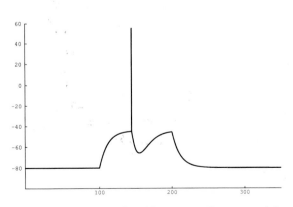

Fig. 2. Passive response of model neurone to direct current injection.

332

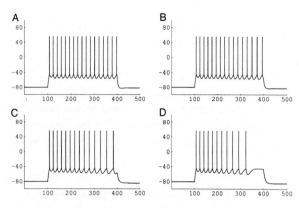

Fig. 3. Responses of single neurone to current injection at 2 x threshold. *A*. Top left, $G_{max}^{A2} = 0.25$ nS. *B*. Top right, $G_{max}^{A2} = 0.5$ nS. *C*. Bottom left, $G_{max}^{A2} = 1.0$ nS. *D*. Bottom right, $G_{max}^{A2} = 1.5$ nS.

tion potential waveform is in effect being "pasted" on for the purposes of display. However, it is the action potential firing of the cell which initiates the AHP conductances, and the effect of these can be seen immediately after the action potential and at the termination of the current pulse.

Fig. 3 shows the responses of the model neurone to a current pulse of 1.4 nA (twice threshold) lasting 300 msec. These responses were used to calibrate the free parameters of the model neurone, so that its behaviour was comparable to the neostriatal cell described by Rutherford et al. (1988), as shown in their fig. 2. In the model, it was assumed that the effect of reducing dopamine was to increase the slow AHP conductance from a low value of G_{max}^{A2} = 0.25 nS to a high value of G_{max}^{A2} = 1.50 nS. In the low G_{max}^{A2} condition shown in Fig. 3*A* (corresponding to a presumed "high – normal" level of dopamine activity) the rate of discharge is highest at the beginning of the current pulse and showed a gradual but relatively slight decrease over 300 msec. As G_{max}^{A2} is increased (Fig. 3*B − D*), the total number of spikes during the current pulse is decreased.

The action potential firing behaviour of a network of 25 model neurones connected into a symmetrical domain (with no feedforward interneurones) is shown in Fig. 4. The network is being driven by excitation from 100 input lines, represent-

ing the corticostriatal afferents. The input is essentially uniform, with symmetry being broken by minor fluctuations brought about by statistical variations in the timing of afferent activity. The neurones are active in bursts of high-frequency firing separated by relatively long periods of inactivity. At any particular moment in time usually only one neurone is active. This is due to the competition occurring among the mutually inhibitory output neurones. Over the 10 sec period shown, the identity of the most active neurone cycles from one neurone to another in a random sequence.

The different patterns of activity in each part of Fig. 4 show the effects of different values of G_{max}^{A2} on the network responses. Fig. 4*A* shows the network response when $G_{max}^{A2} = 0.25$ nS. This low value for the slow AHP conductance (corresponding to high dopamine levels) is associated with an activity pattern in which the most activated neurone suppresses all the other neurones in the domain (after an initial transient). This is essentially the competitive mode of striatal function described by Wickens et al. (1991). A neurone which becomes active in this way tends to fire repetitively until a transition occurs after which the activity shifts to another neurone. The duration of the "bursts" is approximately 900 – 1100 msec. Fig. 4*B* shows the same network under conditions which are identical except for an increased slow AHP conductance ($G_{max}^{A2} = 0.5$ nS). At this still moderately low value for the slow AHP conductance, the duration of the "bursts" becomes shorter (400 – 500 msec). As the slow AHP conductance is increased further (Fig. 4*C*, $G_{max}^{A2} = 1.0$ nS; Fig 4*D*, $G_{max}^{A2} = 1.5$ nS) the episodic firing pattern is disrupted and the bursts become short and irregular. The competitive dynamic breaks down and increasing numbers of instances of coactivation occur.

The response of a smaller network of 9 neurones (no feedforward interneurones) to a patterned stimulus is shown in Fig. 5. This network uses the same set of parameters as in the previous figure, except that the inputs are separated into two subpopulations: 25 "background" and 75 "stimulus" in-

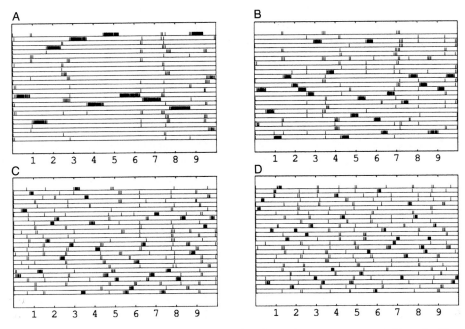

Fig. 4. Activity patterns in a 25 neurone network of medium spiny output neurones with no feedforward interneurones, showing the effects of different slow AHP conductances. Horizontal axis, time (sec). Each neuron in the net receives inputs from 100 excitatory synapses, each 1.25 nS. Each input line is being driven by a Poisson process with mean rate 34 pulses/sec (to represent firing in a much larger number of afferents discharging at a much lower rate).

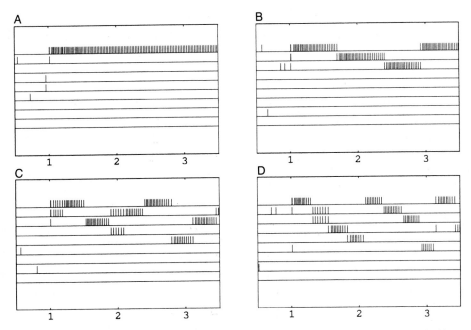

Fig. 5. Activity patterns in a 9 neurone network of medium spiny output neurones with no feedforward interneurones, showing the effects of different slow AHP conductances. Horizontal axis, time (sec). Each neuron in the net receives inputs from 100 excitatory synapses: 25 "background" inputs from $t = 0$ to $t = 1.0$ sec, $G_{max}^{E} = 1.25$ nS, plus 75 "stimulus" inputs started at $t = 1.0$ sec, as described in the text.

puts. The background inputs were statistically uniform (as above). The stimulus inputs were delivered at a higher rate, and the conductance of the excitatory synapses was made to depend on the location of the target neurone. In the figure, the output of neurones receiving higher levels of excitatory input is depicted on the upper traces. The neurone in the topmost trace has the peak conductance of each excitatory synapse set to $G_{max}^{E} = 1.5$ nS. The neurone in the lowermost trace has $G_{max}^{E} = 0.5$ nS. The peak excitatory conductance of the intermediate neurones is set by linear interpolation between these upper and lower bounds.

Figure 5 shows the response of the network to a 1 sec period of background stimulation, followed by a switch to the patterned stimulus at time $t = 1.0$ sec. The patterned stimulus persists for the rest of the period shown. It is clear from Fig. $5B - D$ that some degree of sequential activation occurs when the slow AHP conductance is sufficiently high. There is a simple explanation for this. Intuitively, the first neurone to fire will be the one receiving the strongest excitation. This will become the most active neurone in the network, suppressing the other neurones by its inhibitory collaterals. Repetitive firing by the most active neurone, however, causes the slow AHP to accumulate, until the self-inhibiting effect of the AHP on the most active neurone is greater than the effect of the inhibition it is producing on other neurones. At this point, the next most strongly excited neurone "takes over". This will occur sequentially down the scale of neurones until the point is reached at which the excitation being received by the next most strongly excited neurone is effectively lower than the excitation being received by the most strongly excited neurone, taking into account the effect of the slow AHP conductance.

Despite the intuitive appeal of this mechanism for generating an ordered sequence of activations, it is clear from Fig. 5 that this is not a robust mechanism. Fig. $5B$ shows that at a low – moderate value for the slow AHP ($G_{max}^{A2} = 0.5$ nS) the network produces a short sequence in the manner envisaged. However,

the other parts of Fig. 5 show that the mechanism is prone to several types of error.

First, as shown in Fig. $5A$, it is possible that the neurone receiving the strongest excitation will remain the most active neurone. In this case there can be no sequential activation pattern. This type of error (which may be called "perseveration" by analogy with the performance errors made by animals under the influence of amphetamine) occurs if the slow AHP conductance is too low (in this case, $G_{max}^{A2} = 0.25$ nS) relative to the size of the step change in excitatory conductance to the next most strongly excited neurone.

However, Fig. $5C$ shows that at higher values for the slow AHP conductance, the order of the sequence of activation pattern becomes disrupted in a different way, by transposition errors. One source of transposition errors is unwanted coactivation of some neurones at different stages of the sequence. For example, in Fig. $5C$ there is a period of coactivation in the upper two neurones at the start of the stimulus period. Eventually, the most strongly excited neurone "wins". However, because of the AHP conductance that the second neurone has accumulated, when the transition occurs it is the *third* most excited neurone that is activated. This is followed by another period of coactivation, of the second and fourth neurones.

Another type of error is shown in Fig. $5D$, where an episode of coactivation appears to replace a sequential activation of the second and third neurones. This does not cause a transposition error, but rather a "blend" error, in which the separate items of the sequence occur simultaneously instead of sequentially.

The errors described above usually occur after premature firing of a neurone which the intuitive argument suggests should fire later in the sequence. This disrupts the orderly progression of firing by premature activation of the AHP conductance in these neurones. The network is prone to premature discharges because of the variability in excitatory inputs to individual neurones brought about by the stochastic nature of the excitatory inputs. It is likely that if such a mechanism operates in the neostriatum, it would be prone to the same sort of disruption.

Incorporation of a feedforward inhibitory interneurone into the network model was found to be very helpful in reducing these errors. The responses of a network incorporating a feedforward interneurone are shown in Fig. 6A – D. The bottom trace in these figures shows the activity in the feedforward interneurone. At the onset of the stimulus at time $t = 1.0$ sec, the feedforward interneurone fires a burst of action potentials. This burst silences all of the other neurones in the network for several hundred milliseconds. At the end of the burst, the medium spiny output neurones begin to fire. The effect of having the feedforward interneurone in the circuit is that the medium spiny neurones now fire in an orderly sequence. This is because the effect of any spurious premature discharge has been "cleared" by the prolonged burst of powerful inhibition from the feedforward interneurones. The effect of increasing the slow AHP conductance is now simply

to increase the number of elements in the sequence and decrease the duration of each burst.

Discussion

The computer simulations described above suggest that the neostriatum does contain a mechanism which is able to generate ordered spatiotemporal sequences of action potential activity. However, this conclusion depends on the validity of a number of assumptions about the interactions that occur among medium spiny output neurones and feedforward interneurones, the distribution of corticostriatal afferents, and the properties of a membrane potassium conductance under dopaminergic control.

The organization of the medium spiny output neurones into domains of mutual inhibition is a feature of the striatum that has been noted by several authors (Wilson and Groves, 1980; Groves, 1983; Rolls and Williams, 1986; Wickens et al., 1991). This is an assumption of the model that is, however,

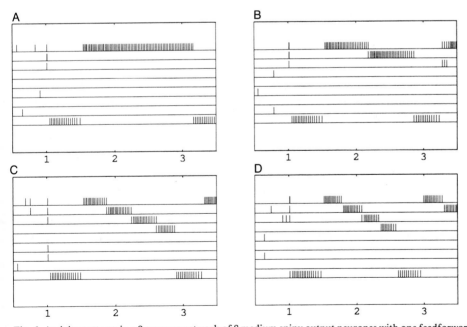

Fig. 6. Activity patterns in a 9 neurone network of 8 medium spiny output neurones with one feedforward interneurone (bottom trace). Horizontal axis, time (sec). Each neuron in the net receives inputs from 100 excitatory synapses: 25 "background" inputs from $t = 0$ to $t = 1.0$ sec, $G^{E}_{max} = 1.25$ nS, plus 75 "stimulus" inputs started at $t = 1.0$ sec, as described in the text.

open to question. There has yet to be a convincing electrophysiological demonstration of reciprocal inhibitory interactions between striatal output neurones. On the other hand, it is not unusual that the anatomy shows collaterals that the electrophysiologists do not see, and the evidence of Katayama et al. (1981) is suggestive. There is also increasing awareness of the importance of a subpopulation of feedforward inhibitory interneurones. The present model proposes an interplay between feedforward and feedback inhibition that improves the performance of the postulated mechanism for generating sequences.

The model predicts that the feedforward interneurones should be activated prior to the beginning of a sequence of movements. The activity of these neurones in the computer simulation is similar to the activity of a subpopulation of movement-related neurones in the putamen, described by Kimura (1990). These neurones, classified as type IIa cells, exhibit burst discharges preceding the first movement of a sequence of repetitive movements but are almost inactive during succeeding movements. A prediction of the model is that the type IIa cells described by Kimura should be GABA (parvalbumin) feedforward interneurones.

In the proposed model the order in which the striatal neurones become active (in response to a fixed input pattern) is determined by the efficacy of the corticostriatal synapses: the most strongly excited neurones become activated first, followed by the next most strongly activated, and so on until the sequence is terminated. An appropriate image for this process is suggested by a ball bouncing down a staircase.

This mechanism for generating serial order is limited to sequences of very few steps. On the other hand, the proposed mechanism allows any arbitrary order of activation to be stored, by a simple adjustment of the corticostriatal synaptic efficacy. Moreover, the dendritic spines upon which the corticostriatal afferents terminate provide a likely site for selective modification of synapses. This could, for example, be achieved by the action of rules for synaptic modification proposed elsewhere (Miller,

1988; Wickens, 1990). Furthermore, different combinations of corticostriatal afferents might produce any possible permutation of the serial order.

The inhibitory synapses between striatal output neurones, in this model, play no role in determining the *order* of the sequence, provided the reciprocal synapses were of approximately equal efficacy. In this respect, the proposed model differs from other possible models for generating serial order. For example, Estes (1972) proposed an interelement inhibition model, in which differences in the strength of inhibitory connections were used to generate a sequence of activations. This idea was developed further by Rumelhart and Norman (1982) who presented a network model which used interelement inhibition to simulate the performance of a skilled typist. In their model, typing a word involved sequential activation of nodes for each letter to be typed. The sequence in which they were activated was determined by the connections between the nodes, which were inhibitory. However, in these connectionist models there is a requirement for selective modification of inhibitory synapses, for which little evidence yet exists.

Definite limits can be placed on the temporal characteristics of the ordered sequences of activity patterns that can be produced by the striatal model. In particular, the assumptions of the model determine the rates at which the elements of a sequence can be produced, and the length of the sequence in terms of the number of elements that can be produced before repetition occurs. In the model, these characteristics were shown to be especially sensitive to the conductance of the slow AHP channels. The effects of dopamine on these channels are therefore of particular interest for future models. Even the present highly simplified model provides some insights into experimental studies on the role of striatal dopamine in the generation of sequences, in particular with regard to the temporal characteristics of the sequences produced by the model, and the way in which these are affected by the presumed effects of changes in dopamine concentration. These will now be considered.

Poizner (1990) has provided an interesting analysis of the signing of a congenitally deaf signer with Parkinson's disease. Compared with a control subject, the parkinsonian signer produced signs of short duration and reduced amplitude. The signs were sometimes incorrectly merged. These errors have some formal similarity to the errors in the sequences produced by the model when the slow AHP conductance is high, as may occur when dopamine concentration is low (as shown in Fig. 5). On the other hand, isolated signs could often be made quite well.

Diseases of the basal ganglia seem to selectively impair the activation or switching of motor sequences rather than disrupt the individual elements in the sequence. This is seen, for example, in patients with Parkinson's disease. In these patients the normal triphasic activation pattern seen in electromyographic recordings during short rapid reaching movements is preserved (Hallet and Marsden, 1979). In these studies the interval between the onset of activity in the biceps muscle and the onset of activity in triceps is of the order of 20 – 30 msec. This suggests that the striatum is unlikely to be involved in generating sequences with interelement intervals of the order of tens of milliseconds.

On the other hand, Benecke et al. (1987) studied longer sequences of activity in which subjects were required to execute a short sequence of movements which involved opposing the thumb and finger, and then flexing the elbow. For the parkinsonian subjects, but not controls, movement times were longer for individual movements when performed sequentially than when executed in isolation. Interonset latencies were slowed in the parkinsonian subjects relative to controls. In controls they were 230 msec while in the parkinsonian subjects they were 400 – 500 msec. This suggests that the striatum may be involved in generating sequences with interelement intervals of the order of hundreds of milliseconds. While it may be coincidental, this intermediate range of interelement intervals appears to be a natural period for the sequences generated by the striatal model proposed.

Acknowledgements

This work was supported by a grant to J.R.W. from the Health Research Council of New Zealand.

References

Akaike, A., Sasa, M. and Takaori, S. (1988) Muscarinic inhibition as a dominant role in cholinergic regulation of transmission in the caudate nucleus. *J. Pharmacol. Exp. Ther.,* 246: 1129 – 1136.

Akins, P.T., Surmeier, D.J. and Kitai, S.T. (1990) Muscarinic modulation of a transient K^+ conductance in rat neostriatal neurons. *Nature,* 344: 240 – 242.

Aronin, N., Chase, K. and DiFiglia, M. (1986) Glutamic acid decarboxylase and enkephalin immunoreactive axon terminals in the rat neostriatum synapse with striatonigral neurons. *Brain Res.,* 365: 151 – 158.

Bargas, J., Galarraga, E. and Aceves, J. (1988) Electrotonic properties of neostriatal neurons are modulated by extracellular potassium. *Exp. Brain Res.,* 72: 390 – 398.

Bargas, J., Galarraga, E. and Aceves, J. (1989) An early outward conductance modulates the firing latency and frequency of neostriatal neurons of the rat brain. *Exp. Brain Res.,* 75: 146 – 156.

Benecke, R., Rothwell, J.C., Dick, J.P., Day, B.L. and Marsden, C.D. (1987) Disturbance of sequential movements in patients with Parkinson's disease. *Brain,* 110: 361 – 379.

Bishop, G.A., Chang, H.T. and Kitai, S.T. (1982) Morphological and physiological properties of neostriatal neurons: an intracellular horseradish peroxidase study in the rat. *Neuroscience,* 7: 179 – 191.

Brotchie, P., Iansek, R. and Horne, M. (1991) A neural network model of neural activity in the monkey globus pallidus. *Neurosci. Lett.,* 131: 33 – 36.

Calabresi, P., Misgeld, U. and Dodt, H.U. (1987) Intrinsic membrane properties of neostriatal neurons can account for their low level of spontaneous activity. *Neuroscience,* 20: 293 – 303.

Calabresi, P., Mercuri, N.B., Stefani, A. and Bernardi, G. (1990a) Synaptic and intrinsic control of membrane excitability of neostriatal neurons. I. An in vivo analysis. *J. Neurophysiol.,* 63: 651 – 662.

Calabresi, P., Mercuri, N.B., Stefani, A. and Bernardi, G. (1990b) Synaptic and intrinsic control of membrane excitability of neostriatal neurons. II. An in vitro analysis. *J. Neurophysiol.* 63: 663 – 657.

Cools, A.R., Jaspers, R., Schwartz, M., Sontag, K.H., Vrijmoed-de Vries, M. and Van den Bercken, J. (1984) Basal ganglia and switching motor programs. In: J.S. McKenzie,

R.E. Kemm and L.N. Wilcock (Eds.), *The Basal Ganglia: Stucture and Function,* Plenum Press, New York and London, pp. 513 – 544.

Estes, W.K. (1972) An associative basis for coding and organization in memory. In: A.W. Melton and E. Martin (Eds.), *Coding Processes in Human Memory,* V.H. Winston, Washington, D.C., pp. 161 – 190.

Fisher, R.S., Buchwald, N.A.. Hull, C.D. and Levine, M.S. (1986) Neurons of origin of striatonigral axons in the cat: connectivity and Golgi markers of somatodendritic architecture. *Brain Res.,* 397: 173 – 180.

Galarraga, E., Bargas, J., Sierra, A. and Aceves, J. (1989) The role of calcium in the repetitive firing of neostriatal neurons. *Exp. Brain Res.,* 75: 157 – 168.

Gerfen, C.R. (1985) The neostriatal mosaic: the reiterated processing unit. In: C. Feuerstein, B. Scatton and M. Sandler (Eds.), *Neurotransmitter Interactions in the Basal Ganglia,* Raven Press, New York, pp. 19 – 30.

Graveland, G.A. and DiFiglia, M. (1985) The frequency and distribution of medium-sized neurons with indented nuclei in the primate and rodent neostriatum. *Brain Res.,* 327: 307 – 311.

Groves, P.M. (1983) A theory of the functional organisation of the neostriatum and the neostriatal control of voluntary movement. *Brain Res. Rev.,* 5: 109 – 132.

Hallet, M. and Marsden, C.D. (1979) Ballistic flexion movements of the human thumb. *J. Physiol. (Lond.),* 294: 33 – 50.

Harrington, D.L. and Haaland, K.Y. (1987) Programming sequences of hand postures. *J. Mot. Behav.,* 19: 77 – 95.

Hull, C., Bernardi, G., Prince, D. and Buchwald, N. (1973) Intracellular responses of caudate neurons to temporally and spatially combined stimuli. *Exp. Neurol.,* 38: 324 – 336.

Jiang, Z.-G. and North, R.A. (1991) Membrane properties and synaptic responses of rat striatal neurones in vitro. *J. Physiol. (Lond.),* 443: 533 – 553.

Jones, E.G., Coulter, J.D., Burton, H. and Porter, R. (1977) Cells of origin and terminal distribution of corticostriatal fibres arising in the sensorimotor cortex of monkeys. *J. Comp. Neurol.,* 173: 53 – 80.

Katayama, Y., Miyazaki, S. and Tsubokawa, T. (1981) Electrophysiological evidence favoring intracaudate axon collaterals of GABAergic caudate output neurons in the cat. *Brain Res.,* 216: 180 – 186.

Kawaguchi, Y., Wilson, C.J. and Emson, P.C. (1989) Intracellular recording of identified neostriatal patch and matrix spiny cells in a slice preparation preserving cortical inputs. *J. Neurophysiol.,* 62: 1052 – 1068.

Kemp, J.M. and Powell, T.P.S. (1971) The connections of the striatum and globus pallidus. *Phil. Trans. R. Soc. B.,* 262: 441 – 457.

Kimura, M. (1990) Behaviorally contingent property of movement-related activity of the primate putamen. *J. Neurophysiol.,* 63: 1277 – 1296.

Kita, H., Kita, T. and Kitai, S.T. (1984) Passive electrical membrane properties of rat neostriatal neurons in an in vitro slice preparation. *Brain Res.,* 300: 129 – 139.

Kitai, H. and Kitai, S.T. (1988) Glutamate decarboxylase immunoreactive neurons in cat neostriatum: their morphological types and populations. *Brain Res.,* 447: 346 – 352.

Lighthall, J.W. and Kitai, S.T. (1983) A short duration GABAergic inhibition in identified neostriatal medium spiny neurons: in vitro slice study. *Brain Res. Bull.,* 11: 103 – 110.

Lighthall, J.W., Park, M.R. and Kitai, S.T. (1981) Inhibition in slices of rat striatum. *Brain Res.,* 212: 182 – 187.

Miller, R. (1988) Cortico-striatal and cortico-limbic circuits: a two tiered model of learning and memory function. In: H. Markowitsch (Ed.), *Information Processing by the Brain: Views and Hypotheses from a Cognitive-Physiological Perspective,* Hans Huber Press, Bern, pp. 179 – 198.

Misgeld, U., Wagner, A. and Ohno, T. (1982) Depolarizing IPSPs and depolarization by GABA of rat neostriatum cells in vitro. *Exp. Brain Res.,* 45: 108 – 114.

Mitchell, I.J., Brotchie, J.M., Brown, G.D.A. and Crossman, A.R. (1991) Modeling the functional organization of the basal ganglia. *Movement Disorders,* 6: 189 – 204.

Park, M.R., Lighthall, J.W. and Kitai, S.T. (1980) Recurrent inhibition in the rat neostriatum. *Brain Res.,* 194: 359 – 369.

Pasik, P., Pasik, T., Holstein, G. and Hamori, J. (1988) GABAergic elements in the neuronal circuits of the monkey neostriatum: a light and electron microscopic immunocytochemical study. *J. Comp. Neurol.,* 270: 157 – 170.

Poizner, H. (1990) Language and motor disorders in deaf signers. In: G.E. Hammond (Ed.), *Cerebral Control of Speech and Limb Movements,* Elsevier Science Publishers B.V. Amsterdam, pp. 303 – 326.

Preston, R.J., Bishop, G.A. and Kitai, S.T. (1980) Medium spiny neuron projection from the rat neostriatum: an intracellular horseradish peroxidase study. *Brain Res.,* 183: 253 – 263.

Rolls, E.T. and Williams, G.V. (1986) Sensory and movement-related neuronal activity in different regions of the primate striatum. In: J.S. Schneider and T.I. Lidsky (Eds.), *Basal Ganglia and Behavior: Sensory Aspects of Motor Functioning,* Hans Huber, Toronto, Lewiston, New York, Bern, Stuttgart, pp. 37 – 60.

Rumelhart, D.E. and Norman, D.A. (1982) Simulating a skilled typist: a study of skilled cognitive-motor performance. *Cogn. Sci.,* 6: 1 – 36.

Rutherford, A., Garcia-Munoz, M. and Arbuthnott, G.W. (1988) An afterhyperpolarization recorded in striatal cells "in vitro". Effect of dopamine administration. *Exp. Brain Res.,* 71: 399 – 406.

Schröder, K.F., Hopf, A., Lange, H. and Thörner, G. (1975) Morphometrisch-statistische Strukturanalysen des Striatum, Pallidum und Nucleus subthalamacus beim Menschen. I. Striatum. *J. Hirnforsch.,* 16: 333 – 350.

Somogyi, P., Bolam, J.P. and Smith, A.D. (1981) Monosynaptic cortical input and local axon collaterals of identified striatonigral neurons. A light and electron microscopy study using the Golgi-peroxidase transport-degeneration procedure. *J.*

Comp. Neurol., 195: 567 – 584.

Stelmach, G.E., Worringham, C.J. and Strand, E.A. (1987) The programming and execution of movement sequences in Parkinson's disease. *Int. J. Neurosci.,* 36: 55 – 65.

Sugimori, M., Preston, R.J. and Kitai, S.T. (1978) Response properties and electrical constants of caudate nucleus neurons in the cat. *J. Neurophysiol.,* 41: 1662 – 1676.

Surmeier, D.J., Bargas, J. and Kitai, S.T. (1988) Voltage-clamp analysis of a transient potassium current in rat neostriatal neurons. *Brain Res.,* 473: 187 – 192.

Updyke, B.V. and Liles, S.L. (1987) The corticostriatal projection in cat: relation between axon terminals and evoked potentials. *Brain Res.,* 402: 365 – 369.

Wickens, J.R. (1990) Striatal dopamine in motor activation and reward-mediated learning: steps towards a unifying model. *J. Neural Transm.,* 80: 9 – 31.

Wickens, J.R., Alexander, M.E. and Miller, R. (1991) Two dynamic modes of striatal function under dopaminergic-cholinergic control: simulation and analysis of a model. *Synapse,* 8: 1 – 12.

Wilson, C.J. and Groves, P.M. (1980) Fine structure and synaptic connections of the common spiny neuron of the rat neostriatum: a study employing intracellular injection of horseradish peroxidase. *J. Comp. Neurol.,* 194: 599 – 616.

Wilson, M.A. and Bower, J.M. (1989) The simulation of large-scale neural networks. In: C. Koch and I. Segev (Eds.), *Methods in Neuronal Modeling: from Synapses to Networks,* MIT Press, Cambridge, MA, pp. 291 – 334.

G.W. Arbuthnott and P.C. Emson (Eds.)
Progress in Brain Research, Vol. 99
© 1993 Elsevier Science Publishers B.V. All rights reserved.

CHAPTER 22

The thorny problem of what dopamine does in psychiatric disease

G.W. Arbuthnott and C.A. Ingham

Preclinical Veterinary Sciences, University of Edinburgh, Summerhall, Edinburgh EH9 1QH, U.K.

Introduction

Dendrites bristling with small protuberances (spines – from spina, the Latin word for a thorn) are characteristic of many classes of neurones in the central nervous system and are best observed in Golgi-impregnated material or in cells filled with other intracellular markers. In the neostriatum the principal output neurones are densely spiny (Fig. 1).

The principal significance of these thorny structures has intrigued neuroscientists since Cajal. What can be the importance of those thorny dendrites? Is the structure as solid as it looks in the picture or do spines change their shape? How can we possibly explore the properties of these strange structures? Mathematical models suggest that they may be capable of controlling the effectiveness of individual synaptic inputs (Wilson, 1984) but the idea is hard to test with current techniques. Recent correlated light and electron microscopic studies in Edinburgh have made us very interested in the neurobiology of spines. Our interest grew from the results of experiments designed to help us to understand the relevance of dopamine for human medicine.

A therapeutic puzzle

The medical problem is a familiar one. How is it that dopamine antagonists whose action on dopamine is instantaneous, still take three weeks to help schizophrenic patients (Casey et al., 1960; Johnstone et al., 1978; Freed, 1988)? One of the most dramatic illustrations of the problem comes from the work of Johnstone et al. (1978) illustrated in Fig. 2 which is modified from their article. The effective enantiomer of flupenthixol is only slightly better than its inactive twin after two full weeks of treatment and only significantly different at three weeks. All the patients improve somewhat from the intensive nursing in the research ward. The drug presumably blocks dopamine receptors in the brain on day one – indeed the same group have evidence that the secretion of prolactin was increased by only the active enantiomer but within the first week (Cotes et al., 1978). The rate of metabolism of the neuroleptics is not an explanation either (Curry, 1974). Does dopamine have nothing to do with the treatment? Is some other action of the neuroleptics changing the brain pathology underlying the disease? There are many possibilities for such an action. In this chapter we want to defend the speculative suggestion that a morphological change might underlie neuroleptic action. This particular heresy arose when our biological results on the action of 6-OH-dopamine (6-OHDA) would not fit into the pattern we predicted.

The localization of dopamine synapses

It all started some time ago when Freund et al. (1984) provided a dramatic anatomical interpretation for

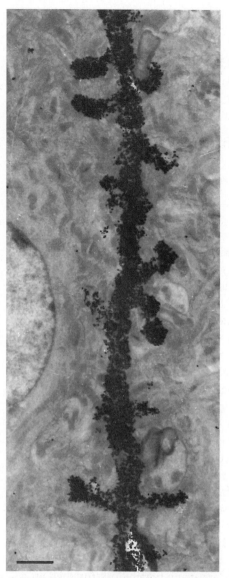

Fig. 1. High-voltage electron micrograph of part of a Golgi-impregnated gold-toned medium size spiny dendrite from rat neostriatum (1 μm thick section). Scale bar, 1 μm. The high-voltage electron microscopy was kindly carried out by the HVEM laboratory (University of Colorado, Boulder, NIH Grant RR00592) in collaboration with C.J. Wilson.

findings which we had understood in a different context (Brown and Arbuthnott, 1983). Our electrophysiology suggested that dopamine acted most potently to modify the action of cortical input on the neostriatal output cells, the medium-sized spiny

neurons of Fig. 1. We had interpreted that as evidence for pre-synaptic D_2 receptors. Freund et al. (1984) demonstrated that 60% of dopamine synapses (tyrosine hydroxylase-like immunoreactivity containing synapses to be precise) were formed on the necks of spines – and that all of these spines which they followed in serial EM sections also had a large asymmetric (probably cortical) synapse on them. Their result was confirmed in the same year by Bouyer et al. (1984). So our ''presynaptic'' action could just as well have been postsynaptic, but localized to the spines where, by modifying the efficiency of the cortical synapse on the head of the spine, dopamine would reduce the neostriatal output to some cortical inputs (Freund et al., 1984; Arbuthnott et al., 1987a). A study of the electrophysiological actions of dopamine in vitro (Rutherford et al., 1988), however, provided us with evidence that dopamine might be very selective in the responses it reduces and might actually increase strong excitatory inputs. These results form a part of the computer simulation in another chapter (Wickens and Arbuthnott, this volume).

The consequences of dopamine removal

We also studied another consequence of the idea that the site of dopamine action was now known at electron microscope resolution. If dopamine usually made synapses on the necks of spines and we destroyed dopamine-containing cells without damaging the striatal output cells (Ungerstedt, 1968; Hökfelt and Ungerstedt, 1969), what would happen to the vacated area on the spine necks? Perhaps, since there is some behavioural (Ungerstedt, 1968; Stricker and Zigmond, 1976) and electrophysiological (Schultz and Ungerstedt, 1978; Arbuthnott et al., 1987b) evidence for recovery from 6-OHDA, *something* replaced the dopamine on the spine-necks and this brought the cortical input back into control. We know, from the work of others (Somogyi et al., 1981; Bouyer et al., 1984) as well as Freund (1984) that non-dopamine-containing terminals also normally make synapses on spine-necks. The local axon collaterals of the output neurones

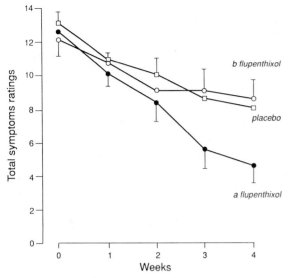

Fig. 2. Clinical assessment of the symptoms of schizophrenia in 45 patients (three groups of 15 each) receiving the treatments shown. Symptoms were estimated on a 0–4 scale and the total score for all nine ratings is shown. As the treatment progressed significant reduction in the scores in the group treated with the active enantiomer of flupenthixol (a flupenthixol) was seen only after three weeks at which point the active drug is significantly better than both placebo and its inactive (on dopamine binding assays) isomer. Further analysis indicates that the drug is most effective on positive symptoms (hallucinations, delusions, thought disorder) and on patients not showing signs of schizoaffective disorder. (Redrawn with permission from Johnstone et al., 1978.)

themselves are one obvious example — would they "replace" dopamine on the vacated spine necks? There was already evidence that such "inappropri-

ate reinnervation" could result from lesions of the hypothalamus (Raisman, 1969; Raisman and Field, 1973). Furthermore there are results from molecular biological (Young et al., 1986) and also from immunocytochemical studies (Voorn et al., 1987) demonstrating that the enkephalin neurones of the striatum do increase their production of enkephalin in response to the loss of dopamine.

Fewer thorns

Our results are surprising and puzzling. It seems likely that *nothing* replaces the dopamine; a proportion of the spines seem to vanish (Ingham et al., 1989, 1993). The output cells seem to be less thorny on the lesion side even a year after the operation which removed their dopamine input (Fig. 3)! To all the other effects of a 6-OHDA lesion we have to add the loss of some of the spines from neostriatal neurones. What happens to the cortical input which was associated with the lost spines? It is possible that along with the spines goes the cortical connection to them. Preliminary counts of asymmetrical synapses in random samples of the neostriatum suggest that they are longer but less common on the lesioned side (Ingham et al., 1991c, 1993).

The converse is certainly true. Kemp and Powell showed in 1971 that removing cortical or thalamic input reduced the number of spines on dendrites in the neostriatum. They carefully suggested that the denervated spines might not have been filled by the

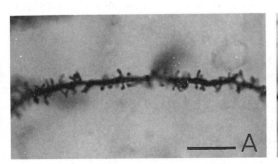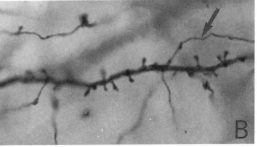

Fig. 3. Light micrographs of Golgi-impregnated, gold-toned medium size spiny neostriatal dendrites. The material was taken from a rat given a unilateral 6-hydroxydopamine lesion into the medial forebrain bundle 12 months previously. A. Dendrite from the contralateral neostriatum. B. An equivalent length of dendrite from the ipsilateral neostriatum. Golgi-impregnated axons (arrow) are also visible. Scale bar, 10 μm.

Golgi precipitate (Kemp and Powell, 1971). We have looked at electron micrographs from the cells whose spines we counted and can find no evidence of unfilled structures continuous with filled dendritic shafts (Ingham et al., 1991a, 1993). It seems possible, then, that removing dopamine disconnects striatal neurones from some of their cortical connections.

An earlier study with a different 6-OHDA model suggested that this might be the case (Hattori and Fibiger, 1982). In the neostriatum a day after the application of 6-OHDA they saw in their electron micrographs degenerating asymmetrical terminals (and the attached spines), endocytosed within glial elements. Thus, damage to dopamine terminals had consequences for both the spine and its cortical synapse. Hattori and Fibiger (1982) warned against the assumption that receptors lost after 6-OHDA lesions were necessarily on the dopamine nerve terminals since so much postsynaptic structure was also lost.

A different explanation?

Meanwhile, Freed (1988, 1989) has also proposed that the close association between dopamine-containing synapses and cortical endings might have functional importance. He too starts from the observation that neuroleptic drugs do not help schizophrenic patients immediately. The therapeutic action takes about three weeks to develop, but dopamine receptors are blocked immediately — indeed parkinsonian side effects are a problem of early neuroleptic treatment, but have usually worn off by the time therapeutic benefit is manifest. The patients in the Johnstone et al. (1978) study were given anticholinergic drugs to mask these motor side effects and thus keep doctors and patients "blind" as to the neuroleptic treatment group. The same researchers (Johnstone et al., 1983) later studied the effects of the anticholinergic action and suggested that it might have reduced the therapeutic action of the neuroleptic.

Freed suggested that the "slow" action of the neuroleptic drugs is a change in glutamate receptor numbers which results from the action of blocking dopamine receptors on the same spines of striatal cells. The mechanism he favours is a receptor — receptor interaction. The receptors, he suggests, are linked so that dopamine receptor supersensitivity results in a reduction in glutamate receptor number, as if there is only "room" for a fixed total number of receptors on each spine. More dopamine receptors mean fewer glutamate ones as a consequence. Evidence for such a change comes from experiments measuring glutamate binding in striatum which decreases by 40% after 6-OHDA lesions (Roberts et al., 1982). A less sensitive response to cortical "information overload" in schizophrenia is then proposed as the therapeutic mechanism of neuroleptic action. Freed supports his idea with behavioural experiments (Freed et al., 1989) which demonstrate that the behavioural consequences of action at glutamate receptors is reduced by previous chronic neuroleptic treatment, but not by acute dopamine receptor block.

A synthesis

Given our results it is tempting to suggest that Freed's idea about the therapeutic action (and his experimental result) could be explained by a physical loss of synapses on the striatal cells. Three weeks is an appropriate length of time for such a morphological change (Raisman and Field, 1973), but we are making a big assumption in suggesting that the action of neuroleptics is similar to a 6-OHDA lesion. However, the removal of dopamine with 6-OHDA is known to result in "up-regulation" of dopamine receptors just as does chronic treatment with neuroleptic drugs (La Hoste and Marshall, 1989). Similarly, in situ hybridization methods have suggested that the molecular biological consequences of the two treatments are related.

Destruction of the dopamine terminals with 6-OHDA results in the striatal cells expressing more mRNA for preproenkephalin and less mRNA for preprotachykinin (Sivam et al., 1987). Recent studies have demonstrated a similar response after neuroleptic treatment (Hong et al., 1979; Young et al., 1986; Shibata et al., 1990), although the drug treatment may not need to be prolonged in every case (Augood et al., 1992).

Our electron microscopic study of the response in enkephalin-containing terminals to 6-OHDA damage of the striatal dopamine innervation, not only demonstrated that the enkephalin fibres did not "replace" dopamine on the spines but also that the enkephalin-containing terminal profiles were larger in area and that their synaptic specialisations were longer after lesions (Ingham et al., 1991b). Although increases in immunoreactive enkephalin levels have been reported after chronic neuroleptic treatment by others (Auchus and Pickel, 1992), we cannot yet be sure that the same ultrastructural changes are also present. Similarly, only an extensive series of experiments will be able to test the idea that the spines are sensitive to chronic treatment with neuroleptics as well as to the total removal of the dopamine input.

An interesting digression provides support of a kind

Meanwhile recent transplant work is also relevant to the discussion. Not to the neuroleptic site of action perhaps, but to the idea that dopamine might be more concerned with the shape of membranes than with their ionic permeability.

After an almost total destruction of adult *neostriatal* cells their "replacement" with a small implant of embryonic striatal precursor cells returns to the animal the skilled use of the contralateral paw which it had lost following the original lesion (Dunnett et al., 1988).

A much smaller lesion − the destruction of dopamine-containing cells in substantia nigra − also deprives the animal of the skilled use of its contralateral paw. Implanting fetal substantia nigra precursor cells into the striatum does help some of the behavioural consequences of the lesion but not the skilled paw use (Dunnett et al., 1987; Montoya et al., 1990). What if adult neostriatal cells cannot regrow those vital spines and re-attach the cortical synapses in spite of the growth of the dopamine

fibres and the existence of similar synaptic patterns in the neostriatum (Freund et al., 1985; Mahalik et al., 1985)? Could it be that striatal neurones from embryonic brain can cause the vital cortical connections to regrow on to spines as well as returning "outputs" to the neostriatum (see, e.g., Rutherford et al., 1988; Wictorin et al., 1989; Xu et al., 1989). There is some direct EM evidence that they can and do attract cortical input (Xu et al., 1989). The same group have also counted spines on spiny neurones in the grafts (Xu et al., 1992). It is clear that the spiny neurones are less spiny in the centre of the graft compared with surviving host spiny neurones in the intact striatum. Neurones in this central area of the graft may have less chance of receiving cortical input. At the border of the grafts where the dendrites of spiny cells were in the "normal" host striatum, they showed nearly normal numbers of spines, which suggests that in the presence of adult cortical axons the spiny cells can make spines if they are themselves neonatal. Perhaps these "border" neurones, with a normal cortical input, carry the cortical influence on to the motor system and thus "repair" the lost motor skill which was the result of the original lesion.

Spine counts have not been done after dopamine replacement by grafting substantia nigra to dopamine depleted striatum. Freund et al. (1985) do see a change in the proportions of dopamine terminals which synapse on spines in grafted animals. Whereas in normal dorsal neostriatum 56% of tyrosine hydroxylase-immunopositive terminals are in synaptic contact with dendritic spines in neostriatum with nigral grafts, only 36% of the immunoreactive terminals make axospinous synaptic contacts (Freund et al., 1985). These data support the idea that fewer spines are available for reinnervation by the dopamine fibres and moreover suggests that the presence of dopamine does not cause sufficient, if any, regeneration of spines on mature neostriatal neurones. Tedious though they are with current technology the decision about the recovery of spine density upon the dendrites of neostriatal neurones could provide evidence for, or against, the idea that the lack of restoration of function is a consequence of the continuing disconnection of striatal cells from cortical (or perhaps thalamic) inputs.

The development of spines

In the striatum we imagine that during development the spines are formed in response to dopamine and to other transmitters interacting with the major excitatory synaptic input to the neurones. They are absent in the earliest filled spiny cells in neonatal rats (Tepper and Trent, this volume) and there is reason to believe that at least some of the dopamine is already present in striatal terminals before postnatal day 7 (Olson et al., 1972; Voorn et al., 1988). The development of the majority of the dopamine innervation is over by day 20, by which time it seems as if the spines are at nearly normal levels (Tepper and Trent, this volume). The development of cortical-type synapses which are asymmetric and have round vesicles, also follows a very similar time course in the rat (Hattori and McGeer, 1973). This close agreement is suggestive that at least the timing is right for a relationship between the interaction of dopamine and cortical input and the formation of spines during development. The full development of cortical responsiveness in the striatal cells is not complete until even later (Tepper and Trent, this volume) and so perhaps something else is necessary for the physiological interaction in addition to spine formation.

Dopamine in retina

Support for an action of dopamine in maintaining morphology in adult nervous tissue was recently summarised by Rogawski (1987). In the retina, dopamine's most important action seems to be a structural one. The changes in morphology resulting from manipulation of dopamine may carry information processing consequences, since the change in shape of the receptor cells and the reduction of gap junction permeability between horizontal cells both alter the extent of surround inhibition. It is perhaps relevant that the computer simulation (Wickens and Arbuthnott, this volume) suggests that a similar information-processing consequence results from

the action of dopamine on the afterhyperpolarization which we recorded in vitro (Rutherford et al., 1989).

Some support from behavioural experiments

The influence of dopamine in adulthood co-operating with the cortical input in maintaining the spine both explains our results with 6-OHDA and allows an easy answer to the dilemma of how difficult it is to return fine motor control to denervated animals. One consequence of this idea is that there should be a similarity between the effects of the loss of dopamine and the results of the loss of cortical input, since we are suggesting that the action of dopamine is to maintain the cortical connections with spiny cells. The prediction that the motor consequences of cortical damage should be similar to loss of dopamine is confirmed at least in the case of paw use in the rat. Although different in extent, the kind of deficit is similar in 6-OHDA-lesioned animals and in animals with motor cortical lesions (Wishaw et al., 1986).

A serious problem

The major argument against this idea seems to be that L-Dopa helps parkinsonian patients to move! To keep the hypothesis alive needs either an effect of L-Dopa (perhaps to preserve spines?) which cannot be achieved by reinnervation, or, an action of L-Dopa *outside* the synaptic area on the spine-necks where after all 40% of the dopamine synapses are normally found in dorsal striatum − the proportion varies in other striatal regions (Zahm, 1992). In fact both of these ideas seem easier to believe than the current dogma that administering a precursor of a transmitter − in the absence of the nerves which usually use the precursor − somehow "replaces" lost synaptic activity. Of course, it is not yet time to discard the hypothesis that dopamine formed from L-Dopa somehow acts at supersensitive dopamine receptors to replace function but a close look at some plausible alternatives seems overdue.

This is especially the case if the explanation also

helps us to understand this mysterious delay in therapeutic action of neuroleptics which has baffled neuropharmacologists for decades. Not only does the suggestion that the major therapeutic result of neuroleptic treatment is on cortico-striatal function (Fig. 4) help resolve the actions of dopamine in neurobiologically testable terms, but it also brings the discussion of what it is that is "wrong" with schizophrenics back into the field of cortical and "cognitive" psychology.

A totally different suggestion for the delay which also emphasises "cognitive" aspects has been proposed by Miller (1987). He suggests that the disease state is characterized by the formation of inappropriate "hyperactive associations" (Miller, 1989) and that the process of recovery depends upon patients relearning appropriate associations, the for-

mation of inappropriate ones having been stopped by the neuroleptic treatment. Such a relearning process might take several weeks. Although at first sight this seems a very different explanation to ours, we do not yet know the morphological consequences of learning. In hippocampus, for instance, after long term potentiation (LTP) – a well studied "model" of learning processes – changes in spine synapses have been reported (Fifkova and Van Harreveld, 1977). Could the changes in spine density, that we propose to underlie the therapeutic action of neuroleptics, be the structural consequence of relearning appropriate associations?

Future alternatives?

Of course the new molecular biology of dopamine

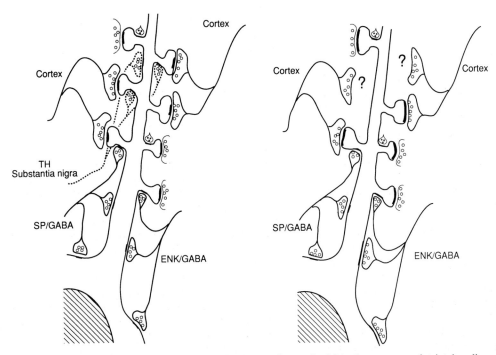

Fig. 4. Diagrams to illustrate the result of dopamine denervation on dendritic ultrastructure of striatal medium-sized densely spiny neurones. On the left is the known pattern of input "before" the lesion. The drawing on the right shows the increased size of the ENK/GABA terminals thought to be recurrent collaterals from other spiny cells, and the loss of spines. The ?'s represent the unsolved problem of what happens to the cortical synapses associated with the lost spines. Could blockage of dopamine receptors produce similar losses of spines and cortical synapses? TH, tyrosine hydroxylase-immunoreactive terminals (containing dopamine); SP/GABA, local collaterals of spiny cells containing substance P as well as GABA; ENK/GABA, local collaterals of spiny cells containing enkephalin as well as GABA.

receptors might lead us off in another direction entirely. Perhaps D_4 receptors will turn out to have a neurobiological action which takes three weeks to come on — but that long a delay in the "second messenger cascade" seems to need some very special second messengers indeed. Should we expect an action of dopamine on one or more of the growing array of "growth factors" as well as the actions which are the focus of the present electrophysiological investigations?

Already, results of repeatedly imaging single dendritic branches in mouse superior cervical ganglion cells (Purves and Hadley, 1985) have clearly shown that even in the adult, dendritic morphology is a much more dynamic thing than was previously supposed. So the idea that dopamine might be necessary for the structural integrity (or even for the shape, see Wilson, 1984) of spines seems less far-fetched than when it first occurred to us.

References

Arbuthnott, G.W., Brown, J.R., MacLeod, N.K., Mitchell, R.P. and Wright, A.K. (1987a) The action of dopamine on synaptic transmission through the striatum. In: M. Sandler, C. Feuerstein and B. Scatton (Eds.), *Neurotransmitter Interactions in the Basal Ganglia,* Raven Press, New York, pp. 71–81.

Arbuthnott, G.W., MacLeod, N.K., Brown, J.R., Wright, A.K., Rutherford, A. and Ryman, A. (1987b) The action of 6-OHDA on the striatonigral cells in the rat. In: N. Chalazonitis and M. Gola (Eds.), *Inactivation of Hypersensitive Neurons,* Alan R. Liss, New York, pp. 223–232.

Auchus, A.P. and Pickel, V.M. (1992) Quantitative light microscopic demonstration of increased pallidal and striatal met[5]-enkephalin-like immunoreactivity in rats following chronic treatment with haloperidol but not with clozapine: implications for the pathogenesis of neuroleptic-induced movement disorders. *Exp. Neurol.,* 117: 17–27.

Augood, S.J., Faull, R.L.M. and Emson, P.C. (1992) Contrasting effects of raclopride and SCH 23390 on the cellular content of preproenkephalin A mRNA in rat striatum: a quantitative non-radioactive in situ hybridization study. *Eur. J. Neurosci.,* 4: 102–112.

Bouyer, J.J., Park, D.H., Joh, T.H. and Pickel, V.M. (1984) Chemical and structural analysis of the relation between cortical inputs and tyrosine hydroxylase-containing terminals in rat neostriatum. *Brain Res.,* 302: 267–275.

Brown, J.R. and Arbuthnott, G.W. (1983) The electrophysiol-

ogy of dopamine (D_2) receptors: a study of the actions of dopamine on corticostriatal transmission. *Neuroscience,* 10: 349–355.

Casey, J.F., Bennett, I.F., Lindley, C.J., Hollister, L.E., Gordon, M.H. and Springer, N.N. (1960) Drug therapy in schizophrenia. *Arch. Gen. Psychiatry,* 2: 210–220.

Cotes, P.M., Crow, T.J., Johnstone, E.C., Barlett, W. and Bourne, R.C. (1978) Neuroendocrine changes in acute schizophrenia as a function of clinical state and neuroleptic medication. *Psychol. Med.,* 8: 657–665.

Curry, S.H. (1974) Metabolism and kinetics of chlorpromazine in relation to effect. In: G. Sedvall, B. Uvnäs and Y. Zotterman (Eds.), *Antipsychotic Drugs: Pharmacodynamics and Pharmacokinetics,* Pergamon, Oxford, pp. 343–352.

Dunnett, S.B., Wishaw, I.Q., Rogers, D.C. and Jones, G.H. (1987) Dopamine-rich grafts ameliorate whole body asymmetry and sensory neglect but not independent limb use in rats with 6-hydroxy-dopamine lesions. *Brain Res.,* 415: 53–78.

Dunnett, S.B., Isacson, O., Sirinathsinghi, D.J.S., Clarke, D.J. and Björklund, A. (1988) Striatal grafts in rats with unilateral neostriatal lesions, III. Recovery from dopamine-dependent motor asymmetry and deficits in skilled paw reaching. *Neuroscience,* 24: 813–820.

Fifkova, E. and Van Harreveld, A. (1977) Long-lasting morphological changes in dendritic spines of dentate granular cells following stimulation of the entorhinal area. *J. Neurocytol.,* 6: 211–230.

Freed, W.J. (1988) The therapeutic latency of neuroleptic drugs and nonspecific postjunctional supersensitivity. *Schizophr. Bull.,* 14: 269–277.

Freed, W.J. (1989) An hypothesis regarding the antipsychotic effect of neuroleptic drugs. *Pharmacol. Biochem. Behav.,* 32: 337–345.

Freed, W.J., Cannon-Spoor, H.E. and Rodgers, C.R. (1989) Attenuation of the behavioral response to quisqualic acid and glutamic acid diethyl ester by chronic haloperidol administration. *Life Sci.,* 44: 1303–1308.

Freund, T.F., Powell, J.F. and Smith, A.D. (1984) Tyrosine hydroxylase immunoreactive boutons in synaptic contact with identified striatonigral neurons, with particular reference to dendritic spines. *Neuroscience,* 13: 1189–1215.

Freund, T.F., Bolam, J.P., Björklund, A., Stenevi, U., Dunnett, S.B., Powell, J.F. and Smith, A.D. (1985) Efferent synaptic connections of grafted dopaminergic neurons reinnervating the host neostriatum: a tyrosine hydroxylase immunocytochemical study. *J. Neurosci.,* 5: 603–616.

Hattori, T. and Fibiger, H.C. (1982) On the use of lesions of afferents to localize neurotransmitter receptor sites in the striatum. *Brain Res.,* 238: 245–256.

Hattori, T. and McGeer, P.L. (1973) Synaptogenesis in the corpus striatum of the infant rat. *Exp. Neurol.,* 38: 70–79.

Hökfelt, T. and Ungerstedt, U. (1969) Electron and fluorescence microscopical studies on the nucleus caudatus putamen of the rat after unilateral lesions of the ascending nigro-neostriatal dopamine neurons. *Acta Physiol. Scand.,* 76: 415–426.

Hong, J.S., Young, H-Y.T., Gilliu, J.C., Di Giulio, A.M., Fratta, W. and Costa, E. (1979) Chronic treatment with haloperidol accelerates the biosynthesis of enkephalins in rat striatum. *Brain Res.,* 160: 192–195.

Ingham, C.A., Hood, S.H. and Arbuthnott, G.W. (1989) Spine density on neostriatal neurons changes with 6-hydroxydopamine lesions and with age. *Brain Res.,* 503: 334–338.

Ingham, C.A., Hood, S.H. and Arbuthnott, G.W. (1991a) Correlated light and electron microscopy of Golgi-impregnated neostriatal neurons after 6-hydroxydopamine lesions in the rat. In: G. Bernardi, M.B. Carpenter and G. DiChiari (Eds.), *Basal Ganglia, III.* Plenum, New York, pp. 21–28.

Ingham, C.A., Hood, S.H., Arbuthnott, G.W. (1991b) A light and electron microscopy study of enkephalin-immunoreactive structures in the rat neostriatum after removal of the nigrostriatal dopaminergic pathways. *Neuroscience,* 42: 715–730.

Ingham, C.A., Hood, S.H., Arbuthnott, G.W., Weenink, A. and Van Maldegem, B. (1991c) Does dopamine loss in the striatum result in changes in synaptic number? *Abstracts of Third IBRO World Congress of Neuroscience,* pp. 22–30.

Ingham, C.A., Hood, S.H., Weenink, A., Van Maldegem, B. and Arbuthnott, G.W. (1993) Morphological changes in the rat neostriatum after unilateral 6-hydroxydopamine injections into the nigrostriatal pathway. *Exp. Brain Res.,* 93: 17–27.

Johnstone, E.C., Crow, T.J., Frith, C.D., Carney, M.W.P. and Price, J.S. (1978) Mechanism of the antipsychotic effect in the treatment of acute schizophrenia. *Lancet,* i: 848–851.

Johnstone, E.C., Crow, T.J., Ferrier, I.N., Frith, C.D., Owens, D.G.C., Bourne, R.C. and Gamble, S.J. (1983) Adverse effects of cholinergic medication on positive schizophrenic symptoms. *Psychol. Med.,* 13: 513–528.

Kemp, J.M. and Powell, T.P.S. (1971) The synaptic organization of the caudate nucleus. *Phil. Trans. R. Soc. B,* 262: 403–412.

La Hoste, G.J. and Marshall, J.F. (1989) Non-additivity of D_2 receptor proliferation induced by dopamine denervation and chronic selective antagonist administration: evidence from quantitative autoradiography indicates a single mechanism of action. *Brain Res.,* 502: 223–232.

Mahalik, T.J., Finger, T.E., Stromberg, I. and Olson, L. (1985) Substantia nigra transplants into denervated striatum of the rat: ultrastructure of graft and host interconnections. *J. Comp. Neurol.,* 240: 60–70.

Miller, R. (1987) The time course of neuroleptic therapy for psychosis: role of learning processes and implications for concepts of psychotic illness. *Psychopharmacology,* 92: 405–415.

Miller, R. (1989) Hyperactivity of associations in psychosis. *Aust. N.Z. J. Psychiatry,* 23: 241–248.

Montoya, C.P., Astell, S. and Dunnett, S.B. (1990) Effects of nigral and striatal grafts on skilled forelimb use in the rat. In: S.B. Dunnett and S.J. Richards (Eds.), *Progress in Brain Research, Vol. 82 – Neural Transplantation from Molecular Basis to Clinical Application,* Elsevier, Amsterdam, pp. 459–466.

Olsen, L., Seiger, A. and Fuxe, K. (1972) Heterogeneity of striatal and limbic dopamine innervation: highly fluorescent islands in developing and adult rats. *Brain Res.,* 44: 283–288.

Purves, D. and Hadley, R.D. (1985) Changes in the dendritic branching of adult mammalian neurones revealed by repeated imaging in situ. *Nature,* 315: 404–406.

Raisman, G. (1969) Neuronal plasticity in the septal nuclei of the adult brain. *Brain Res.,* 14: 25–48.

Raisman, G. and Field, P.M. (1973) A quantitative investigation of the development of collateral reinnervation after partial deafferentation of the septal nuclei. *Brain Res.,* 50: 241–264.

Roberts, P.J., McBean, G.J., Sharif, N.A. and Thomas, E.M. (1982) Striatal glutamatergic function: modifications following specific lesions. *Brain Res.,* 235: 83–91.

Rogawski, M.A. (1987) New directions in neurotransmitter action: dopamine provides some important clues. *Trends Neurosci.,* 10: 200–204.

Rutherford, A., Garcia-Munoz, M., Dunnett, S.B. and Arbuthnott, G.W. (1987) Electrophysiological demonstration of host cortical inputs to striatal grafts. *Neurosci. Lett.,* 83: 275–281.

Rutherford, A., Garcia-Munoz, M. and Arbuthnott, G.W. (1988) An after hyperpolarization recorded in striatal cells "in vitro": effect of dopamine administration. *Exp. Brain Res.,* 71: 399–405.

Schultz, W. and Ungerstedt, U. (1978) Short-term increase and long-term reversion of striatal cell activity after degeneration of the nigro-striatal dopamine system. *Exp. Brain Res.,* 33: 159–171.

Shibata, K., Haverstick, D.M. and Bannon, M.J. (1990) Tachykinin gene expression in rat limbic nuclei: modulation by dopamine antagonists. *J. Pharmacol. Exp. Ther.,* 255: 388–392.

Sivam, S.P., Breese, G.R., Krause, J.E., Napier, T.C., Muller, R.A. and Hong, J.S. (1987) Neonatal and adult 6-hydroxydopamine-induced lesions differentially alter tachykinin and enkephalin gene expression. *J. Neurochem.,* 49: 1623–1633.

Somogyi, P., Bolam, J.P. and Smith, A.D. (1981) Monosynaptic cortical input and local axon collaterals on identified striatonigral neurons. A light and electron microscopy study using the Golgi, peroxidase transport, degeneration procedure. *J. Comp. Neurol.,* 195: 567–584.

Stricker, E.M. and Zigmond, M.J. (1976) Recovery of function after damage to central catecholamine-containing neurons: a neurochemical model for the lateral hypothalamic syndrome. In: J.M. Sprague, and A.N. Epstein (Eds.), *Progess in Psychobiology and Physiological Psychology, Vol. 6,* Academic Press, New York, pp. 121–188.

Ungerstedt, U. (1968) 6-Hydroxydopamine-induced degeneration of central monoamine neurons. *Eur. J. Pharmacol.,* 5: 107–110.

350

Voorn, P., Roest, G. and Groenewegen, J.J. (1987) Increase of enkephalin and decrease of substance P immunoreactivity in the dorsal and ventral striatum of the rat after midbrain 6-hydroxydopamine lesions. *Brain Res.,* 412: 391 – 396.

Voorn, P., Kalsbeek, A., Jorritsma-Byham, B. and Groenewegen, H.J. (1988) The pre- and postnatal development of the dopaminergic cell groups in the ventral mesencephalon and the dopaminergic innervation of the striatum of the rat. *Neuroscience,* 25: 857 – 887.

Wictorin, K. and Björklund, A. (1989) Connectivity of striatal grafts implanted into the ibotenic acid-lesioned striatum. II. Cortical afferents. *Neuroscience,* 30: 297 – 311.

Wictorin, K., Simerly, R.B., Isacson, O., Swanson, L.W. and Björklund, A. (1989) Connectivity of striatal grafts implanted into the ibotenic acid-lesioned striatum. III. Efferent projecting graft neurons and their relation to host afferents within the grafts. *Neuroscience,* 30: 312 – 330.

Wilson, C.J. (1984) Passive cable properties of dendritic spines and spiny neurons in the rat. *J. Neurosci.,* 4: 281 – 297.

Wishaw, I.Q., O'Connor, W.T. and Dunnett, S.B. (1986) The contributions of motor cortex, nigrostriatal dopamine and caudate-putamen to skilled forelimb use in the rat. *Brain,* 109: 805 – 843.

Xu, Z.C., Wilson, C.J. and Emson, P.C. (1989) Restoration of the corticostriatal projection in rat neostriatal grafts: electron microscopical analysis. *Neuroscience,* 29: 539 – 550.

Xu, Z.C., Wilson, C.J. and Emson, P.C. (1992) Morphology of intracellularly stained spiny neurons in rat striatal grafts. *Neuroscience,* 48: 95 – 110.

Young III, W.S., Bonner, T.I. and Brown, M.R. (1986) Mesencephalic dopamine neurons regulate the expression of neuropeptide mRNA's in the rat forebrain. *Proc. Natl. Acad. Sci. U.S.A.,* 83: 9827 – 9831.

Zahm, D.S. (1992) An electron microscopic morphometric comparison of tyrosine hydroxylase immunoreactive innervation in the neostriatum and the nucleus accumbens core and shell. *Brain Res.,* 575: 341 – 346.

Subject Index